AF687545

Salutogenesis: Exploring Mental Health (Volume 1)

Salutogenesis: Exploring Mental Health (Volume 1)

Paul Hoang

AMERICAN
MEDICAL PUBLISHERS
www.americanmedicalpublishers.com

AMERICAN
MEDICAL PUBLISHERS
www.americanmedicalpublishers.com

Cataloging-in-Publication Data

Salutogenesis : exploring mental health (Volume 1) / Paul Hoang.
p. cm.
Includes bibliographical references and index.
ISBN 979-8-88740-446-2
1. Mental health. 2. Clinical health psychology. 3. Mental illness. 4. Psychology, Pathological.
5. Psychiatry. I. Hoang, Paul.
RA790 .S25 2023
616.89--dc23

© American Medical Publishers, 2023

American Medical Publishers,
41 Flatbush Avenue,
1st Floor, New York,
NY 11217, USA

ISBN 979-8-88740-446-2 (Hardback)

This book contains information obtained from authentic and highly regarded sources. All chapters are published with permission under the Creative Commons Attribution Share Alike License or equivalent. A wide variety of references are listed. Permissions and sources are indicated; for detailed attributions, please refer to the permissions page. Reasonable efforts have been made to publish reliable data and information, but the authors, editors and publisher cannot assume any responsibility for the validity of all materials or the consequences of their use.

Trademark Notice: Registered trademark of products or corporate names are used only for explanation and identification without intent to infringe.

Contents

Preface

This book was inspired by the evolution of our times; to answer the curiosity of inquisitive minds. Many developments have occurred across the globe in the recent past which has transformed the progress in the field.

Salutogenesis is an approach to human health that focuses on factors that support human health and well-being rather than on factors that cause disease. It studies the origins of health and also the multidimensional causes of higher levels of health. Different models associated with salutogenesis involve a holistic approach with respect to different aspects such as physical, social, emotional, spiritual, intellectual, vocational, and environmental aspects. Health promotion is based on a salutogenic concept of health, since it aims to empower people and populations to better regulate and manage their health and well-being. The focus of health promotion concentrates on the mechanism of stress management and staying well, thereby having a positive impact on mental health. It also involves increasing this belief in this own potential and building this confidence. The majority of services are health-related, dealing with the treatment, and care of those who are sick. This book unfolds the innovative aspects of salutogenesis which will be crucial for the progress of this field in the future. The topics covered herein offer the readers new insights within this field.

This book was developed from a mere concept to drafts to chapters and finally compiled together as a complete text to benefit the readers across all nations. To ensure the quality of the content we instilled two significant steps in our procedure. The first was to appoint an editorial team that would verify the data and statistics provided in the book and also select the most appropriate and valuable contributions from the plentiful contributions we received from authors worldwide. The next step was to appoint an expert of the topic as the Editor-in-Chief, who would head the project and finally make the necessary amendments and modifications to make the text reader-friendly. I was then commissioned to examine all the material to present the topics in the most comprehensible and productive format.

I would like to take this opportunity to thank all the contributing authors who were supportive enough to contribute their time and knowledge to this project. I also wish to convey my regards to my family who have been extremely supportive during the entire project.

Paul Hoang

Part I

Past and Present of Salutogenesis

1

Salutogenesis: Then and Now

Maurice B. Mittelmark

Part I provides an overview of the development of the field of salutogenesis, as background for the remaining chapters in *The Handbook of Salutogenesis*.

Chapter 2 by Bengt Lindström reviews mileposts in the development of the field from the late 1990s until today. This is a chronology of the meetings, seminars and other events that have provided space and time for the development of salutogenesis as an academic field. This chapter is of historical value and helps describe the global collaborative work that has supported the network of colleagues whose work is in the book.

Chapter 3 by Maurice Mittelmark and Georg Bauer is a revision and expansion of a chapter in the 2017 Edition, meant to convey some of the main ways the term 'salutogenesis' is used today. Antonovsky introduced the term salutogenesis in his 1979 and 1987 books on the Salutogenic Model of Health, but salutogenesis subsequently has come to refer to a core concept in the Model in particular; the sense of coherence. This usage has advanced to the point that some writers have coined the term 'sense of coherence theory'. The term salutogenesis is also frequently used to refer, more generally, to an approach to health theory, research and practice emphasising resources that people may call on to improve health.

Chapter 4 is of particular importance in this Handbook. Written by Aaron Antonovsky's son Avishai Antonovsky, and by one of his closest colleagues and former PhD student, Shifra Sagy, this revised chapter from the 2017 Edition provides the first biography of the founding father of salutogenesis. The authors share their insight regarding the development of the salutogenic idea. They were very close to Aaron Antonovsky for several decades, and their familiarity with his background contributes to understanding the development of salutogenesis.

M. B. Mittelmark (✉)
Department of Health Promotion and Development,
Faculty of Psychology, University of Bergen, Bergen, Norway
e-mail: maurice.mittelmark@uib.no

Chapter 5 by Hege Forbech Vinje, Eva Langeland and Torill Bull is reproduced from the 2017 Edition. The editors are convinced that this summary of Antonovsky's development of the Salutogenic Model of Health is among the best synopses available. While no summary can replace the value of Antonovsky's voluminous productivity on salutogenesis, the reader of this chapter will receive a quite in-depth introduction to Salutogenesis's main lines of development under the guiding hands of its founding theoretician.

Chapter 6 by Georg Bauer provides the reader with a useful description of Salutogenesis meeting places. These are the Society for Theory and Research on Salutogenesis (STARS) and the Global Working Group on Salutogenesis (GWG-Sal) of the International Union for Health Promotion and Education (IUHPE). Bauer also provides information about the Center on Salutogenesis at the University of Zürich in Switzerland. The center is the host organisation of both meeting places. The reader wanting to connect more directly to a global salutogenesis network will find this chapter to be of great practical value.

Finally, Chapter 7 by Lenneke Vaandrager of The Netherlands and colleagues from Spain, Germany, Italy, Norway, the United Kingdom and Poland trace the development of higher education in salutogenesis in Europe, spanning 30 years. At this time, the annual summer schools of the European Training Consortium in Public Health and Health Promotion have trained more than 700 participants from 60 countries. Perhaps the most distinguished member of the summer school's faculty – at least from the perspective of advancing salutogenesis as a theory for health promotion – is Aaron Antonovsky, who participated in the 1992 edition of the course in Gothenburg, Sweden.

The chapters of Part I provide the reader with an overview of the entire scope of development of salutogenesis from its start in 1979 to this day. Just over a mere 40 years, a very rapid eye blink in social science history! Therefore, this book is an introduction to a transdisciplinary field in its infancy. The reader is heartily invited to join in on the 'ground-floor' of the research, theory building and practice that we anticipate will advance salutogenesis to a mature scholastic undertaking. What is the fundamental problem that makes this audacious undertaking worth the effort?

How may we better understand the origins of human health? How may we advance health in a manner considerate of the con-nectedness of health to life generally?

Not just human life, but global life.

2

Development of Salutogenesis: Major Milestones

Bengt Lindström

First Encounter

It was a sunny and windy afternoon in the Spring of 1987. I was waiting for a group of guests of Public Health Officials on the pier of the Nordic School of Public Health. They were arriving quite spectacularly on a 19th-century steamship, "Bohuslän," used at special occasions by the City of Göteborg. The sea was quite rough, and it took a while to dock and land the old, tall, and narrow ship. I had time to scan the many familiar faces of colleagues and friends on board but among them was a new face.

I greeted my friends and walked up to the new person who looked a bit pale and shaky and relieved getting on firm land; he said: "Hi, I am not used to the sea because I come from the middle of the Negeb desert and the Beersheva University in Israel, I am Aaron Antonovsky."

This was my first encounter with Aaron Antonovsky (Fig. 2.1), the father of salutogenesis. As a welcome, he handed me a signed copy of his latest book, fresh from the printers, titled "Unravelling the Mystery of Health." It was the beginning of a friendship that would last until his sudden death seven years later.

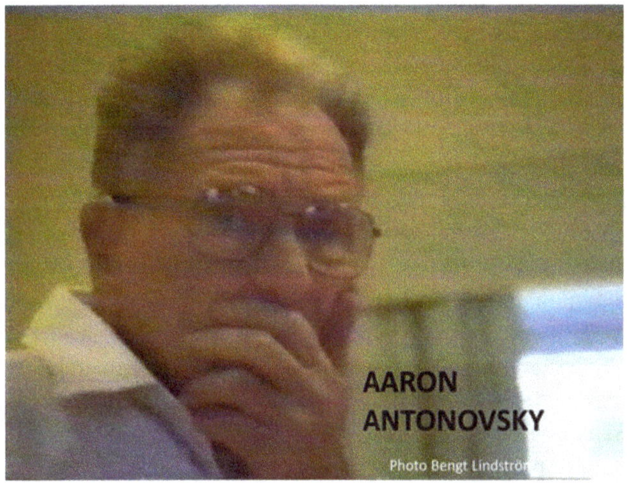

Fig. 2.1 Aaron Antonovsky, teaching at the Nordic School of Public Health in 1992

My Understanding of "Salutogenesis" Before Antonovsky

As for so many others, the salutogenic thought was not completely new to me as such, but we did not have the concepts and words to specify what it was about until Aaron Antonovsky conceptualized his model. My salutogenic journey started before I met with him. I trained as a physician in Finland and specialized in pediatrics; I wished and hoped pediatrics could have been called child health and move beyond the traditional health-disease axis, but this was the late 1960s and early 1970s; in Finland, the prime time for "hardcore biomedical science."

Our teachers were decidedly ignorant of other entry points to medicine and what went on in the community outside of the hospitals. I never understood why you learnt anatomy like reading a telephone book or why you were trained in understanding only the somatic growth of a child, integrating neither the mental and social nor spiritual dimensions into a wholeness. During my specialization, I moved to Sweden, where pediatrics was more open to the community; meaning in your training, you met healthy children and their families in Child Wellbeing Clinics. Also, in Sweden, child mental health services were provided through child and adolescent psychiatry.

Although I loved to work with children and families and was good at it, there was always that longing for a more direct approach to health. Much later, already 10 years into medicine, came the event that finally changed my professional orientation. I was in charge of a group of children with cystic fibrosis, a genetic disease that at that time lead to infections, malnutrition, and usually a premature death due to severe lung infections.

One morning I met a family well-known to me; they had already lost one child to the disease, and this day the younger

B. Lindström (✉)
NTNU Center for Health Promotion Research, Norwegian University of Science and Technology, Trondheim, Norway
e-mail: bengtblind@hotmail.com

sister – 17-year-old Maria[1] – also suffering from cystic fibrosis, was at my surgery. But that day, the front page of her records had a new handwritten note: marked in red were the letters PSEUDOMONAS!!! This meant she had the infection everybody in the care of cystic fibrosis patients feared, an infection we could not master, which would eventually lead to her death. I was young at the time and not yet experienced with death. I was thinking of what to say about her future when she walked into the room. Coughing, wasted and frail she came toward me. I was about to start when I realized her eyes were shining, her cheeks blushing, and she was smiling. I stopped myself and asked "Maria – what is it?" She looked at me, gave me a broad smile and said: "Bengt, I am in love. I want to get married, and I want to have children!"

Because of her sister, she knew very well where everything was going but still, in the face of death, she was talking about life, love and having a family. Eventually, she did not make it, but it left me forever thinking of how this was possible, that what she talked about contradicted all I had learnt in medical school; this is where my journey toward salutogenesis began. Antonovsky would have said, "You idiot (as he said to himself), you were looking in the wrong direction!"

A few years later, because of Maria, I broke out of the Clinics, and in 1984, I went into public health research and training at the Nordic School of Public Health (Nordic School of Public Health), serving five countries in interdisciplinary postgraduate training and research. These were the years when the World Health Organization (WHO) Health for All Strategy was launched; WHO stepped beyond health care into community health and launched the Ottawa Charter for Health Promotion in 1986, which advocated a structural approach to implement health promotion.

My years at Nordic School of Public Health were intensive and rewarding. Of great significance to me, Aaron Antonovsky was a regularly returning visiting scholar at the school from 1987 to 1994, active and engaging in teaching and guiding seminars. It would not take long before he was appointed Honorary Professor at the Nordic School at the same time as Ilona Kickbusch, the then Health Promotion Director of WHO.

I took special care to accompany him during his visits to the School, and I eagerly attended his lectures and seminars, taking detailed notes. As a result, I have a collection of his lectures spanning 7 years and several hours of his presentations on video recordings. I admired the way he presented salutogenesis concepts in the classroom; and ever since, I have tended to emulate his pedagogic approach and his use of drawings to illustrate key ideas.

He was teaching at the European Training Consortium Course at the school when he agreed to read the manuscript of my first publication on salutogenesis, dealing with the amelioration of children experiencing family breakdown. The emphasis was on seeing divorce through the perspective of the child and as a *process,* not as one point-in-time event. Three questions are important from a salutogenic perspective: How do adverse life events affect one over time? How do adverse events (here related to divorce) unfold from the perspective of the target group (here the child)? What is needed to steer a constructive process? My conclusion was that it is not the life event of "divorce" as such that is important. The important thing is what conditions prevail before and after, how the whole process is managed, how does the child perceive it, and how does it make sense to the child?

Discussing my paper, Antonovsky approved of my line of thought. This was 1993; he mentioned he was going to participate in an important meeting at WHO in Copenhagen, where he was to hold a seminar attended by leading health promotion experts, on how salutogenesis could be used as a framework for health promotion. It was a shock when, shortly after the Copenhagen meeting, I received a fax from Aaron reading, *"Dear Bengt, I have a malignant cancer, going into care tomorrow, pray for me."* He died days later. The loss of Antonovsky paralyzed his closest research networks for a long time. It was also the end of his Salutogenesis Newsletters, which at the time were the primary source of news about salutogenesis developments globally.

His WHO presentation was published in *Health Promotion International* after his death (Antonovsky, 1996). This landmark work concluded:

> With great respect for the concept of health promotion (and for those committed to it), I have none the less been highly critical, in emphasizing that the basic flaw of the field is that it has no theory. The salutogenic orientation has been proposed as providing a direction and focus, allowing the field to be committed to concern with the entire spectrum of health ease/dis-ease, to focus on salutary rather than risk factors, and always to see the entire person...

Within a few years, Antonovsky's posthumously published call to action was well heeded. It is not an exaggeration to proclaim this single publication as the catalyst – the milepost – for the burgeoning of salutogenesis scholarship.

A Chronology of Key Developments After 1996

This chronology has a decidedly personal cast since I am aware of salutogenesis developments mainly through my involvement. My first organizational responsibility outside the Nordic School of Public Health was as the Secretary General of the European Society of Social Pediatrics (ESSOP). At the same time, I took a similar position in NOBAB (Nordic Network for Children's rights and needs in

[1]The name has been changed to protect privacy and confidentiality.

health care) concerned with implementing the Convention on the Rights of the Child within Health Care.

One key member of ESSOP whom I worked with for a long time on many health promotion projects was Concha Colomer (1958–2011) from Valencia, Spain. Concha holds a special place in the development of salutogenesis scholarship as a cofounder of a postgraduate training summer course in health promotion that has salutogenesis as a shaping principle. The course is run by the European Training Consortium in Public Health and Health Promotion – ETC-PHHP (the founding partners were the Nordic School of Public Health, the Valencian School of Public Health, the Andrija Stampar School of Public Health in Croatia, and the Liverpool Department of Public Health). Since 1991, 782 students have been trained, coming from over 60 different countries. In a separate chapter in this Handbook, Vaandrager and colleagues describe details of the history and activities of the course.

The autumn following Antonovsky's death, I visited the school of Public Health in Granada, Spain, to participate in a health promotion seminar lead by Erio Ziglio, the WHO European Director of Health Promotion. We discussed the need for greater emphasis on salutogenesis in health promotion research and training, and in 1995, I set up courses on health promotion and salutogenesis at the Nordic School. I was in charge of the course on salutogenesis for over 15 years. In 2007, the salutogenesis course evolved to become the International Seminar on Salutogenesis of the Global Working Group on Salutogenesis – GWG-Sal – which I chaired for a decade (more about GWG-Sal later).

I had the opportunity to introduce salutogenesis at the first Nordic Health Promotion Research Conference at the University of Bergen in 1996, where Maurice Mittelmark was the host. Salutogenesis has featured on the program at all subsequent Nordic conferences, the most recent being the Ninth, held in 2019 at Roskilde University.

About the same time, I was invited to a Swedish Research Council seminar on the status of research on salutogenesis. Attending were Marianne Cederblad and Kjell Hansson, who were among the first to research salutogenesis in Sweden (they also hosted Antonovsky's sabbatical in Lund in 1987). Also participating in the seminar was Olle Lundberg, who together with Maria Nyström Peck had developed the three-question SOC scale. The consensus emerging from the seminar was that research on measuring the SOC was too meager. I wished to contribute to the needed research and recruited Monica Eriksson to work with me on the task. Monica had written her master's thesis on salutogenesis in Finland, where Guy Bäckman had introduced salutogenesis to Finnish academia. With me as her advisor, Monica undertook her PhD at Åbo Akademi University Vasa on the sense of coherence, which resulted in a series of publications that have become classic papers in the field (Eriksson, 2007).

There were many other salutogenesis developments at about the same time. Maurice Mittelmark was the President of the International Union for Health Promotion and Education – IUHPE. He was determined to pave the way for salutogenesis in health promotion, and in 2007, the IUHPE established GWG-Sal, with me as its founding Chair.

A bit earlier, I worked to infuse salutogenesis into a 6-year European Union project to establish a framework for a European Masters in Health promotion (EUMAHP, 1998–2004). The project included many prominent health promotion scholars from the continent, among them was Georg Bauer, who was to succeed me as head of GWG-Sal when I retired in 2017.

In a related EU project aiming to develop health promotion indicators (the EUPHID project), Bauer led the team that constructed an influential framework for research indicators, which had an explicit salutogenesis orientation (Bauer et al., 2006).

In 2005, I became Research Director for Health Promotion at Folkhälsan, an old established Finish NGO that was involved in population health and community development practice and research. Monica Eriksson joined me on the research team. The Folkhälsan position allowed me, for the first time in my career, to pull my thoughts together and focus entirely on my work on salutogenesis.

Monica and I conducted systematic reviews, with rigorous inclusion and exclusion criteria, of research that had used Antonovsky's salutogenesis framework up to that time (Eriksson, 2007). We also built an open-access database on salutogenesis to serve researchers all over the globe. During our 5 years at Folkhälsan, we helped to consolidate international collaboration. For example, we worked closely with two Norwegian collaborators to establish significant salutogenesis infrastructure in Norway. Geir Espnes was the founding director of the Center for Health Promotion Research at the Norwegian University for Science and Technology in Trondheim, and Nina Mjosund reconfigured the Buskerud Regional Psychiatric Services in Norway, resulting in a unique entry point for salutogenesis in mental health care.

From 2007 on, the IUHPE became a principal arena for salutogenesis, which has had a significant place in IUHPE global and regional conferences ever since. This helped to expose health promotion practitioners and researchers to salutogenesis, but a dedicated meeting place was also needed for people immersed in salutogenesis.

Responding to the need, we organized the First International Seminar on Salutogenesis in Helsinki in the Spring of 2008, with about 150 researchers and practitioners participating from Asia, Europe, and North America. Among them was Shifra Sagy (whose PhD advisor in Israel had been

Antonovsky), who gave a brilliant presentation on the early days of salutogenesis.

At the end of 2008, we organized the first meeting of GWG-Sal at Nordic School of Public Health, with founding members Sagy, Mittelmark, Bauer, Lindström, Eriksson, Corey Keyes (United States), Lenneke Vaandrager (the Netherlands), and Jürgen Pelikan (Austria).

The Second International Seminar on Salutogenesis was held in 2009, at Folkhalsan in Helsinki. The same year, the GWG-Sal members participated in a seminar on resilience in London, and as a group, presented salutogenesis and its relationship to resilience to the audience. We also held our second GWG-Sal meeting in London, and at that meeting, we agreed to produce a handbook on salutogenesis, which was published by Springer (Mittelmark et al., 2017).

The Third International Seminar on Salutogenesis was arranged at the IUHPE World Conference in Geneva in 2010, where we launched salutogenesis on a broad scale to the global health promotion community. The same year we introduced our work at the WHO Global Conference on Health Promotion in Nairobi. All IUHPE World Conference scientific programs have since had input from GWG-sal, leading to many salutogenesis subplenary, paper, poster sessions, and workshops, during the 2013, 2016, and 2019 conferences.

In 2010, we published *The Hitchhiker's Guide to Salutogenesis: Salutogenic Pathways to Health Promotion* (Lindström & Eriksson, 2010). This was first published in English, and at the time of writing, the book is available in eight languages: English, Spanish, Catalan, French, Norwegian, Italian, German, and Polish.

In 2011, the International Seminar on Salutogenesis was arranged at University West in Trollhättan, Sweden, where Monica Eriksson was later appointed Professor. The same year, I was appointed Professor of Salutogenesis (the first professorship with this title) at the Norwegian University of Science and Technology in Trondheim, Norway (where I continued until my retirement in 2017). The GWG-Sal operation moved with me to Trondheim, where Geir Espnes had established a new Center for Health Promotion Research. Geir launched a series of International Health Forum biannual conferences (2012–2018), wherein a dedicated part of the scientific program was the International Seminar on Salutogenesis. On my retirement in 2017, Georg Bauer took over the leadership of the GWG-Sal at the newly founded Center on Salutogenesis at the University of Zürich in Switzerland.

Coincident with the inauguration of the Zürich center (by the President of the University), GWG-Sal launched the Society for Theory and Research on Salutogenesis – STARS (www.stars-society.org). The *society* was established as a home for academics interested in salutogenesis, reaching beyond the health promotion discipline to welcome other disciplines in the social science and biomedical sciences communities. The year 2017 was a boom year for salutogenesis; besides the activities just mentioned, the first edition of *The Handbook of Salutogenesis* was published as an open-access publication of Springer Nature, edited by GWG-Sal members. In the short period since its publication, the handbook has risen to the top three Springer open-access publications globally, measured by the number of downloads. It was the popularity of the first edition that gave GWG-Sal members the motivation to start work on this second edition.

Conclusion

The first salutogenesis study was undertaken in the late 1960s and published in Antonovsky's books in 1979 and 1987. With his background in medical sociology, he related his salutogenic framework to the field of health, and he wished to foment a paradigm adjustment, from pathogenesis standing alone to pathogenesis *and* salutogenesis. He reasoned that the field of health promotion was fertile ground for such a shift. Where are we at this point? In a practical sense, the contents of this handbook answer the question. There seems to be no doubt that salutogenesis is thriving in its research, teaching and theory building.

Yet, salutogenesis is still in its infancy, a maturing construct, but with many unanswered questions that are posed in the concluding sections of many of this book's chapters. The final chapter of this handbook, coauthored by its GWG-Sal editors, addresses some of the critical issues that salutogenesis as an academic field must address to advance as transdisciplinary science, and hasten the paradigm adjustment that Antonovsky envisioned (Bauer et al. 2020).

References

Antonovsky, A. (1996). The salutogenic model as a theory to guide health promotion. *Health Promotion International, 11*(1), 11–18.

Bauer, G., Davies, J. K., Pelikan, J., & Euhpid Theory Working Group and The Euhpid Consortium. (2006). The EUHPID Health Development Model for the classification of public health indicators. *Health Promotion International, 21*(2), 153–159.

Bauer, G. F., Roy, M., Bakibinga, P., Contu, P., Downe, S., Eriksson, M., … Mana, A. (2020). Future directions for the concept of salutogenesis: A position article. *Health Promotion International, 35*(2), 187–195.

Eriksson, M. (2007). *Unravelling the Mystery of Salutogenesis*. Folkhälsan Research centre, Research Report 2007:1. Helsinki.

Lindström, B., & Eriksson, M. (2010). *The hitchhiker's guide to salutogenesis: Salutogenic pathways to health promotion*. Folkhälsan Research Center.

Mittelmark, M. B., Sagy, S., Eriksson, M., Bauer, G. F., Pelikan, J. M., Lindström, B., & Arild Espnes, G. (2017). *The handbook of Salutogenesis*. Springer Nature.

3

The Salutogenic Model, Sense of Coherence and the Salutogenic Orientation

Maurice B. Mittelmark and Georg F. Bauer

Introduction

In the health promotion field, the term salutogenesis is associated with various meanings that Aaron Antonovsky introduced in his 1979 book *Health, Stress and Coping*, and that he expounded in many subsequent works. In its most thoroughly explicated meaning, salutogenesis refers to *the salutogenic model of health*, which posits that life experiences help shape one's sense of coherence—an orientation towards life as more or less comprehensible, manageable and meaningful. A strong sense of coherence helps one mobilise resources to cope with stressors and manage tension successfully. Through this mechanism, the sense of coherence helps determine one's movement on the health ease/dis-ease continuum.

In its narrower meaning, salutogenesis is often equated with one part of the *model*, the *sense of coherence*, specifically defined as:

> a global orientation that expresses the extent to which one has a pervasive, enduring though dynamic feeling of confidence that one's internal and external environments are predictable and that there is a high probability that things will work out as well as can reasonably be expected. (Antonovsky, 1979, p. 123).

In its most general meaning, salutogenesis refers to a *salutogenic orientation,* particularly in health promotion research and practice, focusing attention on the origins of health and assets for (positive) health, contra to the origins of disease and risk factors.

These meanings are distinct yet inextricably intertwined. The heart of the salutogenic model is the sense of coherence, a 'global orientation'easily conflated with the 'salutogenic orientation' since the concept of orientation is central to both. A helpful distinction is that 'orientation' in relation to the sense of coherence has relevance for all humans' ability to engage resources to cope with stressors. In contrast, 'orientation' in relation to salutogenesis refers to professionals' interest in the study and promotion of the origins of health and assets for health rather than tackling the origins of disease and risk factors.

This book is about salutogenesis in all these meanings—the salutogenic model, the sense of coherence and the salutogenic orientation. These meanings and their reception in research and practice are taken up in this chapter to set the stage for the chapters that follow. We also briefly discuss salutogenesis in relation to other concepts within and beyond the health arena, with which salutogenesis has important kinship.

The Salutogenic Model

By his own account, the turn in Antonovsky's life from pathogenesis to salutogenesis began to crystallise in the late 1960s. Having worked up to that point as a stress and coping survey researcher with foci on multiple sclerosis, cancer and cardiovascular diseases, he realised that his real interest did not have its starting point in any particular disease. Instead, the starting point was *'the illness consequences of psychosocial factors howsoever these consequences might be expressed'* (Antonovsky, 1990, p. 75). This insight led to research and publications on the ideas of 'ease/dis-ease' (breakdown) and generalised resistance resources. Still, it did not mark the full emergence of salutogenesis in his thinking. At this stage of his career, Antonovsky's focus was still pathogenic (ibid, p. 76). Another decade would pass before

M. B. Mittelmark (✉)
Department of Health Promotion and Development, Faculty of Psychology, University of Bergen, Bergen, Norway
e-mail: maurice.mittelmark@uib.no

G. F. Bauer
Center of Salutogenesis, Division of Public and Organizational Health, Epidemiology, Biostatistics and Prevention Institute, University of Zürich, Zürich, Switzerland
e-mail: georg.bauer@uzh.ch

Antonovsky came to the question *'what makes people healthy?'* and the need to coin the term salutogenesis to convey the thinking mode implied by the question. The time and space to develop these ideas came while he was on sabbatical at Berkeley in 1977 and 1978.

The fruition was Antonovsky's full exposition of salutogenesis in *Health, Stress and Coping* (Antonovsky, 1979), the publication of which completed his turn from pathogenesis to salutogenesis. Antonovsky's illustration of the salutogenic model is reproduced in Fig. 3.1. Up until the 1979 book, no research based on the salutogenic model had been undertaken. The model's core construct, the sense of coherence, had yet to be fully developed, operationalised and measured, and it was to this task that Antonovsky turned his effort. As a result, his book *Unraveling the Mystery of Health* (Antonovsky, 1987) focused a great deal of his attention on the sense of coherence and its role as an independent variable in health research (Eriksson & Lindström, 2006, 2007). Other aspects of the salutogenic model received less attention. Antonovsky's ambitions for further development of the salutogenic model were cut short by his death at age 71, just 7 years following the publication of *Unraveling the Mystery of Health.*

Health professions and disciplines have yet to be powerfully touched by salutogenesis, even if Antonovsky was professionally situated in a medical school during all the years he developed salutogenesis. The venerated *Dorland's Illustrated Medical Dictionary*, in print since 1900 and now in its 33rd Edition, does not even have an entry for salutogenesis, much less the salutogenic model (Dorland, 2020).

The salutogenic model has not yet deeply penetrated social science or medicine; this does not mean that there is no penetration, and the chapters of this book are evidence that certain health-related arenas are captivated. Many scholars who *do* refer to the salutogenic model stray far from its main ideas. Interest in the model's details is watered down by the sweeping generality of the salutogenic orientation, and by the intense interest the sense of coherence awakens. Four aspects of the salutogenic model that require attention are mostly neglected: (a) the origins of the sense of coherence, (b) other answers to the salutogenic question than the sense of coherence, (c) health defined as something other than the absence of disease and (d) processes linking the sense of coherence and health.

The sense of coherence develops from infancy. Antonovsky wrote extensively about the roles of culture in salutogenesis and the development of the sense of coherence (Benz et al., 2014). His writings included attention to the role of culture in shaping life situations, in giving rise to stressors and resources, in contributing to life experiences of predictability, in load balance and meaningful roles, in facilitating the development of the sense of coherence and in shaping perceptions of health and well-being (ibid). With almost the sole exception of work by Israelis, culture is not a theme in salutogenesis research (see, e.g. Braun-Lewensohn & Sagy, 2011; Sagy, 2015). One might protest and point to the plethora of studies that have translated sense of coherence questionnaires. Still, such research is not the study of the cultural forces to which Antonovsky called attention.

Stepping up the salutogenic model's ladder, cultural and historical context is understood as a cauldron generating psychosocial stressors and resistance resources. The processes involved are little studied. Which psychosocial resources are predictably generated by which child-rearing patterns, which social role complexes and their interaction? Is it the case that generalised resistance resources are of prime importance to developing the sense of coherence as Antonovsky maintained, and which are of most importance during which life stages? Do specific resistance resources (SRRs) also play a vital role? How does the experience of stress affect the shaping of resistance resources? Unaddressed questions about the origins of the sense of coherence abound.

Moving on to the issue of *other answers to the salutogenic question than the sense of coherence*, Antonovsky invited others to search for them, even if his interest remained firmly with the sense of coherence. The question is this: What factors (presumably besides the sense of coherence) intervene between the stress/resources complex on the one hand and the experience of health on the other hand? A convenient way to partition the question is with the intra-person/extra-person differentiation. The sense of coherence is an intra-person factor; which other intra-person factors may be important? There are many candidates (hardiness, mastery and so forth), but little effort to compare and contrast their mediating and moderating roles with the sense of coherence *in the same research designs*.

As to extra-person salutary factors, there is at least movement in promising directions. In the work and health literature specifically, and in the settings literature more generally, interest is growing in how physical and social environments can enhance well-being and performance. Such research is attentive to the sociocultural environment, not as a force in shaping the sense of coherence, but as a mediating factor, which may facilitate coping. In the health promotion area, this is referred to as 'supportive environments'. A fundamental precept is that health-enhancing social policy should create supportive environments. An example of a salutary extra-person factor is work and family corporate support policy, which is an SRR related positively to job satisfaction, job commitment and intentions to stay on the job (Butts et al., 2013). Most interestingly, it may be that the perceived availability of support under such policy, rather than the *use* of supports, is the critical factor in good job-related outcomes (ibid). Concerning GRRs at work, Brauchli et al. (2015) identified key job resources relevant for health outcomes across a broad range of diverse economic sectors,

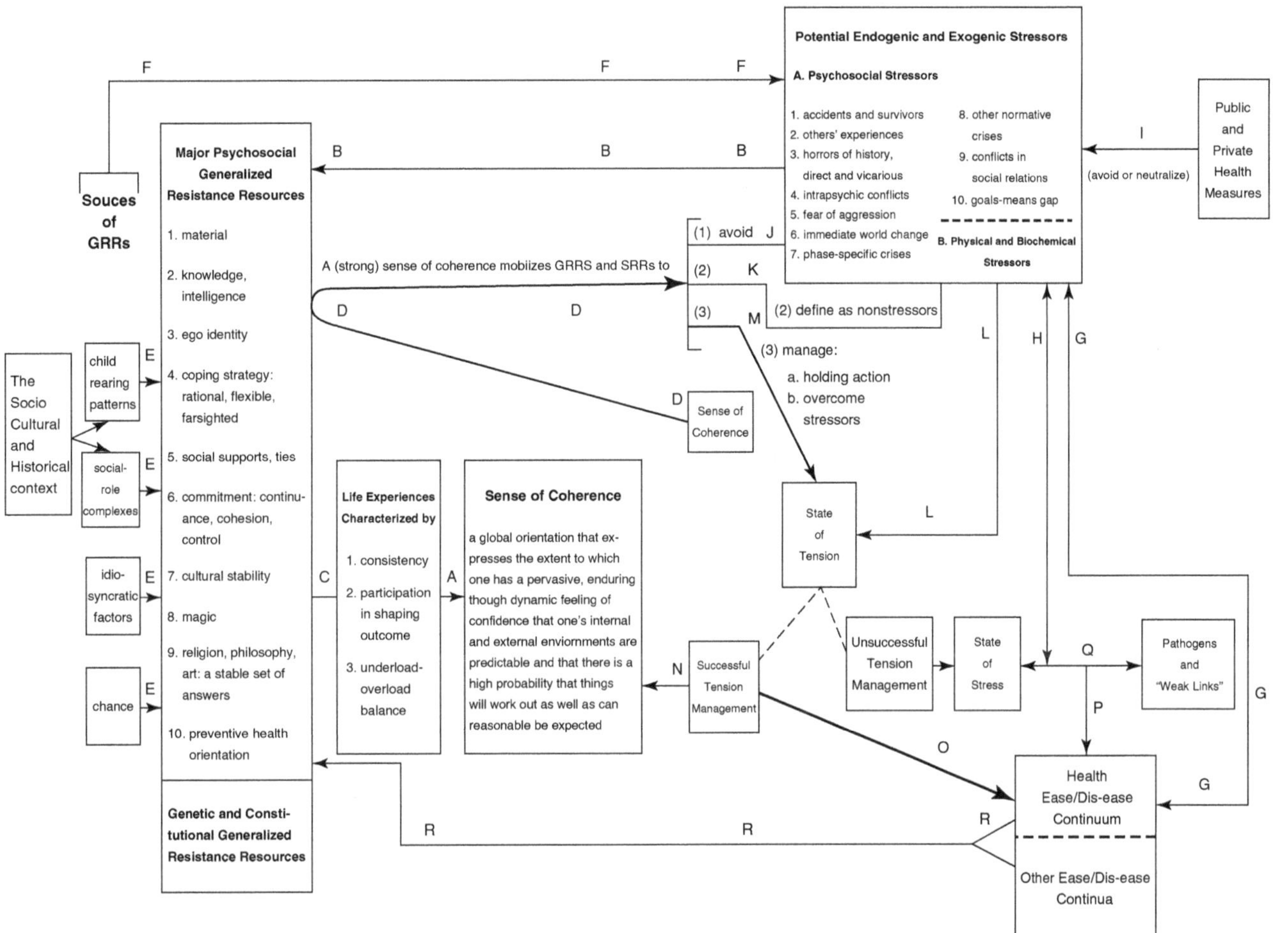

Key to Figure 1

Arrow A: **Life experiences shape the sense of coherence.**

Arrow B: Stressors affect the generalized resistance resources at one's disposal.

Line C: **By definition, a GRR provides one with sets of meaningful, coherent life experiences.**

Arrow D: **A strong sense of coherence mobilizes the GRRs and SRRs at one's disposal.**

Arrows E: **Childrearing patterns,social role complexes,** idiosyncratic factors, and chance **build up GRRs.**

Arrow F: The sources of GRRs also create stressors.

Arrow G: Traumatic physical and biochemical stressors affect health status directly; health status affects extent of exposure to psychosocial stressors.

Arrow H: Physical and biochemical stressors interact with endogenic pathogens and "weak links" and with stress to affect health status.

Arrow I: Public and private health measures avoid or neutralize stressors.

Line J: A strong sense of coherence,mobilizing GRRS and SRRs, avoids stressors.

Line K: A strong sense of coherence,mobilizing GRRS and SRRs,defines stimuli as nonstressors.

Arrow L: **Ubiquitous stressors create a state of tension.**

Arrow M: **The mobilized GRRs (and SRRs) interact with the state of tension and manage a holding action and the overcoming of stressors.**

Arrow N: **Successful tension management strengthens the sense of coherence.**

Arrow O: **Successful tension management maintains one's place on the health ease/dis-ease continuum.**

Arrow P: Interaction between the state of stress and pathogens and "weak links" negatively affects health status.

Arrow Q: Stress is a general precursor that interacts with lhe existing potential endogenic and exogenic pathogens and "weak links."

Arrow R: Good health status facilitates the acquisition of other GRRs.

Note: The statements in bold type represent the core of the salutogenic model.

Fig. 3.1 The salutogenic model of health. (Reprinted from Antonovsky, 1979. Published with permission of © Avishai Antonovsky. All Rights Reserved)

companies and professions. Furthermore, they showed that independent from one's hierarchical position, gender or age, job-related GRRs both protect from negative consequences of work-related stressors (job demands) and directly promote positive health outcomes such as work engagement. The last finding points to the fact that positive health development works not only through the originally postulated salutogenic path of coping but also through GRRs promoting positive health outcomes.

Moving to *health defined as something other than the absence of disease*, the definitions of health evident in the salutogenesis literature are not as specified initially in the salutogenic model of health (Mittelmark & Bull, 2013). Research articles reporting on the relationship of the sense of coherence to a wide range of single disease endpoints fail to note that this is a departure from the salutogenic model's specifications. In contrast, Antonovsky had described the degree of pain, functional limitation, professional prognosis and need for treatment as four broader criteria to assess the movement towards the ease end of the health ease/dis-ease continuum. However, these criteria still define health in negative terms—health is the absence of those four negative qualities. In contrast, health promotion researchers and practitioners applying the salutogenic orientation focus on positive health outcomes—the presence of perceived well-being or fulfilment.

Finally, moving to the issue of *processes linking the sense of coherence and health*, the salutogenic model posits that the sense of coherence helps a person mobilise GRRs and SRRs in the face of psychosocial and physical stressors. This may end with stressors: (1) avoided, (2) defined as non-stressors, (3) managed/overcome, (4) leading to a tension that is managed with success (and enhancing the sense of coherence) or (5) leading to unsuccessfully managed tension. These outcomes impact one's movement on the ease/dis-ease continuum, but what mechanisms link the sense of coherence and movement on the continuum? The sense of coherence is postulated as an orientation towards the appraisal of stimuli, not as a cognitive or emotional mechanism that converts information about stressors and resources into coping responses. What *else* happens in the brain that lies between the sense of coherence and coping responses? This is a little-studied question, surprising since the appraisal of stimuli plays a considerable role in the salutogenic model.

The discussion above suggests some areas of neglected development of the salutogenic model. Why is the model relatively neglected? One obvious answer is its newness and complexity; another is that Antonovsky himself did not pursue the whole complex model's empirical testing. Instead, he focused on the sense of coherence that he considered as the key concept, and even as the ultimate dependent variable in salutogenic thinking. Thus, it is not surprising that many other scholars have followed his inspiring leadership and focused on studying the sense of coherence part of the model. Another explanation might be that the salutogenic model is still incomplete (Bauer et al., 2019). As mentioned above, beyond the coping path, one would need to add a direct path of positive health development leading from generalised promoting (not resistance) resources to positive health outcomes. In his last paper, Antonovsky (1996) introduced the idea of 'salutary factors that actively promote health'. Simultaneously, such an expanded salutogenic model would better capture the salutogenic orientation with its focus on resources/assets and (positive) health outcomes going beyond the absence of disease.

Salutogenesis as the Sense of Coherence

Antonovsky situated salutogenesis as a question: what are the origins of health? His answer was the sense of coherence. The question and this answer comprised the heart of his salutogenic model as just discussed. Antonovsky invited other answers to the salutogenic question while remaining convinced that his answer was fundamental. The way Antonovsky posed and answered the question of salutogenesis was challenging. 'Origins'—he used the plural form—signal the possibility of multiple health-generating determinants and processes. His singular answer—the sense of coherence—suggested a channelling of all salutogenic processes through a particular mental orientation. This answer provides an appealing reduction of complexity compared to the concept of pathogenesis, with its legion of risk factors:

> A salutogenic orientation , I wrote, provides the basis, the springboard, for the development of a theory which can be exploited by the field of health promotion [...] which brings us to the sense of coherence (Antonovsky, 1996).

He considered the sense of coherence as the fundamental concept of the salutogenic model. We say no more about the content of the sense of coherence idea here, referring the reader instead to Part III of this book, which is devoted to the topic. Instead, we focus on why the sense of coherence has been overriding as the answer to the salutogenic question. Why is the sense of coherence equivalent in meaning to salutogenesis for so many scholars?

Firstly, Antonovsky strongly signalled that of all the salutogenic model's aspects, the sense of coherence deserved special attention. In his influential 1996 paper in Health Promotion International, Antonovsky proposed a research agenda consisting *solely* of sense of coherence questions:

- 'Does the sense of coherence act primarily as a buffer, being particularly important for those at higher stressor levels, or is it of importance straight down the line?
- Is there a linear relationship between sense of coherence and health, or is having a particularly weak (or a particularly strong) sense of coherence what matters?
- Does the significance of the sense of coherence vary with age, for example, by the time the ranks have been thinned, and those who survive generally have a relatively strong sense of coherence, does it still matter?
- Is there a stronger and more direct relationship between the sense of coherence and emotional well-being than with physical well-being?
- What is the relationship between the person's movement toward well-being and the strength of his/her collective sense of coherence?
- Does the sense of coherence work through attitude and behaviour change, the emotional level, or perhaps, as sug-

gested by the fascinating new field of PNI (psychoneuroimmunology), from central nervous system to natural killer cells?' (Antonovsky, 1996, pp. 16, 17).

Notably, some of these questions focus on neglected issues discussed in the paragraphs above on the salutogenic model. Antonovsky's focus on the sense of coherence was clear, which undoubtedly influences subsequent generations of salutogenesis researchers' choices.

Besides the importance of Antonovsky's lead, the sense of coherence has the charm of relative simplicity: it suggests that all salutogenic processes are channelled through a measurable global life orientation. Thus, this single, focused concept reduces complexity. Further, the sense of coherence concept has high face validity for both researchers and populations to which it is applied. It makes immediate sense that perceiving life as comprehensible, manageable and meaningful is conducive to health. It is also supposedly more complete and generalisable, and not culture bound, in contrast to concepts such as internal locus of control and mastery. The combination of cognitive, behavioural and motivational components positions the sense of coherence uniquely, and they are all measurable.

This last point that the sense of coherence is appealingly measurable may be the most significant reason for its centre-stage position in the salutogenesis literature. In the prestigious journal *Social Science and Medicine*, Antonovsky (1993) published a paper titled *The Structure and Properties of the Sense of Coherence Scale*, cited as of this writing by over 2500 publications, a momentous achievement. Within just a few years, Antonovsky's sense of coherence scale had been used in 'at least 33 languages in 32 countries with at least 15 different versions of the questionnaire' (Eriksson & Lindström, 2005). The stream of sense of coherence measurement papers has continued unabated (Rajesh et al., 2015).

Thus, it is understandable that, for many, salutogenesis is synonymous with the sense of coherence: it is Antonovsky's answer to the salutogenic question, it was his sole priority for further research and sense of coherence measurement has scientific importance. Still, several lines for future advancement of the SOC concept have been identified (Bauer et al., 2019).

The Salutogenic Orientation

In his last paper, published posthumously, Antonovsky (1996) wrote:

> I was led to propose the conceptual neologism of salutogenesis—the origins of health—(Antonovsky, 1979). I urged that this orientation would prove to be more powerful a guide for research and practice than the pathogenic orientation.

Was Antonovsky predicting a paradigm shift? It is important to note that the 1996 paper cited above was directed at the field of health promotion, which Antonovsky felt had too whole heartedly accepted pathogenesis thinking and disease prevention via risk factor reduction. Expressing his hopes for 'proponents of health promotion,' Antonovsky wrote that the salutogenic orientation might help them 'carve out an autonomous existence—though one undoubtedly in partnership with curative and preventive medicine' (Antonovsky, 1996). Not so much a complete paradigm shift from pathogenesis *to* salutogenesis, Antonovsky wished to foment a shift to salutogenesis as a viable theory basis and an essential supplement to pathogenesis in the health and social sciences (Mittelmark & Bull, 2013). In introducing the salutogenic orientation, Antonovsky referred explicitly to Thomas Kuhn's (1962 and 2012) idea of paradigmatic axioms, which need to change for a paradigm shift to emerge. His thoughts were on:

> ...the axiom ... which is at the basis of the pathogenic orientation which suffuses all western medical thinking: the human organism is a splendid system, a marvel of mechanical organisation, which is now and then attacked by a pathogen and damaged, acutely or chronically or fatally (Antonovsky, 1996).

Challenging this axiom, Antonovsky summarises the essence of the salutogenic orientation in contrast to the pathogenic orientation (Antonovsky, 1996):

- In contrast to the dichotomous classification of pathogenesis into healthy or not, salutogenesis conceptualises a healthy/dis-ease continuum.
- In contrast to pathogenesis' risk factors, salutogenesis illuminates salutary factors that actively promote health.
- In contrast to focusing on a particular pathology, disability or characteristic of a person, salutogenesis might work with a community of persons and relate to all aspects of the person.

We return to our earlier question, slightly rephrased: was Antonovsky calling for a paradigm shift *from* pathogenesis *to* salutogenesis? Certainly not in the sense of salutogenesis as the usurper of pathogenesis. He repeatedly remarked that pathogenesis would remain dominant in the 'health' arena. However, he did hope that salutogenesis would achieve an ascendant position as *the* theory of health promotion. This is not yet achieved but salutogenesis is on the rise. The Health Development Model (Bauer et al., 2006) is a prominent framework for developing health promotion indicators, and it explicitly incorporates aspects of both pathogenesis and salutogenesis. If the paradigm shift concept is not too grand to apply, we could say that the shift is to a paradigm that incorporates pathogenesis and salutogenesis. Even if modest so far, this shift is perhaps the most promising contribution of the salutogenic orientation to the health and social sciences. Compared to other concepts relevant to a search for the origins of health, such as assets, resources, coping and resilience, salutogenesis is in a sense a complete concept, offering a new outlook on health outcomes, health determinants and health development processes. For many health promotion researchers, using the term 'salutogenesis' communicates at a minimum that one pursues an alternative, complementary approach to pathogenesis.

Many health resources and assets concepts (e.g. social support, the sense of coherence, self-efficacy, hardiness and action competency) have kinship under the salutogenesis umbrella (Eriksson & Lindström, 2010). The umbrella also covers diverse positive health conceptions such as quality of life, flourishing and well-being. In this light, salutogenesis might be defined simply as processes wherein individuals' and communities' resources are engaged to further individual and collective health and well-being. Of course, this umbrella concept is a particular view of the salutogenesis aficionado; a self-efficacy researcher might be inclined to place salutogenesis under the umbrella in the company of all the other positive health concepts.

Salutogenesis in Companionship: Comparable Concepts and Developments

The salutogenic model originated as a stress and coping model (Antonovsky, 1979). Antonovsky referred to Selye's (1956) and Lazarus and Cohen's (1977) work as inspirational. As does the salutogenic model, Lazarus and Cohen's transactional model of stress assumes an interaction between external stressors and a person who evaluates stressors based on the resources available to cope. In the domain of working life, the well-established job demand-control model (Karasek, 1979; Bakker et al., 2015), the effort-reward imbalance model (Siegrist et al., 1986; Van Vegchel et al., 2005) and the more generic job demands-resources model (Bakker & Demerouti, 2007) share with the salutogenic model the basic idea of a balance between stressors and resources, and that they have been empirically tested in relation to disease outcomes. In a recent development, an organisational health model has emerged from the explicit linking of the job demand-resource model (Bakker & Demerouti, 2007) with salutogenesis (Bauer & Jenny, 2012; Brauchli et al., 2015).

Salutogenesis as an orientation is an idea in close concert with a broad academic movement towards a positive perspective on human life. There are traces of salutogenesis in philosophy, at least since Aristotle reflected on the hedonic and eudaimonic qualities of (positive) health (Ryan & Deci, 2001). Three decades before *Health, Stress and Coping*, the World Health Organization's constitution pronounced that health is more than the absence of disease. Illich (1976) commented on the medicalisation of life. Social epidemiology has a long tradition of considering broad social determinants of health beyond the proximal disease risk factors (Berkman et al., 2014). More recent developments include research on positive psychology and positive organisational behaviour in organisational psychology (Nelson & Cooper, 2007), on happiness in management research (Judge & Kammeyer-Mueller, 2011), on place as a resource in social ecology (Von Lindern, Lymeus & Hartig, this volume), on promoting strengths in educational sciences (Jensen, Dür & Buijs, this volume) and on pre-conditions for substantially rewarding, satisfying and fulfilling lives in the field of positive sociology (Stebbins, 2009; Thin, 2014). In health promotion, the positive paradigm is evident in the recent literature of two kinds: that which describes protective factors against untoward outcomes (e.g. Boehm & Kubzansky, 2012) and that which describes factors promoting well-being (Eriksson & Lindström, 2014).

Conclusions

This chapter—and this handbook—introduces a broad swath of developments that excite the present generation of salutogenesis scholars. Some of these developments are relevant to the salutogenic model, others are firmly focused on the sense of coherence and yet others are more identifiable with salutogenesis as an orientation. The book also takes up parallel developments in positive psychology, occupational and organisational health sciences, social ecology and educational sciences that may make little explicit reference to salutogenesis and are in evident close kinship with salutogenesis. It is one of the main aims of this book to invite an inclusive, bridging dialogue meant to nourish salutogenesis in all its meanings. The book also aims to introduce salutogenesis researchers to scientific kinfolk who contemplate matters highly relevant to salutogenesis, even if they do so in works of literature not searchable with the keyword 'salutogenesis'.

References

Antonovsky, A. (1979). *Health, stress and coping*. Jossey-Bass.

Antonovsky, A. (1987). *Unraveling the mystery of health—How people manage stress and stay well*. Jossey-Bass.

Antonovsky, A. (1990). A somewhat personal odyssey in studying the stress process. *Stress Medicine, 6*(2), 71–80.

Antonovsky, A. (1993). The structure and properties of the sense of coherence scale. *Social Science and Medicine, 36*(6), 725–733.

Antonovsky, A. (1996). The salutogenic model as a theory to guide health promotion. *Health Promotion International, 11*, 11–18.

Benz, C., Bull, T., Mittelmark, M., & Vaandrager, L. (2014). Culture in salutogenesis: The scholarship of Aaron Antonovsky.

Global Health Promotion, 21(4), 16–23. https://doi.org/10.1177/1757975914528550

Dorland, W. A. N. (2020). *Dorland's illustrated medical dictionary33: Dorland's illustrated medical dictionary*. Elsevier Health Sciences.

Bakker, A. B., & Demerouti, E. (2007). The job demands-resources model: State of the art. *Journal of Managerial Psychology, 22*, 309–328.

Bakker, A. B., van Veldhoven, M., & Xanthopoulou, D. (2015). Beyond the demand-control model. *Journal of Personnel Psychology, 9*(1), 3–16.

Bauer, G., Davies, K. D., & Pelikan, J. (2006). The EUPHID health development model for the classification of public health indicators. *Health Promotion International, 21*, 153–159.

Bauer, G. F., Roy, M., Bakibinga, P., Contu, P., Downe, S., Eriksson, M., Espnes, G. A., Jensen, B. B., Juvinya Canal, D., Lindström, B., Mana, A., Mittelmark, M. B., Morgan, A. R., Pelikan, J. M., Saboga-Nunes, L., Sagy, S., Shorey, S., Vaandrager, L., & Vinje, H. F. (2019). Future directions for the concept of salutogenesis: A position article. *Health Promotion International, 35*, 187.

Bauer, G. F., & Jenny, G. J. (2012). Moving towards positive organisational health: Challenges and a proposal for a research model of organisational health development. In J. Houdmondt, S. Leka, & R. R. Sinclair (Eds.), *Contemporary occupational health psychology: Global perspectives on research and practice* (Vol. 2). Wiley-Blackwell.

Berkman, L. F., Kawachi, I., & Glymour, M. (Eds.). (2014). *Social epidemiology*. Oxford University Press.

Boehm, J. K., & Kubzansky, L. D. (2012). The heart's content: The association between positive psychological well-being and cardiovascular health. *Psychological Bulletin, 138*(4), 655.

Brauchli, R., Jenny, G. J., Füllemann, D., & Bauer, G. F. (2015). Towards a job demands-resources health model: Empirical testing with generalisable indicators of job demands, job resources, and comprehensive health outcomes. *BioMed Research International, 2015*, 959621.

Braun-Lewensohn, O., & Sagy, S. (2011). Salutogenesis and culture: Personal and community sense of coherence among adolescents belonging to three different cultural groups. *International Review of Psychiatry, 23*(6), 533–541.

Butts, M. M., Casper, W. J., & Yang, T. S. (2013). How important are work–family support policies? A meta-analytic investigation of their effects on employee outcomes. *Journal of Applied Psychology, 98*(1), 1.

Eriksson, M., & Lindström, B. (2005). Validity of Antonovsky's sense of coherence scale: A systematic review. *Journal of Epidemiology and Community Health, 59*(6), 460–466.

Eriksson, M., & Lindström, B. (2006). Antonovsky's sense of coherence scale and the relation with health: A systematic review. *Journal of Epidemiology and Community Health, 60*(5), 376–381.

Eriksson, M., & Lindström, B. (2007). Antonovsky's sense of coherence scale and its relation with quality of life: A systematic review. *Journal of Epidemiology and Community Health, 61*(11), 938–944.

Eriksson, M., & Lindström, B. (2010). Bringing it all together: The salutogenic response to some of the most pertinent public health dilemmas. In A. Morgan, E. Ziglio, & M. Davies (Eds.), *Health assets in a global context: Theory, methods, action* (pp. 339–351). Springer.

Eriksson, M., & Lindström, B. (2014). The salutogenic framework for well-being: Implications for public policy. In T. J. Hämäläinen & J. J. Michaelson (Eds.), *Well-being and beyond: Broadening the public and policy discourse: New horizons in management* (pp. 68–97). Edward Elgar.

Illich, I. (1976). *Medical nemesis: The expropriation of health*. Pantheon Books.

Judge, T. A., & Kammeyer-Mueller, J. D. (2011). Happiness as a societal value. *Academy of Management Perspectives, 25*, 30–41.

Karasek, R. A. (1979). Job demands, job decision latitude, and mental strain: Implications for job redesign. *Administrative Science Quarterly, 24*, 285–308.

Kuhn, T. S. (1962). *The structure of scientific revolutions*. The University of Chicago Press.

Lazarus, R. S., & Cohen, J. B. (1977). Environmental stress. In I. Altman & J. F. Wohlwill (Eds.), *Human behavior and environment* (Vol. 2). Plenum.

Mittelmark, M. B., & Bull, T. (2013). The salutogenic model of health in health promotion research. *Global Health Promotion, 20*(2), 30–38.

Nelson, D., & Cooper, C. L. (2007). *Positive organisational behavior*. Sage.

Rajesh, G., Eriksson, M., Pai, K., Seemanthini, S., Naik, D. G., & Rao, A. (2015). The validity and reliability of the sense of coherence scale among Indian university students. *Global Health Promotion.* https://doi.org/10.1177/1757975915572691

Ryan, R. M., & Deci, E. L. (2001). On happiness and human potentials: A review of research on hedonic and eudaimonic well-being. *Annual Review of Psychology, 52*(1), 141–166.

Sagy, S. (2015). Coping, conflict and culture: The salutogenic approach in the study of resiliency. In D. Ajdukovic, S. Kimhi, & M. Lahad (Eds.), *Resiliency: Enhancing coping with crisis and terrorism* (pp. 41–48). Ios Press.

Selye, H. (1956). *The stress of life*. McGraw-Hill.

Siegrist, J., Siegrist, K., & Weber, I. (1986). Sociological concepts in the etiology of chronic disease: The case of ischemic heart disease. *Social Science & Medicine, 22*, 247–253.

Stebbins, R. A. (2009). *Personal decisions in the public square: Beyond problem solving into a positive sociology*. Transaction.

Thin, N. (2014). Positive sociology and appreciative empathy: History and prospects. *Sociological Research Online, 19*(2), 5.

Van Vegchel, N., De Jonge, J., Bosma, H., & Schaufeli, W. (2005). Reviewing the effort–reward imbalance model: Drawing up the balance of 45 empirical studies. *Social Science & Medicine, 60*(5), 1117–1131.

4

Salutogenic Idea and Aaron Antonovsky: The Man and Researcher

Avishai Antonovsky and Shifra Sagy

"Your candle burned out long before your legend ever did" (Bernie Taupin, Candle in the wind).

Introduction

In January 1945, while serving in the American army and stationed in New Guinea, Aaron Antonovsky (hereafter Aaron) wrote a long letter to his younger brother, Carl, who was then 13, ongoing adolescence. Aaron, at the age of 21, expressed two things that would later on become a significant part of his academic character. He wrote: "You don't know the meaning of 'iconoclast'—but you know the idea, because Avraham Aveenu [Abraham, one of the fathers in the Bible] was one. What did he do? He looked all about him, questioned everything, rebelled against everything … and he mercilessly destroyed everything that was false. He broke not only the idols themselves, but the belief he himself had once had in them. He had not yet discovered the great principle of his life, but he had cleared the way for it." Years later, perhaps less dramatically, pathogenesis was "removed" from the agenda to make way for salutogenesis. Toward the end of the letter, Aaron wrote: "… throughout our lives, we must never stop asking questions; but it is most important now." A half a century later, in a tribute to Aaron, Ilona Kickbusch wrote "… there is nothing more practical and efficient than asking the right question …. Aaron Antonovsky consistently had the courage to ask the right question: how is health created?" (1996, p. 5).

Rebelling against the mainstream and searching for the right questions seem to be the two most salient characteristics that bridge between Aaron the scholar and Aaron the man.

In this chapter, we wish to share some insights we have regarding the development of the salutogenic idea, by drawing lines connecting it to the *person* Aaron was. Having been very close to Aaron for several decades, we feel that a certain degree of familiarity with his personal background would contribute to the understanding of the development of the salutogenic theory. Therefore, we wish to shed some light on Aaron's personal experiences, ideological beliefs, and professional development throughout his life, until the crystallization of the salutogenic idea. Being close to him, and knowing what he would prefer, we shall refer to him by first name throughout this chapter (unless quoting others).

But how does one write about Aaron the scholar, without diving too deeply into the world of salutogenesis, which will be discussed thoroughly throughout this book? How does one write about Aaron the man, without becoming too biographically boring? We shall try to accomplish this task by avoiding strict academic writing; instead, following a brief history of his life, we will highlight a few qualities which, we believe, are characteristic of Aaron's scholarly work and his personal life. In doing so, we will quote friends and colleagues of Aaron's who have agreed to contribute their illustrative memories to this chapter.[1] These will be embellished with some unknown, perhaps humorous, anecdotes.

Rebellion and the Importance of Questions

Aaron was born in the United States in 1923, 5 years after the end of World War I and 6 years before the outburst of the Great Depression. His parents and older sister had fled from Russia a few years earlier, arrived in Canada, traveled

A. Antonovsky (✉)
Department of Health and Well-being, Medical Corps, Israel Defense Forces, Ramat-Gan, Israel
e-mail: Antonovsky.soc@gmail.com

S. Sagy
Martin Springer Center for Conflict Studies, Ben-Gurion University of the Negev, Be'er Sheva, Israel

[1]The names of these people are marked in **bold** typeface.

to England, and back to Canada before they finally settled down in Brooklyn, New York. As a child, Aaron's social environment consisted of immigrant families, mostly lower-class Jews and Italians. His father owned a small laundry shop where his wife and two older children spent many hours helping out. Somehow, they managed to survive the difficulties of adapting to a new culture in times of a severe economic depression. Later, in the 1930s, Aaron's parents—for whom education was extremely important (having little or no formal education themselves)—sent him to a prestigious high school, and then to college, until he was drafted into the American army during World War II and sent to the Pacific.

As an adolescent, Aaron was deeply involved in the HaShomer HaTza'ir Jewish youth movement, where he first absorbed a socialistic ideology. As his younger brother **Carl** told us, "Belonging to a Jewish organization was obvious." **Selma Rieff,** a close friend, who met Aaron as a child in the youth movement, remembers those days, of endless ideological discussions, as most important in shaping Aaron's orientation to life.

This was perhaps the first instance of Aaron the rebel because unlike most movement members, he was against Communism. At the age of 26, after the establishment of the State of Israel in 1948, Aaron came to Israel and was a founding member of a kibbutz,[2] where his socialist ideology came into practice.

Upon returning to the United States in the early 1950s, Aaron completed his doctorate in sociology at Yale University. By that time, he had been involved in research and writing about social class, discrimination, inequality, immigration, and ethnic minorities. During this period, we believe, the seeds were planted for what would a quarter of a century later evolve into being the salutogenic model. For Aaron, the two decades between 1955 and 1975 were years of transition: personally, he had married, spent a year in Iran and then came back to Israel (this time to the city of Jerusalem), had a child born, and ended up in the city of Beer Sheva, helping to set up a new medical school. Professionally, Aaron moved back and forth between the sociological studies on immigration, culture, and social class, and the focus on sociology of health. During this period, he was coauthor or coeditor of four books, which are possibly not familiar today to health promotion scholars, but we see them as tied to the salutogenic revolution: *Poverty and health* (1969), *Hopes and fears of Israelis* (1972), *From the golden to the promised land* (1979), and *A time to reap* (1981).

People suffering discrimination, or poverty, or the struggle to adjust to a new country as immigrants (or founding a kibbutz on bare land in the summer heat or the winter cold), are quite obviously prone to physical or mental sickness. Still, many such people maintain good health and well-being. The question that began to arise in Aaron's mind was not why some of these people feel miserable, but rather how some of them manage quite well. This question became more salient following a study of women Holocaust survivors, many of whom were found to be well adapted, despite the excruciating experience in concentration camps and poor life conditions after immigration to Israel.

The answer, which Aaron has termed the sense of coherence, was to follow. But it was the salutogenic *question*—not why does one become sick but how does one move toward the health pole on the ease–dis-ease continuum—that constituted the major philosophical change in thought, from the traditional pathogenic orientation to the salutogenic view of the mystery of health.

The emphasis on asking the right *question*, as a key to relevant answers, is, we believe, crucial to the advancement not only of the study of health and well-being but also of all scientific endeavors. Aaron's mantra "*Ask the right question!*" has been following one of us (AA), first as a teenager, later as a young student, and to these days as a researcher in the social sciences; it is useful in the academia, but no less in solving "simple" daily problems, be it why the TV remote control does not work or where to go on the next vacation.

Asking questions, in itself, is a kind of rebellion. It signifies resistance to blind acceptance. But Aaron wanted more. Aaron put into deeds the words attributed to Mark Twain: "Whenever you find yourself on the side of the majority, it's time to pause and reflect."

From a personal-developmental perspective, we see the roots of Aaron's salutogenic theory in his concrete childhood and adolescence experiences, from which he derived the tendency to question the world and rebel against what he believed was wrong. In a recent conversation, his younger brother **Carl** described him as "very idealistic, striving for a better world, intellectually curious, full of compassion, and having a strong feeling of how things should be done."

Aaron's parents, optimistically tackling the daily hurdles in the time of the Great Depression, served for him as living examples of viewing life as comprehensible, manageable, and meaningful. It is, therefore, clear why he dedicated his book *Unraveling the mystery of health* (1987b) "To my parents ... from whom I learned about the sense of coherence." A good illustration of the strong bond between Aaron and his

[2]A kibbutz (in Hebrew: collection; plural: kibbutzim) is an Israeli unique kind of collective settlement. A person living in a kibbutz is a kibbutznik. There are a few hundred kibbutzim; the first established in 1909. Traditionally based on agriculture, they began as utopian socialist communities, carrying the slogan "From each according to his ability, to each according to his need." Today, many kibbutzim have been privatized, and industry has replaced much of the agriculture.

Antonovsky Aharon Eng English 5I I5

May I3 I940

Remembrances of warmth and life.

The dishes were still on the table.The bright kitchen lights provided a contrast to the darkness all about us.The hissing sound of the radiator reminded us of the fierce frost raging outside. I,a little boy with girls hair ,sat on the chair satisfied to the fullest extent. Eyes and ears wide open,I listened.My mother,the center of my world, sat next to me,the book open on her lap,reading to her little son.

This scene is engraved upon my memory.True,age has put a halo around it,romanticized it,but it stands out clearly in my mind as one of the most beautiful times of my childhood.For several months each evening I would be transported to another world,a world where people lived clean,wonderful lives,and fought against filth and degradation and oppression.Night after night the two of us would sit down after supper and my mother would read.It was "mother " by Gorki that so enchanted the two of us.My mother would read several lines in the Russian and transmit the beauty and idea in them to mein jewish. In spite of the fact that I was far too young to appreciate the entire meaning of the book it was one of the most important things that ever happened to me,

Why? First,it acted as a stimulant in my choice of reading. The beauty and hardness -of reality-of the book provided a basis for shaping my way of thinking and of life of a City child.....discribable only by the smile on the face of a sleeping infant or the joy one experiences when one lives for an hour a day,a yearwith the vibrant smell of the freshness of trees and green grass penetrating one's nostrills- I felt the contentment and warmth of one physically and mentally living a pure,healthy life.

And now when my mother sees me she thinks of the seeds she impregnate within me- the seeds of revolt. A rebellions son faces her.But she does not realize that this is the only way-that it is an immutable law for the son to revolt,to demand to live his own way of life.I am my mother's son.She has taught me thus.Could she but grasp the spark that burns within me,that she herself has planted I would be happy . It has been such a long time that I have written here.Probably the most important part of my life till now has passed during this time.why have I not writing anything. For whom I am I writing? who shall see this?

Fig. 4.1 High school essay by Aaron Antonovsky (yellow markings added by the authors)

mother, his early idealistic thoughts of social justice and health, and his tendency toward rebellion is found in an excerpt from an English essay he wrote in high school at age 16. The original, in Aaron's handwriting, was typewritten by him several years later (see Fig. 4.1). His essay, by the way, earned him a B+ mark.

Warmth and Informality Versus Strictness and Academic Demands

Several colleagues and friends have pointed out two characteristics of Aaron that we know very well, and—we believe—have enabled him not only to make his way to the hearts of other people but also to be a good researcher and health educator: informality, on the one hand, and uncompromising academic demands, on the other.

In a Western professional world where it is a custom to go to work with shoes, a jacket, and a tie, Aaron was known for his appearance with sandals, a short-sleeved shirt, and of course no tie. This habit may have its origin in the kibbutz life, and it was probably very convenient to wear such an outfit in Beer Sheva (where Aaron lived for 18 years while at Ben Gurion University of the Negev).[3] We assume that on very formal occasions abroad (i.e., outside Israel) he would wear a tie, but in our memories (at least for AA), the only time Aaron wore a suit and a bow-tie was for the ceremony in 1993, in which he received an honorary doctorate at the Nordic School of Public Health in Göteborg, Sweden.

An illustration of Aaron's openness, talkativeness, and informality is found in an article by Suzanne C. Ouellette (Kobasa). In 1998, a special issue of *Megamot* ("Trends"—the leading Israeli behavioral sciences journal) was devoted to "Salutogenesis and wellness: Origins of health and well-being." Ouellette, who developed the concept of *hardiness* at about the same time that the idea of the *sense of coherence* was born (e.g., Kobasa, 1979), wrote an article for the special issue, titled "Remembering Aaron Antonovsky: A conversation cherished and one missed." Here are a few excerpts of that article (Ouellette, 1998), back-translated from Hebrew (unfortunately, we were unable to find the original English manuscript, which was translated into Hebrew for the special issue):

> I had only one opportunity to meet Aaron Antonovsky and enjoy a lively, open, and informal conversation about research questions that had interested us. It took place at his parents' apartment in Brooklyn, New York. It was in summer 1982, only a few years after each one of us published, without being introduced to each other, what we had thought were new and unique calls for research about the things that keep people healthy under stress.
>
> In the phone conversation we had before that meeting, Aaron explained that he was visiting his parents and told me a bit about them and his relationship with them. His parents lived during the time of the Holocaust and were now in their old age. His visit was to make sure they are alright. It was also an opportunity for him to gain strength from two people who had been, and still were, key figures for him; an example of how people live, in Aaron's words, a *salutogenic* life.
>
> At the meeting itself I got the impression that Aaron's parents were full of vitality despite their age (his father was over 90 and his mother was approaching 90). They did what was needed to make sure their son's stay in New York would be comfortable and that our meeting would be pleasant for me as well. Aaron was dressed informally: an army-like khaki shirt. I have seen this kind of shirt, but usually in films in a desert area, not in the streets of Brooklyn or Chicago. I wore a suit, but his outfit was more appropriate for the summer heat that day. I looked more or less like I thought that a young lecturer should look like at a meeting with a senior scholar. The clothes remained the only representations of our difference in status. The conversation itself was a free exchange of ideas between two people who had committed themselves to certain questions regarding human behavior, to the search for better-developed theories and for better means to examine such theories.
>
> Much of Aaron's work consisted of simultaneously presenting his own work and the work of others. He developed his ideas by putting them side by side with others' similar ideas. He has given us a lesson on how to work; his intention was not to show that his approach was better; instead, he demonstrated how confrontations between the theoretical and practical ideas of different researchers give rise to new questions, which may bring us closer to a better understanding of human behavior. He showed us that a sense of coherence can be found through the loneliness of writing.

In the same spirit, **Rudolf Moos** of Stanford University has recently written to us about Aaron:

> He loved to engage in discourse with me and several of my colleagues and was always ready and eager to review his ideas and to learn about our comments and criticisms. We had quite a few long conversations about his ideas, which were incisive, original, and rather revolutionary for the time.
>
> Our own work focused heavily on the positive (and negative) influences of the social context on health and behavior and on the specific ways in which individuals could confront and manage stressful life events and life crises.

Regarding the way Aaron related to others' criticisms, **Shifra Sagy** (second author) remembers his openness to critical opinions of other researchers, let them be senior or junior. "He may have not been perceived as such in the academia," says Shifra, "but I knew this characteristic of his very well." She elaborates:

> He always encouraged me to express my opinion and even to argue with him. He liked to tell the story of how I became research coordinator for his big study on sense of coherence and retirees' adjustment. During my first job interview with him, I said he is very wrong, including only retirees in the study, and that to understand their adjustment to retirement he should also have a sample of the retirees' spouses.
>
> I went home and told my husband there is no chance that I got the job. Apparently, I was wrong; and the rest is history.

Deo Strümpfer, a friend and colleague from South Africa, added:

> He was the most supportive colleague and "teacher" a person can ever hope to have. His comments on pre-publication papers were incisive, yet always kind and warm; an amazing aspect was how quickly he responded. He connected persons with similar interests with one another.

Aaron's informality has apparently struck the memories of several other colleagues and students. **Moshe Prywes**, the first Dean of the Beer Sheva medical school (died in 1998), said: "I first met Aaron when he was a fellow at the Guttmann Institute of Applied Social Research at the Hebrew University of Jerusalem. I couldn't help but notice the man who was wearing shorts and sandals." (Prywes, 1996, p. ii). **Asher Shiber**, a medical student and later a colleague, lately recalled that once every week or two, Aaron (and his wife,

[3]Beer Sheva is called the "capital of the Negev." The Negev is a dry, desert-like region in the southern part of Israel. The temperatures range from about 10° (centigrade) in the winter to 35–40° in the summer.

Helen) would invite two or three students to their house for dinner. **Ayala Yeheskel**, a social worker in Beer Sheva in the mid-1980s, told us:

> A while before a meeting with Antonovsky in January 1985, I lost my son, Eldad. At the time I was employed as a social worker in the Department of Psychiatry and in the Department of Family Medicine at the Soroka Medical Center in Beer Sheva, and spent much time teaching about the biopsychosocial approach. Besides that, I was exploring possible topics for my doctoral dissertation at the Hebrew University of Jerusalem, in the context of life stories of Holocaust survivors. About a month after my personal tragedy, emotionally uneasy, I turned to Antonovsky for counseling. With utmost patience and tenderness, he listened, and at the end of the meeting he asked me a question I will never forget: "Ayala, you are now in the midst of your own private holocaust; how will you engage in a subject you are so personally close to? In any case, I will help you and wish you good luck." I felt I had received approval, from an admired and beloved person, of my ability—in spite of my personal circumstances—to carry on with the tasks I had planned for myself.

Aaron's informality and warmth were expressed not only toward his colleagues and students. Several times, while on visits abroad, Aaron was interviewed by local newspapers. One would expect that a serious professor, a well-known scholar in his field, would present himself in formal dress. However, some photos show this was not the case: he was photographed riding a bicycle or wearing short pants because that is what made him comfortable (unfortunately, the authors' attempts to contact the newspapers and obtain permission to use the 30- to 40-year-old photos were unsuccessful).

The Establishment of the Medical School and the "Beer Sheva Spirit"

Although not directly related to salutogenesis or to Aaron's personal characteristics, it seems that a short background on the establishment of the medical school in Beer Sheva is needed in order to put several of the quotes and stories hereafter in context. **Shimon Glick**, professor of internal medicine and former Dean of the Faculty of Health Sciences at Ben Gurion University of the Negev, who worked with Aaron from the first days of the medical school in the early 1970s, described the formation of the "Beer Sheva spirit" and Aaron's contribution to it:

> When Professor Moshe Prywes of Hebrew University and Dr. Haim Doron of Kupat Holim[4] launched the new medical school at Ben Gurion University of the Negev it was not to produce another medical school, but to create an educational institution of another type entirely. This was to be a school which would train humanistic physicians with an orientation to the needs not only of their specific patients but to the needs of the community in which the school is located. These physicians would be sensitive to the psychosocial and cultural aspects of medicine. Wonderful sounding words, but really neither of the two founders of the school, nor hardly any of the existing staff or of the staff recruited to begin to teach at the school had any real concept of how to accomplish this great and important mission. Prywes recruited Aaron to be the spirit and guiding light of the project. Aaron was a scholar in sociology of health, most of it theoretical, as sociology usually is; now here was an amazing challenge and opportunity to apply sociology to the creation of an institution which would train a new kind of physician to serve his/her community in the ideal manner, sensitive to the cultural and psychological needs of the patients and their community. Aaron was not just one of several department heads recruited to join the new medical school, but was perhaps the key individual who contributed to expressing and articulating clearly the school's goals and direction. He was among the handful of individuals who laid the framework for the school. Among the revolutionary concepts were exposure of students in their first school year to patients not just in the hospital, but in their community settings, teaching them how to speak to the patients, how to understand the influence of their surroundings, economic and social conditions on their illness and the like. But first you had to pick the right kind of students who would be open to this kind of educational orientation. So, one had to change the selection process which heretofore depended only on academic achievements.
>
> All of these steps Aaron designed and taught us, step by step. Speaking for me personally, who arrived as professor of internal medicine in 1974 when the school opened, these ideas were new. I had never heretofore read an article in medical sociology, had never even heard of Antonovsky, but quickly became in some way a devoted follower of his. His ideas and concepts resonated with me and we shared fully the goals. He taught us how to interview patients, how to teach students to do so. He also created the admission process to the medical school, helped select the members of the admission committee, trained them and set into motion a unique process that has continued successfully for several decades. His leadership, absolute integrity and idealism permeated the process and made the admission committee a most prestigious and respected unit in the school, trusted by all.
>
> In reality, most physicians and basic scientists at the institution did not really fully comprehend and buy into his philosophy, because their focus and training had been in the traditional biomedical model. But Aaron influenced enough of the key people and had the full support and backing of the medical school leadership. I believe that the so called "Beer Sheva spirit," which characterizes the school and its graduates to this day, is the spirit instilled by Aaron. And in the spirit of salutogenesis that is what keeps the institution on the "right" track often in the face of adversity and administrative and bureaucratic problems.

On a more personal level, **Shimon Glick** mentioned that during almost 20 years of working together with Aaron at the medical school, himself being religious and Aaron growing up in HaShomer Hatza'ir (encompassing great ideological differences and conflicting outlooks), they have always respected one another and had much in common.

Milka Sampson is secretary of the Department of Sociology of Health at Ben-Gurion University, of which Aaron was chairperson. She worked with Aaron from the time she was appointed, in 1984, until he formally retired in

[4] Kupat Holim, literally meaning "sicks' fund," is the Israeli health plan and medical insurance institution.

1993. She described Aaron as "an honest and fair man, from whom I learned so much." She was a beginner secretary in her early 20s and remembers that "Professor Antonovsky" insisted she call him "Aaron." Before Milka, there was a secretary who would always address him as "professor." **Ofra Anson**, who worked with Aaron in the Department of Sociology of Health for almost 20 years, told us in a recent interview that Aaron once said to her in despair, relating to the secretary: "For Heaven's sake, we work together! Why doesn't she stop calling me 'the professor'?!"

Shifra Sagy (second author), who was Aaron's doctoral student and later a colleague in the department, mentioned the "Friday cakes": every Friday, it was someone else's turn to bring a cake to the staff meeting. Aaron had insisted that each one must prepare a cake by him/herself (one time, on his turn, he wanted to bake a fruit cake, but the only fruit he had at home was a grapefruit; so he baked a grapefruit cake ...). In these matters, everyone belonged to the same social status. For example, they would all take turns washing dishes.

The Friday gatherings were devoted not only to professional matters. Actually, this was also an opportunity to discuss a good book someone had read, or to celebrate someone's birthday, or to argue about politics. However, even though Aaron's belief system has probably influenced several of his career choices, he meticulously separated ideology from scientific objectivity. **Zeev Ben-Sira**, a medical sociologist from the Hebrew University of Jerusalem who passed away about a year after Aaron, addressed this issue in an obituary written a short while after Aaron's death (1995, unpublished):

> Aaron was an idealist, believing in the future of a better and just world. He vehemently contended against social injustice, discrimination, and intolerance. However he unpromisingly separated between his beliefs and his scholarly work. He strongly resisted any intrusion of ideologies into scientific objectivity.
>
> Doubtlessly, his beliefs in a better world influenced the choice of the field of his scholarly work, yet did not contaminate the objective, scrupulous and unbiased approach to his research.
>
> Understandably, then, his initial steps in his scientific career and research were devoted to the study of social discrimination, inequality, intergroup and ethnic relations, and of the absorption of immigrants.

Aaron's personal affection was combined with the great importance he ascribed to community medicine. **Aya Biderman**, a family doctor, recollects her meeting with Aaron:

> In 1980 I arrived for internship at the Soroka Medical Center in Beer Sheva, after studying medicine in Jerusalem. During that year I came to know Dr. Aaron Antonovsky, or "Aaron" as he insisted that we call him.
>
> In 1981 I began to specialize in family medicine. The Department of Family Medicine was next door to the Department of the Sociology of Health, of which Aaron was chairperson. Aaron had special feelings toward our profession. He said family medicine was one of the "islands" in which the biopsychosocial model should be applied.
>
> As a young doctor, I conducted a study on the reasons why some patients do not attend their family doctor. I hoped to have it published and thought the data may interest Aaron. I met with him to ask for his help, and he agreed. Thanks to him I had my first publication in the medical literature. Aaron's willingness to help a young doctor, who had no experience in research or writing, was very significant and gave me the push and the enthusiasm toward research and academic practice.
>
> Aaron also agreed to teach a biopsychosocial seminar in our department. It was a great learning experience which we (the young doctors) carried with us for years.

The duality of Aaron the man and Aaron the scholar was also expressed in daily work. Alongside with the warm atmosphere and informal relationships in the department, Aaron was strict about work. The department was quite small (6–7 people), and it was important for Aaron that each one would know what others were working on, as a means of mutual fertilization. He demanded from himself what he asked of others, even when it came to things normally done by junior research assistants, such as counting questionnaires. Shifra recalls that when she was beginning her doctorate, Aaron insisted that she write in English. She then gave him her handwritten draft of part of her work. The next day, Aaron gave it back to her, typewritten and corrected.

Indeed, Aaron gave his students lots of hard work. For Israeli students, most of whom have part-time jobs beside their academic studies, spending hours and hours in the library was not a trivial matter. **Asher Shiber** remembers his basic studies in medical school with Aaron: "The first thing he did was to send me to the library to read and read and read .... As an enthusiastic medical student, I wanted to do medicine, not read about medical research." As the time passed, though, students realized that hard work is productive, and they learned to appreciate Aaron's strictness. Asher sums this point: "With all my appreciation toward Aaron as a professional, the first thing that comes to my mind when I think of him is how much I loved him as a person."

Reading and reading and reading was not only a home work task which Aaron had given his students. Being a bookworm himself, Aaron believed in broadening one's education. **Joel Bernstein**, a neighbor, a friend, and a colleague from the life sciences, wrote to us:

> Our professional backgrounds might not have led to any academic interaction was it not for the connection with Judy.[5] However, from the beginning there were social gatherings and I found myself in the company of a true intellectual. I do not think a visit to the Antonovsky home passed without me reviewing the books lying on the table or in the shelves. The collection was

[5]Judy Bernstein was Aaron's research and teaching assistant and later became a faculty member in the Beer Sheva medical school, where she worked until her premature death in 2001.

> truly eclectic, with a scattering of Yiddish literature (in the original), philosophy, political science (much from the liberal academics of the 1950s and 1960s), and of course sociology and psychology. The Antonovsky abode was no more than 150 meters from ours. They moved in about a year after we did, and like everyone had to install an irrigation system—for which, with only the experience of having done my house, I became the consultant, and occasionally technical assistant.[6]

With Joel's help, Aaron spent several hours working in the garden. The first author of this chapter, having spent much time with Aaron in the garden, thinks it is possible that the seeds Aaron planted in the desert soil around the new house in 1973 were, to some extent, seeds of the salutogenic idea; more than once he would look at a few plants, some dying and some still alive, take a closer look at the green ones, and mumble "I wonder how they survive."

We believe that the importance Aaron saw in informal relationships and in expanding one's knowledge is tied to two unique qualities of the new medical school he had helped to establish, which we touched upon above, quoting Shimon Glick. First, the selection process: unlike at other universities, the main criterion for accepting candidates to medical school was not matriculation grades or psychometric scores, but rather results of two stages of semi-structured interviews. Taking into account criticism on an interview as a selection instrument, it seems that in Beer Sheva they have managed to overcome its disadvantages. As Aaron wrote, "In our case, there has come into being a widespread belief among faculty and students: more humane and responsible, less individualistic and competitive, more compassionate and concerned" (Antonovsky, 1987a).

This quote brings back a story one of us (AA) has heard once from **Dina Ben-Yehuda**, who was one of Beer Sheva's first graduates. Today she is chair of the Department of Hematology at Hadassah Medical Center in Jerusalem and Dean of the Faculty of Medicine at the Hebrew University. The anecdote occurred when Dina was already a senior doctor at Hadassah (forgive us if there are minor inaccuracies). One evening, a senior citizen in his 80s was brought by an ambulance to the emergency room (ER), after having experienced dizziness and weakness. The doctor in charge of the ER that evening, a senior resident, had the patient go through blood tests, a neurological test, and an ECG. After reviewing the results, with no significant findings, the resident doctor ordered the nurse to discharge the guy and send him home. A young intern, who was with the resident, then said: "if I may, I suggest we keep him here for the night." The resident's response was "he's fine, nothing's wrong with him, and we need the bed." The intern replied: "Indeed, he seems to be okay; but he's a widower, no one is waiting for him at home. He would probably be happy to be around people, to have someone make him a cup of tea. I'm sure we can find a bed for him. Why don't we let him spend the night here and send him home tomorrow morning?"

Dina, who was off duty, happened to be in the ER at that time and overheard the conversation. She later approached the intern and said "You studied in Beer Sheva, right?" No doubt, she knew what she was saying…

The second unique quality of the Beer Sheva medical school was the very early stage at which students faced the real world of treating patients. During their first year, students visited community clinics in development towns in the Beer Sheva region, where they met with the poor, the unemployed, and the immigrants who had lost faith in the government's promises for good life. In addition, each student was hospitalized for a few days, without revealing to the medical staff the fact that they were not real patients. They learned that beside anatomy, physiology, and chemistry, it is of utmost importance to learn about doctor-patient relationships.

Ascher Segall, another neighbor, friend, and colleague, and one of the founders of the Beer Sheva medical school, related to the link between Aaron the medical sociologist and Aaron the person:

> One of his most striking characteristics was the ability to maintain complete objectivity as a scholar in parallel with a consistent commitment to the values in which he deeply believed. His development of the theory and practice of salutogenesis attests to his rigor and creativity in research while his focus on the humanistic dimensions of medical education reflected his world view as a human being …. His impact as a teacher at the Ben Gurion School of Medicine went far beyond his formal teaching.

The impact Ascher Segall referred to is also reflected in the words of Aaron's students. For example, in a tribute by Moshe Prywes in a special issue of the *Israel Journal of Medical Sciences* in memory of Aaron, he cited Professor Dina Ben-Yehuda (whom we mentioned earlier), who was a former student of Aaron. Dina was a member of the first class of the Ben Gurion medical school, and 20 years later was Aaron's personal doctor at the Sharet Institute of Oncology in Jerusalem, where he was admitted after being diagnosed with leukemia. Prywes had asked her about Aaron, and she replied: "For Ben Gurion graduates, Professor Antonovsky was not just a name. He was a concept. A concept that contains within it much discussion and debate, all pertaining to the doctor-patient relationship … I took care of Aaron when he was sick and was with him until he died. During that time, he was in full control of all decisions concerning himself. When his condition deteriorated, he called me into his room and asked me to discontinue all treatment, and he took leave of his family and friends. I feel that I have lost the best of my teachers." (Prywes, 1996, p. ii).

The influence Aaron had on students was reciprocal, and so was the respect students and Aaron felt toward each other.

[6]We mourn the sudden death of Joel Bernstein which occurred in 2019.

Aaron's socialist ideology, and his strong belief in all people being equal, may have played a role in the way he prepared the draft for his first book, *Health, stress, and coping* (Antonovsky, 1979), as told by **Leonard Syme**, a colleague from the University of California at Berkeley:

> Aaron wrote me in the spring of 1977 to ask if he could spend a sabbatical year at Berkeley.[7] I said "yes!" immediately of course. When he arrived on campus in the fall of that year, I was able to find him a remarkable office. The office was in the basement of Stephens Hall at the end of a hallway that overlooked Strawberry Creek. It was basically isolated from the rest of the building and looked out over beautiful trees and a babbling little brook.
>
> Then we talked. Aaron said he had this idea about writing a book on something called "salutogenesis." He explained what this word meant and I was captivated. To have one of the world's great scholars come to Berkeley to explore a truly exciting and original idea was one of the great moments in my life. I asked how I could help. He said he would love to give a seminar that fall in which he could explore his ideas. It took two days to recruit an excited class of Social Epidemiology graduate students for the seminar.
>
> What happened next was one of the most amazing things I had ever seen. Aaron welcomed them to the seminar, explained how it would work, and assigned them to critically review a draft chapter that he had written after arriving at Berkeley. The next week, students discussed their assignment and, as they were leaving the room, they were asked to review another new chapter that Aaron had just written during the previous 7 days. This went on for 15 weeks. After the semester ended, Aaron had finished a complete draft of his book and was ready to send it off to a publisher. And the book, was, of course a classic.
>
> What a mind he had! I have thought about this remarkable Antonovsky phenomenon many years since it happened.

In 1983, Aaron returned to Berkeley for another sabbatical, again in an office overlooking the creek. **Guy Bäckman**, from the Åbo Akademi University in Finland, who met Aaron in Berkeley, wrote to us about their acquaintance:

> Unraveling the enigma or mystery of health was at that time a big question and theme among the researchers in Berkeley. Questions of frequent occurrence were "Why are only some of us sick although all of us are, at least in some way, exposed to risks?" and "How do we manage to stay healthy?" I had many fruitful discussions on those themes with Aaron in his office on the Berkeley campus, where, from the window, we could see lots of greenery and running water, which certainly stimulated talk about what it might be that keeps people in good condition and health in changing and sometimes risky and chaotic circumstances.

A Closure and New Horizons

Haim Gunner, an old friend from the days of the youth movement and today a professor of environmental sciences, beautifully summarized the inseparable arenas that made up Aaron's life—the quest for a just world of social equality, and the academic journey toward unraveling the mystery of health:

> The engaged and enthusiastic academic of his later years slips into the image of the devoted kibbutznik and the fields where we shared tractor and plough. And in the evenings, on a crowded balcony with the hills of Galilee facing us, dissected the future with the complete confidence of youth.
>
> Consciously or otherwise, Aaron's life was the model for the salutogenic principle. Two projects dominated his life: initially, the kibbutz and the model society to be derived from it, and always the ongoing fulfillment of the Zionist ideal. And then the building of the medical faculty at Ben Gurion University around the new concept of the family as the arbiter of the individual's health. For the kibbutz, comprehensibility was derived from the perhaps naive, but nonetheless coherent view that Marxism provided. And not only was the project which promised equality and security to be a local event but one which would eventually pervade the entire social structure. Marxism with its dicta and comprehensive weltanschauung made it eminently predictable. Our belief in our skills and the support of the community made it eminently manageable, and our passionate belief, buttressed by juvenile psychoanalytic insights, that it gave meaning to our lives make the kibbutz and its realization the perfect model for the principles of salutogenesis: comprehensibility; manageability and meaningfulness.

We wish we could devote a few paragraphs to the words Aaron's beloved wife, Helen, would have to say for this book. Unfortunately, Helen passed away in 2007. Along the 36 years of marriage to Aaron, she was his greatest supporter, admirer, and critic. There was probably not even one article, lecture, or book of Aaron's that went to press before Helen had read and approved the manuscript. A research psychologist and scholar in her own right, Helen was an inseparable part of the scholar and the man Aaron was.

Shifra Sagy (second author) has been engaged in salutogenic research throughout her academic career, specializing in social-psychological and collective aspects of sense of coherence. She introduced the salutogenic paradigm into the Department of Education, where she headed the educational psychology program for several years. After her retirement, she is still heading the research center of conflict studies at Ben Gurion University of the Negev, under the philosophical agenda of salutogenesis. Avishai (first author) is a social psychologist and grew up in a "salutogenic" household, but until a few years ago salutogenesis has not been a central part of his academic work. However, currently Avishai is leading the implementation of salutogenic thought, as well as the conduction of research, in the Department of Health and Well-being of the Israeli Medical Corps. This promising line of work is described in more detail elsewhere in this book. Aaron would probably be surprised, and hopefully happy, to learn about this new path salutogenesis is marching on. As it appears, salutogenesis has gone way beyond the scope of medical sciences and health, and has become an interdisciplinary area of research and practice.

Aaron passed away in 1994, but his salutogenic vision continues to stimulate theory, research, and policy-making

[7] In 1977, Leonard Syme was chairman of the Department of Biomedical and Environmental Health Sciences in the School of Public Health at the University of California, Berkeley.

worldwide. We hope students and professionals around the world will profit from this comprehensive handbook on salutogenesis, and perhaps some of them will continue to develop salutogenic research and carry it on to new horizons. After all, salutogenesis is not limited to physical or mental health; it is a philosophy of human existence.

References

Antonovsky, A. (1979). *Health, stress, and coping*. San Francisco: Jossey-Bass.

Antonovsky, A. (1987a). Medical student selection at the Ben Gurion University of the Negev. *Israel Journal of Medical Sciences, 23*, 969–975.

Antonovsky, A. (1987b). *Unraveling the mystery of health*. San Francisco: Jossey-Bass.

Kickbusch, I. (1996). Tribute to Aaron Antonovsky—'what creates health'. *Health Promotion International, 11*, 5–6.

Kobasa, S. C. (1979). Stressful life events, personality, and health: An inquiry into hardiness. *Journal of Personality and Social Psychology, 37*, 1–11.

Ouellette (Kobasa), S. C. (1998). Remembering Aaron Antonovsky: A conversation cherished and one missed. *Megamot, 39*, 19–30. (Hebrew).

Prywes, M. (1996). A tribute. *Israel Journal of Medical Sciences, 32*, i–ii.

5

Life Events of Aaron Antonovsky and Development of SMH

Hege Forbech Vinje, Eva Langeland, and Torill Bull

Introduction

> I hope it will become clear in due course that my concern is no mere semantic quibble and that here, as in all of science, how one poses the question is crucial to the direction one takes in looking for the answers (Antonovsky, 1979, p. 12).

When a person thinks seriously about a topic over a period of about three decades, it is a sign of good thinking and personal development if, at the end of that period, he/she is no longer in total agreement with former ideas. Adventures along the road become the germ (to use Antonovsky's own expression) of new ideas and layers of understanding. So was also the case with the development of the salutogenic model of health (SMH), a development described by Antonovsky himself in retrospect as a "personal odyssey" over decades (Antonovsky, 1990). While Chap. 3 portrays Antonovsky, the man and the researcher, this chapter portrays the SMH and its development along with life events of its creator until the untimely death of Antonovsky in 1994. The chapter is based on the authorship of Antonovsky himself. Papers written in his last years, in which he looks back and comments on how his thinking developed, have been of particular value. These papers come in addition to the publications in which he originally introduced his ideas. In the SMH, there are important concepts, the development of which we trace in this chapter: stress, breakdown, resources, sense of coherence (SOC), and health.

Antonovsky departs, in his two major books (Antonovsky, 1979, 1987) from the traditional medical view of homeostasis being the basic human condition, and introduces the fundamental philosophical view of *"the human organism as prototypically being in the state of heterostatic disequilibrium as the heart of the salutogenic orientation"* (Antonovsky, 1987, p. 130). The release of *Health, Stress and Coping* in 1979 was a culmination of 15 years of work, during which he came to understand that disease, illness, and entropy (decline into disorder) are the norm rather than the exception to a rule of otherwise self-regulated homeostatic processes occasionally being disturbed with resulting pathology. He found it to be a futile task to try to understand and control every single factor that might lead to this or that particular disease. A more fruitful approach would be to focus on what he found to be the overall problem of active adaptation to an environment in which stressors are omnipresent and inevitable. He presented the term *negative entropy* (Antonovsky, 1987, p. 9) in which the goal was to search for useful inputs to the sociocultural context, the physical environment, and into the organism down to the cellular level to counter the normal tendency of entropy. So, negative entropy, or *negentropy* as he also termed it, is actually something positive.

In his efforts to study health instead of disease, Antonovsky coined his famous new word: "*salutogenesis*—of the origins *(genesis)* of health *(saluto)*" (Antonovsky, 1979, preface vii), the intriguing question being: what are the origins of health? In the course of his research, Antonovsky correspondingly offered an answer to the question: *"The origins of health are to be found in a sense of coherence"* (Antonovsky, 1979, preface vii). This question and the answer constitute the SMH, the development of which is the focus of this chapter. In his descriptions of the model, most importantly of the process developing it, he points to the struggles it entailed for him, and for other researchers and

H. F. Vinje (✉)
THE FORBECH VINJE ACADEMY (www.forbechvinje.no), Sandefjord, Norway

E. Langeland
Department of Health and Caring Sciences, Faculty of Health and Social Sciences, Western Norway University of Applied Sciences, Bergen, Norway

T. Bull
Department of Health Promotion and Development, Faculty of Psychology, University of Bergen, Bergen, Norway

practitioners, to move from one paradigm to another: *"I have no illusions. A salutogenic orientation is not likely to take over. Pathogenesis is too deeply entrenched in our thinking...."* (Antonovsky, 1996b, p. 171). Antonovsky urged, nevertheless, researchers of different professions, and with use of different methodologies, to work together to bring the knowledge of the origins of health increasingly further.

Antonovsky worked on the SMH for more or less 30 years. The first 15 years resulted in his book *Health, Stress and Coping* in 1979, and the presentation of SMH in its entirety. The next 15 years he was improving, refining, and cultivating the understanding of the model and the elements in it. The release of his 1987 book *Unravelling the Mystery of Health* represented a peak in his career. This release was originally intended to be a revised version of *Health, Stress and Coping*, but ended up being a whole new book, primarily presenting and explaining the concept of sense of coherence, his answer to the salutogenic question. His second book became a huge success and is translated into several languages.

In the preface of his first book, Antonovsky (1979) points out that he offers no easy solutions to the salutogenic question, and that he does not shy away from technical discussions when needed. His writings are directed not only to his colleagues in medical sociology but also to sociologists, psychologists, psychiatric nurses, physicians, healthcare organizers, epidemiologists, architects, community organizers, and even more, who professionally or personally want to understand and enhance the adaptive capacities of human beings (Antonovsky, 1979, preface viii). His rather wide scope of intended audience is also reflected in the cross section of where he finds theoretical and intellectual inspiration. He expresses indebtedness to students, research assistants, and colleagues, without whom he would not have reached as far as he did. Repeatedly he points out the necessity and value of students' and peers' criticism not only for the ideas he took from them but also for the intellectual challenge in the need to explain why. Not only throughout *Health, Stress and Coping* especially but also in *Unravelling the Mystery of Health,* Antonovsky specifies to whom he owes his intellectual debts. He names and credits scholars such as Hans Selye, René Dubos, George Engel, Thomas Holmes, Richard Rahe, John Cassel, and Melvin Kohn. As he believes to have broken new ground, he also claims to see echoes of his ideas everywhere (Antonovsky, 1987, p. 34). Although he says he finds evidence of the influence of great thinkers in his work, he describes a feeling of relative isolation when introducing the concept of salutogenesis and developing the SMH. As he narrates every other researcher of the time focused on the need to explain pathology, his feeling of isolation intensified with the introduction of the sense of coherence, the answer to the salutogenic question (Antonovsky, 1987, p. 33). In developing the SMH, not only did he detach himself from his earlier work but also from the work of just about everyone else at the time. Around the time of the release of *Health, Stress and Coping,* he finds, however, that the salutogenic question is increasingly asked, and he is intrigued to notice that serious research studies at least partly congruent with the SOC concept are being performed. He no longer feels alone as elements, variants, and alternative understandings of health and illness in the social sciences are surfacing (Antonovsky, 1987, p. 34). Antonovsky humbly credits this development primarily to the serious research of colleagues, and not so much to his own work. He dedicates a chapter in his 1987 book to convergences, discrepancies, and disagreements of the research of Suzanne Kobasa, Thomas Boyce, Rudolf Moos, Emmy Werner, and David Reiss and demonstrates once more how his ideas and theories develop in interaction with the theories of other scholars.

In all his writings about the SMH, Antonovsky gives a somewhat personalized account of how he came to work on the subject at hand, he presents challenges he encounters on his way, and he clarifies and explains how he moves ahead and reaches the point at which he stands when writing this particular book or paper. Apparently he learnt this approach from Oriental scholars (Antonovsky, 1979, prologue 1). Being so detailed about his research process makes a very interesting read, and gives the impression of a humble scholar, on his way, inviting other researchers in on his reflections. Antonovsky declares that the SMH is merely one part of the conceptualization of what he finds to be one of the greatest mysteries of the study of human beings: *"How do we manage to stay healthy?"* (Antonovsky, 1979, preface vii). On a hopeful note, in *Health, Stress and Coping* he expresses a wish that the salutogenic question is convincing enough for researchers to take up the gauntlet and develop the model further; of which this book is a clear demonstration.

Stress Research: The Principal Note

At the outset, Antonovsky was not particularly interested in stress (Antonovsky, 1990). In retrospect, however, he singles out research (Hollingshead & Redlich, 1958; Kardiner & Ovesey, 1951; Selye, 1956) causing him to stop a little and reflect upon questions relevant to stress during his training years in the Yale Sumner-Keller anthropological tradition in the 1950s. Nonetheless, at the time, he found them peripheral to his main interests, and he did not believe he would spend most of his career studying the stress process. His major interests during these formative years were in *"culture and personality, stratification and ethnic relations"* (Antonovsky, 1990, p. 71). Growing up as he did in New York, being the son of Jewish parents, one can assume this interest was awakened by his exposure to both Jewish and North-American culture, cultures which he contrasted in several publications (see, e.g., Antonovsky, 1971). In 1955/1956, Antonovsky finished his doctoral dissertation in which he investigated cognitive coping responses to socially structured psychosocial stressors (Antonovsky, 1979). Minority groups and marginal social situations were the focus of his doctoral research. He continued down this path for 6 more years, though his focus shifted to the organizational response on a group level to immigration and the stressors of low income and discrimination (Antonovsky, 1979). This shift was brought on by his work on the history of the Jewish labor movement in the United States (Antonovsky, 1961), and as a director of the New York State Commission Against Discrimination. The organizational response on a group level to the stressors of poverty and immigration became a major concern and he initiated several studies on the consequences of these stressors (Antonovsky & Lorwin, 1959). So although he also worked in a series of projects in the 1950s not connected to his main interests (an experience well known to many a young researcher), stressors and coping responses on both individual and group levels were of particular interest to him. He describes himself as an anthropologically oriented sociologist being interested in understanding the specifics of a society's competence—socioculturally—at coping with stressors it faces (Antonovsky, 1979). In retrospect, in his *Odyssey* article (Antonovsky, 1990), he presents himself as a sociologist of health involved in studying the stress process, and he returns some 25 years describing the starting point as being his work on life stressors.

After migrating to Israel in 1960, Antonovsky's research engagements brought more stimulation for the work he was to pursue for the rest of his life, and put him on the path of becoming a medical sociologist (Antonovsky, 1990, p. 72). He accepted a post at the Israel Institute for Applied Social Research in Jerusalem and begun teaching in the Department of Social Medicine. Together with Judith Shuval he started a research project on the latent functions of healthcare institutions (Shuval et al., 1970), and projects on coronary artery disease, multiple sclerosis, menopause, and series of studies on social class and aspects of health and disease followed (Antonovsky, 1979, the author, xiv). In 1963, he was invited by colleagues in neurology to take part in the design of an epidemiological study on multiple sclerosis, mainly because he had experience in survey research. Antonovsky joined because the study questionnaire included items on this particular area of interest for him—sociocultural factors (Antonovsky et al., 1965; Antonovsky & Kats, 1967). Included among the items was a list of stressors in objective form, such as social class and poor living conditions. This was part of Antonovsky's turn toward a focus on social class, morbidity, and mortality. Studies from this period show his commitment to hypothesizing a direct link between stressors and disease, and especially social class and disease. He defined stressors objectively as those experiences that anyone anywhere would agree were stressors, pointing to going hungry for a long period of time as his illuminating example. His primary concern at this stage was to bring the data of stressors and disease together rather than going deeper and behind the data and ask why? (Antonovsky, 1967a, 1967b, 1968).

In this period, he also coedited the book *Poverty and Health* with his colleagues in the field of sociology (Kosa et al., 1969). Together they pose the question: *"What are the stressors in the lives of poor people that underlie the brute fact that, with regard to everything related to health, illness and patienthood, the poor are screwed?"* (Antonovsky, 1979, p. 3). The why question started forcing itself to the front of his interest. Reflecting about this period of his work, Antonovsky recounts this is the time he starts to depart from what he calls the pathogenic orientation (Antonovsky, 1990). Fueling his pondering was Marc Fried's writings on social differences in mental health in the *Poverty and Health* book. Not only were the stressors important, Fried argued, the poor also had fewer resources to battle these stressors (Antonovsky, 1979, p. 3). The book clearly stated the link between poverty and poorer health, bringing the sociological insight that poorer health was not only due to lower quality of health services to the poor but also due to the conditions to which the poor were exposed. As Antonovsky later wrote, the poorest life class *"had it rough down the line, whatever the dependent variable might be. This was the class which clearly had the highest stress load"* (Antonovsky, 1990, p. 73). In addition, there was another characteristic of the stress of the poor, and the minority groups, that gave insight to the why question, namely the constancy of the stressors.

> The constancy of imposed stressors in such life situations, the continuous emergencies life presents, make it immensely difficult to resolve tension. Life for even the fortunate among us is full of conflict and stressors, but there are many breathing spells (Antonovsky, 1990, p. 74).

To understand the link between stressors and disease, Antonovsky recounts struggling with the methodological problem of getting the right list of life events or stressors to ask about in a survey. Eventually, he came to terms with this not being a methodological but rather a philosophical issue; a result of what he called the pathogenic orientation, or the Parsonian view of social existence, referring to Parsons' sociological theory of the time (Parsons, 1951). At the time, research focusing on stressors tended to assume life as inherently stable and smooth with major stressors only occasionally occurring. Antonovsky (1990) claimed, however, this view not helpful and rather inadequate in understanding the stress process. A more fruitful vision is to see life as turbulent and inherently full of conflicts and stressful. Once again, he drew inspiration from Fried and what he called chronic life strain, referring to long-lasting structural and cultural situations such as poverty, unemployment, marginality, etc., a sad fact of the lives of many persons (Antonovsky, 1990, p. 73). It is important, Antonovsky argued, to understand the ongoing strain of such situations as these are also the sources of many of the major life events, as well as of the daily hassles, which people face.

Continuing undisturbed along this line of reasoning in recapturing Antonovsky's research would, however, make us overlook another important development that came as a result of a parallel development: a study of psychosocial risk factors in coronary artery disease in the form of stressors in immigrants to Israel from North America (Antonovsky, 1967b). Being in fact a respondent in his own study, Antonovsky made the observation that yes, he was exposed to stressors—but they did not result in illness, he was coping successfully. This led him to focus on how specific serious stressors were dealt with (Antonovsky, 1990, p. 74).

> This step marked the germ of the distinction I now make between tension and stress. I had not, and do not now, deny the potential illness consequences of many stressors. Well into the 1970s, I still tended to regard all stressors as unfortunate and pathogenic. But I had begun to ask: What really happens when one encounters a stressor?

The observation was made that exposure to stressors did not invariably lead to stress and illness. Stressors of various kinds created immediate tension in an organism, but if it was resolved it did not result in *stress*, which was the health-damaging condition one needed to avoid. Coping and tension management emerged as important concepts and intervening variables between tension and stress/illness. At this point in his research, there was a decisive change in his thinking, and in his scholarly pondering he turned to both Lazarus (Lazarus & Cohen, 1977) and Selye (1956) for inspiration. In brooding the "why" question, he realized that it is not just the stressors that are vital in this picture, also the poor have fewer resources in order to cope. There will be a difference if two people are exposed to the same stressor and one of them has lots of resources, while the other has practically none. Both the experience and its consequences will be different for the two. Antonovsky's study on cardiovascular disease and stress showed a link between the two. He presented these findings to an audience and was asked a thought-provoking question by Professor J. N. Morris: "*Why just cardiovascular disease, why not cancer or any other disease for that matter?*" (Antonovsky, 1972, p. 537). This set Antonovsky thinking, and the result was his realization that he was not really interested in *any* specific diseases, be it cancer or heart disease. He was interested in the illness consequences of psychosocial stressors, *the breaking down process* taking place no matter how the consequence was expressed (Antonovsky, 1979, prologue 4):

> And then it struck me. By God, Morris is right. I am not interested in heart disease or multiple sclerosis or cancer; I am interested in breakdown. This, then, is the origin of my first major departure from the mainstream.

Antonovsky realized he was interested in a general state, which he wished to call *dis-ease*. However, he found this term impractical because it would be hard, he believed, to achieve a clear enough distinction from *disease*. There are unfortunate examples in publications since Antonovsky, in which "dis-ease" turned into "disease," the hyphen being ignored. Antonovsky's point has then not been communicated. In an effort to help this important distinction come across, we suggest using a slash (dis-ease) instead of a hyphen where needed. Though in this chapter we will stay true to Antonovsky's own choice and use a hyphen. Hence, he landed on the term *breakdown* which Professor Morris had used, and whom he credited in a later paper known as his breakdown paper (Antonovsky, 1972). It was, for technical reasons, not published until 1972, but the main message in this paper was that stressors, unsuccessfully confronted, lead on to breakdown. *"It contained the first answer to the problem posed by the distinction between tension and stress, an answer expressed in the concept generalized resistance resources"* (Antonovsky, 1990, p. 76).

As this outline shows, the late 1960s seem important years to the development of his model. Antonovsky claims 1967 and 1968 as especially vital years in this respect (Antonovsky, 1979, 1990). In the years to come, he was committed to conceptualizing his insights, starting with an explicit focus on resources.

General Resistance Resources (GRRs): A Shift to Another Key

Because people meet such a variety of demands, Antonovsky found it useful to focus on understanding the *generalized resistance resources* (GRRs) because they could be applied to a wide range of demands or stressors. He proposed to distinguish between two kinds of problems: (1) the classical medical problem of why an individual or a group have the disposition for a particular disease, and (2) the problem of experiencing *dis-ease* or *breakdown*, unrelated to diagnosis and disease. The latter of these two became his focus. Further, he theorized that all diseases have something in common and that there are GRRs to counteract all of these (Antonovsky, 1979). Once again he turned to the work of Selye and found particular inspiration in Selye's term *general adaptation syndrome* (Selye, 1956, 1975). Antonovsky (1979, prologue 5) argues: *"it seems imperative to focus on developing a fuller understanding of those generalized resistance resources which can be applied to meet all demands."*

In 1967, Antonovsky made the comment that *"the impact of a given external situation upon a person is mediated by the psychological, social and cultural resources at his disposal"* (Antonovsky & Kats, 1967, p. 16). However, Antonovsky later calls this mentioning of resources essentially a remark made in passing (Antonovsky, 1974, p. 246). In the breakdown paper, he returns to the issue of resources with a clear intent and introduces his most general definition of GRRs: *"any characteristic of the person, the group, or the environment that can facilitate effective tension management"* (Antonovsky, 1972, p. 99). In the same paper, he classifies three large groups of resources: (1) adaptability on the physiological, biochemical, psychological, cultural, and social levels; (2) profound ties to concrete and immediate others; and (3) commitment of and institutionalized ties between the individual and the total community (Antonovsky, 1972, p. 100). Nevertheless, his formal definition of GRRs was not published until 1979 (see Fig. 5.2). In *Health, Stress and Coping,* he also emphasized the importance of *specific resistance resources (SRRs),* as he found them both numerous and frequently beneficial in specific circumstances of tension (Antonovsky, 1979, p. 99):

> They (SRRs) are many and are often useful in particular situations of tension. A certain drug, telephone lifelines of suicide-prevention agencies or an understanding look in the eyes of an audience to whom one is lecturing can be of great help in coping with particular stressors. But these are all too often matters of chance or luck, as well as being helpful only in particular situations.

Summing up, one important observation from this period was that stressors do not have to lead to disease because tension management and coping might function as intervening variables (effect modifiers). The degree to which people were exposed to stress, and the degree to which one had resources to cope, varied. Sure, stressors created tension, but this tension could be successfully resolved. Influenced by René Dubos and his warnings against *the mirage of health* and the escalating wars against every possible disease (Dubos, 1960), Antonovsky moved on to explore the term *adaptability* in psychological, social, and cultural contexts. Antonovsky called it *active adaptation*, and presented is as a complementary term to *the magic bullet* in the pathogenic paradigm; "*Salutogenesis, (…) leads us to focus on the overall problem of active adaptation to an inevitably stressor-rich environment*" (Antonovsky, 1987, p. 9).

In his accounts from 1990, Antonovsky finds himself at this time in his work nonetheless still firmly grounded in pathogenic thinking. He saw stressors as a threat and coping as a mean to prevent illness and disease. However, in 1967–1968 there was yet another important development. Antonovsky was, parallel to the heart disease paper, working on a study of menopausal women (Antonovsky et al., 1971). One finding was that women who had been exposed to severe stressors did poorer in later stages of life. One of the severe stressors given attention in this study was having experienced Holocaust (Antonovsky preferred to call this *a horror*, finding stressor to be a too mundane expression). Most of the women having experienced Holocaust did significantly poorer than other women did. However, a third of them did no poorer at all! This caused Antonovsky to ask, *"What was the miracle?"* (Antonovsky, 1990, p. 76). Here, we see an example of Antonovsky focusing on the deviant case (see section "Harmonizing: SMH's relevance for health promotion" for further comments on this principle). Included in the questionnaire for the menopause study were items on social integration. Antonovsky commented that this study, being prior to the main development of the later so popular concept *social support*, rather asked *how much do you feel you are needed by your spouse, children,* etc. The focus was being turned on its head toward being on the giving end rather than the receiving end of support, and this he commented in recollection was the germ of the *meaningfulness* element of sense of coherence (Antonovsky, 1990, p. 75).

The early 1970s, therefore, sees Antonovsky as having concluded that he was not interested in specific diseases but in a general state of breakdown which comes because of unsuccessful confronting of stressors.

> …breakdown is a result of unresolved disturbance of homeostasis….It is not, then, the imbalance which is pathogenic. It is, rather, the prolonged failure to restore equilibrium which leads to breakdown. When resistance resources are inadequate to meet the demand, to resolve the problem which has been posed, the organism breaks down (Antonovsky, 1972, p. 541).

The dependent variable that interested him was breakdown, and the independent variables of his concern were the GRRs. The level of stressors, whether objectively or subjectively defined, was not at this point of any interest to him (Antonovsky, 1979, prologue 5). A person could cope successfully with stressors through application of resources, called GRRs, thereby preventing the tension caused by stressors being transformed into stress.

To Antonovsky, it was obvious that having resources, being conscious about them, and having ability to use them to counter stressors was an important factor in avoiding disease or breakdown. He had already coined the concept generalized resistance resources (Antonovsky, 1972, p. 99). He also had observed the miracle of people doing well despite horrible experiences. How was that possible (Antonovsky et al., 1971)? Furthermore, he had conducted a community health study in Beersheba, finding a link between GRRs and health, later to be published as a chapter in a book edited by the acknowledged stress researchers, Barbara and Bruce Dohrenwend (Antonovsky, 1974). In 1973, the Beersheba community health study was presented at a large stress research meeting in New York, arranged by the very same Dohrenwend. At this point, GRRs have not yet been carefully defined theoretically. Antonovsky states:

> ... there was some general sense that it referred to some resource which, intuitively, we thought was good to have, an intuition sometimes supported by empirical data. (...) we were all dealing with the lack of GRRs, and hypothesizing that people with high stressor loads who lacked GRRs would become ill (Antonovsky, 1990, p. 76).

Though elements of the SMH were taking shape, Antonovsky was still not ready to formulate the full model. He describes a development over 10 years from 1968 (Antonovsky, 1990, p. 76):

> By 1968, as I have indicated, I had realised that I was interested in dis-ease, not in diseases. But it took almost another decade, involved in the growing awareness of the ubiquitousness of stressors and a greater focus on resistance resources, before I was able to take the next step.

One of the important happenings during this decade was that he moved from Jerusalem to Beersheba in 1973. Helping to set up a community- and primary care-oriented medical school there had the consequence that he thoroughly thought about the kind of doctors he and they wanted to educate (Antonovsky, 1990, p. 76). Starting by turning to the GRRs concept, still not properly defined, he was inspired to formulate his research findings and theoretical ideas into a fuller picture as he developed the curriculum. He chose to call the new department within the school *The Sociology of Health* (not medical sociology, which was commonly used in the field elsewhere). As an indication of the zeitgeist, he recounts that the Research Committee of the International Sociological Association needed 13 years to change its name from Medical Sociology to the Sociology of Health (ibid, p. 76). Bringing forth the illustration of *the river of life* and the bias of the downstream focus that was debated at the time, Antonovsky wanted to educate doctors who devoted their energies to prevent people from being pushed into the river, rather than pulling them out at the downstream end. Over time, however, Antonovsky's perspective on stress and health developed, and he came to acknowledge that there are no people on the river banks—all are in the river, as all are exposed to stressors and illness. *"Of course we differ on how close we are to drowning. But as my friend and colleague Rose Coser has taught me, 'we are all terminal cases'"* (Antonovsky, 1990, p. 76).

This differentiated his view on health and illness from that of colleagues—we are not all well and occasionally fall ill, we are all on a continuum with different degrees of health (Antonovsky, 1990, p. 76):

> It was at this point that I began to see the work of my colleagues in stress research as being characterized by a pathogenic orientation. They were asking: 'What makes people have a heart attack? Develop cancer? And so on?' I had earlier moved to the question 'What makes people sick?' But now I took a decisive further step. It was not only a matter of standing the question on its head and asking 'What makes people healthy?' I proposed asking, rather, 'What moves people toward the health end of the health ease/dis-ease continuum?

Because he was not a clinician himself, he argued, he was not in the habit of categorizing people as healthy or sick. Moreover, he understood that his formation of stressors and GRRs moved him much further than the preventive medicine perspective (Antonovsky, 1990). He discussed the need to exceed the traditional medical dichotomy of sick/healthy in the pathogenic paradigm. From the perspective of heterostasis and entropy, it was obvious to him that every one of us, as long as we live, is in part healthy and in part sick (Antonovsky, 1979, prologue 5). He called this *the health ease/dis-ease continuum*, or *breakdown continuum*, and he defined the construct operationally in a mapping sentence (Fig. 5.1).

He became, however, increasingly more reluctant in using the word breakdown:

> I used the term breakdown (in 1972). I then indicated that I would have preferred to use dis-ease.....The term breakdown seems to have caught on, and I shall continue to use it, asking the reader to bear with me and to keep in mind that the fully appropriate term is the ease/dis-ease continuum. (Antonovsky, 1979, p. 57)

In 1979, Antonovsky recollects, however, that the very use of the term breakdown points to the fact that he in the early 1970s had a pathogenic orientation, *"Like everyone else,"* he adds (Antonovsky, 1979, prologue 5). The realization of the "health ease/dis-ease continuum" extended his interest from Holocaust survivors to all humans. As some were doing better than others were, he finally in the mid-1970s formulated the question: *"What moves people toward the health end of the health ease/dis-ease continuum?"* He needed a term for this—for the movement toward the health end of the continuum—and landed on salutogenesis, which he had himself used in another context 10 years earlier. In recollection, he remarks (Antonovsky, 1996b, p. 171): *"I did not really depart from the mainstream until I coined the term salutogenesis in 1978."* Later in this chapter, we focus more on Antonovsky's development of the health concept, but for now we follow Antonovsky to Berkeley, where important developments took place. In the *Odyssey* (Antonovsky, 1990), he narrates that he leaves for his sabbatical with a nagging sense of discontent. While being satisfied with posing the radically new salutogenic question in the mid-1970s, he was not completely happy with his tentative answer, GRRs.

Fig. 5.1 Mapping sentence definition of health ease/dis-ease continuum. (Reprinted from Antonovsky, 1979, p. 65. Published with permission of © Avishai Antonovsky. All Rights Reserved)

Breakdown is any state or condition of the human organism that is felt by the individual to be

A. Pain

{ 1. not at all / 2. mildly / 3. moderately / 4. severely } painful;

that is felt by him/her to be

B. Functional Limitation

{ 1. not at all / 2. mildly / 3. moderately / 4. severely } limiting for the performance of life activities self-defined as appropriate;

that would be defined by the professional health authorities as a

C. Prognostic Implication

{ 1. not acute or chronic / 2. mild, acute, and self-limiting / 3. mild, chronic, and stable / 4. serious, chronic, and stable / 5. serious, chronic, and degenerative / 6. serious, acute, and life-threatening } condition;

and that would be seen by such authorities as requiring

D. Action Implication

{ 1. no particular health-related action / 2. efforts at reduction of known risk factors / 3. observation, supervision, or investigation by the health care system / 4. active therapeutic intervention } .

Sense of Coherence (SOC): Successive Notes of the Scale

With many ideas in his luggage, he left for a sabbatical at Berkeley in 1977. During this year, he wrote *Health, Stress and Coping* published in 1979 and which: *"contained the first full statement of what I call the salutogenic model and its core concept, the sense of coherence"* (Antonovsky, 1990, p. 77). He approached the salutogenic question, and knew he already had part of the answer: GRRs. Working on his data using a technique called *smallest space analysis*, which renders a graphic map of variables, he constantly saw *a factor X* turning up, being closer to health than any of the other GRRs were. Was it a common element of all GRRs? What did GRRs have in common that led to health? Antonovsky knew social support was a GRR, and that Cassel (1976) theorized that social support worked through providing various kinds of feedback. Antonovsky theorized that all GRRs provide feedback of some kind, *"... sending messages like: Here is the right track; you can handle things; you are of worth"* (Antonovsky, 1990, p. 78). He was now in the position where he could formally define GRRs (Fig. 5.2).

Furthermore, he could also now describe factor X that operated at a different level than the other GRRs, revealing a phenomenon about a specific orientation to life. Repeated and consistent messages of the kind described just above led one to become high on X, while confusing and negative messages led one to become low on X. He called X *sense of coherence* (*SOC*) and defined it the following way (1979, p. 123):

> A global orientation that expresses the extent to which one has a pervasive, enduring though dynamic, feeling of confidence that one's internal and external environments are predictable and that there is a high probability that things will work out as well as can reasonably be expected.

In the preface of *Unraveling the Mystery of Health*, Antonovsky credits his wife Helen as the one who proposed the term *the sense of coherence.* Being a developmental psychologist with anthropological training, she was able to grasp exactly what he wished to say, and he considered her a most competent professional critic (Antonovsky, 1987, preface xviii). Antonovsky could now depict the model in full, and Fig. 5.3 shows how it was rendered in the 1979 book. In 1990, Antonovsky comments that stressors were in the periphery in his 1979 model because he at that time had had his focus on resources. This shows how Antonovsky himself did not see the model as fixed once it had been described, but opened up for further developments along with new insights.

Antonovsky was now eager to test the new concept SOC empirically, and after his return to Beersheba, he developed

Fig. 5.2 Mapping sentence definition of GRRs. (Reprinted from Antonovsky, 1979, p. 103. Published with permission of © Avishai Antonovsky. All Rights Reserved)

A GRR is a {1. physical; 2. biochemical; 3. artifactual-material; 4. cognitive; 5. emotional; 6. valuative-attitudinal; 7. interpersonal-relational; 8. macrosociocultural} characteristic of an {1. individual; 2. primary group; 3. subculture; 4. society} that is effective in {1. avoiding; 2. combating} a wide variety of stressors

and thus preventing tension from being transformed into stress.

a 29-item instrument that he felt was good. With this, he returned to Berkeley in 1983 for a second sabbatical aiming to test the questionnaire. In the meantime, he had gotten a request to write a second edition of *Health, Stress and Coping*, which had been well received. He proposed rather to add an epilogue chapter—which turned into a completely new book: *Unravelling the mystery of health* (Antonovsky, 1987). This book has a deeper treatment of the sense of coherence, and we can see the definition being expanded (Antonovsky, 1987, p. 19):

> The sense of coherence is a global orientation that expresses the extent to which one has a pervasive, enduring though dynamic feeling of confidence that (1) the stimuli deriving from one's internal and external environments in the course of living are structured, predictable, and explicable; (2) the resources are available to one to meet the demands posed by these stimuli; and (3) these demands are challenges, worthy of investment and engagement.

In 1990, Antonovsky still remains with this definition and comments that elements (1) *comprehensibility* and (2) *manageability* were present in the 1979 definition, but that element (3) *meaningfulness* is new, and that this element grew steadily more important in his thinking (Antonovsky, 1990, p. 78). He also commented that the second definition, therefore, has less of a cognitive emphasis than the initial one. The process of operationalizing the concept to be able to test the model leads Antonovsky to become aware of its inadequacies. He narrates that he also at the time had become aware of the works of Moos (Moos, 1984, 1985), Kobasa (1979, 1982), and Victor Frankl (Frankl, 1975), which he believed, in his terms, were working on the salutogenic problem (Antonovsky, 1990). In the 1979 version of the SOC definition, he was clearly influenced by systems theory and ideas of order and disorder, and he gave much room to outlining the first component *comprehensibility*. A person could not deal with a stressor unless one felt one had a clear understanding of the character of the problem at hand. In delineating the second component *manageability,* he was inspired by the work on mastery and coping, particularly locus of control (Rotter, 1966). As he continued to deepen his understanding of coping, it became, in *Unraveling the mystery of health*, important to him to underline that the crucial thing about *manageability* is the sense that adequate resources to cope with stressors are to be found either: *"...in one's own hands or in the hands of legitimate others"* (Antonovsky, 1990, p. 79). The third component *meaningfulness* is new and delineated fully in the 1987 book. It had been mentioned only briefly in 1979, and phrases such as *the world makes sense* were primarily used to describe a cognitive perception of order. Inspired by the work of, for instance, Victor Frankl, Antonovsky now understands meaningfulness in the emotional sense as a way of looking at life as worth living, providing the motivational force: *"...which leads one to seek to order the world and to transform resources from potential to actuality"* (Antonovsky, 1990, p. 79).

Antonovsky used the terms *entropy* and *negative entropy* (*negentropy*) to explore and describe the connection between chaos and order, and he argued that systems theory certainly is a valuable theoretical framework for understanding sense of coherence as an answer to the quest creating order out of chaos. Throughout *Health, Stress, and Coping,* Antonovsky's concern was the SOC of individuals, he only loosely suggested that the concept could be employed at the social level. In *Unravelling the Mystery of Health*, he questioned this assumption and discussed the SOC as a group property more in depth. Rhetorically he asks (Antonovsky, 1987, p. 170): *"Is it too grandiose an ambition to set as a goal moving closer to an integrated theory that proposes how any system copes with its reality?"* Antonovsky discussed relevant preconditions, or dimensions for it to be meaningful to

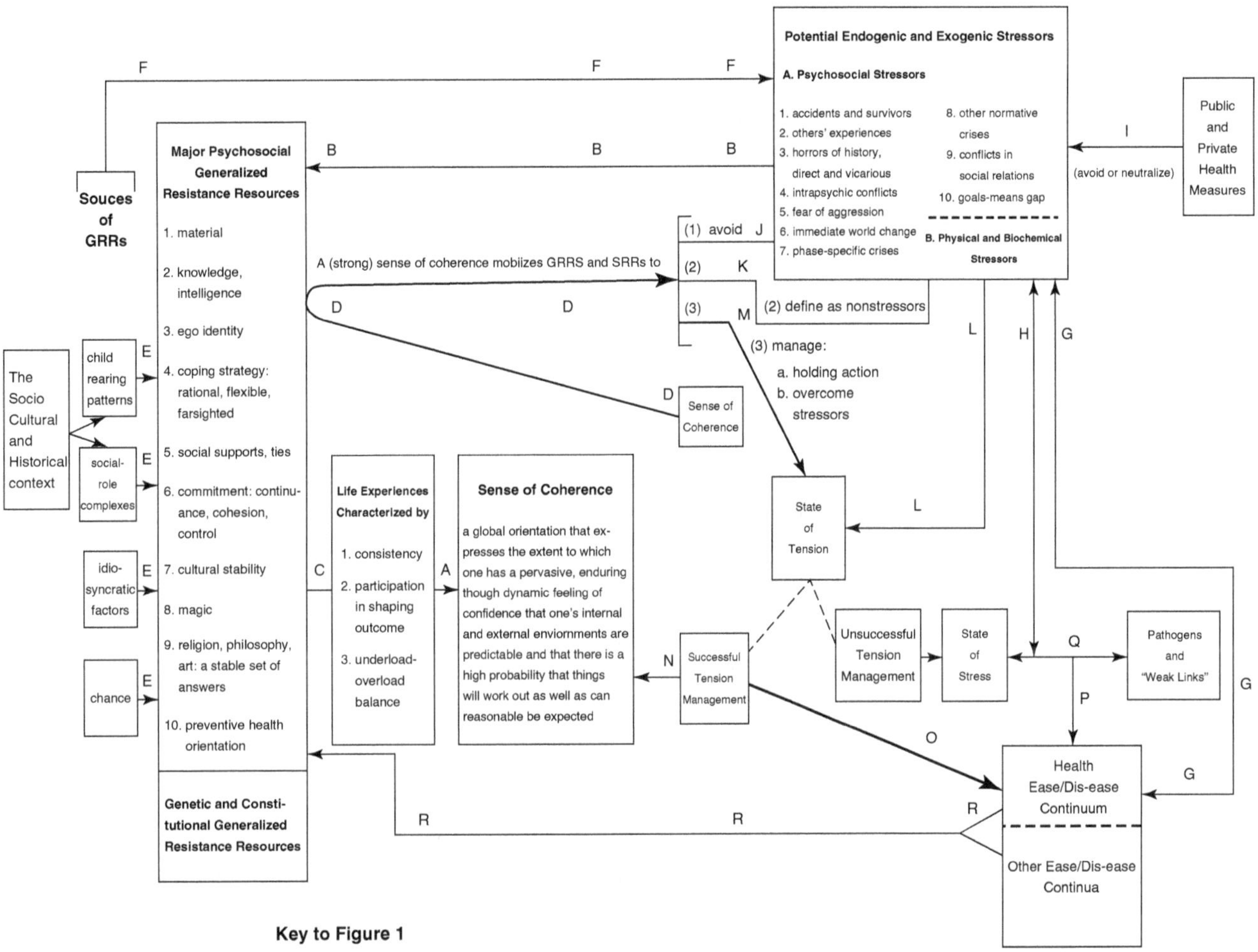

Key to Figure 1

Arrow A: **Life experiences shape the sense of coherence.**

Arrow B: Stressors affect the generalized resistance resources at one's disposal.

Line C: **By definition, a GRR provides one with sets of meaningful, coherent life experiences.**

Arrow D: **A strong sense of coherence mobilizes the GRRs and SRRs at one's disposal.**

Arrows E: **Childrearing patterns,social role complexes,** idiosyncratic factors, and chance **build up GRRs.**

Arrow F: The sources of GRRs also create stressors.

Arrow G: Traumatic physical and biochemical stressors affect health status directly; health status affects extent of exposure to psychosocial stressors.

Arrow H: Physical and biochemical stressors interact with endogenic pathogens and "weak links" and with stress to affect health status.

Arrow I: Public and private health measures avoid or neutralize stressors.

Line J: A strong sense of coherence,mobilizing GRRS and SRRs, avoids stressors.

Line K: A strong sense of coherence,mobilizing GRRS and SRRs,defines stimuli as nonstressors.

Arrow L: **Ubiquitous stressors create a state of tension.**

Arrow M: **The mobilized GRRs (and SRRs) interact with the state of tension and manage a holding action and the overcoming of stressors.**

Arrow N: **Successful tension management strengthens the sense of coherence.**

Arrow O: **Successful tension management maintains one's place on the health ease/dis-ease continuum.**

Arrow P: Interaction between the state of stress and pathogens and "weak links" negatively affects health status.

Arrow Q: Stress is a general precursor that interacts with lhe existing potential endogenic and exogenic pathogens and "weak links."

Arrow R: Good health status facilitates the acquisition of other GRRs.

Note: The statements in bold type represent the core of the salutogenic model.

Fig. 5.3 The salutogenic model of health. (Reprinted from Antonovsky, 1979, pp. 184–185. Published with permission of © Avishai Antonovsky. All Rights Reserved)

talk of a group SOC. He considered size as the most crucial parameter, and he was quite assured that SOC would be an emergent group property in primary groups such as the family, a small local community, a work or a friendship group, or the like. However, he felt increasingly less confident about whether SOC *"...is applicable to a large-scale, complex, diversified collectivity"* (1987, p. 175). He made a distinction, however, between collectivities that are social categories, and collectivities that are associational in character, arguing that there must be a sense of group consciousness, a subjectively identifiable collectivity, before it makes sense, or is even possible to talk of a group SOC. Still,

Antonovsky emphasized that the size of the group and a sense of group consciousness will not indicate whether the group has a weak or a strong SOC. He suggested that a group with a strong SOC would be characterized by (Antonovsky, 1987, p. 174): *"A group whose individual members tend to perceive the collectivity as one that views the world as comprehensible, manageable, and meaningful, and among whom there is a high degree of consensus in these perceptions."* Describing it like this, one has to move beyond the mere aggregation of data on the SOC of individuals in a group, and take into account the perceptions by individual members of the group of how the group sees the world. In addition, he claimed one also has to consider the extent of the consensus of the perceptions by looking at the variance of individual scores.

Antonovsky (1987, p. 176) brought forth yet two relevant dimensions for group SOC: (1) the duration of the existence of an identifiable collectivity, and (2) that membership in the collectivity is of overriding centrality in the life of each member, and to such an extent that the self and the social identity are deeply interwoven. His argument about the duration of the existence of the group is closely tied to his hypothesis that SOC is a rather stable property for an individual, and that one's location on the continuum will not change much after one has reached the age of 30. He, thus, argued that it would be difficult to imagine a group SOC, strong or weak, if the social context and conditions were not relatively stable and consistent over several years. The prerequisite of a year-long group duration implies that there most likely will be turnover among the individual members of the group. However, the turnover must not unsettle the stability and consistency of the collectivity. The subjectively identifiable group must remain (Antonovsky, 1987, p. 176). A final important possibility of the group SOC raised by Antonovsky is whether it makes a difference to an individual's health to belong to a group or groups with a weak or strong SOC. He asks (Antonovsky, 1996a, p. 17): *"What is the relationship between the movement of the person toward wellbeing and the strength of his/her collective SOC?"* His hypothesis is that, yes, it makes a difference in terms of health prediction, beyond merely knowing the SOC level of the person. First, because of the importance of the social environment in giving experiences that are decisive to the development of a strong or weak SOC. He emphasized that groups with a strong SOC tend to structure situations and, thus, provide experiences that over time will enhance the SOC of the group's individual members. Second, and even more importantly, he believes that in order to cope with some stressors, interventions are required by collectivities rather than by individuals, pointing to working life as an illustrative example (Antonovsky, 1987, p. 178). Some stressors stem from conditions deeply rooted in organizations, and/or in the structure of society, and confront the entire collectivity, and therefore call for group resources to be properly dealt with. It is about the group's ability to mobilize and activate its collective resources to confront the problem and relieve tension, more than the person needing the group to confront a stressor that he/she cannot deal with alone. In such cases, the individual SOC is relevant and important in regulation of emotion. In coping with the collective stressor directly, Antonovsky claims (1987, pp. 178–179):

> ...it is what the group does that matter...Only individuals are more or less healthy, depending, among other things, on how well they manage tension, but in the face of collective stressors, the strength of the group, rather than of the individual, SOC is often decisive in tension management.

Through his arguing, Antonovsky tried to make sense of SOC as a group property by use of quantitative measures, which of course reflects his training and the dominant way of doing science at the time. Yet, he claimed that the ontological beliefs of entropy and negentropy and the search for order out of chaos require multiple approaches across disciplines. His idea of taking into account the perceptions by individual members of the group points in the direction of qualitative research. His suggestion to move beyond aggregated individual SOC data and to deal with the cultural production of the group as a source of data for understanding group SOC does the same. He advocated observing collective behavior such as myths, rituals, humor, language, ceremonies, and so on of the group (Antonovsky, 1987, p. 176), and by that, as we understand it, he is calling for a variety of methodological approaches. This is a call, which possibly has better circumstances to be answered in our time than in his.

Tuning the Model: General Resistance Resources—General Resistance Deficits

Another of the elements in the SMH which he did change his conceptualization of in the 1987 book was *stressors*. In 1979, he was quoting Lazarus and Cohen (1977, p. 109) and defined stressors as: *"A stimulus which poses a demand to which one has no ready-made, immediately available and adequate response"* (Antonovsky, 1979, p. 72). The strength of this definition, according to Antonovsky, was that one could classify stimuli without knowing the consequences—whether tension is transformed into stress or not. However, in 1987, he linked the definition of stressors to resources. He claimed that the absence of a GRR could become a stressor (Antonovsky, 1987, p. 28). One illustrative example here could be the absence of money (authors' comment). Such an absence of resources he called *Generalized Resistance Deficit (GRD)*. He suggested that the total stressor-resource situation (GRR-GRD) could be captured by a continuum, with many potential subcontinua (Antonovsky, 1987, p. 28):

> I propose then, that we can speak of 'major psychosocial generalized resistance resources—resistance deficits' (GRR-RDs) as one unified concept. In each case—wealth, ego strength, cultural stability, and so on—a person has can be ranked on a continuum. The higher one is on the continuum, the more likely is it that one will have the kind of life experiences that are conducive to a strong SOC; the lower one is, the more likely is it that the life experiences one undergoes will be conducive to a weak SOC. A stressor, in sum, can be defined as a characteristic that introduces entropy into the system—that is, a life experience characterized by inconsistency, under—or overload, and exclusion from participation in decision-making.

Thus, any phenomenon can be characterized by the degree to which it creates these three important life experiences: *consistency, load balance, and participation in decision-making.* These are the life experiences conducive to SOC, and every individual can be placed on a continuum for each of these life experiences. If an experience is toward the fortunate end of these continua it indicates the existence and use of GRRs, if it is toward the unfortunate end it indicates the lack of GRRs and, thus, a GRD. Antonovsky was optimistic for the utility of this new reconceptualization of stressors (Antonovsky, 1987, pp. 30–31):

> Subsuming the stressors , and particularly chronic, endemic stressors , under the overarching concept of GRR-RDs provides a theoretical basis for constructing a measurement tool that links the resources and stressors —would that I could coin a single word!—through the SOC to health outcome.

This highlights Antonovsky's understanding of not focusing on stressors alone, not focusing on resources alone, but focusing on their combined effect to create life experiences that are characterized by consistency, load balance, and participation in decision-making. Such experiences are conducive to a high SOC and, therefore, move a person toward health.

The SMH demonstrates that sense of coherence and different resistance resources work together in a mutual interplay. The more resistance resources people are conscious of and are able to mobilize and make use of, the higher SOC. A higher SOC will in turn help people mobilize more of their resources, leading to better health and well-being. Thus, SOC is flexible rather than being constructed around a fixed set of dominant strategies such as the classic coping strategies (Antonovsky, 1987, 1992, 1993). Antonovsky lists a spectrum of ways in which SOC affects health (Antonovsky, 1990, p. 78):

- SOC leads one to engage in health-promoting behavior, for instance, through attitudes.
- SOC influences one's process of defining a stimulus as a stressor-nonstressor. Some stimuli might rather be seen as neutral, or even salutary.
- SOC leads one to interpret a stressor as ordered.
- SOC leads one to search one's repertoire for GRRs that are appropriate for the specific situation, including the resources available through one's network, thereby giving a flexible rather than rigid pattern of response.
- SOC-induced response patterns cause the brain to send messages to activate appropriate bodily resources.
- SOC opens one up to analysis of the results of one's behavior and makes one ready to redesign response as needed.
- SOC makes one aware of the need to cope both instrumentally as well as emotionally.

In Chap. 5, *Unraveling the Mystery of Health,* Antonovsky writes he believes that it is in early adulthood that one's location on the SOC continuum becomes more or less fixed. He claims that SOC developed in this period of life stabilizes and remains at this level and that only rarely might experiences in life improve the level of SOC afterward (Antonovsky, 1996b, p. 175):

> I have often committed myself, orally and in writing, to the hypothesis that the strength of a person's SOC is more or less stabilized by roughly the age of 30, that is, when one has been in the normal work and family situation of one's culture and subculture for a number of years.

His hypothesis is based on him arguing there are no major changes in the quality of the experiences that affect the SOC after the age of 30 (Antonovsky, 1987, p. 123):

> For the middle-aged adult, the new marriage, new job, new country, new social climate, or new therapist can only at best (or at worst) begin to initiate change, insofar as this stimulus provides a different long-range set of life experiences characterized by different levels of consistency, load balance, and participation in socially valued decision making.

However, he emphasized that his position is a hypothesis based on theoretical considerations and is not based on empirical evidence (Antonovsky, 1996b). Further, he maintained that it is important to clarify what is meant by a major strengthening of the SOC and claims that if a substantial number of people experience a given mode of therapy and improve their SOC score by 5 points on the average, *"this is not to be sneezed at"* (Antonovsky, 1996b, p. 176). Moreover, he also suggests that practitioners can arrange for SOC-enhancing experiences and he writes, *"this would be true for any therapeutic mode that facilitates a long-lasting, consistent change in real life experiences that people undergo"* (Antonovsky, 1987, p. 126).

Health and Well-Being: In or Off Key?

One of Antonovsky's deviations from pathogenesis was to reject the dichotomization into categories of sick or well. Through extensive use of statistics, he argued that it is very rare indeed to be completely healthy (Antonovsky, 1979).

We are rather all more or less ill or well at any given point in time—located on a health ease/dis-ease continuum from maximally ill (dis-ease pole of continuum) to maximally well (ease pole of continuum). The important point is to focus on what moves an individual toward the ease pole of the continuum, regardless of where he/she was initially located. This is the process of salutogenesis (Antonovsky, 1979, preface xiv–xv):

> …I am persuaded that the salutogenic orientation, that thinking in terms of the mystery of movement toward the ease pole of the ease/dis-ease continuum, is a significant and radically different approach to the study of health and illness than the pathogenic orientation.

What lies at the ease pole of the continuum is a question we will return to later. However, before moving on we will linger a bit on Antonovsky's writings on illness and disease, and on whether or not it is ok to study illness within the salutogenic paradigm. While Antonovsky stated that his thinking is greatly indebted to Dubos' work on adaptive capacity and adaptive coping, he nevertheless criticized Dubos for not going explicitly beyond the concept of multiple causation of specific diseases, though Dubos claimed this to be his main agenda. Antonovsky stated, however (Antonovsky, 1972, p. 538): *"…his (Dubos') focus on adaptive capacity is certainly congenial to the concept of breakdown."* It seems as though Antonovsky introduced the term breakdown to have a phrasing for the process of departing (Antonovsky, 1972, p. 537): *"from the social norm we call health."* Whether Antonovsky meant by this that breakdown will result in various kinds of diseases and thus be, in fact, nearly synonymous with disease, or that breakdown is merely a description of the subjective experience of not feeling well (being ill)—and thus a movement toward dis-ease— is unclear. In outlining the salutogenic philosophy of life, Antonovsky claimed that entropy is the norm and that experiences of disease and illness are to be considered requisite to the human condition. Illness, being the subjective experience of not feeling well is thus a larger and a more holistic experience than a specific disease, is it not? Inferring, one can indeed experience disease and or illness without being diagnosed with a disease. Breakdown may or may not include having a particular disease, but will it not always include experiences of dis-ease and illness?

Despite Antonovsky's intention of going beyond the dichotomy of healthy/sick in the pathogenic paradigm, it is as though he remained within the paradigm when using the terms illness and disease interchangeably. Did he mean that the movement toward the ease pole is a salutogenic movement, whereas the movement toward the dis-ease pole is a pathogenic one (Antonovsky, 1979, p. 69):

> Inevitably, both because I have been conditioned as well as everyone else by the question of pathogenesis and because the overwhelming part of the data available asks this question, I too shall slip into asking, Why are people located on—or why do they move down toward the dis-ease end of the continuum? I shall seek to avoid doing so and ask the reader to join me in this effort.

Alternatively, did he find it worthwhile and relevant to study movements toward the dis-ease pole of the ease/dis-ease continuum *within* the salutogenic orientation (Antonovsky, 1979, p. 37): *"Salutogenesis asks, what are the factors pushing this person towards this end or towards that end of the continuum."* Engaging in this effort has perhaps nothing to do with pathogenesis as such. Maybe it is of importance for understanding health-promoting processes. As apparent from the two quotations above, Antonovsky seemed unclear and to contradict himself on this. Taking Antonovsky's own critique of Dubos into account, it is tempting to root for breakdown being the salutogenic paradigm's counterpart to disease in the pathogenic paradigm; namely the subjective experience of being ill, including periods of having diseases in a pathogenic sense. However, this remains unclear in Antonovsky's own texts, and there are examples in the literature of different interpretations of his writings on this topic.

A second deviation from the pathogenic orientation was the rejection of the medical expert as the judge of who is sick or well, through the focus on disease and diagnosis. Such an approach, Antonovsky stated (1979, p. 36): *"blinds us to the subjective interpretation of the state of affairs of the person who is ill."* In the health ease/dis-ease continuum, we find this expressed in the hyphen in dis-ease: dis-ease infers the subjective experience of illness, possibly including periods of being sick and diagnosed in the pathogenic sense. This is also evident from the operationalization of health that is found in Fig. 5.1, which clearly demonstrates that Antonovsky advocated for a health concept that included subjective judgment. Thus, to understand health in the salutogenic paradigm, we seem to need to define illness explicitly and differently than being sick because of diagnosis. Given the focus on subjective interpretation of health and a movement in a positive direction, it could easily (and mistakenly) be assumed that Antonovsky was a proponent for the concept of *positive health.* Quite opposite to this, he stated that (1979, p. 52): *"the resemblance between the focus on positive health and the problem of salutogenesis is quite superficial."* He strongly opposed the WHO definition of health that states, *"Health is a state of complete physical, mental and social well-being and not merely the absence of disease or infirmity"* (WHO, 1948). Antonovsky gave several reasons for his opposition to this definition of health: it cannot be operationalized and, therefore, cannot be measured; it is too optimistic without dynamic reference to the struggles of life; and most importantly, it opens up for *"medical imperialism"* (Antonovsky, 1979, p. 53). This is a point Antonovsky felt strongly about (1979, pp. 53–54):

> Whatever the powers that be do not like enters the proper sphere of medicine: political dissent, whatever the social system, has led to locking people up "for their own good"; and sex education, family planning and abortion, divorce and homosexuality, along with underachievers and overachievers, dropouts and jocks and grinds—all these and many more fall within the province of health with the blessings of WHO.

The skepticism to WHO's broad health concept that necessitates value judgment (including social and mental well-being in the wider sense) made Antonovsky advocate for a more precise definition of health. A more limited definition of health would be measurable and, therefore, useful in empirical research, and not less importantly limit the scope of the "proper sphere of medicine" and the possibilities of the power abuse which history warns us about. His operationalization of the health ease/dis-ease continuum (Fig. 5.1) demonstrates this wish for a rather precise definition of health, avoiding the imprecision of a positive dimension. A closer look at this figure reveals that a maximum state of health according to Antonovsky is a score of 1 on each of the components (1-1-1-1): no pain (by subjective judgment), no functional limitation (by subjective judgment), no medically defined condition (by health authority judgment), and no treatment needed (by health authority judgment). This is a negative definition of health, in that it is based on absence of certain characteristics—it is not more than "the absence of disease or infirmity."

However, still in 1979, he made one interesting comment on what can potentially be found at the maximum ease pole of the health ease/dis-ease continuum. He acknowledges that this continuum seems to formulate the most desirable health category in negative terms. And he opens for a possibility of going beyond the negative even if he does not take great interest in this himself because *"the salutogenic orientation is not concerned primarily with explaining how people reach perfect health - at best, a heuristic notion"* (Antonovsky, 1979, p. 67) and continues:

> Yet it may be valuable, if we are to study really healthy people, few as they are, to have some way of identifying them beyond the 1-1-1-1 category. To this end, I would propose an additional question, to be asked after the first four questions have been answered with the first alternative in each case: "You have said that your state of health is not painful and imposes no limitations. The doctor's report gives you a clean bill of health. But these are negative things. Would you say that your state of health goes beyond this, that you feel an abundance of energy, that you are what people call a picture of perfect health?

Did Antonovsky stick to this understanding of health throughout his authorship, or did his view develop after these early statements in 1979? As late as in 1995 (in a paper published a few months after his death), he repeated the arguments from 1979, warning against a value-based definition of health. In this paper, he used Nazi doctors as an example of how alleged deviants were tortured not only for the sake of other peoples' health but sometimes even for their own good. He wrote about his wish for research that would define health relatively narrowly and *"far from coextensively with all of well-being or happiness"* (Antonovsky, 1995, p. 10). He believed this was vital to avoid blurring the line between SOC and health, to distinguish health from other aspects of well-being, and to protect against using salutogenesis to pressure people to live moral lives. He warned against the danger of assuming that *"the morally good is salutary"* (ibid, p. 11). The morally good might be quite the opposite of salutary, as in the sacrifice of one's own health for the good of others. Moreover, the salutary might be morally repugnant, as in the case of persons who harm others, with the help of their strong SOC. He pointed out, however, that he often found himself in a bind as a teacher of medical students. In spite of his above-mentioned arguments, he thought (Antonovsky, 1979, p. 67): *"it is crucial that they learn to see health in a broad context going far beyond the physiological level."* He emphasized that seeing health in a broad context entailed moving beyond a post-Cartesian dualism and taking into account fantasy, love, playing, meaning, will, and the social structures that promote these (Antonovsky, 1987).

Antonovsky did write about well-being. However, he warned about confusing well-being with the definition of health (Antonovsky, 1979, p. 197):

> I have insisted that the health ease/dis-ease continuum is not to be regarded as coextensive with the entire realm of well-being. Other ease/dis-ease continua exist (...) a nod has (then) been made in their direction; they are highly relevant to and intertwined with health, but they are distinct (...) If our interest are in understanding health, then location on the family-relations or social-relations or material-resources ease/dis-easee continua can usefully be viewed as a GRR.

One possible interpretation of this is that Antonovsky was of the opinion that only physiological health was captured under the health ease/dis-ease continuum and part of his operationalization thereof. He warned against dangers related to classifying mental and social well-being as elements of health, as that would open up for medical imperialism. However, he was positive to the concept of well-being as something wider (*"the entire realm of well-being"*), of which health as he defined it was only one dimension. That could be why he so often specified it as the *health* ease/dis-ease continuum—other continua exist. Regarding social well-being, Antonovsky seems quite willing to classify a variety of social ease/dis-ease continua as GRRs, for instance, for family relations and social relations (see quotation above, 1979, p. 197).

When it came to mental health, however, Antonovsky contradicted himself, and admitted to it. He wrote (Antonovsky, 1985, p. 274):

> Mental health, as I conceive it, refers to the location, at any point in the life cycle, of a person on a continuum which ranges from excruciating emotional pain and total psychological malfunctioning at one extreme to a full, vibrant sense of psychological wellbeing at the other.

Antonovsky describes the movement on the continuum toward better mental health as shifting and continues:

> ...from the use of unconscious psychological defense mechanisms toward the use of conscious coping mechanisms...from the rigidity of defensive structures to the capacity for constant and creative inner readjustment and growth...from a waste of emotional energy toward its productive use...from emotional suffering toward joy...from narcissism toward giving of oneself...from exploitation of others toward reciprocal interaction.

Later he commented on himself that this was a value-based definition (Antonovsky, 1995, p. 9):

> I have made an attempt in print to formally define mental health (...). Was I not, by definition, requiring that to be mentally healthy, a person be someone whom I (or even most others) liked, respected, admired?

While Antonovsky's treatment of the concept of health is extensive and at times bewildering, it seems safe to conclude that his main messages remained the same throughout his authorship. Health is part of a larger realm of well-being. Health is best understood as a continuum, not as a dichotomy. Health must be narrowly defined to facilitate for empirical research and to avoid value-based definitions that might open up for the abuse of power. Further, although unclear, he seemed to believe that salutogenesis is about focusing on the movement toward the ease pole of the health ease/dis-ease continuum—regardless of how far into the positive that continuum might stretch. While advocating a narrow physiological definition of health when debating health and moral, in other texts he broadens the scope and writes (Antonovsky, 1996a, p. 13): *"It (the SMH) is, however, not a theory which focuses on keeping people "well". Rather, (...) it is a theory of the health of that complex system, the human being,"* indicating an ecological understanding of health. This understanding is apparent also in citations as the following (Antonovsky, 1994, p. 10):

> The study of the macrosocial is essential to understanding movement toward health ... (but) a sensitivity to the macrosocial is only a point of departure. What is required is a systematic framework within which structural sources of health can be understood.

These quotations make us leave the presentation of health and well-being on a somewhat uncertain and off-key note. Nevertheless, the very same statements demonstrate that the SMH and Antonovsky were in tune with the core values of health promotion.

Harmonizing: SMH's Relevance for Health Promotion

In *Unraveling the mystery of health,* Antonovsky starts with a detailed and explicit explanation of why he is persuaded that the salutogenic orientation is a radically different approach than the pathogenic orientation. Through six different aspects, he illustrates the distinction between salutogenesis and pathogenesis as he sees it (Fig. 5.4). He claims these aspects have implications for research, for understanding health and illness, and for clinical practice. Antonovsky's fundamental philosophical assumption is that all human beings are in the river of life. Nobody stays

SALUTOGENIC ORIENTATION	PATHOGENIC ORIENTATION
Heterostasis	Homeostasis
1. Health ease/dis-ease continuum	1. Healthy/sick dicotomy
2. The history of the person	2. The person's disease/diagnosis
3. Salutary factors	3. Risk factors
4. Stressors and tension might be pathogenic, neutral or salutary	4. Stress is pathogenic
5. Active adaptation	5. The magic bullet
6. The "deviant" case	6. Hypothesis confirmation

Fig. 5.4 A summary of six main aspects of the salutogenic and the pathogenic orientation as presented by Antonovsky in *Unravelling the Mystery of Health.* The authors' illustration. (Adapted from Antonovsky, 1987. Published with permission of © Avishai Antonovsky. All Rights Reserved)

on the shore. Much of the river is polluted, literally and figuratively. There are forks in the river that leads to gentle streams or to dangerous rapids and whirlpools and the crucial questions is *"What shapes one's ability to swim well?"* (Antonovsky, 1987, p. 90). This metaphor illustrates that heterostasis and not homeostasis is *the* prototypical characteristic of the living organism. The daily structures in which we are all embedded are unavoidably and unendingly stressful.

The first aspect Antonovsky asserts as important to health promotion is understanding health as a continuum, and not as a dichotomy between sick and healthy people. He emphasizes that in order to explain health one will have to study the movement toward the ease pole of the health ease/dis-ease continuum. His focus is on the dynamic interaction between health-promoting factors and stressors in human life, and on how people may move to the healthy end of the health ease/dis-ease continuum. A sense of coherence is proposed to be the significant variable in effecting this movement (Antonovsky, 1985).

The second aspect is to focus on people's own story and not only the diagnosis. He emphasizes that to listen to a person's own story (Antonovsky, 1987, p. 5):

> ...it does not guarantee problem solution of the complex circularities of people's lives, but at the very least it leads to a more profound understanding and knowledge, a prerequisite for moving toward the healthy end of the continuum.

Further, in the third aspect, he underscores the importance of salutary factors when focusing on promoting movement toward better health, his claim being that salutary factors contribute directly to health (Antonovsky, 1996a, p. 14):.

> Posing the salutogenic question, namely, 'how can we understand movement of people in the direction of the health end of the continuum?'—note all people, wherever they are at any given time, from the terminal patient to the vigorous adolescent—we cannot be content with answer limited to 'by being low on risk factors'... To answer the question requires another neologism: **salutary** factors. I will not quarrel with 'health-promoting' factors or any other term, as long as the concept is clear: factors which are negentropic, actively promote health, rather than just being low on risk factors.

Health is, thus, according to Antonovsky, much more than being low on risk factors. In the fourth aspect, he explains the view on stress and claims that stress might be pathogenic, neutral, or salutogenic. Because stress is ubiquitous, salutogenesis opens up for the rehabilitation of stressors in human life. The fifth aspect is related to the view on therapy. In salutogenesis, the ideal in therapy is the person's (he does not use the word patient) ability to actively adapt and not the magic bullet meaning that based on the right diagnosis you search to find the right cure as in medication or surgery. To underline the significance of active adaptation as ideal in therapy, he writes (Antonovsky, 1987, p. 9):

> When one searches for effective adaptation of the organism, one can move beyond post-Cartesian dualism and look to imagination, love, play, meaning, will, and the social structures that foster them.

The last and sixth aspect is about the focus in research and Antonovsky asks whether we are looking for the *deviant case* or *hypothesis confirmation*. He uses an example to illustrate his point: a confirmed hypothesis is that depression is predictive of cancer mortality. However, the difference between the depressed and nondepressed who died of cancer is, respectively, 7.1% and 3.4%, inferring that the great majority did not die of cancer and this is the deviant case. Consequently, he claims, it is possible to generate hypotheses to explain salutogenesis (Antonovsky, 1987).

In a paper from 1996, he argued that the salutogenic orientation can be a basis for health promotion and, in being so, it (Antonovsky, 1996a, p. 14) *"directs both research and action efforts to encompass all persons, wherever they are on the continuum, and to focus on salutary factors."* A third weighty inference of embracing a salutogenic orientation in health promotion, he continued, is the orientations' focus on the history of the person and not on the persons' diagnosis and disease. He claims this to be a moral stance, and it to be (ibid.): *"impermissible to identify a rich, complex human being with a particular pathology, disability or characteristic."* Whereas those working within the pathogenic orientation are pressured to forget the complexity of the human being, the health promoter is, and should be, pressured to relate to all aspects of the person (or collective) to help him/her move toward the ease end of the continuum. Consequently, this issue is not only moral but it is also scientific (Antonovsky, 1996a). Antonovsky firmly asserted that a salutogenic orientation offers direction and focus for health promotion, and he stated that the salutogenic model could be a foundation for the development of a theory that will be productive in this specific field (Antonovsky, 1996a, p. 18): *"The salutogenic model, I believe, is useful for all fields of health care. In its very spirit, however, it is particularly appropriate to health promotion."*

Conclusions

Diving into Antonovsky's writings, trying to provide an overview of his salutogenic model of health has been not only challenging but also utterly worthwhile. Overall, it has been an interesting and, for most parts, salutary learning process. We feel safe and supported by Antonovsky when we urge you all to keep reflecting, researching, and further developing the SMH. Antonovsky claims that one of the advantages of the model is just that, that it allows us, indeed even stimulates us, to ask questions, whatever the answers turn out to be.

We want to wrap this chapter up the way we started, with Antonovsky's own words (1987, preface xvii):

> If I have been motivated by one purpose to write this volume, it is to reinforce those who are already at work—to spark ideas in the minds of those colleagues who share with me the enchantment with the mystery of health.

References

Antonovsky, A. (1961). *The early Jewish labor movement in the United States*. YIVO Institute for Jewish Research.

Antonovsky, A. (1967a). Social class and illness: A reconsideration. *Sociological Inquiry, 37*, 311–322.

Antonovsky, A. (1967b). Social class, life expectancy and overall mortality. *Milbank Memorial Fund Quarterly, 45*, 31–73.

Antonovsky, A. (1968). Social class and the major cardiovascular diseases. *Journal of Chronic Diseases, 21*, 65–106.

Antonovsky, A. (1971). Social and cultural factors in coronary heart disease. An Israel-North American sibling study. *Israel Journal of Medical Sciences, 7*(12), 1578–1583.

Antonovsky, A. (1972). Breakdown: A needed fourth step in the conceptual armamentarium of modern medicine. *Social Science & Medicine, 6*(5), 537–544. https://doi.org/10.1016/0037-7856(72)90070-4

Antonovsky, A. (1974). Conceptual and methodological problems in the study of resistance resources and stressful life events. In B. Dohrenwend & B. Dohrenwend (Eds.), *Stressful life events: Their nature and effects*. Wiley.

Antonovsky, A. (1979). *Health, stress, and coping*. Jossey-Bass.

Antonovsky, A. (1985). The life cycle, mental health and the sense of coherence. *Israel Journal of Psychiatry and Related Sciences, 22*(4), 273–280.

Antonovsky, A. (1987). *Unraveling the mystery of health: How people manage stress and stay well*. Jossey-Bass.

Antonovsky, A. (1990). A somewhat personal odyssey in studying the stress process. *Stress Medicine, 6*(2), 71–80.

Antonovsky, A. (1992). Can attitudes contribute to health? *Advances, 8*(4), 33–49.

Antonovsky, A. (1993). The implications of salutogenesis: An outsider's view. In A. P. Thurnbull, J. M. Patterson, S. K. Behr, D. L. Murphy, J. G. Marquis, & M. J. Blue-Banning (Eds.), *Cognitive coping, families and disability* (pp. 111–122). Brooks.

Antonovsky, A. (1994). A sociological critique of the "well-being" movement. *Advances, 10*(3), 6–12.

Antonovsky, A. (1995). The moral and the healthy: Identical, overlapping or orthogonal? *The Israel Journal of Psychiatry and Related Sciences, 32*(1), 5–13.

Antonovsky, A. (1996a). The salutogenic model as a theory to guide health promotion. *Health Promotion International, 11*(1), 11–18.

Antonovsky, A. (1996b). The sense of coherence—An historical and future perspective. *Israel Journal of Medical Sciences, 32*(3–4), 170–178.

Antonovsky, A., & Kats, R. (1967). The life crisis history of a tool in epidemiological research. *Journal of Health and Social Behavior, 8*(1), 15–21. https://doi.org/10.2307/2948487

Antonovsky, A., Leibowitz, U., Smith, H. A., Medalie, J. M., Balogh, M., Kats, R., et al. (1965). Epidemiologic study of multiple sclerosis in Israel. An overall review of methods and findings. *Archives of Neurology, 13*, 183–193.

Antonovsky, A., & Lorwin, L. (1959). *Discrimination and low incomes*. New York State Commission Against Discrimination.

Antonovsky, A., Maoz, B., Dowty, N., & Wijsenbeek, H. (1971). Twenty-five years later: A limited study of the concentration camp experience. *Social Psychiatry, 6*(4), 186–193.

Cassel, J. (1976). The contribution of the social environment to host resistance. *American Journal of Epidemiology, 104*(2), 107–123.

Dubos, R. J. (1960). *The mirage of health*. Allen & Unwin.

Frankl, V. (1975). *The unconscious god*. Simon & Schuster.

Hollingshead, A. B., & Redlich, F. C. (1958). *Social class and mental illness: A community study*. Wiley.

Kardiner, A., & Ovesey, L. (1951). *A psychosocial study of the American Negro*. Norton.

Kobasa, S. C. (1979). Stressful life events, personality, and health. *Journal of Personality and Social Psychology, 37*(1), 1–11.

Kobasa, S. C. (1982). The hardy personality: Toward a social psychology of stress and health. In G. S. Sanders & J. Suls (Eds.), *Social psychology of health and illness*. Erlbaum.

Kosa, J., Antonovsky, A., & Zola, I. K. (1969). *Poverty and health: A sociological analysis*. Harvard University Press.

Lazarus, R. S., & Cohen, J. B. (1977). Environmental stress. In I. Altman & J. F. Wohlwill (Eds.), *Human behavior and environment*. Plenum.

Moos, R. H. (1984). Context and coping: Toward a unifying conceptual framework. *American Journal of Community Psychology, 12*(1), 5–25.

Moos, R. H. (1985). Creating healthy human contexts: Environmental and individual strategies. In J. C. Rosen & L. J. Solomon (Eds.), *Prevention in health psychology*. University Press of New England.

Parsons, T. (1951). *The social system*. Free Press.

Rotter, J. B. (1966). Generalized expectancies for internal versus external control of reinforcement. *Psychological Monograph: General and Applied, 80*(1), 1–28.

Schuval, J. T., Antonovsky, A., & Davies, A. M. (1970). *Social functions of medical practice: Doctor-patient relationships in Israel*. Jossey-Bass.

Selye, H. (1956). *The stress of life*. McGraw-Hill.

Selye, H. (1975). Confusion and controversy in the stress field. *Journal of Human Stress, 1*(2), 37–44.

WHO. (1948). *WHO definition of health: Preamble to the constitution of the World Health Organization as adopted by the International Health Conference, New York, 19–22 June 1946; signed on 22 July 1946 by the representatives of 61 States (official records of the World Health Organization, no. 2, p. 100) and entered into force on 7 April 1948*. Retrieved March 19, 2014, from http://www.who.int.

6

Society for Theory and Research on Salutogenesis

Georg F. Bauer

Introduction

Salutogenesis is a rapidly expanding academic field of research relevant to theory, practice, and policy (Bauer et al., 2020). This chapter presents the Society for Theory and Research on Salutogenesis (STARS). It also describes two other organizations that are closely involved with the society (Fig. 6.1):

- The Global Working Group on Salutogenesis (GWG-Sal) of the International Union for Health Promotion and Education (IUHPE).
- The Center of Salutogenesis of the University of Zürich in Switzerland (Center), which hosts and coordinates the two aforementioned groups, alongside its research activities.

We, the Editors of this handbook, extend an invitation to you to join STARS, which is transdisciplinary and open to all persons who are interested in salutogenesis. Indeed, the key message of this chapter is that **your** involvement in STARS will extend your professional network, open new avenues for research and publishing, and help achieve a vision of "salutogenesis for thriving societies" (see Chap. 61).

If you are working in the field of health promotion, membership in the IUHPE is also cordially invited – visit www.iuhpe.org. As an IUHPE member, you will have direct access to – and the possibility to be elected to – the GWG-Sal. Aside from its vital coordinating function as shown in Fig. 6.1, the Center is significant due to its work organizing international salutogenesis conferences and publishing material such as this handbook, available to all as a free, open-access publication due to financial support from the Center.

G. F. Bauer (✉)
Center of Salutogenesis, Division of Public and Organizational Health, Epidemiology, Biostatistics and Prevention Institute, University of Zürich, Zürich, Switzerland
e-mail: georg.bauer@uzh.ch

Society for Theory and Research on Salutogenesis (STARS)

STARS aims to advance and promote the science of salutogenesis. These principles guide it:

- Transdisciplinary: STARS connects scholars from diverse disciplines, who share an interest in the science of salutogenesis.
- Open membership: STARS welcomes anyone with an interest in the science of salutogenesis! Having published salutogenesis articles is not a condition of membership. Students are especially welcome. Joining is easy, and it is free of charge.
- Sharing: STARS members are encouraged to announce their publications, news, and events on the STARS website, download free materials such as research questionnaires and books, join discussion groups, and participate in STARS-sponsored conferences.

At www.stars-society.org (Fig. 6.2), you can follow recent news and events on salutogenesis, get informed about recent publications on salutogenesis (including new language editions of The Hitchhiker's Guide to Salutogenesis) (Lindström & Eriksson, 2010), learn about upcoming conferences, and interact with colleagues in the discussion forum. Further, you get free access to the Sense of Coherence (SOC) Scales, and you can freely download the classic books by Aaron Antonovsky. In the membership database, you can search for colleagues working in your country or specific subfield of salutogenesis research and can get connected to regional networks on salutogenesis.

STARS organizes regular, international conferences on salutogenesis. Recently, we added an overview of current salutogenesis research of STARS members related to the COVID-19 crisis. To become engaged in STARS, visit the website, follow us on Twitter (@stars_society), sign up for our newsletter, and become a member now

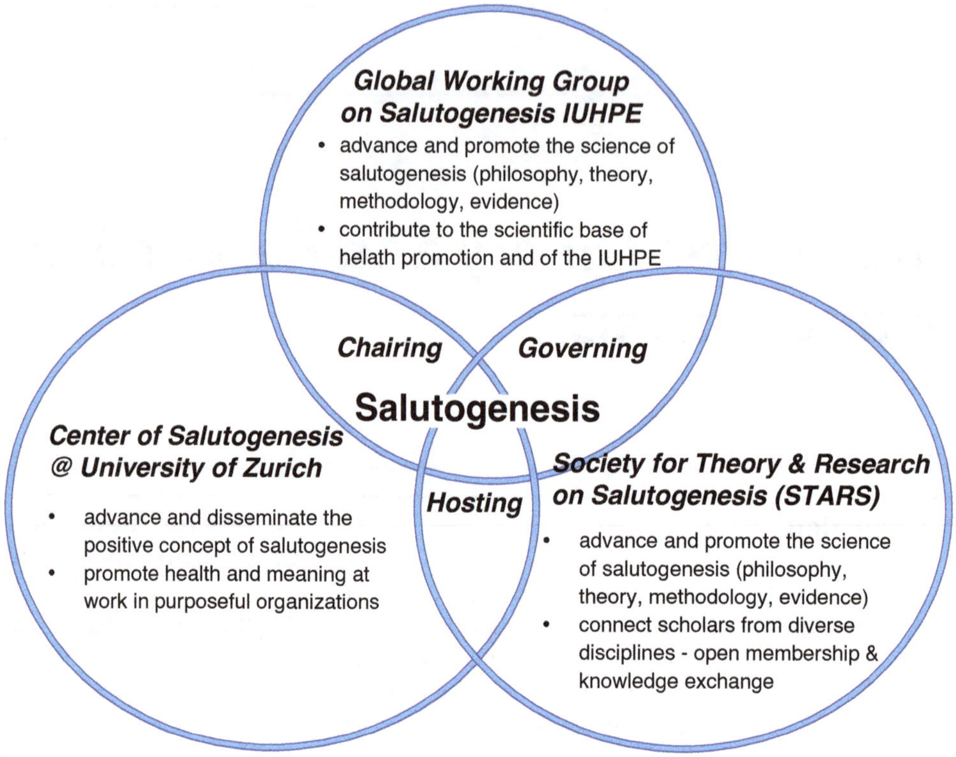

Fig. 6.1 Salutogenesis meeting places and their relationships

and share your perspectives and expertise. Together, we will advance our vision of "salutogenesis for thriving societies!"

Global Working Group on Salutogenesis (GWG-Sal)

GWG-Sal was established in 2007 by the IUHPE, and it has since been crucial for broadening the foundation of salutogenesis in the academic field of health promotion. Not least, the GWG-Sal initiated the first edition of The Handbook of Salutogenesis. This second edition of the Handbook is a joint effort of STARS, GWG-Sal, and the Zürich Center. These major writing projects bring together academics from across the Globe. We cordially invite readers to suggest content for, and contribute to, future editions of the handbook.

The Mission of the GWG-Sal is "to advance and promote the science of salutogenesis (philosophy, theory, methodology, evidence) and thus to contribute to the scientific base of health promotion and the IUHPE" (www.iuhpe.org/index.php/en/global-working-groups). It does this by:

- Salutogenesis agenda setting for, within and beyond, the IUHPE.
- Infusing salutogenesis in IUHPE activities.
- Engaging with key (regional) research fields and stakeholders for capacity-building regarding salutogenesis.

The GWG-Sal is an international group of more than 20 academics representing different world regions and research areas in salutogenesis. GWG-Sal elects new members from the IUHPE, seeking to include underrepresented geographical areas, emerging research themes, and experts willing to work for our mission proactively. We self-apply salutogenesis to our group through considering principles of the Ottawa Charter; assuring inclusiveness regarding regions, gender, and age; following a coherent work plan; and voluntary engagement through joyful experience. The GWG-Sal pursues the following strategies specified in regularly updated action plans:

- We meet regularly to review developments in the field of salutogenesis, health promotion and public health, and to agree on action needed to advance salutogenesis.
- We regularly contribute keynotes, symposia, and workshops to scientific conferences and seminars related to salutogenesis.
- We contribute to the written academic discourse through compilation and regular updates of The Handbook of Salutogenesis as well as through joint position papers on general advancements of salutogenesis (Bauer et al., 2020) and on the specific contribution of salutogenesis in times of COVID-19 and other crises (Maas et al., forthcoming).
- We promote networking and exchange of the academic community of salutogenesis through the initiation and support of the activities of STARS, including regular international conferences.

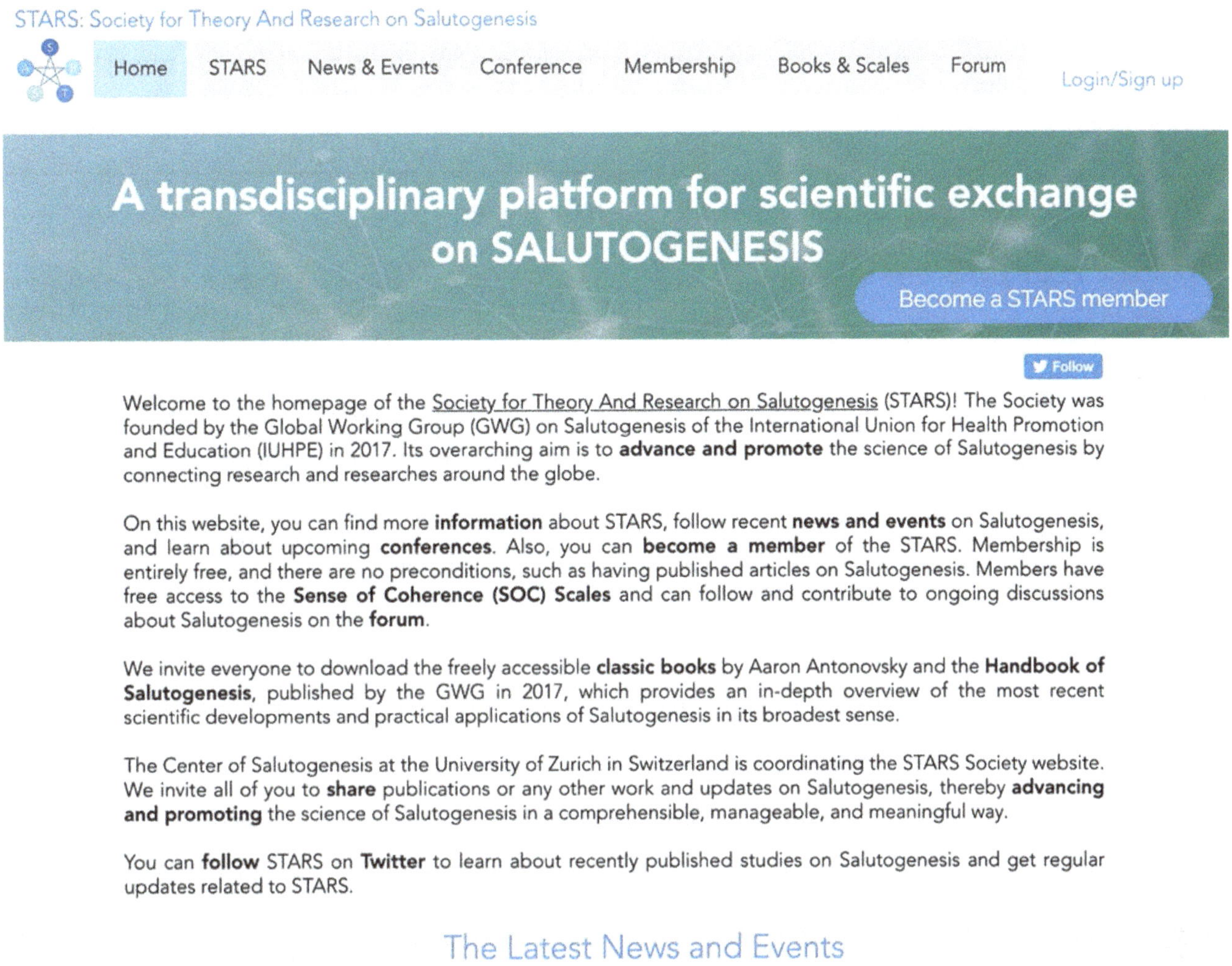

Fig. 6.2 The STARS website (www.stars-society.org)

- We are working to connect salutogenesis-related research initiatives across Europe and beyond to advance our vision of coherence-rich, thriving societies that master societal challenges in a humanistic way. Such challenges include pandemics, racism, rising inequalities, eroding democracies, and planetary health. Our goal is to investigate the role of coherence and value systems in the development of new equilibria of individuals, groups, organizations, and societies in the face of crisis.

Center of Salutogenesis, University of Zürich

The first coordinating center for salutogenesis was organized and run by Bengt Lindström in the period 2005–2012, at the Folkhalsan Health Promotion Research Center in Helsinki, Finland (another important center of activity on salutogenesis, established by Monica Eriksson and Bengt Lindström, serves Swedish researchers and is located at University West in Sweden).

In 2012, the international coordinating center moved from Helsinki to the Norwegian University of Science and Technology in Trondheim, Norway, where Lindström held the first-ever Professorship in Salutogenesis.

On Lindström's retirement in 2016, Georg Bauer initiated to take over the international coordinating center role. In 2017, the President of the University of Zürich formally launched the Center of Salutogenesis, financially supported by a philanthropic foundation. The Center aims to advance and disseminate the powerful, positive concept of salutogenesis in the fields of public health, health promotion, economics, and beyond. Our research systematically applies salutogenesis to the specific context of working life and organizations – facilitating the testing and advancement of the general theory of salutogenesis. Currently, the Center focuses on the following research and development themes:

- «Stress reduction + Meaning-making»: Employees' proactive, resource-oriented crafting of the dynamic working and private life to reduce stress and to create meaningfulness

- «Salutogenic organizational change»: Leader and team development to improve working conditions, collaboration, and meaningfulness
- «Purposeful organizations»: Mind map and participatory approaches to creating purposeful organizations that make a difference for society
- «Positive health»: Developing concepts and indicators of positive health at work and in organizations (happiness, well-being, meaningfulness, and purpose)

Conclusion

Because you are reading this chapter, I know you have a serious interest in salutogenesis! You are welcome and needed as an active participant in the salutogenesis meeting places described in this chapter. Join STARS for free, for access to a global salutogenesis network, research materials such as questionnaires, books by Aaron Antonovsky and other scholars, involvement in discussion groups, and news about salutogenesis.

References

Bauer, G. F., Roy, M., Bakibinga, P., Contu, P., Downe, S., Eriksson, M., … Mana, A. (2020). Future directions for the concept of salutogenesis: A position article. *Health Promotion International, 35*(2), 187–195.

Lindström, B., & Eriksson M. (2010). *The hitchhiker's guide to salutogenesis: Salutogenic pathways to health promotion.* Folkhälsan research center, Health Promotion Research.

Maass, R., Meier Magistretti C., Roy M., Mana A., Shorey S., Vaandrager V., Sagy S., Antonovsky A., Saboga-Nunes L., Juvinya Canal D., Contu P., Bakibinga P., Lindström B., Bauer G.F. (under review). Salutogenesis: Promoting health during the COVID-19 pandemic and beyond.

7

Post-Graduate Education and the Impact of Salutogenesis

Lenneke Vaandrager, Anna Bonmatí-Tomàs, Arnd Hofmeister, Carlos Alvarez-Dardet, Paolo Contu, Maria Koelen, Gaby Ortiz-Barreda, Giuseppe Masanotti, Gwendolijn Boonekamp, Lynne Kennedy, Giancarlo Pocetta, Dolors Juvinya Canal, Patrizia Garista, Bengt Lindström, and Magdalena Wrzesińska

Introduction

In 2021, the European Training Consortium in Public Health and Health Promotion (ETC-PHHP) will celebrate the 30th anniversary of its summer school in Valencia, Spain. This is the founding place for the first summer school, which was organised by Concha Colomer, Spanish co-founder of ETC-PHHP. Since 1991, 782 participants from over 60 different countries across multidisciplinary disciplines have participated in these annual summer schools.

Today, the consortium consists of 13 higher education partners from across Europe: University of Zagreb (Croatia); University of Chester (UK); University of Bergen (Norway); Wageningen University (The Netherlands); University of Perugia (Italy); University of Girona (Spain); HAN University of Applied Sciences (the Netherlands); Norwegian University of Science & Technology NTNU (Norway); University of Cagliari (Italy); The University of Alicante (Spain); Nexus Institute (Germany); University of Lodz (Poland) and the Lebanese International University

L. Vaandrager (✉)
Department of Social Sciences, Health and Society, Wageningen University and Research, Wageningen, The Netherlands
e-mail: lenneke.vaandrager@wur.nl

M. Koelen
Department of Social Sciences, Health and Society Group, Wageningen University, Wageningen, The Netherlands

A. Bonmatí-Tomàs
University of Girona, Faculty of Nursing, Girona, Spain

A. Hofmeister
Nexus Institute, Berlin, Germany

C. Alvarez-Dardet
The Public Health Research Group, University of Alicante, Alicante, Spain

P. Contu
Department of Medical Sciences and Public Health, University of Cagliari, Cittadella Universitaria, Monserrato-Cagliari, Italy

G. Ortiz-Barreda
Department of Health Promotion and Development, Faculty of Psychology, University of Bergen, Bergen, Norway

G. Masanotti
Experimental Research Centre for Health Promotion and Education (CeSPES), University of Perugia, Perugia, Italy

G. Boonekamp
HAN University of Applied Sciences, School of Sport and Exercise, Nijmegen, The Netherlands

L. Kennedy
College of Natural and Health Science, Zayed University, United Arab Emirates, and University of Chester, Chester, UK

G. Pocetta
Department of Medicine and Surgery and Experimental Research Centre for Health Promotion and Education (CeSPES), University of Perugia, Perugia, Italy

D. J. Canal
Nursing Department, Faculty of Nursing, University of Girona, Girona, Spain

P. Garista
National Institute of Documentation, Innovation and Educational Research, University of Perugia, Perugia, Italy

B. Lindström
NTNU Center for Health Promotion Research, Norwegian University of Science and Technology, Trondheim, Norway
e-mail: bengtblind@hotmail.com

M. Wrzesińska
Department of Psychosocial Rehabilitation, Medical University of Lodz, Lodz, Poland

(Lebanon). Each year a different partner organises the summer school.

Today, the network consists of these 13 higher education partners and 725 alumni participants from over 50 different countries, representing a broad range of disciplines from across the fields of public health and health promotion.

ETC was first founded to advance health promotion capacity following the publication of the Ottawa Charter (WHO, 1986). It emerged as a leader in helping practitioners translate and implement the somewhat ethereal theoretical nature of the key concepts of health promotion into everyday practice.

The starting point for ETC is to view health as a resource for life and living. In the 1992 ETC course, Aaron Antonovsky presented his research on the salutogenic approach as a theoretical framework on how to promote health through resilience and flourishing as opposed to the avoidance or prevention of disease. Since then, the salutogenic approach has been a key element of the ETC summer schools not only as a theory but also as a way of thinking, which permeates the planning, facilitation and evaluation of the summer school.

Unique to the ETC programme is the fusion of professionals, who exchange ideas on the salutogenic model of health in a trusting, safe environment. The deeper learning occurs through the process of exploring, listening, reflecting and engaging in dialogue with other professionals (participants and tutors) from diverse social and cultural backgrounds. Moreover, the summer school offers participants insight and skills in being able to work across many different languages and cultures, to master the real demands of working collaboratively on salutogenic principles.

ETC aims to advance health promotion capacity at masters and doctoral level, and practitioners, with several years of experience in health promotion. This level of seniority provides for an experienced, high-level exchange of rich and culturally diverse experiences in health promotion. This chapter outlines how salutogenesis shapes our way of working in post-graduate education.

Competence Development

The first summer schools in the 1990s for academic and non-academic professionals were oriented to the introduction of the new public health and health promotion approach (Ashton & Seymour, 1988). At that time, the field of health promotion theory and research was in its infancy; the evidence base for health promotion practice was limited, so fundamental health promotion ideas for capacity building needed to be developed. The salutogenic perspective offered a useful and inspiring theory to stimulate discussions and created a vibrant atmosphere to which we often refer to as the 'ETC spirit'.

In the 2000s, the field of health promotion had expanded rapidly, and much had been written about health promotion theory and practice. We realised that most participants had a rather solid understanding of health promotion and salutogenesis. However, they did not always apply this knowledge in their research, policy and practice. The content of the course was, therefore, adapted to reflect this. The process not only remained the same but also evolved: the emphasis shifted away from knowledge transfer to competence development; based on the principles that all learning elements should be (1) comprehensible, manageable and meaningful; (2) participatory and democratic so that students can influence the programme; (3) support learning and (4) co-creating knowledge.

The salutogenic environment created in the course facilitates learning by doing and experiencing for both participants and tutors. Participants of the summer schools get an opportunity to collaborate in an international context and together design international projects and programmes which are based on salutogenic principles.

Each summer school has an overall theme that is chosen by the host (see Table 7.1 with titles of all courses since 1991). Throughout the summer school, the focus is on creating a programme that fosters interaction and participation between participants and tutors. This lifelong learning experience is a key strength of ETC.

Based on the pedagogic principles of cooperative and interdisciplinary learning (Hernandez, 2002; Morse et al., 2007), we focus on student-centred participatory methods. Learning occurs through the process of (self-)exploring, listening, reflecting and engaging in dialogue with other professionals (participants and tutors) with broad and diverse social and cultural backgrounds. ETC-PHHP promotes an approach to facilitate learning that applies the salutogenic model of health to practice (ETC-PHHP Team 2016).

The Summer School Programme

The summer school is structured in two parts: a preparatory distance learning element and a 2-week residential summer school.

On average, 30 participants and 10 tutors are involved (a total group of 40 persons). The distance learning element was introduced in the 2000s. During this time, the distance learning element focused primarily on knowledge, knowledge application and critical appraisal. In the second decade with our shift towards competences, we started to integrate critical reflections of personal and professional experiences and perspectives linked to conceptual discussions and best practice analyses. The results of the distance-learning assignments are then discussed in small groups during the residential summer school to support the meaningfulness of

Table 7.1 Topics addressed in the summer schools (1991–2020)

1991	Valencia: Healthy lifestyle
1992	Gothenburg: Promoting the health of children and youth in Europe
1993	Valencia: Settings for health promotion
1994	Liverpool: Strategies for health in Europe
1995	Prague: Networks and collaboration for health promotion
1996	Prague: Innovation in education and training for the new public health
1997	Cagliari: Health promotion and research
1998	Wageningen: Participatory methods in health promotion
1999	Liverpool: Health and health care
2000	Zagreb: Back to the future: From principles to practice, from practice to visions
2002	Valencia: From public health to new public health and health promotion
2003	Cagliari: Community participation and intersectoral collaboration[a]
2004	Galway: European perspectives on promoting health and well-being[a]
2005	Perugia: Rethinking health promotion in a changing Europe[a]
2006	Zagreb: Sailing across new seas – Capacity building for health promotion action[a]
2007	Wageningen & Dusseldorf: Reducing health inequalities – Evidence for community action[a]
2008	Bergen: Health in all policies[a]
2009	Cagliari: Exploring salutogenic pathways to health promotion
2010	Magdeburg: Building civil society for health[a]
2011	Croatia: Strategies for health in Europe: Health in a lifecourse perspective
2012	Wrexham: Assets for health
2013	Girona: Building bridges – Creating synergy for health
2014	Rennes: Mobilising local health promotion systems for equity
2015	Cagliari: Creating salutogenic environments: Health promoting universities, schools, hospitals, cities & workplaces
2016	Wageningen: Health & place: Connecting people, environment and health
2017	Alicante: Public health assets: Mapping and mobilising health assets
2018	Perugia: Lifecourse health development: Empowering people and settings
2019	Girona: Implementing sustainable development goals for healthy local governance
2020	Lodz: People centred health promotion from local, national and European perspectives[b]

[a]in collaboration with Europan Master in Health Promotion project (EUMAHP)
[b]Cancelled due to COVID-19. As an alternative, an online Concha Colomer symposium was held on the 20th of July 2020

this learning activity. A total of 8 European Credit Transfer and Accumulation System (ECTS) credits can be earned: 4 for the distance learning and 4 for the residential summer school.

Since 2011, the residential part starts with the 'Concha Colomer Symposium', a local conference or seminar open to a broader audience of professionals and academics in the field of health promotion. Concher Colomer is one of the founders of ETC and was Director of the Valencian IVESP (Valencian Institute of Public Health Studies, currently known as the Valencian School of Public Health (EVES)). She passed away in April 2011. The annual symposium is a tribute to her contribution to ETC and the field of health promotion. It sets the scene for the 2-week residential summer school. The symposium provides international participants with the opportunity to connect with the local public health and health promotion experts, politicians and international guest speakers. The symposium consists of a few keynote lectures as well as open space sessions to discuss the summer school's theme with public health and health promotion experts from the hosting country also.

The residential summer school programme is divided into morning and afternoon sessions. The mornings consist of plenaries and the afternoons of group work. In the plenary sessions, we give short lectures followed by activities that stimulate discussions and interaction to enable the integration of knowledge and experience of both tutors and participants.

Knowledge is understood as the result of a constant co-production of everybody involved. The afternoon sessions are dedicated to group work. Here, participants work collaboratively on an international project in heterogeneous groups. Group members differ in gender, age, home country and experience. The combination of learning activities enhances comprehensive learning, understanding and the development of core skills in health promotion practice.

At the end of the first week, a local field visit is organised to experience and discuss local health promotion projects in practice. In 2019, we, for instance, visited the town Torroella de Montgrí, which shared how they work with an asset-based approach and how they were experts in asset mapping.

Following the Principles of Health Promotion

One of the five principles of health promotion is to actively involve the population (Ashton & Seymour, 1988). For this reason, during the summer course, the voice of the participants is included in all the sessions, especially in country profile presentations and the photovoice session.

In the country profile presentations, the participants, grouped by countries, present the state of the art of health promotion in their countries and illustrate this with examples of their research or practice. This inductive approach starting with personal experiences leads students to general concepts, content and knowledge (Hofmeister, 2011). The discussion about these experiences during the face-to-face summer school with fellow students integrates this personal approach in a wider international and social context.

Since the 2015 summer course experience in the United Kingdom, the consortium decided to integrate the everyday life of the communities of the town, which hosts the summer school through a photovoice session. Photovoice is defined as 'a process by which people can identify, represent and enhance their community through a specific photographic technique' (Wang et al., 2000). Participants are asked to take a picture in the host city representing an asset which, according to them, promotes health. They also are asked to describe their perspectives or feelings about the picture in one sentence. This activity helps participants to see and observe similarities and differences between their community and that of another country using the lens of a health promoter. Usually, the pictures are presented in an exhibition for the local municipality or community as a gratitude for their hospitality. For the municipality, the results of the photovoice activity bring them international feedback on their local health promotion policies.

Another important goal of health promotion is to make it easier for people to make healthy choices. Several barriers, both within individuals and within their physical and social environment, can hamper the possibilities to make such healthy choices. This goal is not only facilitated by the host of the summer school offering healthy food, sports facilities and sustainable transport but also by participants who organise social activities such as walks after lunch, physical exercises during sessions or salsa classes to show some examples to facilitate healthful choices that can be applied in their home institutions. Also, the field visits usually provide examples in this respect.

Salutogenesis

Salutogenesis introduces two fundamental concepts: the general resistance resources (GRRs) and the sense of coherence (SOC). GRRs are those resources that help a person or a system to avoid or to counteract a wide variety of stressors (Antonovsky, 1979; 1987). GRRs can be found not only within people as resources bound to their person and capacity but also within their immediate and distant environment, and can be both material and non-material (Lindström & Eriksson, 2010).

Health promotion professionals are expected to play an important role in helping people to learn how to recognise and use their GRRs and available SRRs to cope with stressors, and to strengthen their SOC (Super et al., 2015). This is central to the course, especially when some difficulties appear during the course, such as the feeling of time pressure to finish the group work or difficulties because of cultural differences in the way of working. The tutors and also the participants develop skills and abilities to talk about these difficulties and cope with challenges to mobilise the resources of the individuals or the group. These reflection processes strengthen the SOC of groups as well as of individuals.

If people can identify such resources in themselves or their immediate surroundings at their disposal, there is a better chance for them to deal successfully with the challenges of life. GRRs open up the possibility for people to construct coherent life experiences. More important than the resources themselves, however, is that the individual has developed the ability or capacity to recognise, use and re-use the resources for the intended purpose, which helps to improve health and well-being. A strong SOC facilitates this ability.

According to Lindström, the salutogenic model could become a lens for reading and co-constructing a learning/teaching process. Following this perspective, the course design is developed following the idea that students are active and participating subjects, who shape their lives and learning experiences through their SOC. As a consequence, a salutogenic learning model not only demands methods that support the acquisition of health promotion knowledge and competence but also other competencies in navigating lifelong learning, such as narrative skills, problem-solving, guidance and reorientation, self-assessment and the communication of emotions. In other words, learning experiences should balance previous experiences with what is learned and what could be shifted into future practice (Garista et al., 2019). This salutogenic course design privileges learning and teaching methods capable of giving voice to all aspects of human experience. Visual and expressive methods support the use of verbal techniques to balance cognition and embodied cognition in knowledge building, from team-building activities to participatory evaluation sessions. During the long story of ETC, several methods have been explored and then introduced into the course, showing all possible dimensions that could generate knowledge about health and quality of life: narratives, art performances, senso-biographic walking, drawings and cinema. All these methods become useful and make sense only within a meaningful relationship between tutors and students. A salutogenic approach for learning requires not only the general competencies of the tutors but also the co-creation with the participants (Eriksson, 2019). During the summer school, the synergies between all participants permit to create a collective sense of coherence. Participants, for example, present tools they work within their own country and discuss what the use of these tools in another context can mean. Taking into account the dimensions of SOC, it is possible to establish some parallels with the creation of this salutogenic ambiance of learning. Comprehensibility is related to a person's capacity to transform stimuli into information about what is being experienced or perceived that is meaningful, orderly, consistent, structured and clear. The ETC summer school offers a participatory and transparent type of management, gives clear and detailed explanations of the programme and activities to the participants and looks for creative strategies to solve problems. Manageability refers to the individual's perception of the available resources and their adequacy to meet daily demands. During the summer school, mutual trust between participants and tutors is key. There is a relaxed atmosphere that everything will be fine, and knowledge and resources contributed by each person are considered to support the course. However, the most fundamental idea is the thought that difficulties are not considered an individual problem but a collective opportunity that requires collective solutions. Meaningfulness indicates the extent to which a person feels that life makes sense emotionally and, despite the problems and difficulties, is sufficiently motivated to put effort into confronting them. The ETC consortium has a vision based on human rights and equity, which gives the overall activity a high level of meaningfulness. Personal involvement, strong motivation and team building create group synergy. Apart from a team-building session, the morning sessions include activities to increase the feeling of belonging.

While developing the programme for each summer school, including the distance learning element, we aim for a high level of coherence. Each element is discussed in its relevance for the overall theme and how it is connected to other parts of the programme so that the result is a comprehensible, manageable and meaningful narrative for participants, tutors and the hosting community.

Assets

Salutogenesis focuses on health rather than on disease. Morgan and Ziglio (2007) defined assets as any factor or resource that enhances the capacity of individuals, communities and populations to maintain health and well-being. It highlights the positive abilities of each person and their capacities to identify problems and enable solutions to increase self-esteem and leadership in individuals or communities (Morgan et al., 2010). The summer school has an asset orientation; that is to say, the course draws on all those assets provided by the host, the city, the participants and the tutors. Therefore, the first competence that the summer course aims to train is to be attentive to discover the assets of oneself and of other people from different communities, spaces and places. After this, the aim is to develop the competence of creativity to discover where this asset can fit for the benefit of the collective. For this reason, it is a dynamic and flexible course that can adapt to the interest, needs and assets of the members of it.

The assets of the participants are mobilised through a tools session, in which they present useful tools, the country profiles and the group work. Group work can be considered as 'cooperative learning' or 'team learning'. It is about the creation of cooperative structures that are effective in promoting high-level thinking and learning in a group (Kennedy & Vaandrager, 2011). Effective group learning is based on the principles of using the power of the team to encourage students to accomplish the learning objectives (Hernandez, 2002). In all these activities, the participants use their assets, are empowered and discover other assets to mobilise them for the team effort. Simultaneously, these activities develop a sense of community and usually a collective asset mobilisation.

The assets of the hosts are also mobilised. The summer school is organised in a different place every year as each host has different assets to explore. These assets include the multiple and diverse connections to the locality, or regional structures and the stakeholders involved in the course but especially in the Concha Colomer Symposium and the field visit. The Concha Colomer Symposium includes a theoretical introduction of the summer school's theme and, at the same time, some good practices of the host community. The field visit allows participants to observe how to apply the theme in reality and discover new visions or different ways of working with and for the community.

The competences, knowledge and skills of tutors and especially their experience are essential assets for the course. Their assets are shared during formal sessions or taking a coffee break in the canteen, or walking to the accommodation. Participants and tutors are equal, the course is transversal and this fact permits co-creation. This way of working and how things are addressed is appreciated by participants and the host institution, and facilitates salutogenic practice, research and policy.

References

Antonovsky, A. (1979). *Health, stress and coping*. Jossey-Bass.

Antonovsky, A. (1987). *Unravelling the mystery of health*. Jossey-Bass.

Ashton, J., & Seymour, H. (1988). *The new public health*. Open University Press.

Eriksson. (2019). Research supervision as a mutual learning process: Introducing salutogenesis into supervision using 'The Collegial Model'. *HPI, 34*(6), 1200–1206.

ETC-PHHP Team 2016. (2016). *Twenty-five Years of Capacity Building: The ETC 'Healthy Learning' Process*. Wageningen: European Training Consortium in Public Health and Health Promotion (ETC-PHHP) and the Wageningen University, Health and Society Group.

Garista, P., Pocetta, G., & Lindström, B. (2019). Picturing academic learning, Salutogenic and health promoting perspectives on drawings. *HPI, 34*(4), 859–868. https://doi.org/10.1093/heapro/day027

Hernandez, S. A. (2002). Team learning in a marketing principles course: Cooperative Structures that facilitate active learning. *Journal of Marketing Education, 24*(1), 73–85.

Hofmeister, A. (2011). From knowledge and facts to reflections – The turn to competence orientation in distance learning. In G. Pavlekovic, K. D. Pluemer, & L. Vaandrager (Eds.), *Twenty years of capacity building. Evolution of salutogenic training: The ETC' healthy learning' process* (pp. 37–46). ETC-PHHP and Andrija Štampar School of Public Health.

Kennedy, L., & Vaandrager, L. (2011). Experimental learning stimulates partnership working for health promotion. In G. Pavlekovic, K. D. Pluemer, & L. Vaandrager (Eds.), *Twenty years of capacity building. Evolution of salutogenic training: The ETC' healthy learning' process* (pp. 27–36). ETC-PHHP and Andrija Štampar School of Public Health.

Lindström, B., & Eriksson, M. (2010) *The hitchhikers guide to Salutogenesis*. Folkhalsan Research Center, Research report 2010:2, Helsinki.

Morgan, A., Davies, M., & Ziglio, E. (2010). *Health assets in a global context: Theory methods action*. Springer.

Morgan, A., & Ziglio, E. (2007). Revitalising the evidence base for public health: An assets model. *Promotion & Education*, (Suppl 2), 17–22.

Morse, W. C., Nielsen-Pincus, M., Force, J., & Wulfhorst, J. (2007). Bridges and barriers to developing and conducting interdisciplinary graduate-student team research. *Ecology and Society, 12*(2), 8.

Super, S., Wagemakers, M. A. E., Picavet, H. S. J., Verkooijen, K. T., & Koelen, M. A. (2015). Strengthening Sense of Coherence: Opportunities for theory building in health promotion. *Health Promotion International*. https://doi.org/10.1093/heapro/dav071

Wang, C. C., Cash, J. L., & Powers, L. S. (2000). Who knows the streets as well as the homeless? Promoting personal and community action through photo voice. *Health Promotion Practice, 1*, 81–89.

World Health Organization. (1986). *Ottawa Charter of health promotion*. WHO.

Part II

Salutogenic Model of Health: Major Ideas

8

Major Ideas in the Salutogenic Model of Health

Monica Eriksson

Part II starts with a description of the theoretical framework of the salutogenic model of health, with special focus on the key concepts and reflection on the ontological and epistemological background of the health model, which so far is little explored and described (Chap. 9). Essential in the salutogenic model of health is the understanding of health as a process in a continuum, the health ease/dis-ease continuum. This is described and explained in the chapter. Some evidence of the relationship between sense of coherence (SOC) and health is presented.

In Chap. 10, the focus is on how the SOC influences stressor appraisal, positively as well as negatively. The processes of stimulus appraisal have a central place in salutogenic theory, even if they have received relatively little theoretical and empirical attention since Aaron Antonovsky's extensive treatment of stimulus appraisal in *Unraveling the mystery of health: How people manage stress and stay well.* The chapter aims to elevate researchers' appreciation of stimulus appraisal as Antonovsky's little-tested answer to three key questions: How does the SOC concept link to coping behavior, what is the mechanism that makes the connection, and what is the black box in between?

In Chap. 11, measurement issues are addressed concerning Antonovsky's original SOC questionnaires of 29 items and of 13 items, as well as several modified translations applicable at the individual, the family, the organization, and the community levels. Validity (face, construct, consensual, criterion, and predictive) and reliability issues (test-retest and internal consistency) of the scales are discussed. Criticism of the original scales is deliberated.

Chapter 12 presents and discusses theoretical considerations and empirical findings regarding the concepts: generalized resistance resources (GRRs) and generalized resistance deficits (GRDs). Recent research findings are presented, showing how these resources or deficits impact the SOC. Suggestions for future research directions (e.g., individuals' differential susceptibility to environmental effects and eudaimonia/hedonia perspectives) and interventional implications are presented.

Chapter 13 discusses conceptual and concrete differences between generalized and specific resistance resources in the salutogenic model of health. It is important to distinguish between the two types of resistance resources to ensure that health promotion pays attention to both types. Specific resistance resources have as much or more relevance to health promotion practice as do generalized resistance resources. By drawing attention to the nature of specific resistance resources, one also draws attention to what should be a main aim of health promotion.

The part editor has devoted herself not only to producing overviews of salutogenic research but also to deepening knowledge of how the theory and the model of health developed subsequent to Antonovsky's seminal contributions. Salutogenesis has become the air I breathe! Certain trends in salutogenic research are evident:

- The translation and validation of the SOC questionnaires to languages other than English.
- The use of the SOC questionnaires in studies with an ever widening range of endpoints.
- An increasing appreciation that the salutogenic model has utility at the level of social theory (something more than a model).
- A growing interest in developing interventions aiming to strengthen the SOC among patients and professionals.
- The use of SOC questionnaires in evaluating the effectiveness of interventions.

Perhaps the most obvious trend is the burgeoning interest in salutogenic research as judged by the expanding literature. A search in PubMed (January 2020) using the terms salutogenesis and/or sense of coherence identified about 3000 pub-

M. Eriksson (✉)
Department of Health Sciences, Section of Health Promotion and Care Sciences, Center on Salutogenesis, University West, Trollhättan, Sweden
e-mail: monica.eriksson@hv.se

lished papers. Searching in the largest online library, WorldCat, more than 1200 doctoral dissertations on salutogenesis were identified. Most of the research effort has included a focus on the measurement of the SOC using the long and short versions of Antonovsky's Orientation to Life Questionnaire in a broad range of patient groups, community samples, and samples of age groups from young to old. As interest in using the SOC questionnaires has steadily increased, they have been translated into many different languages worldwide (see Chap. 11, Fig. 11.2), and this trend continues today.

The SOC questionnaires are used today in a much wider range of research areas compared to the early years. Examples of new areas are oral health, health behavior, and work and organizational life.

A particularly welcoming trend is the tendency to move from only measuring the SOC to applying salutogenic principles in health promotion practice, and in programs and interventions in various community settings.

Also notable is the trend in recent years to use SOC questionnaires to evaluate the effectiveness of interventions and health promotion programs. In many studies, an increase in SOC scores has been interpreted as due to successful intervention. Such conclusions are overly not really warranted as yet because we do not know the degree to which an increase in the magnitude of SOC scores may be due in part to normal fluctuations in the SOC, or other as-yet-unmeasured confounding factors.

There is much progress, but still, much work to do. There is an urgent need for new salutogenic instruments measuring human resources, which in turn could contribute to the development of the theory. Salutogenesis can be seen as an umbrella concept, and here a completely new world opens up to explore the relationship between related concepts and the SOC. Finally, educational sciences have the challenge to explore how an education approach can foster the strengthening of the SOC at the levels of the individual and in social groups.

9

Theoretical Framework of Salutogenesis

Monica Eriksson

Introduction

The aim of this chapter is to describe briefly the theoretical framework of salutogenesis with a focus on the key concepts, the sense of coherence, and the generalized and specific resistance resources. This chapter begins with reflection on the ontological and epistemological background of salutogenesis, which is not particularly described and explained to any significant extent in the publications by Antonovsky (1979, 1987). Next, health as a process is described by starting from Antonovsky's definition of salutogenesis as a movement toward the health end of a health continuum. The chapter ends with some evidence of how the sense of coherence impacts health and well-being.

The Ontological Background

Ontology is the study of reality (Heil, 2005). What do we know about the ontological background of salutogenesis? In his second book, *Unraveling the Mystery of Health* (1987), Antonovsky described how he perceived the world. Two important things stand: (1) he saw man in interaction with his environment and (2) chaos and change is a normal state of life. The former calls for system theory thinking where the focus is on the individual in a context (Antonovsky, 1985). By the latter, he perceived daily life as constantly changing; a heterostatic as opposed to a homeostatic state. For the individual, the challenge is to manage the chaos and find strategies and resources available for coping with the changes in everyday life. As a medical sociologist, this was a natural way for Antonovsky to perceive the world: seeing humans as part of a larger context.

At the beginning of the 1990s, Aaron Antonovsky published an article about the six C's: complexity, conflict, chaos, coherence, coercion, and civility (Fig. 9.1). Here, he expressed how he looked at society and the human being in that context (Antonovsky, 1993a). As a medical sociologist, he distinctly expressed systems theory thinking. He saw the individual in interaction with the environment and context. He stressed that the salutogenic theory and its key concept, sense of coherence, can be applied at a collective level, and not only with a focus on the individual level.

Complexity, according to Antonovsky, related to how a system is organized:

> Complexity refers to the level of organization of a system. This level both sets the problems and provides the potential, interacting with sub and suprasystem, for the system to maintain a dynamic steady state. Such a steady state is one way of defining health. (Antonovsky, 1993a, p. 969)

Complexity may lead to conflicts, the greater the complexity, the deeper the conflicts. He especially mentioned conflict between civilizations:

> Conflict refers to internal tensions of the human being, to tensions between persons, to tensions between the individual and the suprasystems of which she or he is a part, and to tensions between or among such suprasystems. (Antonovsky, 1993a, p. 970)

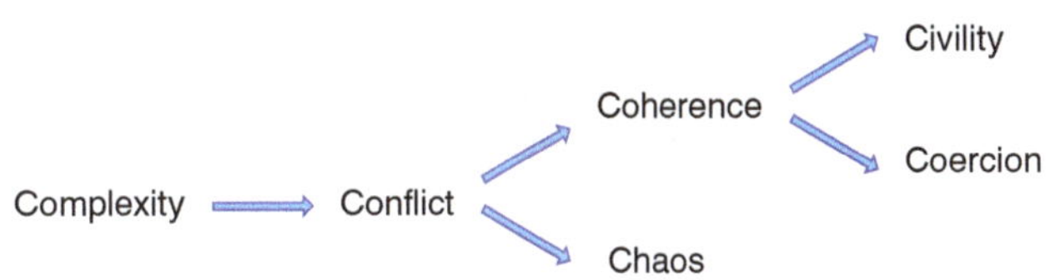

Fig. 9.1 The six C's—an ontological perspective on salutogenesis. (Reprinted from Antonovsky (1993a), with permission from Elsevier. https://www.sciencedirect.com/journal/social-science-and-medicine. All rights reserved)

M. Eriksson (✉)
Department of Health Sciences, Section of Health Promotion and Care Sciences, Center on Salutogenesis, University West, Trollhättan, Sweden
e-mail: monica.eriksson@hv.se

Complexity also offers opportunities for different and flexible choices, possibilities for adapting to change, and possibilities for systems (communities) to reorganize themselves. Conflict leads to tension; therefore, how a community deals with this tension and avoids stress is crucial. Chaos can be exemplified as violence and war, and the image of young men and women equipped with weapons trying to solve conflicts with even more violence, senseless and unpredictable violence (Antonovsky, 1993a, p. 972). The difficulties in resolving conflicts go from a societal level to the group level, to families torn apart, and where children, women, and the elderly are particularly vulnerable. As opposed to this chaos, Antonovsky raised another way to go, to coherence. Sense of coherence is the term he introduced as an opportunity to manage and adapt to a life of chaos. Two important dimensions in Fig. 11.1 remain to be explained: civility and coercion.

Civility is one of the values of salutogenesis, a value that informs how we relate to other people, how we look at them as either people with different strengths and abilities or people with flaws and shortcomings. Civility is about respect toward other people and about the humanity we communicate. Antonovsky discussed humanity and values in terms of respect toward other people, or to use his own words, "*The key lies in a society and in people who care about each other*" (Antonovsky, 1993c, p. 2). The opposite of civility and respect is coercion. A society based on respect for people also requires restrictions against domination, oppression, and poverty (Antonovsky, 1993a, p. 973). More recent research in the salutogenic field highlights a new concept of reasonableness (Boström et al., 2014; Kaplan & Kaplan, 2003, 2011), which brings together the supporting factors in the environment of perceived health and well-being in a particular model, the reasonable person model. Kaplan and Kaplan (2003) describe how people are more respectful, cooperative and more contented in situations where the environment supports their basic information needs. The model focuses on how people are interdependent. It emphasizes three dimensions that contribute to civility, namely a curiosity to explore and understand, meaningful activities, and recovery. The concept of reasonableness has similarities with the dimensions of the sense of coherence: comprehensibility, meaningfulness, and manageability.

The Epistemological Background

Epistemology is the study of knowledge (Audi, 2011). Going back to Antonovsky's two books, *Health, Stress and Coping* and *Unraveling the Mystery of Health*, one can find little insight into how he considered knowledge and learning. As far as this author knows, he did not manifest an epistemological basis for salutogenesis, neither describing his view of how knowledge in general arises nor how learning is meaningful in the salutogenic framework. It appears that he was preoccupied with examining and describing how a strong sense of coherence may have an impact on perceived health. A search in different databases provides little response. However, others have focused on knowledge and learning aspects of salutogenesis related, for example, to the education of children with special needs (Lindström, 1999) and children with learning difficulties (Lackaye & Margalit, 2006; Margalit & Efrati, 1996).

More generally, Nilsson and Lindström (1998) describe how learning can be considered a health promotion process, not only to learn about health but that the learning process also promotes health. By combining educational theories and salutogenesis, they describe "the salutogenic school" (Antonovsky, 1993c, p. 5), achieved by creating meaningful learning situations, clear structures for curricula and the school work, with dedicated teachers supporting each other and the students, and being role models.

Boström and Lassen (2006) point out the importance of giving space for individual ways of learning and different learning strategies. Individual learning styles create opportunities for students to find meaning in school. A new concept that describes learning as a health promotion process is "healthy learning" (Lindström & Eriksson, 2011). This can be applied in research supervision, exemplified through "The Collegial Model," as a mutual learning process (Eriksson, 2018). It means to move on from traditional health education through to increased health awareness (health literacy), and on to learning which promotes health (Lindström & Eriksson, 2011; Quennerstedt, 2006; Quennerstedt et al., 2010). As an example, the curriculum for health education in Australia has recently been revised and now adopts a strength-based (salutogenic) approach (Macdonald, 2013; McCuaig, Quennerstedt, & Macdonald, 2013). The curriculum focuses on promoting sound health habits instead of the earlier focus on avoiding health risks. Health is understood as a multidimensional concept including physical, social, mental, and spiritual health. Health is regarded as a lifelong dynamic process with people as active participants in a context. Finally, health is seen not as an end in itself but as a means to live a good life (McCuaig et al., 2013, p. 113). As another example, from Germany, an attempt to apply salutogenesis didactically in education is the "team ombuds model" (tOm) (Mayer & Boness, 2011), developed to promote the sense of coherence and cross-cultural competence among students and teachers.

More recent research has explored the moderating and mediating roles of learning within the relationship between sense of coherence and generalized resistance resources among employees working in the healthcare sector in the Netherlands (Pijpker et al., 2018). They found that the relationship between SOC and the GRRs seems to be strengthened or explained by instrumental and social learning. Instrumental learning moderated the relationship between job control and SOC.

Epistemologically, salutogenesis can be conceived as a constant learning process (Fig. 9.2), supporting movement toward health (and other desired aspects of one's existence) via improving health literacy: knowledge supports health literacy, which supports development in the ways one relates to one's world. The process of relating to others produces learning, and the knowledge gained from practice expands one's area of knowledge. In the course of daily life, this integrated learning process is continuous. The concept of work integrated learning (WIL) is a new concept describing distinctive aspects of pedagogics and learning processes in healthcare settings (Pennbrant & Svensson, 2018).

Health as a Process

According to Antonovsky, health is movement on a continuum of ease and dis-ease (Antonovsky, 1993b). He referred to the ability to comprehend the whole situation, and the capacity to use the resources available, as the sense of coherence. This capacity was a combination of peoples' ability to assess and understand the situation they were in, to find a meaning to move in a health-promoting direction, also having the capacity to do so—that is, comprehensibility, meaningfulness, and the manageability, to use Antonovsky's own terms (Lindström & Eriksson, 2005). In such an approach, no one is categorized as healthy or diseased. Since we are all somewhere between the imaginary poles of total wellness and total illness, the whole population becomes the focus of concern. Even the fully robust, energetic, symptom-free, richly functioning individual has the mark of mortality: he or she wears glasses, has moments of depression, comes down

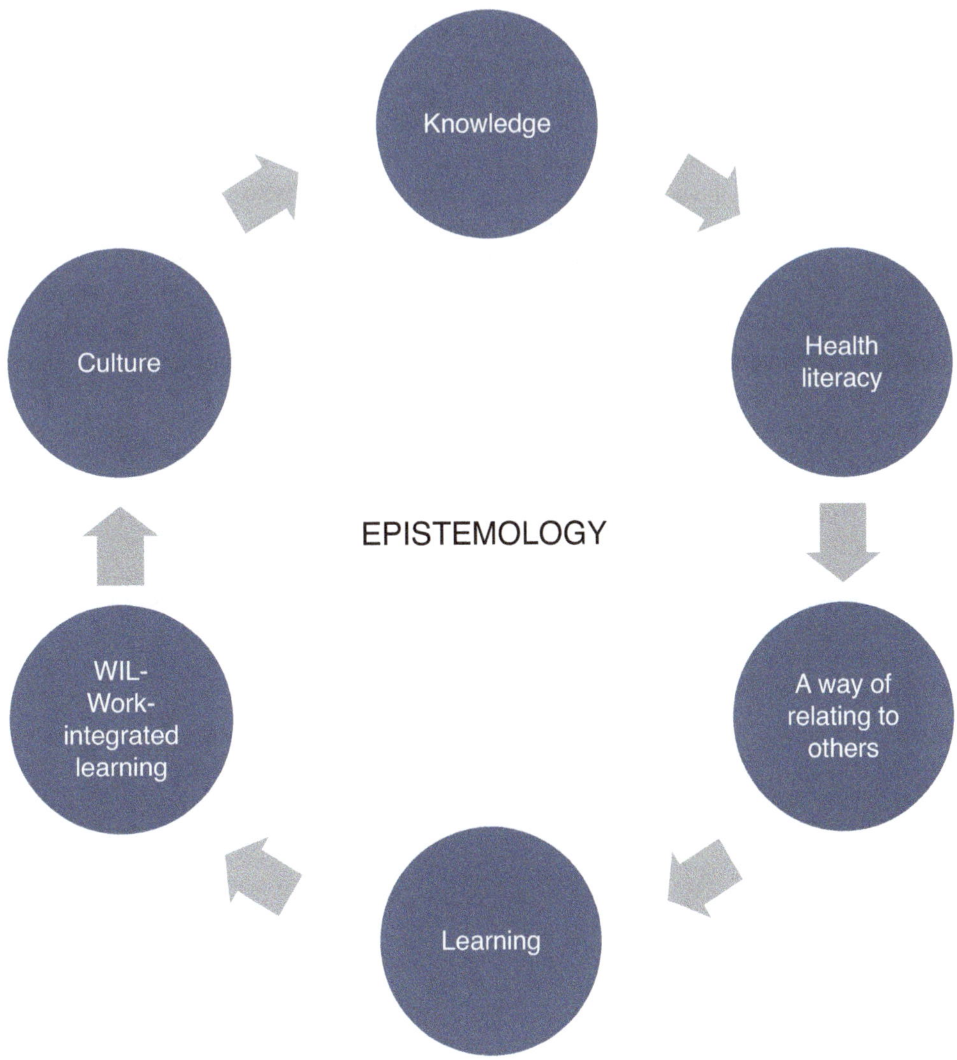

Fig. 9.2 Salutogenesis from an epistemological perspective

with flu, and may also have as-yet nondetectable malignant cells. Even the terminal patient's brain and emotions may be fully functional. The majority of us are somewhere between the two poles. Priority in health service is justly given to those at the sicker end of the continuum. However, in our thinking and our research, we should ask: "How does a person—wherever he or she is on the continuum—move toward the healthy pole?" (Sagy et al., 2015). The idea of movement along an ease/dis-ease continuum is illustrated in Fig. 9.3.

Antonovsky assumed that we continuously are exposed to changes and events that may be considered as stressors. This may involve major life events such as when someone in the family falls ill, changes in the family (e.g., a divorce), or changes in the workplace (organizational changes or unemployment). Previous research shows that such major life events affect health (Folkman, 1984). They can reduce health temporarily but can also in the longer-term strengthen us in a way that makes it possible for us to manage stress. The adverse life events have even given us experiences that can be used in other similar situations.

Antonovsky discussed the theories behind stress and coping extensively. He particularly rejected the thoughts behind Lazarus' cognitive theory on stress and coping as well as theories of life events (Lazarus & Folkman, 1984). According to Antonovsky, the assumption behind these theories was life in balance, that is, a homeostatic life. A disturbance was assumed to damage the balance and damage health and well-being, that is, a pathogenic view of life. Furthermore, traditional theories on stress and coping are mainly focused on the concept of control. In salutogenesis, the emphasis is on the person's ability to use generalized resistance resources, both internal and external, at disposal to manage ubiquitous stressful situations. The actual starting point, according to Antonovsky, is that life is a chaos in which we must constantly relate to change. It becomes vital how we can manage this chaos. This is the salutogenic view of stress and coping, according to Antonovsky:

> *... life is inherently full of stressors, with life-situation stressor complexes by far deserving most of our attention of we wish to understand either health or disease. Focusing on health, I expressly rejected the implicit assumption that stressors are inherently pathogenic. Their health consequences can only be understood if we understand the coping process.* (Antonovsky, 1992, p. 48)

Three potential reactions and outcomes of stress are as follows: (1) being neutral against the stressors, (2) being able to manage stress for the movement toward the health end, and (3) being unable to manage stress which leads to a breakdown expressed in terms of diseases and death (Antonovsky, 1987). In the case of events that do not concern us as much, that is, daily hassles to use the words by Antonovsky (1987), we can remain neutral to them, since they do not affect health in any significant way. However, if it is a question of events that we cannot manage, we become ill, or we mobilize internal and/or external resources around us, allowing us to deal with what happened and move in the direction of health.

Generalized and Specific Resistance Resources

Along with the sense of coherence, a key concept in the salutogenic model is resistance resources (Antonovsky, 1979, 1987), including generalized resources (potentially available for engagement in a wide range of circumstances) and specific resources (particular resources relevant to particular circumstances). Since the subject of resistance resources is dealt with in detail in several chapters in Part II of this book,

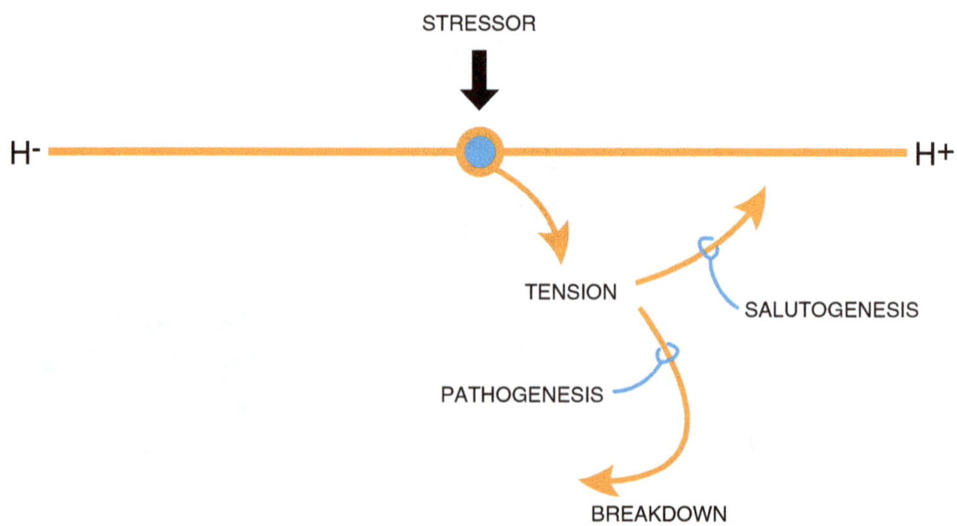

Fig. 9.3 The ease/dis-ease continuum (Antonovsky, 1979, 1987). Graphic: Bengt Lindström, Monica Eriksson, Peter Wikström (Lindström & Eriksson, 2010)

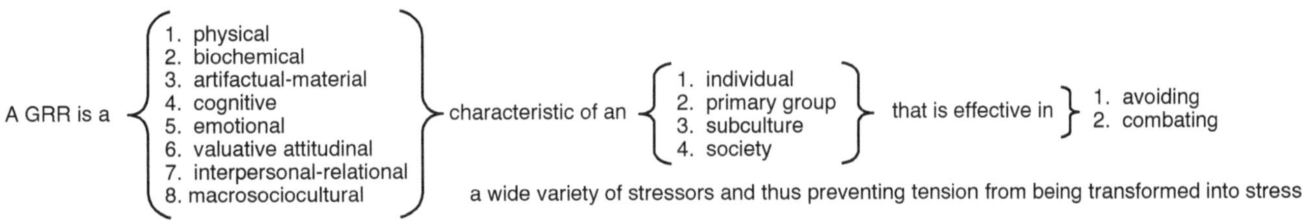

Fig. 9.4 The definition of generalized resistance resources. (Antonovsky, 1979, s. 103)

only a few comments are offered here, with particular attention to the relevance of resistance resources to the main subject of this section "Sense of Coherence".

Generalized resistance resources are the cornerstones in the development of a strong sense of coherence. They are diverse: genetic and constitutional, psychosocial, cultural, spiritual, material, and a preventive health orientation (Lindström & Eriksson, 2005). Resistance resources exist at the individual, the group (family), the subculture, and the whole society levels (Antonovsky, 1979, p. 103). Antonovsky's formal definition of generalized resistance resources is given in Fig. 9.4.

Research on the role of generalized resistance resources in building the sense of coherence is still scarce. Early research (Antonovsky, 1991, cited in Sagy & Antonovsky, 1999, p. 256) showed that three factors seemed to be particularly important for developing a strong sense of coherence: consistency, balance between under- and overload, and the opportunity to participate in decision-making affect one's situation. The question of which resistance resources are involved in building the sense of coherence has received some attention:

- A Finnish study examined the importance of generalized resistance resources such as cognitive ability, marital status, level of family income, the length of formal education, and physical activity for the development of a strong sense of coherence among Finns aged 65–69 years (Read et al., 2005). The results showed that cognitive ability and physical activity were related to the sense of coherence, which in turn was associated with good social and mental health.
- A qualitative Swedish study of caregivers to older adults aimed to illuminate generalized and specific resistance resources against caregiver stress; it identified the panoply of negative and positive experiences of caring for a relative as a particularly salient resource—"caregivinghood," as in the sense of "parenthood" (Wennerberg et al., 2012; Wennerberg et al., 2016; Wennerberg et al., 2018; Wennerberg et al., 2019).
- Through a thematic analysis of the work by Antonovsky and more recent research, Griffiths, Ryan, and Foster (2011, p. 170) identified 15 general resistant resource themes: (1) structure in life, (2) predictability in life, (3) social support, (4) coping strategies, (5) life meaning, (6) responsibility, (7) comprehension, (8) expression of confidence, (9) challenges worth investing time and effort, (10) health/illness, (11) future orientation, (12) past orientation, (13) positive, solution-focused outlook, (14) emotional connection, and (15) ensuring that you are justly treated. No resource-related theme emerged that did not fit the sense of coherence concept.

Sense of Coherence

Antonovsky initiated a study among different ethnic groups of women in Israel to investigate their menopausal symptoms, that is, a traditional epidemiological study from a risk perspective (Antonovsky, 1987). He interviewed them about perceived health, and also about various life events affecting them, such as losing their eyesight, loss of husband/wife, amputation of the leg/arm, or to have suffered a serious illness (Antonovsky, 1983). After analyzing the interviews, he found that 29% of the women reported good health, although they survived the Holocaust. Antonovsky raised the question of how it could be possible that women may experience good health despite experiencing the Holocaust. It led him to focus on this small number of respondents, and a search for their health resources. This was the start of Antonovsky's paradigm shift from pathogenesis to salutogenesis.

Based on the interviews with the Israeli women, an important factor emerged: the sense of coherence. The sense of coherence reflects a person's view of life and capacity to respond to stressful situations. It is a global orientation to view life as structured, manageable, and meaningful. It is a personal way of thinking, being, and acting, with an inner trust, which leads people to identify, benefit, use, and reuse the resources at their disposal (Eriksson & Lindström, 2006). Sense of coherence consists of three elements: comprehensibility, manageability, and meaningfulness. The original definition by Antonovsky (1987) is as follows:

> a global orientation that expresses the extent to which one has a pervasive, enduring though dynamic feeling of confidence that (1) the stimuli from one's internal and external environments in the course of living are structured, predictable, and explicable;

> (2) the resources are available to one to meet the demands posed by these stimuli; and (3) these demands are challenges, worthy of investment and engagement. (p. 19)

It is also about one's own ability to identify one's internal and external resources and use them in a way that promotes health and well-being (Eriksson & Lindström, 2006). Further, it is a way of thinking in terms of peoples' resources, and even a way to work, to meet and treat other people. It is also important to understand why and how resources work. This has been further examined in a Norwegian qualitative study using a grounded theory approach (Maass et al., 2017). They investigated how neighborhood resources may contribute to the development of a strong SOC. They found that a strong SOC can be described as a deeper understanding of how and why resources work, which allows for more flexible use of resources. According to Antonovsky, sense of coherence is a life orientation. Koltko-Rivera (2004) defines life orientation as follows:

> ... a way of describing the universe and life within it, both in terms of what is and what ought to be. A given worldview is a set of beliefs that includes limiting statements and assumptions regarding what exists and what does not. ... A worldview defines what can be known or done in the world, and how it can be known or done. ... What goals can be sought in life ... defines what goals should be pursued.

It is to the nature of the life orientation that is termed "the sense of coherence" that this part of the book is devoted. Inevitably, the sense of coherence is also a theme, major or minor, in virtually every chapter of this book. The sense of coherence was Antonovsky's main interest in his study of salutogenesis, even if he encouraged research on all aspects of the salutogenic model. Following Antonovsky's wholehearted lead, succeeding generations of scholars have focused so much on the study of the sense of coherence that the salutogenic model is sometimes referred to as the "sense of coherence theory." While Antonovsky did not himself define the sense of coherence as a theory, it was his answer to the salutogenic question: what are the origins of health? He encouraged a search for other answers, but as this book reveals, most salutogenesis researchers have chosen to follow the path to the sense of coherence, the path that Antonovsky himself so doggedly trod. A new concept is suggested, sense for coherence (SFC), useful in connection with the implementation of salutogenesis in practice (See chapter Part VII Sense for coherence: An emerging concept for salutogenesis practice?).

Sense of Coherence and the Relationship to Health

A search in the Medline database as of September 17, 2019, shows that more than 1700 studies using some version of the SOC scale have been performed. The results show that a strong SOC is associated with perceived good health, particularly mental health. A systematic review of studies using the SOC questionnaire during 1992–2003 showed that a strong SOC protected against anxiety, depression, burnout, and hopelessness; was strongly and positively related to health resources such as optimism, hardiness, control, and coping; and predicted good health and QoL from childhood to adulthood. In other words, the stronger the SOC, the fewer the symptoms of mental illnesses (Eriksson & Lindström, 2006, 2007). The correlation with health ranges in general from slight to good, using instruments such as the General Health Questionnaire, the Health Index, the Hopkin's Symptom Checklist, and the Mental Health Inventory, with such health measures explaining up to 66% of the variance in the SOC-29 (Eriksson & Lindström, 2005). Galletta et al. (2019) examined the relationship between SOC and physical health-related quality of life in patients (n = 209) with chronic illnesses, focusing on the mediating role of the mental component of quality of life. The results showed that SOC was mainly associated with the mental health component of the quality of life, and after that, the physical component. Mediating analysis confirmed that SOC was directly related to the mental health component, but not to the physical one. They conclude that the findings give evidence for SOC as a psychological process that impacts mental health status, which in turn affects physical health.

The SOC is not a coping strategy but a coping resource dealing with stress connected to work-related stress (Palm & Eriksson, 2018), adverse life events, such as family breakdown (Richardson & Ratner, 2005; Ristkari et al., 2008), being a victim of sexual abuse (Priebe et al., 2010; Nilsson et al., 2015), violence in the form of bullying (Birkeland Nielsen et al., 2008), political violence (Abu-Kaf et al., 2017; Abu-Kaf & Braun-Lewensohn, 2019), and war (Veronese & Pepe, 2017; Braun-Lewensohn & Al-Sayed, 2018).

References

Abu-Kaf, S., Braun-Lewensohn, O., & Kalagy, T. (2017). Youth in the midst of escalated political violence: Sense of coherence and hope among Jewish and Bedouin Arab adolescents. *Child and Adolescent Psychiatry and Mental Health, 11*, 42. https://doi.org/10.1186/s13034-017-0178-z

Abu-Kaf, S., & Braun-Lewensohn, O. (2019). Coping resources and stress reactions among Bedouin Arab adolescents during three military operations. *Psychiatry Research, 273*, 559–566.

Antonovsky, A. (1979). *Health, stress and coping*. Jossey-Bass.

Antonovsky, A. (1983). The sense of coherence: Development of a research instrument. In *Newsletter Research Report* (Vol. 1, pp. 11–22). Schwartz Research Center for Behavioral Medicine, Tel Aviv University.

Antonovsky, A. (1985). The life cycle, mental health and the sense of coherence. *Israel Journal of Psychiatry & Related Sciences, 22*(4), 273–280.

Antonovsky, A. (1987). *Unraveling the Mystery of Health. How people manage stress and stay well*. Jossey-Bass.

Antonovsky, A. (1991). The structural resources of salutogenic strengths. In C. L. Cooper & R. Payne (Eds.), *Personality and stress: Individual differences in the stress process*. L. Wiley.

Antonovsky, A. (1992). Can attitudes contribute to health? *Advances, The Journal of Mind-Body Health, 8*(4), 33–49.

Antonovsky, A. (1993a). Complexity, conflict, chaos, coherence, coercion and civility. *Social Science & Medicine, 37*(8), 969–981.

Antonovsky, A. (1993b). The structure and properties of the sense of coherence scale. *Social Science & Medicine, 36*(6), 725–733.

Antonovsky, A. (1993c). *Some salutogenic words of wisdom to the conferees*. NHV, Göteborg. [Electronic] http://www.angelfire.com/ok/soc/agoteborg.html

Audi, R. (2011). *Epistemology. A contemporary introduction to the theory of knowledge*. Routledge.

Birkeland Nielsen, M., Matthiesen, S. B., & Einarsen, S. (2008). Sense of coherence as a protective mechanism among targets of workplace bullying. *Journal of Occupational Health Psychology, 13*(2), 128–136.

Boström, A., Kaplan, R., & Kaplan, S. (2014). Creating supportive environments to foster reasonableness and achieve sustainable well-being. In T. J. Hämäläinen & J. Michaelson (Eds.), *Well-being and beyond. Broadening the public and policy discourse*. Edward Elgar.

Boström, L., & Lassen, L. M. (2006). Unraveling learning, learning styles, learning strategies and meta-cognition. *Education & Training, 48*(2/3), 178–189.

Braun-Lewensohn, O., & Al-Sayed, K. (2018). Syrian adolescent refugees: How do they cope during their stay in refugee camps? *Frontiers in Psychology, 9*, 1258. https://doi.org/10.3389/fpsyg.2018.01258

Eriksson, M. (2018). Research supervision as a mutual learning process: Introducing salutogenesis into supervision using "the collegial model". *Health Promotion International*. https://doi.org/10.1093/heapro/day088

Eriksson, M., & Lindström, B. (2005). Validity of Antonovsky's sense of coherence scale: A systematic review. *Journal of Epidemiology and Community Health, 59*(6), 406–466.

Eriksson, M., & Lindström, B. (2006). Antonovsky's Sense of Coherence Scale and the relation with health: A systematic review. *Journal of Epidemiology & Community Health, 60*(5), 376–381.

Eriksson, M., & Lindström, B. (2007). Antonovsky's sense of coherence scale and its relation with quality of life – A systematic review. *Journal of Epidemiology and Community Health, 61*(11), 938–944.

Folkman, S. (1984). Personal control and stress and coping processes: A theoretical analysis. *Journal of Personality and Social Psychology, 46*(4), 839–852.

Galletta, M., Cherchi, M., Cocco, A., Lai, G., Manca, V., Pau, M., Tatti, F., Zambon, G., Deidda, S., Origa, P., Massa, E., Cossu, E., Boi, F., & Contu, P. (2019). Sense of coherence and physical health-related quality of life in Italian chronic patients: The mediating role of the mental component. *BMJ Open*. https://doi.org/10.1136/bmjopen-2019-030001

Griffiths, C. A., Ryan, P., & Foster, J. H. (2011). Thematic analysis of Antonovsky's sense of coherence theory. *Scandinavian Journal of Psychology, 52*, 168–173.

Heil, J. (2005). *From an ontological point of view*. Clarendon.

Kaplan, S., & Kaplan, R. (2003). Health, supportive environments, and the reasonable person model. *American Journal of Public Health, 93*, 1484–1489.

Kaplan, R., & Kaplan, S. (2011). Well-being, reasonableness, and the natural environment. *Applied Psychology: Health and Well-Being, 3*(3), 304–321.

Koltko-Rivera, M. E. (2004). The psychology of worldviews. *Review of General Psychology, 8*, 3–58.

Lackaye, T. D., & Margalit, M. (2006). Comparisons of achievement, effort, and self-perceptions among students with learning disabilities and their peers from different achievement groups. *Journal of Learning Disabilities, 39*(5), 432–446.

Lazarus, R., & Folkman, S. (1984). *Stress, appraisal and coping*. Springer.

Lindström, B. (1999). The salutogenic model as a tool for quality of life enhancement for children with special needs. *Exceptionality Education Canada, 9*(1/2), 105–109.

Lindström, B., & Eriksson, M. (2005). Salutogenesis. *Journal of Epidemiology and Community Health, 59*(6), 440–442.

Lindström, B., & Eriksson, M. (2010). *The hitchhiker's guide to salutogenesis: Salutogenic pathways to health promotion*. The IUHPE Global Working Group on Salutogenesis. Helsinki: Folkhälsan research center, Health promotion research, Research report: 2010:2.

Lindström, B., & Eriksson, M. (2011). From health education to healthy learning: Implementing salutogenesis in educational science. *Scandinavian Journal of Public Health, 39*(Suppl 6), 85–92.

Maass, R. E. K., Lindström, B., & Lillefjell, M. (2017). Neighborhood-resources for the development of a strong SOC and importance of understanding why and how resources work: A grounded theory approach. *BMC Public Health, 17*(1), 704–717.

Macdonald, D. (2013). The new Australian health and physical education curriculum: A case of/for gradualism in curriculum reform? *Asia-Pacific Journal of Health, Sport and Physical Education, 4*(2), 95–108.

Margalit, M., & Efrati, M. (1996). Loneliness, coherence and companionship among children with learning disorder. *Educational Psychology, 16*(1), 69–80.

Mayer, C.-H., & Boness, C. (2011). Interventions to promoting sense of coherence and transcultural competences in educational contexts. *International Review of Psychiatry, 23*(6), 516–524.

McCuaig, L., Quennerstedt, M., & Macdonald, D. (2013). A salutogenic, strengths-based approach as a theory to guide HPE curriculum change. *Asia-Pacific Journal of Health, Sport and Physical Education, 4*(2), 109–125.

Nilsson, L., & Lindström, B. (1998). Learning as a health promoting process: The salutogenic interpretation of the Swedish curricula in state education. *Internet Journal of Health Promotion*. [Elektronic]. http://www.diva-portal.org/smash/record.jsf?searchId=2&pid=diva2:696903

Nilsson, D., Nordenstam, C., Green, S., Wetterhall, A., Lundin, T., & Svedin, C. G. (2015). Acute stress among adolescents and female rape victims measured by ASC-Kids: A pilot study. *Nordic Journal of Psychiatry, 69*(7), 539–545.

Quennerstedt, M. (2006). *Learning health*. [Doctoral thesis]. Örebro: Örebro University.

Palm, K., & Eriksson, A. (2018). Understanding salutogenic approaches to managing intensive work: Experiences from three Swedish companies. *Work, 61*(4), 627–637.

Pennbrant, S., & Svensson, L. (2018). Nursing and learning – Healthcare pedagogics and work-integrated learning. *Higher Education, Skills and Work-Based Learning, 8*(2), 179–194.

Pijpker, R., Vaandrager, L., Bakker, E. J., & Koelen, M. (2018). Unravelling salutogenic mechanisms in the workplace: The role of learning. *Gaceta Sanitaria, 32*(3), 275–282.

Priebe, G., Hansson, K., & Svedin, C. G. (2010). Sexual abuse and associations with psychosocial aspects of health. A population-based study with Swedish adolescents. *Nordic Journal of Psychiatry, 64*(1), 40–48.

Quennerstedt, M., Burrows, L., & Maivorsdotter, N. (2010). From teaching young people to be healthy to learning health. *Utbildning & Demokrati, 19*(2), 97–112.

Read, S., Aunola, K., Feldt, T., Leinonen, R., & Ruoppila, I. (2005). The relationship between Generalized Resistance Resources, Sense of Coherence, and health among Finnish people aged 65–69. *European Psychologist, 10*(3), 244–253.

Richardson, C. G., & Ratner, P. A. (2005). Sense of coherence as a moderator of the effects of stressful life events on health. *Journal of Epidemiology and Community Health, 59*, 979–984.

Ristkari, T., Sourander, A., Rønning, J. A., Nikolakaros, G., & Helenius, H. (2008). Life events, self-reported psychopathology and sense of coherence among young men – A population-based study. *Nordic Journal of Psychiatry, 62*(6), 464–471.

Sagy, S., & Antonovsky, H. (1999). Factors related to the development of the sense of coherence (sense of coherence) in adolescents. A retrospective study. *Polish Psychological Bulletin, 30*(4), 255–262.

Sagy, S., Eriksson, M., & Braun-Lewensohn, O. (2015). The salutogenic paradigm. In S. Joseph (Ed.), *Positive psychology in practice: Promoting human flourishing in work, health, education, and everyday life* (2nd ed., pp. 61–80). Wiley.

Wennerberg, M. M. T., Lundgren, S. M., & Danielson, E. (2012). Using the salutogenic approach to unravel informal caregivers' resources to health: Theory and methodology. *Aging & Mental Health, 16*(3), 391–402.

Wennerberg, M. M. T., Eriksson, M., Danielson, E., & Lundgren, S. M. (2016). Unravelling Swedish caregivers' generalized resistance resources. *Scandinavian Journal of Caring Sciences, 30*, 602–613.

Wennerberg, M. M. T., Eriksson, M., Lundgren, S. M., & Danielson, E. (2018). Unravelling Swedish informal caregivers' generalized resistance resources. *Scandinavian Journal of Caring Sciences, 32*, 186–196.

Wennerberg, M. M. T., Lundgren, S. M., Eriksson, M., & Danielson, E. (2019). Me and you in caregivinghood – Dyadic resistance resources and deficits out of the informal caregiver's perspective. *Aging & Mental Health, 23*(8), 1041–1048.

Veronese, G., & Pepe, A. (2017). Sense of coherence as a determinant of psychological well-being across professional groups of aid workers exposed to war trauma. *Journal of Interpersonal Violence, 32*(13), 1899–1920.

10

Appraising and Reacting to Stressors: Impact of SOC

Maurice B. Mittelmark

Introduction

An extensive literature shows that the sense of coherence (SOC) is related statistically to a host of behaviours with implications for illness and health (Eriksson & Lindström, 2006, 2007; Mittelmark et al., 2017). To make sense of the statistical associations, we require research on the *mechanisms* by which the SOC is involved in health development (Super et al., 2016). What makes the connection? What is in the black box?

This chapter is about Aaron Antonovsky's answer: the SOC influences how a person *appraises and reacts to stressors*. This process occupies a critical place along the pathway from the SOC to behaviour.

We begin with definitions of two key terms (Antonovsky, 1979, p 72):

- A routine *stimulus* is one to which the organism can respond more or less automatically, which poses no problem in adjustment.
- A *stressor* is a stimulus making a demand from an organism's internal or external environment that upsets its homeostasis, restoration of which depends on a nonautomatic and not readily available energy-expending action.

Research reveals that the SOC develops during the entire life course (Silverstein & Heap, 2015), influenced by the accumulating experience of encountering, appraising and reacting to stressors, and experiencing sequela. How one experiences stressors today is, therefore, affected by how one experienced stressors previously. Which stressors one encounters, how one appraises them and how one reacts is recursive. For example, one's first encounter with a dog as a child can help determine if and how dogs will tend to be encountered in the future (one might be inclined to seek the companionship of dogs with joy, to shun them with fear or to ignore them). One's appraisal of and reactions to dogs, and the reactions of dogs, adds to one's accumulating experience. Feedback from experience is a critical factor in shaping one's future appraisals.

The resources one was able to engage while experiencing one's first dog (perhaps a parent's encouraging words) impacts one's appraisal, adds to one's accumulating coping resources and ultimately influences the development of one's SOC. One's store of general and specific resistance resources (GRRs and SRRs, see Chaps. 12 and 13) and one's ability to engage them in coping also develop. One's growing experience using resources affects the development of the SOC.

The Central Role of the Brain

Appreciative of the role of the brain in coping with stressors, Antonovsky wrote:

> Whether the source of the stressors is the internal or external environment, whether they are daily hassles, acute or chronic and endemic, whether they are imposed upon one or freely chosen, our lives are replete with stimuli to which we have no automatic, adequate adaptive response and in the face of which we must respond. The message to the brain… is clear: You have a problem. The nature of the problem is dual, consisting of (a) the problem-solving or instrumental issue and (b) the issue of the regulation of emotion. Tension, then, reflects the recognition in the brain that some need one has is unfulfilled, that a demand on one has to be met, and that one must do something if one is to realise a goal. (Antonovsky, 1990a, p. 35)

By 'problems', Antonovsky meant exposure to both unpleasant *and* pleasant stimuli that are salient enough to evoke appraisal (Antonovsky, 1990a, p 136):

- The worker just informed that she is to be laid off.
- The woman enduring sexual harassment from her boss.
- The woman giving birth to her first child.
- The person just promoted to a much more responsible position at work.
- The couple planning their wedding.

M. B. Mittelmark (✉)
Department of Health Promotion and Development, Faculty of Psychology, University of Bergen, Bergen, Norway
e-mail: maurice.mittelmark@uib.no

Unpleasant or pleasant, a salient problem induces one to appraise one's situation.

As Antonovsky understood it, the appraisal process may be conscious, barely conscious and even subconscious, with multiple considerations simultaneously unfolding in a jumble, often with great rapidity:

> Although it has taken me many words to discuss the processes… this does not necessarily reflect the time span involved in confronting a stressor from its appearance until the moment one acts (or does not act) directly to deal with it. Nor is the process anywhere near as rational or cognitive as it may sound. The process may be most rapid and very largely unconscious. (Antonovsky, 1990a, p. 43)

The appraisal process leads to an appraisal outcome; do nothing or do something. We are bombarded continuously by stimuli that are salient enough to warrant appraisal, which is the nature of living (Antonovsky, 1987). What is meant by 'bombarded'? Consider the woeful student worrying over the exam next hour while cycling anxiously along a busy and dangerous thoroughfare to the university, uneasy about the threatening and lightning-filled storm clouds approaching from the horizon and feeling desperate about covering the week's rent, overdue for several days already.

A description of the student's appraisal processes defies neat arrow and box diagrams. A description of the student's appraisal *outcomes* is more feasible, and this is the subject of extensive stress and coping literature spanning three decades (Lazarus & Cohen, 1977; Lazarus & Folkman, 1984; Lazarus, 1984; Scherer et al., 2001; Feldman et al., 2004; Aldwin & Park, 2004; Cheng & Cheung, 2005; Sideridis, 2006; Searle & Auton, 2015). This rich and fascinating literature was an important background for Antonovsky's work, and he brought to it his unique perspective on the role of the SOC in coping with stressors.

Stimulus and Stressor Appraisal on the Pathway to Health

Antonovsky proposed that on the pathway to health, relatively strong- compared to weak-SOC persons tend to appraise and react to stimuli and stressors differently. In his writings, Antonovsky offered arguments for a series of propositions about how the strength of the SOC affects appraisal (Antonovsky, 1987, 1990a, 1990b, 1990c, 1992). In the section below, I refer to his propositions as hypotheses.

Antonovsky's most extensive treatment of pathways leading to health appeared in Chap. 6, *Unraveling the Mystery of Health* (1987). In a later chapter, he revised and updated material from the 1987 book (Antonovsky, 1990a). Here, we rely most on the 1990 publication, as it was Antonovsky's most advanced exposition on the role of the SOC in stimulus and stressor appraisal.

The idea of *stimulus and stressor appraisal stages* is of core importance in the stress and coping literature. Antonovsky's central contribution to this literature was to discuss how the strength/weakness of the SOC affects appraisal, action and reaction to feedback, at primary, secondary and tertiary stages (see Table 10.1). The right-hand column in Table 10.1 presents snapshots of Antonovsky's expectations (hypotheses) about how the SOC affects stimulus and stressor appraisal, and this is discussed in detail below.

H1 'The person with a strong SOC is more likely to define stimuli as nonstressors, and to assume that he or she can adapt automatically to the demand than one with a weak SOC. In this way, the former will not experience tension, nor see it transformed into stress'. (Antonovsky, 1990a, p 37)

Table 10.1 The role of strong compared to weak SOC in stimulus and stressor appraisal, action and reaction to feedback

Appraisal stage	Appraisal and coping processes	The strong-SOC person is more likely to…
Primary appraisal I Stimulus encountered that calls for focused consideration	Non-stressor (does not pose demands that exceed resources) or. Stressor (state of tension created).	Experience the stimulus as non-stressor. Assume that stimulus demands can be met 'automatically'.
Primary appraisal II Stimulus perceived as a stressor	Endangering one's well-being. Being positive. Being benign/irrelevant.	Experience the stressor as benign/irrelevant/ positive. Feel confident that the tension will soon dissipate.
Primary appraisal III Stressor perception and regulation of stressor-induced emotion	Happy, non-conflictual and not dangerous. Unhappy, conflictual or/and dangerous.	Understand the instrumental coping challenge. Experience the stressor as happier, less conflictual and less dangerous.
Secondary appraisal Coping	Moves from perception to action.	Mobilise the most appropriate GRRs / SRRs.
Tertiary appraisal Feedback and learning	Experiences coping attempts and outcomes. Exposed to direct and indirect feedback.	Elicit feedback and assess it. Attend to signals. Be willing to change course. Experience that GRRs are strengthened. Experience that the SOC is 'fortified'.

Primary Appraisal I

H1 has hardly received empirical scrutiny. It is hard to conceive how quantitative research on the SOC and appraisal behaviour could uncover findings that support or refute H1. It seems that only qualitative research could produce the needed data, using in-depth interviews to document strong- and weak-SOC persons' lifelong experience, including instances of encountering stimuli that might, but do not necessarily provoke appraisal of a stimulus as a stressor. It is easy to think up a long list of such stimuli, but it is not easy to imagine how the researcher could account for context effects. Consider, for example, two drivers encountering a very busy roundabout while driving in heavy city traffic. Regardless of SOC, the driver on a casual Sunday drive might blithely disregard the potential stress in the situation, while the driver delivering his labouring wife to the hospital might well break out in a cold sweat. Regardless of what differences the researcher might find regarding SOC levels, the probable conclusion would likely depend on the context. If this cautious analysis has merit, we might just as well dismiss H1 as untestable.

H2 'The strong-SOC person, having considerable experience in encountering stimuli that initially seem to be stressors but soon turn out not to be problematic, without any particular investment of energy on his or her part, is more likely, at the primary appraisal-II stage, to define a stressor as benign or irrelevant, to feel confident that the tension will quickly dissipate" (Antonovsky, 1990a, p 37).

Primary Appraisal II

Primary appraisal II is invoked when stimuli are perceived as stressors

> '...endangering one's well-being, positive, benign or irrelevant... to perceive a stressor as benign or irrelevant is to define it as of little consequence for one's life... it is assumed that the tension will soon be dissipated'. (Antonovsky, 1990a, p 37)

However, Antonovsky warned of a potential downside of a strong-SOC person's tendency to define a stressor as benign or irrelevant. He mentioned delay in seeking medical treatment (a problem of global proportion, see Wechkunanukul et al., 2017) writing, *'there is a danger that the strong-SOC person will at times deceive himself or herself'*. Antonovsky equivocates, suggesting that self-deception is in some instances *less* likely to be the case for the strong-SOC, compared to the weak-SOC person, with the former tending to be more realistic in not worrying about tension-arousing stimuli (like chest and other pains that can be a warning of a heart attack).

This equivocation is equivalent to saying 'it depends' and complicates any effort to examine empirically H2. To the degree that a person's previous experience is a factor at the appraisal II stage, the researcher would wish to know the person's history. As a methodological issue, this suggests the importance of qualitative approaches to the study of Antonovsky's appraisal hypotheses to uncover information about the respondent's encounters with stressors that did and did not induce coping (see Chap. 54).

Antonovsky concludes his discussion of appraisal I and II provocatively, writing *that 'if, then, the strong-SOC person is advantaged..., such advantage is relatively unimportant'* because life is filled with stressors that cannot be shrugged aside.

Regarding the availability of data suitable to test H2 and the feasibility and importance of testing H2, we might well come to the same conclusion as for H1. It seems stress researchers have little interest in instances where a person can shrug off a stressor lightly. We might as well agree with Antonovsky that the proposition behind this hypothesis is 'relatively unimportant'.

Or we may wish to follow Amirkhan and Greaves (2003) in exploring Antonovsky's writings for new theoretical ideas about primary appraisal mechanisms that might explain the link between the SOC and health. They discuss three possibilities: perceptual, cognitive and behavioural mechanisms. As to perception, they suggest that:

> '...while all people sort stimuli according to intensity, size, shape, and other properties, perhaps those with a strong SOC also classify according to the perceived meaningfulness of the stimulus. When confronted with problems, then, strong SOC individuals might view some or all of these as coherent, while other people might simply not attend to this property'. (ibid, p 33)

They do not speculate how the differential perception of a stimulus by strong- and weak-SOC people might lead to different primary appraisal outcomes. However, they do discuss the possibility of a reciprocal relationship with the SOC influencing stimulus perception that influences the SOC that influences perception, and so on. As a result, over the long term, strong-SOC persons may be more likely to perceive coherence and meaningfulness *and* experience SOC strengthening.

Regarding cognition, Amirkhan and Greaves (2003) point out the possible relevance of attribution theory (Weiner, 2010), suggesting that attributes of stimuli are important in differentiating strong- and weak-SOC persons' appraisals. They mention the possibility that one attribution dimension is the degree of coherence of a stimulus' causes. Compared to weak-SOC persons, strong-SOC persons encountering a stressor may have the knack of analysing the degree of coherence among causes behind the stressor. Stressors judged to have coherent causes may produce less emotional distress or more motivated responses.

Regarding behaviour, Amirkhan and Greaves (2003) point to the possibility that the SOC's strength determines at least partly coping choices, independent of the effects of appraisal processes. In other words, perhaps strong-SOC persons have a more marked propensity to focus on and rectify problems compared to weak-SOC persons.

A series of laboratory and field studies undertaken to explore these mechanisms revealed

> '...a perceptual process, that was pervasive and yet subtle in nature. A strong SOC seems to work much like rose-colored glasses that one has grown accustomed to wearing: Although not conscious of their presence, one still benefits by the pleasant tint that they provide'. (Amirkhan & Greaves, 2003)

Amirkhan and Greaves' (2003) idea about rose-coloured glasses indicates a subconscious level of stimuli engagement and not the conscious and near-subconscious levels that held Antonovsky's attention. This suggests a line of inquiry that may prove illuminating, although not directly relevant to this chapter's theme.

Even if the work just discussed does not directly address Antonovsky's hypotheses about stimulus appraisal, it may illuminate ways to improve coping effectiveness. Amirkhan and Greaves' (2003) ideas about perceptual, cognitive and behavioural primary appraisal mechanisms, and subconscious processing, are certainly deserving of further exploration.

Regardless of the SOC's strength, health benefits might accrue if one learns to deploy coping responses in a manner consonant with that of strong-SOC persons.

H3 The strong-SOC person is 'more likely to appraise a stressor as happier, as less conflictful, or less dangerous than one with a weak SOC'. (Antonovsky, 1990a, p 39–40).

Primary Appraisal III

Primary appraisal III is focused on how the strong-SOC person perceives and regulates the emotion induced by a stressor and apprehends the instrumental challenge of coping with the stressor.

This is a compound statement (happier, less conflictual and less dangerous); are underlying dimensions thought to link these appraisal possibilities? The answer seems to be no. One can easily imagine a questionnaire in which the respondent is asked to consider a particular stressor and rate it on three separate dimensions: happy-unhappy, conflictual-not conflictual and dangerous-not dangerous.

Antonovsky describes how a 'happy' stressor may arouse different emotions: two widowers meet attractive women; the widower with a strong SOC feels hope and excitement, while the widower with a weak SOC feels hopelessness and apathy. The differences in emotion feed differences in reacting instrumentally. Meeting the attractive woman is, in SOC terms, more meaningful to the strong- than to the weak-SOC widower, or as Antonovsky writes:

> 'The strong-SOC person perceives the same problems, but with greater clarity, more specificity, and more precise differentiation. The problems...are seen as more comprehensible and manageable...[and] as challenges rather than as burdens... The strong-SOC person, encountering a stressor, is more likely to be capable of introducing order and meaning into the situation... The strong-SOC person... has a head start. Before taking action, he or she has mobilised resources to confront the stressor. By contrast, the weak-SOC person, confused and devoid of the desire to cope, tends to give up at the outset'. (Antonovsky, 1990a, p 40-41).

Brady (2017) undertook a meticulous examination of appraisal *à la* H3. She studied 591 American graduate students with paid employment alongside studies and adults who were full-time employees working at least 34 hours per week. Brady administered the SOC-29 Orientation to Life Questionnaire (Antonovsky, 1993) and the Work-Related Sense of Coherence (Work-SOC) of Bauer and Jenny (2007). She also assessed the prevalence of 17 stressors in a participant's workplace, and administered scales measuring primary appraisal propensities (Searle & Auton, 2015) and threat (Feldman et al., 2004):

- *Challenge appraisal* of a stressor that opens for personally meaningful gain having the potential to engage the person (Cavanaugh et al., 2000).
- *Hindrance appraisal* of a stressor perceived to restrict or obstruct opportunities for personally meaningful gains or to interfere with work achievement (Cavanaugh et al., 2000).
- *Threat appraisal* of a stressor perceived as holding risk for personal harm or loss (Tuckey et al., 2015).

Challenge appraisal is somewhat akin to Antonovsky's happiness dimension. Hindrance appraisal is akin to Antonovsky's conflict dimension. Threat appraisal is to a reasonable degree akin to Antonovsky's danger dimension. Therefore, the measures of challenge, hindrance and threat appraisal in Brady's research are of some utility in exploring H3.

Brady hypothesised that (a) there is a positive relationship between SOC and tendency to appraise work stressors as challenges; (b) there is a negative relationship between SOC and tendency to appraise work stressors as hindrances and (c) there is a negative relationship between SOC and tendency to appraise work stressors as threats.

Her analysis of correlation coefficients among the SOC and the appraisal variables confirmed the hypotheses, both for the SOC-29 and the work-SOC measures. She concluded:

> ...stronger SoC are more likely to appraise stressors as challenges and that individuals with a weaker SoC are more likely to appraise stressors as hindrances and threats. Similarly, the initial results suggest that individuals with a stronger Work-SoC are more likely to appraise stressors as challenges and individuals with a weaker Work-SoC more likely to appraise stressors as hindrances and threats.

Brady's structural equation modelling with the same data revealed thought-provoking findings on the SOC components comprehensibility, manageability and meaningfulness:

- Individuals who viewed their world as more comprehensible were less likely to appraise stressors in their work environment as challenges and as threats.
- Individuals who viewed their world as more manageable were more likely to appraise stressors in their work environment as hindrances.
- Individuals who viewed their world as more meaningful were less likely to appraise stressors in their work environment as threats.

These results on the SOC components are provocative since they do not take cognisance of Antonovsky's assertion that, from a theoretical standpoint, the SOC components are linked inextricably. Still, the findings on comprehensibility and meaningfulness seem to offer support to H3, while the finding on manageability does not. The overall pattern of results from this study does seem to support H3.

This study is of particular value because it included targeted stimuli appraisal measures, rare in the stress and coping and the salutogenesis literatures.

Other findings relevant to H3 come from a series of studies in Israel and Greece:

- Braun-Lewensohn et al. (2011) measured cognitive appraisal – feelings of danger – in 138 teenagers living in Southern Israel cities and villages in January 2009, a period of violent hostilities and missile attacks on the teenagers' communities.
- Braun-Lewensohn and Al-Sayed (2018) measured appraisals of danger in 110 Syrian adolescents, boys and girls, living in a European refugee camp for between 6 months and 2 years. Besides the experience of severe social disruption in Syria that resulted in relocation, these youth suffered the trials and tribulations of living an extended period as refugees.
- Braun-Lewensohn et al. (2019) measured cognitive appraisal (feelings of danger) in 110 Syrian refugee women (ages 19–70) living in a camp in Greece. In this study, individual SOC and community SOC (Braun-Lewensohn et al., 2011) were assessed.

The three papers just cited reported extensive and noteworthy findings on coping strategies and adaptation. But for the present purposes, the as-yet unpublished findings of relevance are these: in all three samples of youth and adults living in distressful condition, strong-SOC participants reported significantly lower levels of feeling danger than weak-SOC participants (Braun-Lewensohn, personal communication).

These studies are of particular interest because they do not focus on the appraisal of specific instances of experiencing a stimulus but rather a backdrop of stress-inducing stimuli over an extensive period. The findings in all samples – that SOC level differentiated cognitive appraisal (feeling danger) – add a new dimension to the test of H3. Antonovsky's analysis and proposition about primary appraisal III referred to one's experience of 'a stressor', not a widespread pattern of social stress (a context of stress). These studies not only provide support for H3; they extend our consideration of primary appraisal III to contextual stress. Braun-Lewensohn et al. (2019) conclude:

> ... it is very important to strengthen the SOC and ComSOC [community SOC] of refugee women, to enable them to better adapt when confronted with a variety of stressful situations. It is also important that women be integrated into societal processes, in order for them to feel in control of their lives and to strengthen their senses of manageability and comprehensibility.

H4 The person with a strong SOC 'chooses from the repertoire of generalised and specific resistance resources at his or her disposal what seems to be the most appropriate combination... it is in the actual mobilisation of what seems to be the most appropriate resource or combination of resources in the face of the given stressor that the true advantage of the strong-SOC person [over the weak-SOC person] comes to the fore." (Antonovsky, 1990a, p 42).

Secondary Appraisal

Antonovsky moves from stressor perception to *action* with this question: How does the strong-SOC person resolve the instrumental problem? With this, we come to the subject of coping, and as Antonovsky adamantly states, in the salutogenic model, coping does not refer to a specific coping *style* (italics his). Stressors are many and varied, and so is coping.

A test of H4 would require the researcher to gather information on respondents' GRRs and SRRs, and which of these resources were mobilised in the past in response to particular stressors. The researcher would also need to make judgements about the most appropriate resource or combination of resources in each respondent's armamentarium that the respondent could have called on in the face of the given stressors. This would need to be followed by comparing strong- and weak-SOC respondents' actual engagement of resources.

As far as I am aware, no such study has been reported in the literature. This is not surprising since it is hard to conceive a practical research methodology to collect the needed data. At the very least, the researcher would need to gather copious amounts of interview data from each respondent, then conduct within-case analyses, followed by cross-case analyses. The research effort would be strenuous indeed, and conclusions would be decidedly tenuous. We might just as well conclude that such studies are infeasible, or at least too demanding, to be worth the effort to investigate H4.

H5 'The person with a strong SOC… will tend to focus on the instrumental parameters of the problem, and will see as the challenge the question of what resources can be mobilised to meet the problem… The person with the weak SOC, seeing the stressor only in its burdensome aspects, will tend to focus on the emotional parameters, on handling the anxiety and unhappiness brought into being by the stressor." (Antonovsky, 1990a, p 43).

H5 receives some support. In research by Gambetta-Tessini et al. (2016), 2049 oral health professional students in Australia, New Zealand and Chile completed the SOC-13 and Brief Coping Orientation for Problems (COPE) Questionnaires in English and Spanish (Chile). COPE gathers self-report data on coping strategies that the respondents have engaged in, categorised as adaptive coping (e.g. active coping, planning, positive reframing and seeking support) or maladaptive coping (e.g. denial, venting and substance abuse). Compared to weak-SOC respondents, strong-SOC respondents reported significantly more adaptive coping strategies (active coping $r = 0.14$, and positive reframing $r = 0.13$). Conversely, compared to weak-SOC respondents, strong-SOC respondents reported significantly fewer maladaptive coping strategies (self-distraction $r = -0.12$; denial $r = -024$; substance use $r = -0.22$; behavioural disengagement $r = -026$; venting $r = -0.24$ and self-blame $r = -0.0.38$). These results suggest that strong-SOC young people are perhaps more inclined to choose adaptive coping strategies than avoiding maladaptive strategies. While there is some evidence supporting H5, the most significant pattern in the data supports a moderating effect of the SOC on coping, but in a manifestation not precisely in synchrony with H5.

Several studies highly relevant to H5 have been undertaken in Poland.

Konaszewski and Kwadrans (2020) studied the relationship between SOC and coping styles in 210 juveniles in probation centres in Poland. SOC was measured using the Orientation to Life Questionnaire. Coping strategies were measured using a 48-item inventory measuring three coping styles: task oriented, emotion oriented and avoidance oriented. In the probation sample, a strong SOC was significantly positively associated with a task-oriented style ($r = 0.29$) and significantly negatively associated with an emotion-oriented style ($r = -0.27$). Analyses of SOC components (comprehensibility, manageability and meaningfulness) revealed the same pattern of results. Thus, there is support for H5 and consistency with Gambetta-Tessini et al. (2016) results. This adds weight to the earlier suggestion for a corollary to H5 – the hypothesis that strong-SOC persons are more inclined to avoid maladaptive strategies than weak-SOC persons.

Konaszewski et al. (2019), using the same instruments as above, observed that strong-SOC university students were significantly more likely than weak-SOC students to report using a stress coping style focused on tasks ($r = 0.38$) and significantly less likely to use a style focused on emotions ($r = -0.62$).

Kotowska and Weber-Nowakowska (2019) compared coping styles in 50 orthopaedic surgery patients and 50 healthy controls. In both groups, strong-SOC participants were significantly more likely than weak-SOC participants to report active coping, acceptance of the problem, positive reframing and planning, and significantly less likely to report self-distraction, denying problems, discharging frustration, ceasing activity and engaging in self-blame. The study also examined styles of coping for the SOC components and found the same pattern. The two study groups did differ (regardless of SOC strength) in some coping styles, but the overall pattern noted above was the dominant finding.

Also in Poland, Andruszkiewicz et al. (2017) studied 188 adults aged 60–89 years with diagnoses of chronic illness and accompanying pain. Participants with a strong SOC were significantly less likely than weak-SOC participants to report using a catastrophising coping style. In contrast, the strong- and weak-SOC participants did not differ in their reported use of distraction or turning to prayer/hope.

In yet another Polish study, Krok (2016) enrolled 212 adults aged 65–79 years and measured SOC and coping styles (task oriented, emotion oriented and avoidance oriented). Strong- compared to weak-SOC participants were significantly more likely to report task-oriented coping and significantly less likely to report emotion-oriented coping. There was no difference in the use of avoidance-oriented coping.

Moving to The Netherlands, Polhuis et al. (2020) collected SOC and interview data from 17 Dutch respondents with type 2 diabetes mellitus to explore how and why their eating practices developed after encountering turning points (stressors) for developing unhealthy or healthy eating. Examples of turning points for unhealthy eating were child neglect, losing a job and losing a parent. Examples of turning points for healthy eating were confrontations with ill health, becoming a parent and getting married. In this study, most strong-SOC respondents who had experienced a confrontation with ill health intended to engage in active coping (adhering to dietary guidelines). The qualitative study design did not permit statistical analysis of strong- compared to weak-SOC respondents' active coping. These findings are not consistent with an alternative expectation; strong-SOC persons may deny symptoms and delay taking action on medical problems. Antonovsky was well aware of this possibility but maintained that such self-deception was more likely to be the case for the weak- than for the strong-SOC person (Antonovsky, 1987, p 134).

In Sweden, Kristofferzon et al. (2018) enrolled 348 seriously ill chronic disease patients with a mean age of 69 and measured the SOC and two coping styles, emotion focused and problem focused. Strong- compared to weak-SOC participants were significantly less likely to report using problem-focused coping ($r = -0.24$) and emotion-focused coping ($r = -0.45$). This is consistent with H5 because the negative relationship between SOC and emotion-focused coping was stronger than the negative relationship between SOC and problem-focused coping.

Finally, Ngai (2019) enrolled 201 women in Hong Kong, ages 40–60, who underwent the menopausal transition. Ngai measured the SOC and coping styles, including adaptive coping (acceptance and humour) and maladaptive coping (venting, behavioural disengagement, self-distraction, self-blame, substance use and denial). Strong- compared to weak-SOC respondents were more likely to report using an adaptive coping style ($r = 0.41$) and significantly less likely to report using a maladaptive coping style ($r = -0.51$).

H6 "The person with a strong SOC, long familiar with looking for feedback, will both elicit it and be capable of assessing it. With a weak SOC, once one's course is set, one tends to disregard signals that contradict the wisdom of the action chosen. There is no motivation to relinquish a course leading to a dead end and search for alternative courses of action. One goes on one's way blindly." (Antonovsky, 1990a, p 48)

Tertiary Appraisal

We come, then, to the final stage of the appraisal and coping process as the salutogenic model has it; that of applying resources to meet a stressor and the process of receiving and apprehending feedback and making course corrections. As for several of the other hypotheses discussed above, H6 seems to have attracted little attention from salutogenesis researchers. In the cases of H1, H2 and H4, this chapter has pondered reasons for researchers' neglect, such as methodological difficulties that seem to preclude the possibility of hypothesis testing. In the case of H6, the lack of data is disappointing. At a theoretical level, tertiary appraisal seems to be an essential aspect of learning to cope with stressors. Feedback should lead to strengthened SOC and the accumulation of GRRs and SRRs. The failure to engage in tertiary appraisal (not learning from experience) would, in theory, have opposite results: weak SOC and meagre access to resources. As Antonovsky put it,

> The person with a strong SOC, long familiar with looking for feedback, will both elicit it and be capable of assessing it. With a weak SOC, once one's course is set, one tends to disregard signals that contradict the wisdom of the action chosen. There is no motivation to relinquish a course leading to a dead end and search for alternative courses of action. One goes on one's way blindly. (Antonovsky, 1990a, p 48)

Literature searches using Google Scholar and PubMed in 1979–2020 uncovered just one study directly relevant to H6 (Pijpker et al., 2018). This seminal report from the Netherlands recruited 481 Dutch nurses and caregivers in four residential care settings and one healthcare-related Dutch Facebook group. SOC was measured using the Dutch 13-item Orientation to Life Questionnaire. Feedback was measured using the Workplace Learning Processes Questionnaire (WLPQ). The investigators used factor analysis of the WLPQ to identify a scale measuring feedback (social learning), with these four items: reflecting with my colleagues on my actions, asking colleagues for advice, observing my colleagues and developing new ideas with my colleagues. The study also gathered data on GRRs in three categories: social support, meaning attached to work and job control. Strong SOC participants had significantly higher feedback scores compared to weak-SOC participants ($r = 0.10$ $p < 0.05$). Based on the results of moderating and mediating analyses, the investigators concluded that a strong SOC fosters behaviour (learning) via feedback, a conclusion in line with H6.

Discussion

The salutogenesis literature abounds with the finding that the SOC's strength is related significantly to a plethora of proximal (behaviours) and distal (disease, health and well-being) endpoints. Researchers' conclusions are almost all in the form of 'persons with a strong-SOC are better off than persons with a weak-SOC'. One implication is that interventions to strengthen the SOC are needed. This handbook includes several chapters that describe ways to strengthen the SOC.

Regrettably, there is a lack of thinking and research about how to shape stressor appraisal to foster better health, regardless of SOC strength. Because stressor appraisal is theorised as the most proximal factor connecting the SOC and behaviour, this chapter alerts salutogenesis researchers to the idea that stressor appraisal, and not just the SOC, should be in focus in our intervention research.

Antonovsky's main ideas about strong versus weak SOC and appraisal of stimuli are summarised in the six hypotheses discussed in this chapter. Though Antonovsky writes about strong and weak SOC, he presumes the reader understands this is shorthand for referring to the SOC continuum's poles. He also assumes that the reader understands the enormous importance of culture and context in accessing resources and the possibility of their activation. He cautions that few people have a very strong SOC (conversely, we should understand that few people have a very weak SOC). Finally, he has warned against any tendency to assume that a strong SOC is good in and of itself, noting that a Nazi may well have a strong SOC (Antonovsky, 1986).

With these caveats in the back of our minds, what may we conclude from the present literature analysis?

Regarding H1 – At the stage when stimuli are appraised as non-stressors or stressors, no evidence of the importance of the SOC was uncovered in my search. H1 remains speculative, and I think it must remain so. It seems infeasible to study one's daily bombardment of stimuli and connect one's SOC strength to judgements about which stimuli are stressors. How a researcher might trace and record all relevant stimuli during a respondent's daily life is a mystery. H1 is interesting but untestable.

Regarding H2 – at the stage when stimuli are appraised as stressors, no evidence was uncovered supporting H2 that strong-SOC persons will be more likely to define a stressor as benign or irrelevant, to feel confident that the tension will quickly dissipate. Indeed, after considering it extensively, Antonovsky concluded that primary appraisal is relatively unimportant to the subject of coping because even if a strong-SOC person is advantaged, life is filled with stressors that cannot be shrugged aside. We may conclude that H2 is perhaps testable, but not very interesting.

Regarding H3 – Antonovsky believed that the strong-SOC person is more likely to appraise a stressor as (a) happier, (b) less conflictful or (c) less dangerous than one with a weak SOC. I discovered no study intending to measure all three appraisal outcomes. But Brady's (2017) findings in the USA on challenge, hindrance and threat appraisal are consistent with the predictions of H3, and all three studies by Braun-Lewehsohn and her colleagues (2011, 2018, 2019) provide support for the danger dimension in H3.

So, there is some evidence supportive of H3, but only indirectly so. The measures used by Brady (2017) and Braun-Lewehsohn and colleagues (ibid) were not selected explicitly to test H3. But it may be that indirect tests are all that can be expected. Antonovsky's writings about pathways connecting the SOC and health-related behaviour have not aroused much interest in the research community, for reasons already discussed in the Introduction. This is as true for his writings underlying H4, H5 and H6 as for H3.

Regarding H4, I briefly summarise what was stated earlier in this chapter. No research relevant to a test of H4 was uncovered in a literature search conducted for this chapter. Besides needing data on available GRRs and SRRs and those used in the past to address stressors, a researcher would also need to make judgements about the most appropriate resource or combination of resources in each respondent's armamentarium that the respondent could have called on in the face of given stressors. It is hard to conceive a practical research methodology that would facilitate collecting the needed data. We must conclude that such studies are infeasible, or at last, too demanding to be worth the effort to investigate H4.

Regarding H5, there is more evidence relevant to this hypothesis alone than for all the other five hypotheses taken together. In studies from Australia, New Zealand, Chile, Poland, the Netherlands, Sweden and Hong Kong, the findings were consistent. Strong-SOC respondents faced with stressors were significantly more likely than weak-SOC respondents to engage in adaptive coping and were significantly less likely to engage in maladaptive coping. The issue of quite selective study samples deserves some discussion. The Australian, New Zealand and Chilean samples were oral health professionals (Gambetta-Tessini et al., 2016). The Polish samples were youth in probation centres (Konaszewski & Kwadrans, 2020) and the elderly and surgery patients (Krok, 2016; Kotowska & Weber-Nowakowska, 2019; Andruszkiewicz et al., 2017). The Dutch sample was composed of type 2 diabetes mellitus patients (Polhuis et al., 2020), the Swedish sample was elderly chronically ill patients (Kristofferzon et al., 2018) and the Hong Kong sample were composed of older women undergoing menopausal transition (Ngai, 2019).

What is needed, therefore, is research with *population-based samples* that crosscut society. Antonovsky was adamant that salutogenic processes were equally relevant in all persons regardless of age, sex, culture, societal position or the severity and acuteness of their stressor experiences. It is the 'universality' of salutogenesis that distinguishes the salutogenic model from the resilience model of coping:

> The special interest of resilience scholarship is to assist people living in particularly adverse conditions to do well. Adverse conditions in this sense are exemplified by the experience of poverty, unemployment, violence, crime, family breakdown, and substance abuse. In salutogenesis scholarship, extreme conditions like this cause deep consternation, but the main thrust of the theory is the notion that all people live in the rough and tough river of life from birth to death. (Mittelmark, 2021)

Finally, H6 has attracted little attention from salutogenesis researchers. It posits that through the experience of feedback, learning occurs, facilitating the acquisition of GRRs and SRRs, strengthening the SOC, which encourages adaptive coping, which in turn supports health-promoting behaviour. In other words, feedback processes are held by Antonovsky to be essential for salutogenic development. The research discussed earlier by Pijpker et al. (2018) shows that the study of feedback processes in salutogenesis is feasible. Two health promotion priorities seem evident for H6: research is needed on how people can be encouraged to *elicit* useful feedback, and research is called for on how they can be helped to *learn* from feedback.

Intervention research is needed with a focus on the tertiary stressor appraisal stage, to enhance feedback and learning processes that strengthen GRRS and fortify the SOC:

- *boost skill at eliciting and assessing feedback*
- *learn to be more attentive to signals about how one is coping*
- *improve judgement and skill on how and when to alter course*

A Role for Health Promotion

What is the role for health promotion, in the presence of an uncountable number of stress management programmes, advice columns in magazines and newspapers and best-selling books? Health promotion's role is *not* to add yet more to the plethora of advice on offer. Instead, can we not conduct and apply research on integrating adaptive stimulus and stressor appraisal skills into the home, neighbourhood, educational, work, worship and recreation settings? As many chapters in this handbook testify, it is feasible to integrate health promotion practice into community settings wherein health is not the primary concern, such as schools and workplaces. Therefore, the call here is for health promotion research and practice that fosters a strong-SOC pattern of stressor appraisal in communities *generally*. This is suggested as an adjunct to, and not a replacement for, SOC strengthening as discussed in other parts of this handbook.

Moving Forward

As mentioned in the Introduction, Antonovsky did not use the term 'hypothesis' in stating his predictions about how the SOC affects stimulus appraisal. Why are his predictions cast – by this author – as hypotheses? The aim is to elevate researchers' appreciation of *stimulus and stressor appraisal* as Antonovsky's little-tested answer to the questions posed at the beginning:

- How does the SOC concept link to coping behaviour?
- What are the mechanisms that make the connection?
- What is the black box between?

Antonovsky's absorbing proposals have been discussed in this chapter, and some empirical findings support his contentions. Yet, inevitably, I conclude as the reader might expect – more research is needed. Even more pointedly, salutogenesis researchers should increase their attention to stressor appraisal, action and reaction processes, both conscious and subconscious. We should develop, test and disseminate interventions to help people improve their capacity to engage in adaptive stressor appraisal, as we are all compelled to swim in the river of life – in its constant stream of challenges.

References

Aldwin, C. M., & Park, C. L. (2004). Coping and physical health outcomes: An overview. *Psychology & Health, 19*(3), 277–281.

Amirkhan, J. H., & Greaves, H. (2003). Sense of coherence and stress: The mechanics of a healthy disposition. *Psychology and Health, 18*(1), 31–62.

Andruszkiewicz, A., Basińska, M. A., Felsmann, M., Banaszkiewicz, M., Marzec, A., & Kędziora-Kornatowska, K. (2017). The determinants of coping with pain in chronically ill geriatric patients–the role of a sense of coherence. *Clinical Interventions in Aging, 12*, 315–323.

Antonovsky, A. (1979). *Health, stress, and coping*. Jossey-Bass.

Antonovsky, A. (1986). Intergenerational networks and transmitting the sense of coherence. In N. Datan, A. L. Green, & H. W. Reese (Eds.), *Life-span developmental psychology: Intergenerational relations* (pp. 211–222). Lawrence Erlbaum Associates.

Antonovsky, A. (1987). *Unraveling the mystery of health: How people manage stress and stay well*. Jossey-Bass.

Antonovsky, A. (1990a). Pathways leading to successful coping and health. In M. Rosenbaum (Ed.), *Learned resourcefulness: On coping skills, self-control, and adaptive behavior* (pp. 31–63). Springer Publishing.

Antonovsky, A. (1990b). Personality and health: Testing the sense of coherence model. *Personality and Disease, 7*, 155–177.

Antonovsky, A. (1990c). A somewhat personal odyssey in studying the stress process. *Stress Medicine, 6*(2), 71–80.

Antonovsky, A. (1992). Can attitudes contribute to health? *The Journal of Mind-Body Health, 8*(4), 33–49.

Antonovsky, A. (1993). The structure and properties of the sense of coherence scale. *Social Science & Medicine, 36*(6), 725–733.

Bauer, G. F., & Jenny, G. J. (2007). Development, implementation and dissemination of occupational health management (OHM): Putting salutogenesis into practice. In J. Houdmont & S. McIntyre (Eds.), *Occupational health psychology: European perspectives on research, education and practice* (pp. 219–250). ISMAI Publications.

Brady, L. L. (2017). *The role of sense of coherence in stressor appraisal*. The University of Tennessee at Chattanooga. https://doi.org/10.1037/e507482017-001; Corpus ID: 151688631.

Braun-Lewensohn, O., Sagy, S., & Roth, G. (2011). Coping strategies as mediators of the relationship between sense of coherence and stress reactions: Israeli adolescents under missile attacks. *Anxiety, Stress, & Coping, 24*(3), 327–341.

Braun-Lewensohn, O., & Al-Sayed, K. (2018). Syrian adolescent refugees: How do they cope during their stay in refugee camps? *Frontiers in Psychology, 9*, 1258. https://doi.org/10.3389/fpsyg.2018.01258

Braun-Lewensohn, O., Abu-Kaf, S., & Al-Said, K. (2019). Women in refugee camps: Which coping resources help them to adapt? *International Journal of Environmental Research and Public Health, 16*(20), 3990. https://doi.org/10.3390/ijerph16203990

Cavanaugh, M. A., Boswell, W. R., Roehling, M. V., & Boudreau, J. W. (2000). An empirical examination of self-reported stress among U.S. managers. *Journal of Applied Psychology, 85*, 65–74.

Cheng, C., & Cheung, M. W. (2005). Cognitive processes underlying coping flexibility: Differentiation and integration. *Journal of Personality, 73*(4), 859–886.

Eriksson, M., & Lindström, B. (2006). Antonovsky's Sense of Coherence Scale and the relation with health: A systematic review. *Journal of Epidemiology & Community Health, 60*(5), 376–381.

Eriksson, M., & Lindström, B. (2007). Antonovsky's sense of coherence scale and its relation with quality of life – A systematic review. *Journal of Epidemiology and Community Health, 61*(11), 938–944.

Feldman, P. J., Cohen, S., Hamrick, N., & Lepore, S. J. (2004). Psychological stress, appraisal, emotion and cardiovascular response in a public speaking task. *Psychology & Health, 19*(3), 353–368.

Gambetta-Tessini, K., Mariño, R., Morgan, M., & Anderson, V. (2016). Coping strategies and the salutogenic model in future oral health professionals. *BMC Medical Education, 16*(1), 1–8.

Konaszewski, K., Kolemba, M., & Niesiobędzka, M. (2019). Resilience, sense of coherence and self-efficacy as predictors of stress coping style among university students. *Current Psychology*. https://doi.org/10.1007/s12144-019-00363-1

Konaszewski, K., & Kwadrans, Ł. (2020). Sense of coherence and resilience for coping with stress in the group of juveniles referred to probation centres by family courts. *Kwartalnik Pedagogiczny, 1*(255), 134–159.

Kotowska, J., & Weber-Nowakowska, K. (2019). Sense of coherence, its meaning and coping with stress among people after orthopedic surgery. *Journal of Education, Health and Sport, 9*(4), 459–467.

Kristofferzon, M. L., Engström, M., & Nilsson, A. (2018). Coping mediates the relationship between sense of coherence and mental quality of life in patients with chronic illness: A cross-sectional study. *Quality of Life Research, 27*(7), 1855–1863.

Krok, D. (2016). Sense of coherence mediates the relationship between the religious meaning system and coping styles in Polish older adults. *Aging & Mental Health, 20*(10), 1002–1009.

Lazarus, R. S., & Cohen, J. B. (1977). Environmental stress. In I. Altman & J. E. Wohlwill (Eds.), *Human behavior and environment* (Vol. 2). Plenum.

Lazarus, R. S. (1984). Puzzles in the study of daily hassles. *Journal of Behavioral Medicine, 7*, 375–389.

Lazarus, R. S., & Folkman, S. (1984). *Stress, appraisal, and coping*. Springer.

Mittelmark, M. B., Sagy, S., Eriksson, M., Bauer, G. F., Pelikan, J. M., Lindström, B., & Arild Espnes, G. (2017). *The Handbook of Salutogenesis*. Springer Nature. E-book, open access.

Mittelmark, M. B. (2021). Resilience in the salutogenic model of health. In M. Ungar (Ed.), *Multisystemic resilience*. Oxford University Press. https://doi.org/10.1093/oso/9780190095888.003.0009

Ngai, F. W. (2019). Relationships between menopausal symptoms, sense of coherence, coping strategies, and quality of life. *Journal of the North American Menopause Society, 26*(7), 758–764.

Pijpker, R., Vaandrager, L., Bakker, E. J., & Koelen, M. (2018). Unravelling salutogenic mechanisms in the workplace: The role of learning. *Gaceta Sanitaria, 32*, 275–282.

Polhuis, C. M. M., Vaandrager, L., Soedamah-Muthu, S. S., & Koelen, M. A. (2020). Salutogenic model of health to identify turning points and coping styles for eating practices in type 2 diabetes mellitus. *International Journal for Equity in Health, 19*, 1–20.

Scherer, K. R., Schorr, A., & Johnstone, T. (2001). *Appraisal processes in emotion*. Oxford University Press.

Searle, B. J., & Auton, J. C. (2015). The merits of measuring challenge and hindrance appraisals. *Anxiety, Stress, and Coping, 28*(2), 121–143.

Sideridis, G. D. (2006). Coping is not an 'either' 'or': The interaction of coping strategies in regulating affect, arousal and performance. *Stress and Health, 22*(5), 315–327.

Silverstein, M., & Heap, J. (2015). Sense of coherence changes with aging over the second half of life. *Advances in Life Course Research, 23*, 98–107.

Super, S., Wagemakers, M. A. E., Picavet, H. S. J., Verkooijen, K. T., & Koelen, M. A. (2016). Strengthening sense of coherence: Opportunities for theory building in health promotion. *Health Promotion International, 31*(4), 869–878.

Tuckey, M. R., Searle, B. J., Boyd, C. M., Winefield, A. H., & Winefield, H. R. (2015). Hindrances are not threats: Advancing the multidimensionality of work stress. *Journal of Occupational Health Psychology, 20*(2), 131–147.

Wechkunanukul, K., Grantham, H., & Clark, R. A. (2017). Global review of delay time in seeking medical care for chest pain: An integrative literature review. *Australian Critical Care, 30*(1), 13–20.

Weiner, B. (2010). The development of an attribution-based theory of motivation: A history of ideas. *Educational Psychologist, 45*, 28–36.

11

Challenges of Measurement in SOC

Monica Eriksson and Paolo Contu

Introduction

Antonovsky (1987) developed a questionnaire to measure the sense of coherence. The original form, the Orientation to Life Questionnaire, consists of 29 items, 11 items measuring comprehensibility, 10 items measuring manageability, and 8 items measuring meaningfulness. The response alternatives are a semantic scale of 1 point to 7 points, where 1 and 7 indicate extreme feelings about questions (and statements) about how one's life is experienced (e.g., the question "when you talk to people, do you have the feeling that they do not understand you?" is scored from 1 = never have this feeling to 7 = always have this feeling). The questionnaire is a summed index with a total score ranging from 29 to 203 points for the original scale of 29 questions (SOC-29). A shorter version of 13 questions (SOC-13) of the original form was developed by Antonovsky (1987), where the score ranges between 13 and 91 points. Antonovsky intended that the sense of coherence scales be scored with a single total score and not component scores (Fig. 11.1) since he theorized that it was the sense of coherence in its totality that influenced movement along the ease/dis-ease continuum. This issue is taken up again later in this chapter.

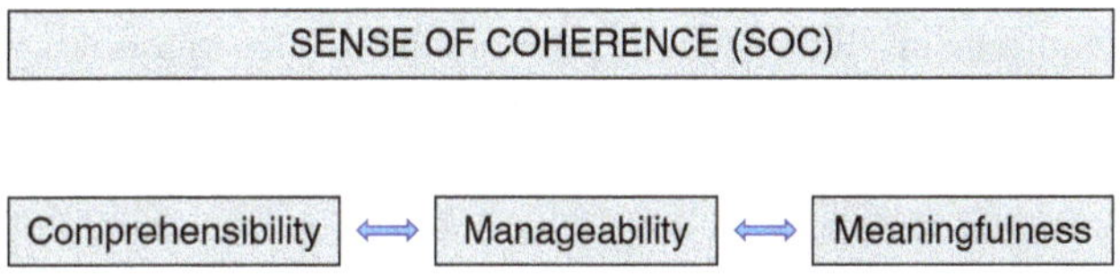

Fig. 11.1 The original view of the sense of coherence and its three dimensions

Examples of items measuring the comprehensibility dimension are as follows (Antonovsky, 1987, p. 190ff.):

- When you talk to people, do you have a feeling that they don't understand you? (from 'never have this feeling' to 'always have this feeling')
- Do you have a feeling that you are in an unfamiliar situation and don't know what to do? (from 'very often' to 'very seldom or never')

The following items are examples that measure manageability:

- When something unpleasant happened in the past your tendency was: (from 'to eat yourself up about it' to 'to say "ok that's that, I have to live with it" and go on')
- When you do something that gives you a good feeling: (from 'it's certain that you'll go on feeling good' to 'it's certain that something will happen to spoil the feeling')

Meaningfulness is measured with items like these:

- Doing the things you do every day is: (from 'a source of deep pleasure and satisfaction' to 'a source of pain and boredom')
- When you think about your life, you very often: (from 'feel how good it is to be alive' to 'ask yourself why you exist at all')

M. Eriksson (✉)
Department of Health Sciences, Section of Health Promotion and Care Sciences, Center on Salutogenesis, University West, Trollhättan, Sweden
e-mail: monica.eriksson@hv.se

P. Contu
Department of Medical Sciences and Public Health, University of Cagliari, Cittadella Universitaria, Monserrato-Cagliari, Italy

Comprehensibility, the cognitive dimension, refers to the extent to which one perceives internal and external stimuli as rationally understandable, and as information that is orderly, coherent, clear, structured rather than noise—that is, chaotic, disordered, random, unexpected, and unexplained (Antonovsky, 1987, p. 17). The ability to create structure out of chaos makes it easier for us to understand one's context and one's part in it, for example, one's role in the family or the workplace. A prerequisite to being able to cope with a stressful situation is that one can, to some extent, understand it. What one comprehends is easier to manage.

Manageability, the instrumental or behavioral dimension, defined as the degree to which one feels that there are resources at one's disposal that can be used to meet the requirements of the stimuli one is bombarded by Antonovsky (1987, p. 17). Formal resources include, for example, social services and care staff in public and private organizations. Informal resources include, for example, family, a circle of friends, colleagues, and significant others, in other words, people who are trusted and who can be relied on difficult situations. Coping also requires that one is motivated to solve the problems that cause stress, is willing to invest energy to solve the problem, and finds meaning in being able to manage the situation. This leads to the third dimension of the sense of coherence, meaningfulness.

Meaningfulness, the motivational dimension, refers to the extent to which one feels that life has emotional meaning, that at least some of the problems faced in life a face are worth commitment and dedication, and are seen as challenges rather than only as burdens (Antonovsky, 1987, p. 18). One needs to have a clear desire to resolve difficulties and willingness to invest energy to get through experiences of stress that have the potential to cause distress.

The Validity and Reliability of the Sense of Coherence

Face validity: The sense of coherence scales has been empirically tested in different cultures, both Western and cultures in Africa and Asia. Studies have been conducted on different samples: general populations, different professions, in persons with disabilities, different patient groups as well as in children, adolescents, adults, and elderly, in families, in organizations, and also on a societal level. A systematic research review shows that as of 2003, the SOC-29 and SOC-13 had been used in at least 33 different languages in 32 different countries (Eriksson & Lindström, 2005). An update shows that another 16 languages can be added: Albanian (Roth & Ekblad, 2006), Croatian (Singer & Brähler, 2007), Brazilian (Bonanato et al., 2009), Hungarian (Biro et al., 2010), Korean (Han et al., 2007), Lingala (Bantu language spoken in parts of Africa) (Pham et al., 2010), Persian, Swahili (Rohani et al., 2010) as well as local languages in Africa Afar, Bilein, Hidareb, Kunama people, Nara, Saho, Tigre, and Tigrinya (Almedom et al., 2007; Getnet & Alem, 2019). An update per 2019 at least additional languages can be found: Portuguese (Encarnação et al., 2018) and Slovenia (Stern et al., 2019).

Since 2003, the SOC-29 and the SOC-13 have been used in further 13 countries (Eriksson, 2014): Eritrea (Almedom et al., 2007), Croatia (Pavicic Bosnjak et al., 2012), Hungary (Biro et al., 2010), India (Suraj & Singh, 2011), Iran (Rohani et al., 2010), Italy (Sardu et al., 2012; Ciairano et al., 2010), Korea (Han et al., 2007), Kosovo, the Democratic Republic of Congo (Pham et al., 2010), Spain (Virues-Ortéga et al., 2007), Sudan (Abdelgadir et al., 2009), Taiwan (Tang & Li, 2008), and Turkey (Öztekin & Tezer, 2009). More recent research shows three additional countries: Austria (Mautner et al., 2014), Estonia (Höjdahl et al., 2015), and Malaysia (Rostami et al., 2014). An update per 2019 shows further expansion: Ethiopia (Getnet & Alem, 2019), Ireland (Groarke et al., 2018), Portugal (Encarnação et al., 2018), and Slovenia (Stern et al., 2019).

In sum, the SOC questionnaires have been used in at least 51 different languages in at least 51 different countries around the world (Fig. 11.2).

The translation process: As shown above, SOC-13 has been translated and used in many countries and different populations. Translation of scales and questionnaires requires explicit attention since translation may influence validity (Naaldenberg et al., 2011). According to Fawcett (1997) and the Curitiba Statement on Health Promotion (Sotgiu et al., 2018), several translation techniques have to be used: calque, literal translation, transposition, modulation, reformulation, and adaptation. Transposition means rearranging a sentence's word sequence in order to satisfy grammatical rules; modulation is replacing original phrases with a set phrase, which has the same significance; reformulation is to express the same concept in a completely different manner; and, finally, adaption explains a concept in the source and target languages in a completely unique way, so it is appropriate to the culture of the recipients.

A critical term is the word "feelings." In English, the word "feeling" means both "something that you feel through the mind or the senses like hunger, sadness" and "the emotions of a person." A problem arose in the process of translation of SOC-13 from English to Italian. In Italian, two

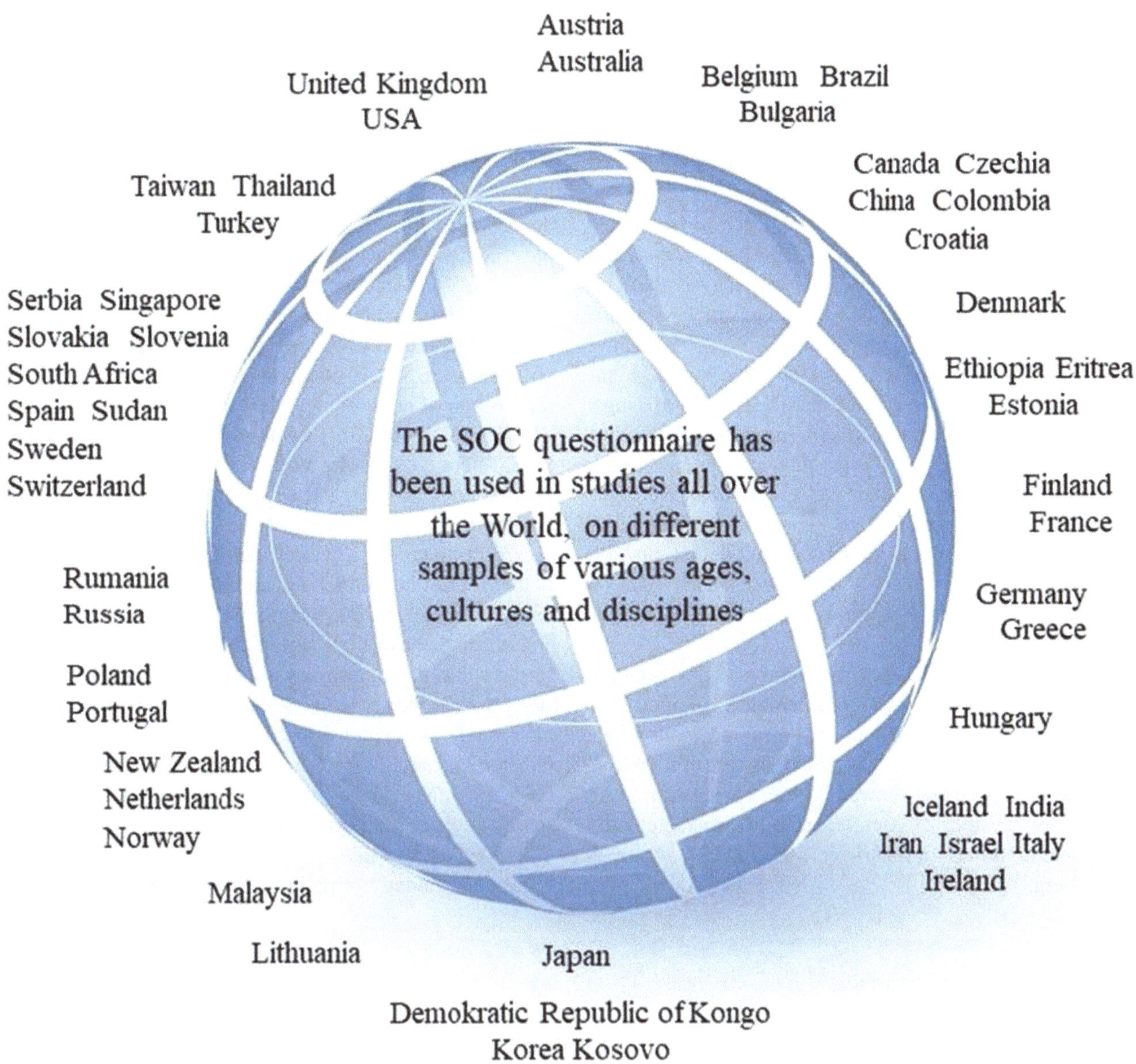

Fig. 11.2 The distribution of studies using the sense of coherence scale 1992–2019 in a global context © Monica Eriksson 2017. (All Rights Reserved)

concepts are expressed, respectively, with the words "sensazione" and "emozione."

The translation of the question, "Many people – those with even a strong character – sometimes feel like sad sacks (losers) in certain situations. How often have you felt this way in the past?," revealed a minor difficulty of idiomatic equivalence. In the Italian version, it was necessary to eliminate the idiom "sad sacks" for which there is no corresponding expression. The significance of the question is still guaranteed by the translation of the word "losers."

Construct validity: The structure of the sense of coherence is complex. Recent research shows that the sense of coherence seems to be a multidimensional construct rather than a unidimensional as proposed by Antonovsky (1987), with all three dimensions continually interacting with each other and together to form a collective, overarching factor, sense of coherence. Following that, Antonovsky maintained that on theoretical grounds, one should avoid lifting out individual dimensions in order to examine them separately.

Nevertheless, recent research has focused on the study of the structure and content of the sense of coherence. There are studies that support Antonovsky's idea of the sense of coherence as a general factor with three dimensions (Antonovsky, 1993; Drageset & Haugan, 2015; Klepp et al., 2007; Rajesh et al., 2015; Söderhamn & Holmgren, 2004; Söderhamn et al., 2015; Spadoti Dantas et al., 2014), but these dimensions do not fully fit with comprehensibility, manageability, and meaningfulness. Söderhamn et al. (2015) found evidence in a confirmatory factor analysis that confirmed the SOC-29 as one theoretical construct with three dimensions, comprehensibility, manageability, and meaningfulness. In a cross-sectional survey among Norwegian cognitively intact nursing home residents, Drageset and Haugan (2015) found that the three-factor model fit their data. Lajunen (2019) examined the psychometric properties and the cross-cultural impact of the SOC-13 questionnaire among Australian, Finnish, and Turkish young adults. The findings from all the three countries suggested that the first- and second-order three-factor models fit the data better than the single-factor model. Nor cultural differences in SOC scale scores were found.

Other models obtained with factorial analysis, although three-dimensional and with considerable explained variance, are not related to the traditional dimensions of the SOC. This is in agreement with previous research on SOC factorial dimension that showed different results not fitting with the dimensions of comprehensibility, manageability, and meaningfulness (Togari et al., 2008; Larsson & Kallenberg, 1999).

A high correlation between item "Has it happened in the past that you were surprised by the behavior of people whom you thought you knew well?" and item "Has it happened that people whom you counted on disappointed you?" has been found in several studies (Naaldenberg et al., 2011; Sardu et al., 2012), and was explained by interviewees perceiving these questions as similar. Drageset and Haugan (2015) defined this correlation as "especially troublesome": the people whom we know well usually also embody the ones we trust or rely on, which is a central focus in OLQ3; you are not supposed to be disappointed by people you trust. Therefore, it seems theoretically reasonable that OLQ2 and OLQ3 share error variance. Nevertheless, including correlated error terms for this pair of items did not yield a good fit with the present data. Lerdal et al. (2017) found psychometric limitations of the 13-item SOC scale using Rasch analysis. Two items demonstrated poor fit, and once they were deleted from the scale, the remaining 11-item scale (SOC-11) demonstrated acceptable item fit. However, neither the SOC-13 nor the SOC-11 met the criteria for unidimensionality or person-response validity. While both the SOC-13 and SOC-11 were able to distinguish three groups of SOC, none of the subscales could distinguish any such groups. Recent research suggests that the sense of coherence seems to be a multidimensional concept consisting of many different dimensions rather than a single factor (Eriksson & Lindström, 2005; Feldt, 2007; Naaldenberg et al., 2011). Figure 11.3 shows the sense of coherence as a multidimensional construct.

Sandell et al. (1998) examined the sense of coherence instrument among a sample of Swedes and could not find

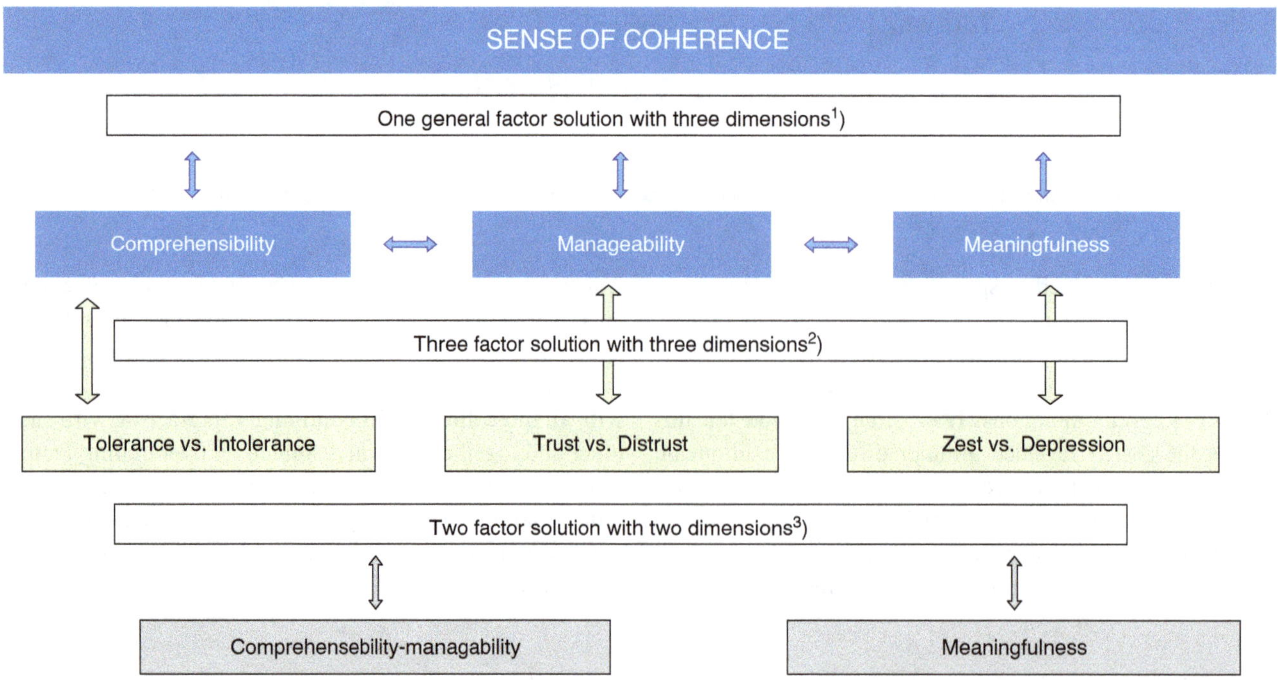

Fig. 11.3 The sense of coherence as a multidimensional construct. (1) Antonovsky, 1987, (2) Sandell et al., 1998, (3) Sakano & Yajima, 2005

support for a common factor, nor the three dimensions of comprehensibility, manageability, and meaningfulness. Three more or less stable dimensions emerged, where lust and depression were two extremes which could best be referred to the dimension of meaningfulness. Antonovsky's concept comprehensibility could in this study be seen in the form of tolerance versus intolerance. The third factor, manageability, was reflected by trust and distrust (Sandell et al., 1998, p. 701).

In the model reported by Larsson and Kallenberg (1999) in Sweden, the first factor appears to measure mainly anxiety and inner tension, although they partly also reflect one's ability to manage these emotions, the second factor covers comprehension regarding social perception, and the third factor appears to measure sense of personal meaningfulness and satisfaction. Also in the Sardinian general population, the model obtained with factorial analysis, although three-dimensional and with considerable explained variance, is not related to the traditional dimensions of SOC represented in more than one factor (Sardu et al., 2012. The same model was substantially confirmed in samples of students and persons affected by chronic diseases.

Although a clear structure based on the three components was never obtained, three more or less stable dimensions emerged in most of the studies that have explored SOC-13 dimensions. The main factor normally involves most of the questions related to Antonovsky's comprehensibility component (items 6, 8, 9,11) but also items related to manageability (13 and sometimes 5). The Antonovsky's meaningfulness component (items 12, 1, 4, 7) is mainly represented in the second factor but also shows relevant correlations with the first one (in Sardinia all these items are combined with comprehensibility in the first factor). In the Sardinian study, question 10 (manageability dimension) does not show a stable pattern (Sardu et al., 2012). So one factor identified the comprehensibility component, and a second factor correlated very strongly with meaningfulness. The third factor was related to questions B and C that, as previously discussed, are part of different dimensions, yet are strongly correlated.

On the basis of the present findings, one may conclude that the factorial structure of the SOCS is sufficiently stable across different samples, although the emerging factors are not related to the traditional Antonovsky's dimensions of SOC. Sandell et al. (1998) conclude that these patterns are clouded by the fact that the items are indeed not "cleanly" referring to one or the other component, as Antonovsky endeavored (Table 11.1).

Consensual validity is a term that indicates the extent to which various scientists agree on the properties of an instrument (Cooper, 1998). The consensual validity is somewhat weak. While many researchers use either the SOC-29 or the SOC-13, there are also many different modified versions in use, with different numbers of questions and different possibilities of response options. Most of the modified versions have partially abandoned the original scale of 1–7 points (but the wording of the questions is usually the same as in the SOC-29 and SOC-13). Results from a research review 1992–2003 showed that there were at least 15 different modified forms consisting of only 3 questions to 28 questions (Eriksson & Lindström, 2005). This includes the particular version adapted for families (FSOC) (Antonovsky & Sourani, 1988; Sagy & Antonovsky, 1992), for children (Margalit & Efrati, 1996), and a version for a school context (Nash, 2002). The Children's Orientation to Life Scale consists of 16 questions plus 3 distracters (Idan & Margalit, 2014; Margalit & Efrati, 1996). The response options follow a scale of 1–4, where 4 indicates the highest degree of sense of coherence. There are also two variants of the FSOC, the original with 26 questions and a shorter version with 12 questions (Antonovsky & Sourani, 1988; Sagy, 2008; Sagy & Antonovsky, 1992). The questions are the same as in the original form but tailored to the child or a family context. Table 11.2 provides a summary of some of the other sense of coherence scales in the literature, demonstrating a range of items from 3 to 16, and intended for use by various sociodemographic groups.

Antonovsky (1979) originally described the sense of coherence as an individual property. He later widened the perspective (Antonovsky, 1987) with sense of coherence also conceived at the family level. Recent research shows that the sense of coherence concept and measurement also can be applied in organizations such as a workplace (Bauer & Jenny, 2012; Bringsén, 2010; Bringsén et al., 2009; Forbech & Hanson, 2013; Graeser, 2011; Mayer & Krause, 2011; Mayer & Boness, 2011; Nilsson et al., 2012; Orvik & Axelsson, 2012; Vogt et al., 2013).

Research that examines and discusses salutogenesis and the sense of coherence at a societal level is sparse. Braun-Lewensohn and Sagy (2011) report findings from studies using an instrument adapted for the societal sense of coherence (Sense of Community Coherence), which contains seven questions describing how the individual experiences the society in terms of comprehensibility, manageability, and meaningfulness. Comprehensibility at the societal level addresses the experience of society as more or less organized in a way that makes life somewhat predictable, that the structure of society can be more or less understood, and that society is perceived as more or less safe and secure. Manageability is a state in which the individual experiences a society with resources that support individuals, for example, in emergencies or critical situations. Societal support includes, for example, programs to support young people's mental health and initiatives to create conditions so that people from different generations can meet each other. Meaningfulness refers to the experience that society supports people to experience

Table 11.1 Factorial structure (factor loadings) in a number of European populations

		General population 1			University students 2			High school students 2			University hospital 2			General population 3			Non-institutionalized people (>64) 4						General population 5		
		Sardinia-Italy			Sardinia-Italy			Sardinia-Italy			Sardinia-Italy			Romania			Netherlands			Netherlands (11 items)			Sweden		
Question		1	2	3	1	2	3	1	3	2	1	3	2	1	2	3	1	3	2	1	3	2	1	3	2
F	C	**0.69**	0.03	0.06	**0.64**	0.15	0.08	**0.65**	0.08	−0.02	**0.70**	−0.11	0.11	**0.48**	**0.43**	0.14	**0.51**	0.16		**0.46**	0.12	0.17	**0.42**	**0.24**	
H	C	**0.69**	**0.34**	0.03	**0.67**	**0.39**	−0.05	**0.75**	−0.01	0.05	**0.72**	0.16	−0.11	**0.77**	0.16	0.33	**0.82**			**0.85**			**0.76**		
I	C	**0.64**	0.19	0.19	**0.68**	0.21	0.20	**0.78**	−0.18	0.19	**0.68**	0.28	0.02	**0.76**	0.18	0.32	**0.79**			**0.71**		0.10	**0.76**		
K	C	**0.51**	−0.07	−0.05	**0.65**	−0.11	0.02	**0.48**	−0.45	−0.05	**0.48**	−0.20	0.05	**0.62**	0.12	−0.10	**0.26**	**0.33**		**0.28**	**0.27**		**0.28**		
M	MA	**0.67**	0.26	−0.02	**0.67**	0.31	0.06	**0.72**	−0.09	0.16	**0.70**	0.17	0.17	**0.66**	0.29	0.04	**0.63**	0.18		**0.62**	0.21		**0.66**		
E	MA	**0.62**	−0.19	**0.25**	**0.38**	0.22	**0.21**	**0.55**	0.04	0.15	**0.57**	−0.13	**0.34**	0.15	**0.48**	**0.46**	**0.29**	0.10	0.20	0.16		**0.37**	**0.34**	**0.32**	
J	MA	**0.47**	**0.31**	0.20	**0.40**	**0.37**	0.11	**0.53**	0.14	**0.46**	**0.47**	0.17	**0.37**	**0.37**	**0.47**	0.30	**0.36**		**0.30**	**0.14**		**0.58**	**0.28**		0.23
L	ME	**0.60**	**0.43**	−0.11	**0.53**	**0.51**	−0.05	**0.74**	0.14	−0.06	**0.74**	0.14	−0.01	**0.37**	**0.63**	0.10	0.11	**0.70**		0.17	**0.73**		**0.39**	**0.39**	
A	ME	**0.58**	−0.17	−0.05	−0.02	**0.69**	0.25	0.21	**0.77**	0.16	0.18	**0.80**	0.17	−0.02	**0.63**	0.13		**0.41**			**0.41**		0.05	**0.26**	0.22
D	ME	**0.30**	**0.72**	0.12	**0.62**	0.02	−0.01	**0.60**	0.27	−0.14	**0.68**	−0.09	−0.14	**0.32**	**0.59**	−0.05	0.13	**0.35**	−0.22				0.10	**0.58**	
G	ME	**0.31**	**0.71**	−0.02	*0.19*	**0.75**	−0.06	**0.43**	**0.55**	0.07	**0.47**	**0.57**	−0.02	*0.23*	**0.69**	0.04	*0.14*	**0.41**		*0.12*	**0.37**	0.13	*0.15*	**0.38**	
B	C	0.16	0.04	**0.86**	0.05	0.05	**0.90**	0.25	0.06	**0.79**	0.17	0.13	**0.85**	0.18	−0.05	**0.83**			**0.75**						**0.76**
C	MA	0.27	0.06	**0.83**	0.11	0.08	**0.89**	0.37	0.13	**0.76**	0.22	0.00	**0.85**	0.18	−0.05	**0.84**			**0.88**	-0.15		**0.67**			**0.71**

References: (1) Sardu et al., 2012; (2) Data from Cagliari University; (3) Vasiliu et al., 2015; (4) Naaldenberg et al., 2011; (5) Larsson & Kallenberg, 1999

Table 11.2 A selection of different versions of the sense of coherence instrument

Authors	Country	Sample	N	Number of items	Response options	Cronbach's alpha
Agardh et al. (2003)	Sweden	Healthy middle-aged women	4821	SOC-3	3	
Schumann et al. (2003)	Germany	General population	3515	SOC-3 BASOC Brief Assessment—SOC	3	0.45
Bayard-Burfield et al. (2001)	Sweden	Immigrants/refugees Swedes	4981	SOC-3	7 - Likert	
Kivimäki et al. (2002)	Finland	Women employed in municipalities	433	SOC-6	7 - Likert	0.76
Toft Würtz et al. (2015)	Denmark	Pupils	773	SOC-7	7 - Likert	0.77
Forsgärde et al. (2000)	Sweden	Health professional	354	SOC-9	3 - Likert	0.60–0.69
Klepp et al. (2007)	Norway	Adults	1062	SOC-9	7 - Likert	0.79
Li et al. (2014)	China	Patients in hospitals	491	SOC-9	7 - Likert	
Mayer and Thiel (2014)	Germany	Elite sports	698	SOC-L9Leipzig Short Scale	2	0.82
Naaldenberg et al. (2011)	Netherlands	Elderly people ≥ 65	1361	SOC-11	7 - Likert	
Kanhai et al. (2014)	Finland	Adults	848	SOC-12	7 - Likert	0.85
Sagy (1998)	Israel	School children and their parents	399	SOC-12Family-SOC	7 - Likert	0.81
Margalit & Efrati (1996)	Israel	Children with learning disabilities	324	SOC-16 + 3Childrens'-SOC	7 - Likert	0.72
Suominen et al. (1999)	Finland	General population	3115	SOC-16	4 - Likert	0.84
Sagy and Antonovsky (1992)	Israel	Retirees and their relatives	214	SOC-26Family-SOC	7 - Likert	0.88

fulfillment, to develop their abilities, and to feel satisfied with life (Braun-Lewensohn & Sagy, 2011, p. 535).

The relevance of salutogenesis and the sense of coherence to the building of healthy public policy has also been a focus of theorizing and research (Eriksson et al., 2007; Lindström & Eriksson, 2009). To develop a social policy based on the salutogenic framework means to identify resources for health and welfare of the society, in the past as well as in the present, including risks of illnesses, and how this knowledge and the most effective measures can be used to resolve the current challenges. The core of such policy is to create coherence and synergies, from individuals to groups and organizations in the local community, and finally to the whole of society (Eriksson & Lindström, 2014; Lindström & Eriksson, 2009).

Criterion validity: Eriksson and Lindström (2005) present information about the relation between the SOC-29 and other instruments measuring health, perceived self, stressors, quality of life, well-being, attitudes, and behaviors. The correlation with health ranges in general from slight to good, using instruments such as the General Health Questionnaire, the Health Index, the Hopkin's Symptom Checklist, and the Mental Health Inventory, with such health measures explaining up to 66% of the variance in the SOC-29. There seems to be an overlap between the sense of coherence and the Big Five (Kase et al., 2018). Neuroticism was here negatively correlated, and extraversion was positively correlated with comprehensibility (r –0.47, 0.35), manageability (r –0.44, 0.26), and meaningfulness (r –0.28, 0.30). These correlations were strong, and the overlap between the two scales was about 36 percent. Also, there are a number of studies on the relation between SOC and quality of life and well-being. In general, they show that a high SOC is related to a high quality of life Eriksson and Lindström (2005).

Predictive validity: The ability of an instrument to predict how, for example, health develops in the future is called predictive validity (Abramson & Abramson, 1999). The predictive validity of the sense of coherence questionnaire seems to be relatively good, based on a review of longitudinal studies (Eriksson & Lindström, 2005). There are studies that support predictive ability (Lundman et al., 2010; Luutonen et al., 2011; Poppius et al., 2006; Surtees et al., 2003), whereas other studies have not done so (Norekvål et al., 2010). It seems that the time for follow-up is an important factor for the predictive ability of the instrument. The results of a study among elderly persons, the Umeå 85+ study, show that the sense of coherence predicted mortality at 1-year follow-up, but not at follow-up after 4 years (Lundman et al., 2010).

Reliability: SOC-29 test–retest correlations range from 0.69 to 0.78 (1 year), 0.64 (3 years), 0:42 to 00:45 (4 years), 0:59 to 0.67 (5 years), and finally 0:54 after the 10-year follow-up (Eriksson & Lindström, 2005). More recent research provides support for the stability over time, in 1- to 3-year perspective (Lindblad, Sandelin, Petersson et al., 2016). The *internal consistency* measured by Cronbach's alpha ranges from 0.70 to 0.95 using SOC-29 (124 studies) and 0.70 to 0.92 (127 studies) using SOC-13 (Eriksson & Lindström, 2005, p. 463). The sense of coherence scale shows high internal consistency overall. However, there are other results reported. Among Swedish nurses working at hospitals, the internal consistency, measured by Cronbach's alpha, was as low as 0.63 (Eriksson et al., 2019). An inter-item-correlation test indicated that item 5 "Do you have the feeling that you're being treated unfairly?" and item 6 "Do you have the feeling that you are in an unfamiliar situation and don't know what to do?" decreased the internal consistency.

Critique of the SOC-29 and SOC-13

One indirect form of criticism has practical roots: as mentioned earlier, various senses of coherence measures have been developed that are shorter than even the SOC-13, as short as just three items. This reflects the reality that in many health survey applications, questionnaires must be very short. More directly, the SOC-29 and SOC-13 have been criticized based on supposed shortcomings in the instruments' psychometric properties (Korotkov, 1993; Larsson & Kallenberg, 1999; Schnyder et al., 2000). It is also asserted that the sense of coherence concept does not deal adequately with emotional aspects of life experience (Flannery & Flannery, 1990; Flensborg-Madsen et al., 2006c; Korotkov, 1993; Korotkov & Hannah, 1994). Inconsistent evidence about the lability/stability of the sense of coherence over the life course has also been noted by critics (Geyer, 1997). Criticism of salutogenesis generally includes implicit doubt about efforts to measure the sense of coherence via any means (Bengel et al., 1999; Kumlin, 1998). The leveling of such criticism is welcome as part of the healthy evolution of a "living" theory or model, and responses to the critics are published (Eriksson, 2007; Lindström & Eriksson, 2010).

In the limits of this chapter, we focus on just the critical ideas of Flensborg-Madsen et al. (2005a). The critique stems from their conclusion that the SOC-29 and SOC-13 are only moderately to weakly related to various measures of physical health (Flensborg-Madsen et al., 2005a), leading them to construct and test a new measure of the sense of coherence, intended to overcome limitations in the SOC-29 and SOC-13 (Flensborg-Madsen et al., 2006a, 2006b). Their critique can be summarized in this way:

- Antonovsky presumed that one's internal and external environment has to be predictable in order for a person to have a high sense of coherence.
- Predictability should not be included in conceptualizing and measuring the sense of coherence, because lack of predictability is not necessarily unhealthy.
- Instead, unpredictability is what makes life matter in the first place; it can provide a state of initiative, energy, and positive attitudes.

Since the SOC-29 includes several items that have to do with predictability, Flensborg-Madsen et al. (2005b) regard the instrument as flawed and they developed an alternative 9-item measure that excluded the concept of predictability, but that otherwise was purportedly built, as they write, on the same idea, theory, and conceptualization used by Antonovsky (Flensborg-Madsen et al., 2006a, 2006b).

Their conclusion about a weak association between the SOC-29 and SOC-13 and physical health is based on a review of about 50 studies (2005a). They categorize the health instruments in the reviewed studies as having foci on physical health, biological measures, psychological measures, health measures incorporating psychological aspects, stress, and behavioral aspects. They conclude that the SOC scales are unable to explain health that is measured only in physical terms (Flensborg-Madsen et al., 2005a, p. 665). As a solution, Flensborg-Madsen et al. (2006c) propose the concept of "emotional coherence" in relation to physical health and "mental coherence" in relation to psychological health. This is supported by Endler et al. (2008).

Such fragmentation of the concept of the sense of coherence into physical and mental components breaks significantly from Antonovsky's fundamental notion of an "orientation to life" (1979, 1987). Such fragmentation also reinforces the physical health/mental health divide in modern health care (and in the public's imagination), which has been challenged vigorously (WHO, 2001).

We move on to the issue of excluding predictability in the sense of coherence measurement; to do so is to depart emphatically from "the same idea, theory and conceptualization" used by Antonovsky, who wrote:

> From the time of birth, or even earlier, we constantly go through situations of challenge and response, stress, tension, and resolution. The more these experiences are characterized by consistency, participation in shaping outcome, and an underload-overload balance of stimuli, the more we begin to see the world as being coherent and predictable. When, however, one's experiences all tend to be predictable, one is inevitably due for unpleasant surprises that cannot be handled, and one's sense of coherence is weakened accordingly. Paradoxically, then, a measure of unpredictable experiences-which call forth hitherto unknown resources—is essential for a strong sense of coherence. One then learns to expect some measure of the unexpected. When there is little or no predictability, there is not much one can do except seek to hide until the storm (of life) is over, hoping not to be noticed. Or else one strikes out blindly and at random until exhaustion sets in. No defense mechanisms can be adequate. We must note an implicit assumption here. If a strong sense of coherence is to develop, one's experiences must be not only by and large predictable but also by and large rewarding, yet with some measure of frustration and punishment. (Antonovsky, 1979, p. 187)

As this extended passage makes clear, reasonable predictability functions inextricably with many other aspects of experience to shape the sense of coherence.

Sense of Coherence Develops Over Time

According to Antonovsky (1987), sense of coherence develops until the age of about 30 years. After that, the sense of coherence was estimated to remain relatively stable until retirement, after which a decrease was expected. This assumption finds no support in subsequent empirical research. The sense of coherence seems to be relatively stable over time, but not as stable as Antonovsky assumed. Research shows that sense of coherence develops over the entire life cycle and increases with age (Feldt, Lintula, et al., 2007; Feldt, Metsäpelto, et al., 2007; Nilsson et al., 2010). Nilsson and co-authors were able to demonstrate on a sample of 43,500 Swedish respondents, aged 18–85 years, that sense of coherence increases with age in both men and women. Support for a corresponding development of the sense of coherence over time could also be seen in a longitudinal study of more than 18,000 Finns, in the Health and Social Support Study, where the sense of coherence continuously increased with age. A strong sense of coherence initially appears to determine its development over time (Feldt et al., 2011). There is a lack of longitudinal studies with long-term follow-up. The most extended follow-up is that of 13 years (Hakanen et al., 2007). Table 11.3 shows findings from longitudinal studies with different follow-up periods.

Table 11.3 The development of the sense of coherence over time, based on a sample of longitudinal studies

1 → 2 year	0.8 points	SOC-13	Bergman et al. (2012)
1 → 3 year	14.2 points	SOC-28	Kuuppelomäki and Utriainen (2003)
1 → 3 year	0.1 points	SOC-13	Honkinen et al. (2008)
1 → 5 year	1.6 points	SOC-13	Volanen et al. (2007)
1 → 5 year	1.8 points	SOC-13	Bergman et al. (2012)
1 → 5 year	3.6 points	SOC-13	Lövheim et al. (2013)
1 → 9 year	0.1 points	SOC-13	Luutonen et al. (2011)
1 → 10 year	2.7 points	SOC-13	Kalimo et al. (2003)
1 → 12 year	0.3 points	SOC-29	Holmberg and Thelin (2010)
1 → 13 year	0.4 points	SOC-13	Hakanen et al. (2007)

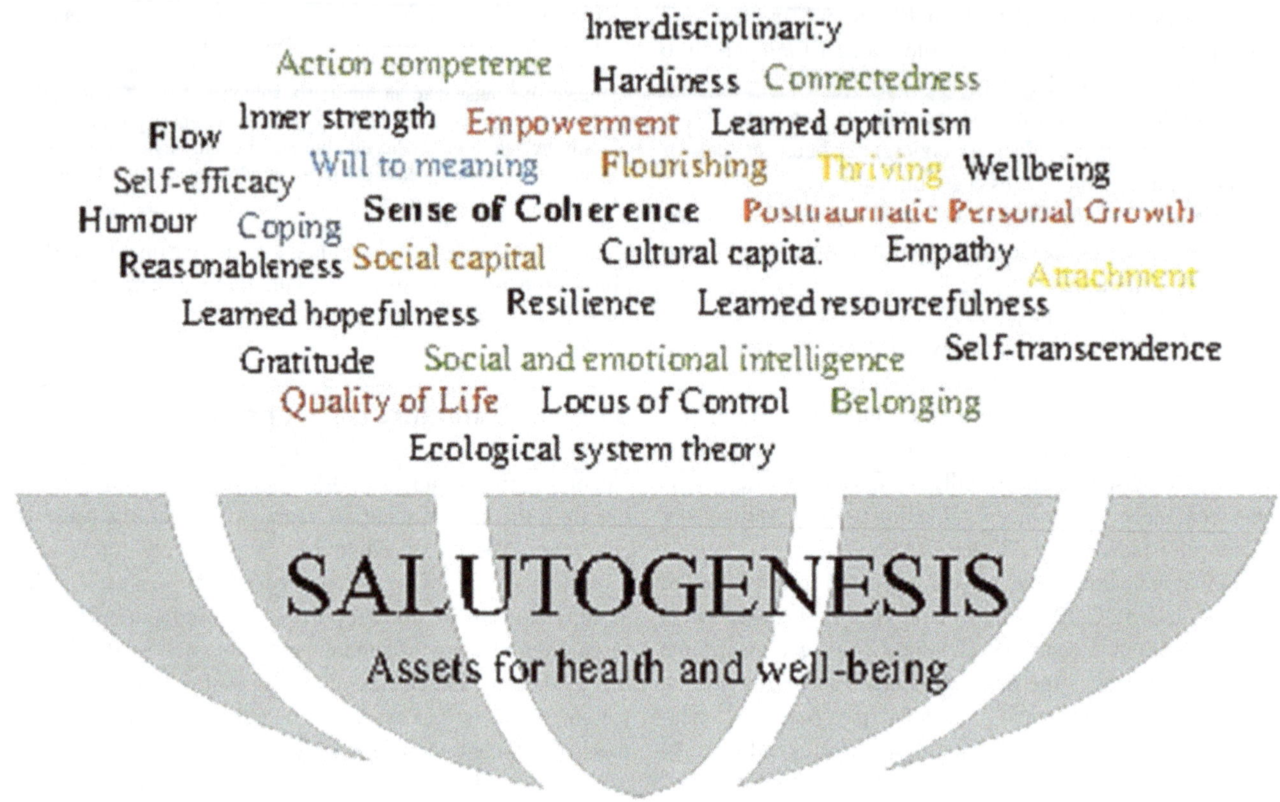

Fig. 11.4 The salutogenic umbrella, salutogenesis as an umbrella concept © Monica Eriksson 2017. (All rights reserved)

Salutogenesis Is More than the Measurement of the Sense of Coherence

Salutogenesis, focusing on health and people's resources, is something more than the measurement of the sense of coherence. Today, we can talk about salutogenesis as an umbrella concept with many different theories and concepts with salutogenic elements and dimensions (Lindström & Eriksson, 2010). There is extensive research that focuses on the resources of individuals, groups, and communities. All this and more can be accommodated under the common umbrella. Figure 11.4 shows some related concepts to the sense of coherence collected under an umbrella.

References

Abdelgadir, M., Shebeika, W., Eltom, M., Berne, C., & Wikblad, K. (2009). Health related quality of life and sense of coherence in Sudanese diabetic subjects with lower limb amputation. *Tohoku Journal of Experimental Medicine, 217*, 45–50.

Abramson, J. H., & Abramson, Z. H. (1999). *Survey methods in community medicine. Epidemiological research programme evaluation clinical trials* (5th ed.). Churchill Livingstone.

Agardh, E. E., Ahlbom, A., Andersson, T., et al. (2003). Work stress and low sense of coherence is associated with type 2 diabetes in middle-aged Swedish women. *Diabetes Care, 26*(3), 719–724.

Almedom, A. M., Tesfamichael, B., Mohammed, Z. S., Mascie-Taylor, C. G. N., & Alemu, Z. (2007). Use of "Sense of Coherence (SOC)" scale to measure resilience in Eritrea: Interrogating both the data and the scale. *Journal of Biosocial Science, 39*(1), 91–107.

Antonovsky, A. (1987). *Unraveling the mystery of health. How people manage stress and stay well.* Jossey-Bass Publishers.

Antonovsky, A. (1993). The salutogenic approach to aging. *Lecture held in Berkeley*, January 21, 1993.

Antonovsky, A. (1979). *Health, Stress and Coping: New Perspectives on Mental and Physical Well-Being*. San Francisco: Jossey-Bass.

Antonovsky, A., & Sourani, T. (1988). Family sense of coherence and family adaptation. *Journal of Marriage and Family, 50*, 79–92.

Bauer, G., & Jenny, G. J. (2012). Moving towards positive organizational health: Challenges and a proposal for a research model of organizational health development. In J. Houdmondt, S. Leka, & R. R. Sinclair (Eds.), *Contemporary occupational health psychology: Global perspectives on research and practice* (Vol. 2). Wiley-Blackwell.

Bayard-Burfield, L., Sundquist, J., & Johansson, S.-E. (2001). Ethnicity, self-reported psychiatric illness, and intake of psychotropic drugs in five ethnic groups in Sweden. *Journal of Epidemiology and Community Health, 55*, 657–664.

Bengel, J., Strittmatter, R., & Willman, H. (1999). *What keeps people healthy? The current state of discussion and the relevance of Antonovsky's salutogenic model of health.* Federal Centre for Health Education (FCHE).

Bergman, E., Årestedt, K., Fridlund, B., Karlsson, J.-E., & Malm, D. (2012). The impact of comprehensibility and sense of coherence in the recovery of patients with myocardial infarction: A long-term follow-up study. *European Journal of Cardiovascular Nursing, 11*(3), 276–283.

Biro, E., Balajti, I., Adany, R., & Kosa, K. (2010). Determinants of mental well-being in medical students. *Social Psychiatry and Psychiatric Epidemiology, 45*, 253–258.

Bonanato, K., Paiva, S. M., Pordeus, I. A., Ramos-Jorge, M. L., Barbabela, D., & Allison, P. J. (2009). Relationship between mothers' sense of coherence and oral health status of preschool children. *Caries Research, 43*, 103–109.

Braun-Lewensohn, O., & Sagy, S. (2011). Salutogenesis and culture: Personal and community sense of coherence among adolescents belonging to three different cultural groups. *International Review of Psychiatry, 23*(6), 533–541.

Bringsén, Å. (2010). *Taking care of others—What's in it for us? Exploring workplace-related health from a salutogenic perspective in a nursing context.* Doctoral thesis. Lund: Lund University.

Bringsén, Å., Andersson, I. H., & Ejlertsson, G. (2009). Development and quality analysis of the Salutogenic Health Indicator Scale (SHIS). *Scandinavian Journal of Public Health, 37*(1), 13–19.

Ciairano, S., Rabaglietti, E., Roggero, A., & Callari, T. C. (2010). Life satisfaction, sense of coherence and job precariousness in Italian young adults. *Journal of Adult Development, 17*, 177–189.

Cooper, H. (1998). *Synthesizing research. A guide for literature review*. Sage.

Drageset, J., & Haugan, G. (2015). Psychometric properties of the Orientation to Life Questionnaire in nursing home residents. *Scandinavian Journal of Caring Sciences*. https://doi.org/10.1111/scs.12271

Encarnação, P., Oliveira, C. C., & Martins, T. (2018). Psychometric properties of the suffering assessment questionnaire in adults with chronic diseases or life-threatening illness. *Scandinavian Journal of Caring Sciences, 32*(4), 1279–1287.

Endler, C. P., Haug, T. M., & Spranger, H. (2008). Sense of Coherence and physical health. A "Copenhagen interpretation" of Antonovsky's SOC concept. *The Scientific World Journal, 8*, 451–453.

Eriksson, M. (2007). *Unravelling the Mystery of Salutogenesis. The evidence base of the salutogenic research as measured by Antonovsky's Sense of Coherence Scale.* [Doctoral thesis]. Åbo Akademi University, Department of Social Policy. Folkhälsan Research Centre, Health Promotion Research Programme, Research Report 2007:1. Turku: Folkhälsan.

Eriksson, M. (2014). The salutogenic framework for health promotion and disease prevention. In D. I. Mostofsky (Ed.), *The handbook of behavioral medicine*. Hoboken.

Eriksson, M., Kerekes, N., Brink, P., Pennbrant, S., & Nunstedt, H. (2019). The level of sense of coherence among Swedish nursing staff. *Journal of Advanced Nursing, 00*, 1–7. https://doi.org/10.1111/jan.14137

Eriksson, M., & Lindström, B. (2005). Validity of Antonovsky's sense of coherence scale—A systematic review. *Journal of Epidemiology & Community Health, 59*(6), 460–466.

Eriksson, M., & Lindström, B. (2014). The salutogenic framework for well-being: Implications for public policy. In T. J. Hämäläinen & J. Michaelson (Eds.), *Well-being and beyond. Broadening the public and policy discourse* (pp. 68–97). Edward Elgar.

Eriksson, M., Lindström, B., & Lilja, J. (2007). A sense of coherence and health. Åland, a special case. *Journal of Epidemiology and Community Health, 61*(8), 684–688.

Fawcett, P. (1997). *Translation and language: Linguistic theories explained.* St Jerome Publishing.

Feldt, T., Metsäpelto, R.-L., Kinnunen, U., & Pulkkinen, L. (2007). Sense of coherence and five-factor approach to personality. Conceptual relationships. *European Psychologist, 12*(3), 165–172.

Feldt, T., Leskinen, E., Koskenvuo, M., Suominen, S., Vahtera, J., & Kivimäki, M. (2011). Development of sense of coherence in adulthood: A person-centered approach. The population-based HeSSup cohort study. *Quality of Life Research, 20*(1), 69–79.

Feldt, T., Lintula, H., Suominen, S., Koskenvuo, M., Vahtera, J., & Kivimäki, M. (2007). Structural validity and temporal stability of the 13-item sense of coherence scale: Prospective evidence from the population-based HeSSup study. *Quality of Life Research, 16*(3), 483–493.

Flannery, R. B., & Flannery, G. J. (1990). Sense of coherence, life stress, and psychological distress: A prospective methodological inquiry. *Journal of Clinical Psychology, 46*(4), 415–420.

Flensborg-Madsen, T., Ventegodt, S., & Merrick, J. (2005a). Sense of coherence and physical health. A review of previous findings. *The Scientific World Journal, 5*, 665–673.

Flensborg-Madsen, T., Ventegodt, S., & Merrick, J. (2005b). Why is Antonovsky's sense of coherence not correlated to physical health? Analyzing Antonovsky's 29-item Sense of Coherence Scale (SOC-29). *The Scientific World Journal, 5*, 767–776.

Flensborg-Madsen, T., Ventegodt, S., & Merrick, J. (2006a). Sense of coherence and physical health. Testing Antonovsky's theory. *The Scientific World Journal, 6*, 2212–2219.

Flensborg-Madsen, T., Ventegodt, S., & Merrick, J. (2006b). Sense of coherence and physical health. A cross-sectional study using a new scale (SOC II). *The Scientific World Journal, 6*, 2200–2211.

Flensborg-Madsen, T., Ventegodt, S., & Merrick, J. (2006c). Sense of Coherence and physical health. The Emotional Sense of Coherence (SOC-E) was found to be the best-known predictor of physical health. *The Scientific World Journal, 6*, 2147–2157.

Forbech, V. H., & Hanson, A. L. (2013). Salutogenic presence supports a health-promoting work life. *Journal of Social Medicine, 6*, 890–901.

Forsgärde, M., Westman, B., & Nygren, L. (2000). Ethical discussion groups as an intervention to improve the climate in inter-professional work with the elderly and disabled. *Journal of Interprofessional Care, 14*(4), 351–361.

Getnet, B. & Alem, A. (2019). Construct calidity and factor structure of sense of coherence (SoC-13) scale as a measure of resilicence in Eritrean refugees living in Ethopia. *Conflict and Health*, 13, 3.

Geyer, S. (1997). Some conceptual considerations on the sense of coherence. *Social Science & Medicine, 44*(12), 1771–1779.

Government Offices of Sweden. (2006). *The convention of the rights of the child.* [Elektronic]. Retrieved December 30, 2015, from http://www.regeringen.se/content/1/c6/04/09/98/b8de24c7.pdf

Government Offices of Sweden. (2008). *UN:s convention on the Rights of Persons with disabilities.* [Elektronic]. Retrieved December 30, 2015, from http://www.regeringen.se/content/1/c6/10/19/18/516a2b36.pdf

Government Offices of Sweden. (2011). *United Nations. The Universal Declaration of Human Rights.* [Elektronic]. Retrieved December 30, 2015, from http://www.regeringen.se/content/1/c6/18/37/41/3014596d.pdf

Graeser, S. (2011). Salutogenic factors for mental health promotion in work settings and organizations. *International Review of Psychiatry, 23*(6), 508–515.

Groarke, A. M., Curtis, R., Walsh, D. M. J., & Sullivan, F. (2018). What predicts emotional response in men awaiting prostate biopsy? *BMC Urology, 18*, 27. https://doi.org/10.1186/s12894-018-0340-9

Hakanen, J. J., Feldt, T., & Leskinen, E. (2007). Change and stability of sense of coherence in adulthood: Longitudinal evidence from the Healthy Child Study. *Journal of Research in Personality, 41*, 602–617.

Han, K., Lee, P., Park, E., Park, Y., Kim, J., & Kangh, H. (2007). Family functioning and mental illness a Korean correlational study. *Asian Journal of Nursing, 10*, 129–136.

Holmefur, M., Sundberg, K., Wettergren, L., & Langius-Eklöf, A. (2015). Measurement properties of the 13-item sense of coherence scale using Rasch analysis. *Quality of Life Research, 24*, 1455–1463.

Höjdahl, T., Magnus, J. H., Mdala, I., Hagen, R., & Langeland, E. (2015). Emotional distress and sense of coherence in women completing a motivational program in five countries. A prospective study. *International Journal of Prisoner Health, 11*(3), 169–182.

Holmberg, S., & Thelin, A. G. (2010). Predictors of sick leave owing to neck or low back pain: A 12-year longitudinal cohort study in a rural male population. *Annals of Agricultural and Environmental Medicine, 17*(2), 251–257.

Honkinen, P. L., Suominen, S., Helenius, H., Aromaa, M., Rautava, P., Sourander, A., et al. (2008). Stability of the sense of coherence in adolescence. *International Journal of Adolescent Medicine and Health, 14*(4), 587–600.

Idan, O., & Margalit, M. (2014). Socioemotional self-perceptions, family climate, and hopeful thinking among students with learning disabilities and typically achieving students from the same classes. *Journal of Learning Disabilities, 47*(2), 136–152.

Kanhai, J., Harrison, V. E., & Suominen, A. L. (2014). Sense of coherence and incidence of periodontal disease in adults. *Journal of Clinical Periodontology, 41*, 760–765.

Kalimo, R., Pahkin, K., Mutanen, P., & Toppinen-Tanner, S. (2003). Staying well or burning out at work: Work characteristics and personal resources as long-term predictors. *Work & Stress, 17*(2), 109–122.

Kase, T., Ueno, Y., & Oishi, K. (2018). The overlap of sense of coherence and the Big Five personality traits: A confirmatory study. *Health Psychology Open*, 1–4. https://doi.org/10.1177/2055102918810654

Kivimäki, M., Elovainio, M., Vahtera, J., et al. (2002). Sense of coherence as a mediator between hostility and health. Seven-year prospective study on female employees. *Journal of Psychosomatic Research, 52*, 239–247.

Klepp, O. M., Mastekaasa, A., Sørensen, T., Sandanger, I., & Kleiner, R. (2007). Structure analysis of Antonovsky's sense of coherence from an epidemiological mental health survey with a brief nine-item sense of coherence scale. *International Journal of Methods in Psychiatric Research, 16*(1), 11–22.

Korotkov, D. (1993). An assessment of the (short-form) sense of coherence personality measure: Issues of validity and well-being. *Personal and Individual Differences, 14*(4), 575–583.

Korotkov, D., & Hannah, E. (1994). Extraversion and emotionality as proposed superordinate stress moderators: A prospective analysis. *Personal and Individual Differences, 16*(5), 787–792.

Kumlin, T. (1998). *Sense of coherence in theory, empiri and criticism.* [In Swedish]. (Vol. 9). Stockholm: The Swedish Research Council.

Kuuppelomäki, M., & Utriainen, P. (2003). A 3 year follow-up study of health care students' sense of coherence and related smoking, drinking and physical exercise factors. *International Journal of Nursing Studies, 40*(4), 383–388.

Lajunen, T. (2019). Cross-Cultural Evaluation of Antonovsky's Orientation to Life Questionnaire: Comparison Between Australian, Finnish, and Turkish Young Adults. *Psychological Reports, 122*(2), 731–747.

Larsson, G., & Kallenberg, K. (1999). Dimensional analysis of sense of coherence using structural equation modelling. *European Journal of Personality, 13*, 51–61.

Lerdal, A., Opheim, R., Gay, C. L., Moum, B., Fagermoen, M. S., & Kottorp, A. (2017). Psychometric limitations of the 13-item Sense of Coherence Scale assessed by Rasch analysis. *BMC Psychology, 5*(1), 18. https://doi.org/10.1186/s40359-017-0187-y

Li, W., Leonhart, R., Schaefert, R., et al. (2014). Sense of coherence contributes to physical and mental health in general hospital patients in China. *Psychology, Health & Medicine*. https://doi.org/10.1080/13548506.2014.952644

Lindblad, C., Sandelin, K., Petersson, L.-M., Rohani, C. & Langius-Eklöf, A. (2016). Stability of the 13-item sense of coherence (SOC) scale: a longitudinal prospective study in women treated for breast cancer. Quaility of Life Research, 25, 753–60.

Lindström, B., & Eriksson, M. (2009). The salutogenic approach to the making of HiAP/healthy public policy: Illustrated by a case study. *Global Health Promotion, 16*(1), 17–28.

Lindström, B., & Eriksson, M. (2010). *The Hitchhiker's Guide to Salutogenesis. Salutogenic pathways to health promotion.* Folkhälsan and IUHPE Global Working Group on Salutogenesis.

Lövheim, H., Graneheim, U. H., Jonsén, E., Strandberg, G., & Lundman, B. (2013). Changes in sense of coherence in old age—A 5-year follow-up of the Umeå 85+ study. *Scandinavian Journal of Caring Sciences, 27*, 13–19.

Lundman, B., Forsberg, K. A., Jonsén, E., Gustafson, Y., Olofsson, K., Strandberg, G., et al. (2010). Sense of coherence (SOC) related to health and mortality among the very old: The Umeå 85+ study. *Archives of Gerontology and Geriatrics, 51*(3), 329–332.

Luutonen, S., Sohlman, B., Salokangas, R. K. R., Lehtinen, V., & Dowrick, C. (2011). Weak sense of coherence predicts depression: 1-year and 9-year follow-ups of the Finnish Outcomes of Depression International Network (ODIN) sample. *Journal of Mental Health, 20*(1), 43–51.

Margalit, M., & Efrati, M. (1996). Loneliness, coherence and companionship among children with learning disorder. *Educational Psychology, 16*(1), 69–80.

Mautner, E., Ashida, C., Greimel, E., Lang, U., Kolman, C., Aalton, D., & Inoue, W. (2014). Are there differences in the health outcomes of mothers in Europe and East-Asia? A cross-cultural health survey. *BioMed Research International*. https://doi.org/10.1155/2014/856543

Mayer, C. H., & Boness, C. (2011). Concepts of health and Well-being in managers. An organizational study. *International Journal of Qualitative Studies on Health and Well-being, 6*. https://doi.org/10.3402/qhw.v3406i3404.7143

Mayer, C.-H., & Krause, C. (2011). Promoting mental health and salutogenesis in transcultural organizational and work contexts. *International Review of Psychiatry, 23*(6), 495–500.

Mayer, J., & Thiel, A. (2014). Health in elite sports from a salutogenic perspective: Athletes' sense of coherence. *PLOS One, 9*(7), 1–11.

Naaldenberg, J., Tobi, H., van den Esker, F., & Vaandrager, L. (2011). Psychometric properties of the OLQ-13 scale to measure Sense of Coherence in a community-dwelling older population. *Health and Quality of Life Outcomes, 23*(9), 37. https://doi.org/10.1186/1477-7525-9-37

Nash, J. K. (2002). Neighborhood effects on sense of school coherence and educational behavior in students at risk of school failure. *Children & Schools, 24*(2), 73–89.

Nilsson, P., Andersson, I. H., Ejlertsson, G., & Troein, M. (2012). Workplace health resources based on sense of coherence theory. *International Journal of Workplace Health Management, 5*(3), 156–167.

Nilsson, K. W., Leppert, J., Simonsson, B., & Starrin, B. (2010). Sense of coherence and psychological well-being: Improvement with age. *Journal of Epidemiology and Community Health, 64*(4), 347–352.

Norekvål, T. M., Fridlund, B., Rokne, B., Segadal, L., Wentzel-Larsen, T., & Nordrehaug, J. E. (2010). Patient-reported outcomes as predictors of 10-year survival in women after acute myocardial infarction. *Health and Quality of Life Outcomes, 8*, 140.

Orvik, A., & Axelsson, R. (2012). Organizational health in health organizations: Towards a conceptualization. *Scandinavian Journal of Caring Sciences, 26*(4), 796–802.

Öztekin, C., & Tezer, E. (2009). The role of sense of coherence and physical activity in positive and negative affect of Turkish adolescents. *Adolescence, 44*, 421–432.

Pavicic Bosnjak, A., Rumboldt, M., Stanojevic, M., & Dennis, C. L. (2012). Psychometric assessment of the Croatian version of the breastfeeding self-efficacy scale-short form. *Journal of Human Lactation, 28*(4), 565–569.

Pham, P. N., Vink, P., Kinkodi, D. K., & Weinstein, H. M. (2010). Sense of coherence and its association with exposure to traumatic events, posttraumatic stress disorder, and depression in the eastern Democratic Republic of Congo. *Journal of Traumatic Stress, 23*, 313–321.

Poppius, E., Virkkunen, H., Hakama, M., & Tenkanen, L. (2006). The sense of coherence and incidence of cancer - role of follow-up time and age at baseline. *Journal of Psychosomatic Research, 61*, 205–211.

Rajesh, G., Eriksson, M., Pai, K., Seemanthini, S., Naik, D. G., & Rao, A. (2015). The validity and reliability of the Sense of Coherence scale among Indian university students. *Global Health Promotion*. https://doi.org/10.1177/1757975915572691

Rohani, C., Khanjari, S., Abedi, H. A., Oskouie, F., & Langius-Eklöf, A. (2010). Health index, sense of coherence scale, brief religious coping scale and spiritual perspective scale: Psychometric properties. *Journal of Advanced Nursing, 66*, 2796–2806.

Rostami, R., Lamit, H., Khoshnava, S. M., & Rostami, R. (2014). The role of historical Persian gardens on the health status of contemporary urban residents: Gardens and health status of contemporary urban residents. *EcoHealth, 11*(3), 308–321. https://doi.org/10.1007/s10393-014-0939-6

Roth, G., & Ekblad, S. (2006). A longitudinal perspective on depression and sense of coherence in a sample of mass-evacuated adults from Kosovo. *Journal of Nervous and Mental Disease, 194*, 378–381.

Sagy, S. (1998). Effects of personal, family, and community characteristics on emotional reactions in a stress situation. *Youth & Society, 29*(3), 311–330.

Sagy, S. (2008). *Sense of Coherence in a family context.* The International Seminar on Salutogenesis and The 1st Meeting of the IUHPE Thematic Working Group on Salutogenesis, Helsinki Finland, 12–13 May, 2008.

Sagy, S., & Antonovsky, A. (1992). The family sense of coherence and the retirement transition. *Journal of Marriage and Family, 54*(4), 983–994.

Sakano, J., & Yajima, Y. (2005). Factors structure of the SOC scale 13-item version in Japanese university students. *Japanese Journal of Public Health, 52*(1), 34–45.

Sandell, R., Blomberg, J., & Lazar, A. (1998). The factor structure of Antonovsky's sense of coherence scale in Swedish clinical and nonclinical samples. *Personality and Individual Differences, 24*(5), 701–711.

Sardu, C., Mereu, A., Sotgiu, A., Andrissi, L., Jacobson, M. K., & Contu, P. (2012). Antonovsky's sense of coherence scale: Cultural validation of SOC questionnaire and socio-demographic patterns in an Italian population. *Clinical Practice & Epidemiology in Mental Health, 8*, 1–6.

Schnyder, U., Büchi, S., Sensky, T., & Klaghofer, R. (2000). Antonovsky's sense of coherence: Trait or state? *Psychotherapy and Psychosomatics, 69*, 296–302.

Schumann, A., Hapke, U., Meyer, C., et al. (2003). Measuring Sense of Coherence with only three items: A useful tool for population surveys. *British Journal of Health Psychology, 8*, 409–421.

Singer, S., & Brähler, E. (2007). Die "sense of coherence scale". In *Testhandbuch zur deutschen Version*. Vandenhoeck & Ruprecht.

Sotgiu, A., Demurtas, A., Cannas, N., Sias, E., & Tobarra-López, A. (2018). The Curitiba Statement on Health Promotion and Equity: Italian version and analysis of criticalities. *Annali d'giene, 30*, 181–190.

Spadoti Dantas, R. A., Silva, F. S., & Ciol, M. A. (2014). Psychometric properties of the Brazilian versions of the 29- and 13-item scales of the Antonovsky's Sense of Coherence (SOC-29 and SOC-13) evaluated in Brazilian cardiac patients. *Journal of Clinical Nursing, 23*(1–2), 156–165.

Stern, B., Socan, G., Rener-Sitar, K., Kukec, A., & Zaletel-Kragelj, L. (2019). Validation of the Slovenian version of the short sense of coherence questionnaire (SOC-13) in multiple sclerosis patients. *Zur Varst, 58*(1), 31–39.

Söderhamn, O., & Holmgren, L. (2004). Testing Antonovsky's sense of coherence (SOC) scale among Swedish physically active older people. *Scandinavian Journal of Psychology, 45*, 215–221.

Söderhamn, U., Sundsli, K., Cliffordson, C., & Dale, B. (2015). Psychometric properties of Antonovsky's 29-item Sense of Coherence scale in research on older home-dwelling Norwegians. *Scandinavian Journal of Public Health, 43*(8), 867–874.

Suominen, S., Blomberg, H., Helenius, H., et al. (1999). Sense of coherence and health—does the association depend on resistance resources? *Psychology and Health, 14*, 937–948.

Suraj, S., & Singh, A. (2011). Study of sense of coherence health promoting behaviour in north Indian students. *Indian Journal of Medical Research, 134*, 645–652.

Surtees, P., Wainwright, N., Luben, R., Khaw, K.-T., & Day, N. (2003). Sense of coherence and mortality in men and women in the EPIC-Norfolk United Kingdom prospective cohort study. *American Journal of Epidemiology, 158*(12), 1202–1209.

Tang, S. T., & Li, C.-Y. (2008). The important role of sense of coherence in relation to depressive symptoms for Taiwanese family caregivers of cancer patients at the end of life. *Journal of Psychosomatic Research, 64*, 195–203.

Toft Würtz, E., Fonager, K., & Tølbøll Mortensen, J. (2015). Association between sense of coherence in adolescence and social benefits later in life: a 12-year follow-up study. *BMJ Open*. https://doi.org/10.1136/bmjopen-2014-006489

Togari, T., Yamazaki, Y., Takayama, T. S., Yamaki, C. K., & Nakayama, K. (2008). Follow-up study on the effects of sense of coherence on well-being after two years in Japanese university undergraduate students. *Personality and Individual Differences, 44*(6), 1335–1347. https://doi.org/10.1016/j.paid.2007.12.002

Virues-Ortéga, J., Martinez-Martin, P., Del Barrio, J. L., Lozano, L. M., & Grupo Espanol, E. (2007). Cross-cultural validation of Antonovsky's Sense of Coherence Scale (OLQ-13) in Spanish elders aged 70 years or more. *Medicina Clinica, 128*, 486–492.

Vasiliu, D., Marinescu, D.-A., Marinescu, G., & Rizeanu, S. (2015). *Assessing sense of Coherence. Psychometric properties for the sense of coherence scale: SOC-13*. May 2015. Conference: Sesiunea de comunicari stiintifice a Universitatii Hyperion At: Hyperion University, Bucharest, Romania.

Vogt, K., Jenny, G. J., & Bauer, G. F. (2013). Comprehensibility, manageability and meaningfulness at work: Construct validity of a scale measuring work-related sense of coherence. *South African Journal of Industrial Psychology, 39*(1), 8.

Volanen, S. M., Suominen, S., Lahelma, E., Koskenvuo, M., & Silventoinen, K. (2007). Negative life events and stability of sense of coherence: A five-year follow-up study of Finnish women and men. *Scandinavian Journal of Psychology, 48*(5), 433–441.

WHO. (2001). *The World health report 2001: Mental health: New understanding, new hope*. World Health Organization.

12

Salutogenic Model: Role of GRRs

Orly Idan, Monica Eriksson, and Michal Al-Yagon

Introduction

This chapter reviews and integrates conceptual and empirical research focusing on the role of generalized resistance resources (GRRs) within the salutogenic model. In particular, this chapter discusses findings regarding the conceptual and empirical progress seen in the study of GRRs at the individual, family, and community ecological levels in understanding individual differences in sense of coherence (SOC). Each of the latter attempts to relate to the lifespan in its childhood, adolescent, and adult developmental phases. Specifically, the present chapter uniquely focuses on variables that may contribute to the understanding of individuals' level of SOC within the salutogenic model, in contrast to previous reviews that focused primarily on SOC's role in understanding individuals' affective functioning, such as well-being, resilience, and coping strategies.

The term *generalized resistance resource* (GRR) was coined by Antonovsky (1979, 1987) and refers to the resources of a person, a group, or a community that facilitate the individual's abilities to cope effectively with stressors and contribute to the development of the individual's level of SOC. As proposed by Antonovsky (1987), the GRRs refer to "phenomena that provide one with sets of life experiences characterized by consistency, participation in shaping outcomes and an underload-overload balance" (Antonovsky, 1987, p. 19). According to Antonovsky (1979, 1987), such resources may include the following factors: (1) material resources (e.g., money), (2) knowledge and intelligence (e.g., knowing the real world and acquiring skills), (3) ego identity (e.g., integrated but flexible self), (4) coping strategies, (5) social support, (6) commitment and cohesion with one's cultural roots, (7) cultural stability, (8) ritualistic activities, (9) religion and philosophy (e.g., stable set of answers to life's perplexities), (10) preventive health orientation, (11) genetic and constitutional GRRs, and (12) individuals' state of mind (see Horsburgh & Ferguson, 2012 for a review).

In an attempt to develop a more parsimony model, Antonovsky (1987) merged the concept of the GRRs with his earlier concept of the "stressors" and combined them into one concept—*Generalized Resistance Resources—Resistance Deficits* (GRRs-RDs). Accordingly, each of these GRRs was presented on a continuum. Thus, an individual who is higher on the continuum tends to have consistent, balanced life experiences and high participation in decision-making. In contrast, an individual who is lower on the continuum tends to have inconsistent, low balanced life experiences and low participation in decision-making. In line with these assumptions, among individuals who are higher on the continuum, the GRR-RDs are viewed as GRRs, and among individuals who are lower on the continuum the GRR-RDs are viewed as GRDs. Based on these assumptions, both GRRs and GRDs contribute to the development of an individual's SOC.

Importantly, although the salutogenic model presumes that individuals develop strong SOC through successful applications of GRR-RDs across the lifespan, this model also proposed a reciprocal and dynamic relationship between SOC and GRR-RDs. Thus, GRR-RDs may contribute to an individual's level of SOC, and an individual's level of SOC may contribute to mobilizing GRRs for enhancing tension management. However, as suggested by Antonovsky (1987),

O. Idan (✉)
School of Psychology, Interdisciplinary Center (IDC), Herzliya, Israel
e-mail: oidan@idc.ac.il

M. Eriksson
Department of Health Sciences, Section of Health Promotion and Care Sciences, Center on Salutogenesis, University West, Trollhattan, Sweden

M. Al-Yagon
Department of School Counseling and Special Education, Constantiner School of Education, Tel Aviv University, Tel Aviv, Israel

when GRRs or GRDs may become chronic and built into the life situation of the person, they are viewed as the primary determinants of the strength of an individual's level of SOC.

In general, the initial GRR resources (Antonovsky, 1979) may be perceived as manifested within the life experiences as proposed by Antonovsky (1991). Thus, three types of life experiences are assumed to contribute to the SOC developmental process: consistency, load balance, and participation in shaping outcomes. The fourth dimension—emotional closeness—was added later by Sagy and Antonovsky (2000). The first of these life experiences—*consistency*—refers to the extent to which, during growing up, messages were clear, and there were order and structure rather than chaos in one's environment. As suggested by Antonovsky (1991), experiences of consistency in an individual's life provide the basis for the comprehensibility component of the SOC. The other life experience—*load balance*—refers to the extent to which, during growing up, one experienced overload or underload in the balance between the demands made upon one and one's resources. Such load balance is important for the SOC's manageability component. The third life experience—*participation in shaping outcomes*—refers to the extent to which one had a significant part in deciding her/his fate and was not an object of the power and whims of others. Participation in shaping outcomes provides the basis for the meaningfulness component. Sagy and Antonovsky (1996) selected the mentioned three life experiences in their qualitative analysis of the narratives of two women whose life histories were similar in their historical and social contexts. However, their life orientation as expressed in their stories and their levels of SOC were different. The fourth life experience (Sagy & Antonovsky, 2000)—*emotional closeness*—refers to the extent to which one felt consistent emotional bonds and a sense of belonging in social groups of which one was a member. Similar to the *participation in shaping outcomes*, the *emotional closeness* resource was assumed as relevant to the meaningfulness component.

Generalized Resistance Resources: The Individual Level

Emotional Closeness and Attachment Relationships

As mentioned above, *emotional closeness* is one of the four types of life experiences assumed to contribute to the SOC developmental process (Sagy & Antonovsky, 2000). Close emotional relationship with significant others has been conceptualized primarily within the framework of attachment theory (Bowlby, 1973; Grossmann et al., 2006; Mikulincer & Shaver, 2007). Overall, Bowlby's attachment theory (Bowlby, 1973; Bowlby, 1982/1969) underscored the role of early interactions with significant others in explaining individual variations in a variety of emotional, social, and behavioral adjustments (Cassidy & Shaver, 2008; Grossmann et al., 2006). To be noted, although this theory focused on early interactions with significant others, studies have pinpointed that attachment theory is a lifespan developmental theory (see Mikulincer & Shaver, 2007 for a review). Accordingly, researchers have underscored how adults' attachment representations (Bowlby, 1973, 1982/1969) contribute to a variety of psychological resources such as coping with distress and affect regulation (Bernier & Matte-Gagne, 2011; Collins & Ford, 2010; Mikulincer & Shaver, 2004, 2007).

Briefly, attachment theory emphasizes that during the first year of life, infants develop a specific and enduring relationship with their primary caretakers (Ainsworth & Wittig, 1969). Infants' strong tendency to seek proximity to caregivers is the overt manifestation of the inborn attachment behavioral system, which is designed to restore or maintain proximity to support others in times of need. Proximity to an available, supportive, and responsive caregiver ("attachment figure") provides the infant with a sense of "secure base," which refers to a set of expectations about others' availability and responsiveness in times of stress. As emphasized by this theory, attachment figures play a central role in the infant's cognitive, social, and emotional development as well as in the development of a sense of self (Bowlby, 1982/1969; Waters & Cummings, 2000). Children's experiences with attachment figures are internalized into "working models of attachment"—mental representations of significant others and the self. These result in unique attachment styles, that is, stable patterns of cognitions as well as behaviors that are manifested in other close relationships and social interactions across the lifespan. Following these assumptions, infants of available and supportive attachment figures are more likely to develop a sense of security and trust. In contrast, infants of unavailable, inconsistent, and/or unresponsiveness attachment figures are more likely to perceive the world as unpredictable, threatening, or rejecting.

In examining the relations between patterns of attachment and youngsters' well-adjusting functioning, the vast majority of attachment research studies indicated that securely attached children and adolescents revealed better mental health and functioning and higher levels of psychological well-being, than did children and adolescents with an insecure style (see Allen, 2008; Grossmann et al., 2006 for a review). Data from such studies also suggested the role of youngsters' attachment relationships with significant others in understanding their level of SOC. For example, Al-Yagon (2010) investigated the possible role of children's attachment with mothers in understanding variance in children's SOC in a sample of 205 mother–child dyads: 107 mothers and their children with specific learning disabilities

(SLD), and 98 mothers and their typically developing children. Utilizing structural equation modeling, this study's outcomes indicated that among both groups, children with and without SLD, children's attachment toward the mother significantly explained the variance in the children's SOC. Thus, children who felt more securely attached to the mother revealed a higher SOC level than did children who felt less securely attached to the mother. Similar findings emerged in examining the role of children's attachment with their fathers in explaining their level of SOC (Al-Yagon, 2011). Accordingly, for both groups (children with and without SLD), the variable of children's attachment toward the father significantly explained variance in children's SOC. Children who felt more securely attached to the father revealed a higher SOC than did children who felt less securely attached to the father.

Interestingly, in exploring the differences in the role of attachment with the fathers and the mothers, Al-Yagon (2014a) reported that in the model modified for elementary school children with SLD, a higher number of significant paths emerged between child–mother attachment relationships and internalizing measures than for child–father attachment. Data also showed that attachment with fathers contributed mainly to children's coping resources (i.e., SOC, hope, and effort), whereas attachment with mothers contributed to a broader range of internalizing adjustment measures including not only SOC but also self-reported loneliness and parent-rated internalizing problems. In other words, regarding attachment to fathers, those children with SLD who viewed themselves as more securely attached with the father reported a higher tendency to see the world as comprehensible, manageable, and meaningful (i.e., higher SOC) compared to children with SLD who viewed themselves as less securely attached.

The role of attachment relationships with significant others in understanding SOC has been less examined among adolescents and adults. However, such studies indicated similar findings to those reported for younger children. For example, in examining three groups of Chinese American college students, Ying et al. (2007) highlighted the important role of close attachment relationships with both parents and peers in explaining these individuals' development of SOC. Specifically, this study's outcomes yielded that for the groups of early and late Chinese immigrants, both parent and peer attachment enhanced their level of SOC. Thus, these college students' ability to comprehend, manage, and find meaning in their world was contributed both by their parents who may have served as an anchor in their cross-cultural transition, and their peers who facilitated an understanding and mastery of the American environment. As suggested by Ying and his colleagues (Ying et al., 2007), such close relationships may be of particular importance for these college students due to the Chinese cultural values of stigma and privacy, which may reduce their likelihood to utilize campus mental health services.

Likewise, attachment studies on adults also highlighted the contribution of adults' attachment to their level of SOC. For instance, Mikulincer and Shaver (2005) reported that lower scores on attachment anxiety and avoidance (i.e., higher levels of attachment security) were associated with higher levels of meaning and SOC in life. Also, in examining the role of adults' anxiety and avoidance attachment in exploring differences in SOC among parents of children with and without Learning Disabilities (LD), Al-Yagon (2014b) highlighted the potential role of parents' attachment anxiety in explaining their coping strategies. Specifically, for fathers from the two populations studied, a high level of anxiety in close attachment relationships, as reflected by a hyperactivation of negative emotions and rumination on distress-related thoughts (Mikulincer & Shaver, 2004), significantly contributed to fathers' low SOC. Similar findings emerged for mothers of children with SLD and mothers of children with typical development, indicating that a high level of anxiety in attachment relationships significantly contributed to these mothers' low SOC. This study also underscored the role of high parental level avoidant attachment, as reflected by a lower tendency to adopt attachment-deactivating strategies (Mikulincer & Shaver, 2004) in contributing to parents' high SOC.

Along with the attachment framework, studies have also utilized a variety of other measures to explore the role of emotional closeness in understanding differences in the individual's level of SOC. For example, in investigating the role of parent–child relationships in adolescents' SOC, García-Moya et al. (2013) and García-Moya et al. (2012) indicated that the quality of parent–child relationships (i.e., perceived affection, ease of communication with parents, parental knowledge, and satisfaction with family relationships) emerged as the main predictors of adolescents' (aged 13–19) level of SOC. Focused on adulthood, findings from Volanen et al. (2004) suggested that for both men and women the quality of a close relationship with their spouse significantly contributed to their level of SOC. Thus, an individual's poor close relationship with a partner was a significant threat in predicting their level of SOC. Furthermore, a study (Daoud et al., 2015) on styles of marriage (polygamous versus monogamous) as predictors of SOC found that Bedouin women in polygamous marriages demonstrated higher levels of SOC than women in monogamous marriages, when controlling for socioeconomic factors, sociodemographic factors, and social support.

These findings suggested that the patterns of attachment relationships and the quality of close relationships with significant others contributed to variation in individuals' coping resources and abilities (i.e., SOC), across the lifespan (see Mikulincer & Shaver, 2007 for a review). Accordingly, these outcomes highlighted that securely attached individuals appraised themselves as able to cope effectively with stressors, whereas individuals with insecure attachment manifested deficiency in these coping resources. Furthermore, as assumed by attachment researchers, patterns of secure attachment and high qualities of emotional closeness may enhance support-seeking in constructive and effective ways, whereas patterns of insecure attachment and low qualities of emotional closeness may increase inhibition or interference with effective support-seeking (Florian et al., 1995; Seiffge-Krenke & Beyers, 2005).

Personal Characteristics and Resources

Studies have also explored the possible role of the individual's characteristics and resources in facilitating his/her level of SOC. For example, Volanen et al. (2004) examined the effect of childhood living conditions on SOC levels among men and women aged 25–64. Specifically, childhood living conditions comprised family long-lasting economic difficulties, alcohol problems of a family member, an individual's fear of family a member, and family conflicts. Outcomes of this study reported that childhood living conditions showed a strong association with men's and women's SOC. As suggested by those researchers, poor childhood living conditions may affect adult SOC in various ways such as the negative impact on self-esteem and positive life attitudes that may contribute to low levels of SOC.

Studies have also explored the role of another demographic feature—marital status—in understanding the SOC. For instance, Read et al. (2005) examined a sample of Finnish participants aged 65–69 years. Outcomes from their study yielded that for men, unlike women, marital status has an important impact as a GRR. Accordingly, for men, being married or cohabiting was positively associated with SOC and, SOC, in turn, contributed to physical, social, and psychological health. As suggested by these researchers, marriage may enhance health in several ways such as influencing the physical and psychosocial environment in which the individual lives. These results were similar to those reported by several other studies demonstrating the beneficial effect of marriage in buffering against morbidity and mortality, especially for men (see Read et al., 2005 for a review). Several explanations were proposed regarding these results, such as the possibility that men may profit more than women from marriage as a GRR because healthy lifestyle and behaviors are more encouraged by wives than husbands, due to the women's tendency to value health more than men (Read et al., 2005).

In these contexts of personal characteristics and resources, Al-Yagon (2014b) explored the role of parents' emotional resources (attachment anxiety/avoidance and negative/positive affect) in explaining differences in their coping resources (child-related active/avoidant coping and SOC). Results from this study highlighted the potential role of parental positive and negative affect in explaining their SOC, especially among parents of children with SLD. Thus, higher levels of positive affect such as feelings of "energetic" or "happy" significantly contributed to parents' higher SOC levels in both groups of fathers and mothers of children with SLD. In contrast, higher negative affect such as feeling anxious, tense, agitated, or worried significantly contributed to lower levels of parental SOC.

A high level of negative parental affect was a significant risk factor for lower SOC, and a high level of positive affect was a significant protective factor for higher SOC. This study suggested several directions for interventions, such as teaching parents to become more attuned to their emotional functioning, learn how their feelings influence parenting, and learn strategies to regulate emotions (Al-Yagon, 2014b).

Of particular importance, studies of personal characteristics and resources among individuals in the "third age" emphasize the contribution of psychological resources on SOC. Weismann and Hannoch (2011) examined salutogenic predictors of multiple health behaviors in a sample of healthy "third age" individuals and, consistent with Antonovsky's (1987) hypothesis, found that meaningfulness was the most distinguishing among the SOC components. Moreover, the aging individuals reported that their lives made sense and were worthy of commitment and engagement. SOC components were significantly associated with multiple health behaviors and were also significantly interrelated. Consistent with the salutogenic theory, the strong correlations among the components explained their overlapping and yet distinct character. Furthermore, meaningfulness mediated self-esteem and self-efficacy influences on multiple health behaviors, and advanced age was associated with a greater extent of comprehensibility of the world. The latter supported the salutogenic assumption that psychological resources such as self-esteem and self-efficacy created life experiences that contributed to the individual's meaningful world.

In this context of self-perception, studies have also examined the possible role of an individual's self-reported health; this refers to an individual's view of his/her health irrespective of one's actual health and predicts the comprehensibility component of SOC (Solcova et al., 2017).

Individuals' Social Support

In general, studies on social support investigated individuals' resources from a variety of approaches such as contextual, emotional, and cognitive perspectives and also highlighted that the presence of others in stressful situations enhances one's mental health (see Srensen et al., 2011 for a review). Such studies focused on several dimensions of social support like the availability of support, irrespective of the extent of the support, provision of emotional support, information, tangible care, or material assistance from one's social network (Cohen, 2004). In examining the possible influence of social support on the development of SOC, Antonovsky and Sagy (1986) proposed that stable social support may reflect living in a stable community and therefore may enhance the development of a stronger SOC.

Consequently, several studies have examined such assumptions. For example, data from research studies among children and adolescents emphasized the contribution of social support provided by classmates and teachers at school (Bowen et al., 1998; Natvig et al., 2006), as well as from friends in the peer group (Evans et al., 2010; Marsh et al., 2007) for individuals' level of SOC. Similarly, these studies also demonstrated the role of aspects of neighborhood social support, such as neighborhood social cohesion (Marsh et al., 2007; Nash, 2002).

Studies have also explored the possible role of social support among adults. For example, Volanen et al. (2004) reported that among men and women aged 25–64, the ability to receive social support and their satisfaction with this support contributed to the level of SOC among both sexes. At the same time, Volanen et al. (2004) raised the possibility of reciprocal relationships between these two variables suggesting that a high level of social support may contribute to SOC, and a strong SOC may help gain social relationships.

Genetic Factors

According to the salutogenic model, two major subgroups of variables are essential for the GRRs. First, major psychosocial GRRs extensively described previously and second genetic and constitutional GRRs (Antonovsky, 1979). For example, in exploring the psychological factors, in the late 1990s Cohen conducted a study among 74 women (mean age 35) in which she examined which variables, sociological or personality factors, best explained the development of SOC (Cohen, 1997). The relationship between a narcissistic personality trait and the SOC was explored. The results showed that narcissistic elements made a more significant contribution to the SOC than the sociodemographic factors did. Here, especially items from the Narcissistic Personality Questionnaire linked to feelings of entitlement and self-satisfaction made the most significant contribution to SOC. A few years later, the question of the SOC as a state or personality trait was raised (Schnyder et al., 2000). The main aim of this longitudinal study was to investigate the stability of the SOC over 6–12 months and how SOC was associated with depression and anxiety (n = 156). The results showed that SOC could be seen as a relatively stable trait. It was negatively associated with depression and anxiety. The authors concluded that SOC was not merely a proxy measure of psychopathology, but rather a partially independent, general measure of a person's worldview.

Research exploring genetic factors has been conducted with twins. However, research on the association between genetic factors and SOC is sparse. Hansson et al. (2008) conducted the Twin Mother's Study with the specific aim to explore individual resilience factors from a genetic perspective among 326 Swedish twin pairs (150 monozygotic and 176 dizygotic). The study was the first one to investigate how genes and the environment influence resiliency/salutogenic factors. The results showed that nonshared environmental components were of principal importance in individual resiliency/salutogenic factors, but noted that genetic influences were important. They found that 35% of SOC was due to genetic effects and 57% was due to nonshared environmental effects (environmental differences between the twins). More recently, published research confirmed the results of the Swedish Twin Mother's Study. Silventoinen and colleagues analyzed the effects of genetic and environmental factors on the SOC in young adulthood among 3193 Finnish twins (Silventoinen et al., 2014). The twins and their parents rated their emotional family environment independently when the twins were 12 years of age. The findings showed that genetic factors explained 39% of the variation of SOC in males and 49% in females. The rest of the variation was explained by environmental factors unique to each twin individually. For the dimensions of SOC, the highest genetic correlation was found between comprehensibility and manageability (0.90 in males and 0.97 in females). These studies emphasize the possible role of genetic factors as well as environmental factors in understanding individual SOC.

Generalized Resistance Resources: The Family Level

Parental Resources

As observed in many studies, parents' psychological resources, as well as their developmental histories, may influence the quality of their childrearing and, through parenting, child development outcomes (Arteche & Murray, 2011; Belsky & Pluess, 2012). Such studies investigated diverse parental personal resources, including variables such as parents' psychopathology and well-being (Campbell, 2003; Goodman & Gotlib, 2002), parents' personality (Belsky & Barends, 2002), and parents' patterns of attachment (Mikulincer & Shaver, 2007). In light of these studies' assumptions, the current section will review research studies focusing on the possible role of parental personal resources in understanding children's SOC.

For example, outcomes from Al-Yagon (2008) reported on the unique value of the maternal level of SOC to her offspring's level of SOC. As suggested by this study, one may assume that mothers with high coherence levels, who tend to perceive stressful situations as less threatening and as more manageable, may provide their children with a more secure, consistent, and calm environment and may model effective strategies to cope with stressors as well. Similarly, Idan (2010) examined the role of parental SOC, hope, and family climate in explaining the coping resources, such as SOC, of high school students with severe and persistent LD, and reported that parental and family resources (parents' cohesion, SOC, hope, and effort) predicted their children's coping resources (children's cohesion, SOC, hope, and effort).

Research has also highlighted the contribution of fathers' emotional resources (i.e., attachment and affect) in explaining their offspring's SOC. For instance, Al-Yagon (2011) reported that among school-age children with SLD or with typical development, fathers' high positive affect and low level of avoidance in attachment relationships as reflected by a lower tendency to adopt attachment-deactivating strategies (Mikulincer & Shaver, 2004) contributed to children's high level of SOC.

Other studies of parental resources have investigated the possible influence of parenting style. For example, in a longitudinal study, Feldt et al. (2005) showed that parental child-centeredness, which refers to an accepting and emotionally warm parental attitude toward the child combined with parents' supervision, was the only adolescents' variable that contributed to these participants' high SOC in adulthood.

Together, these studies suggested that in order to provide optimal care and a more consistent and load-balanced environment, which in turn might enhance children's level of SOC, parents must possess sufficient psychological and coping resources such as regulating impulses, taking others' perspectives, perceiving stressful situations as more manageable, and providing a model for effective coping with stressors (Belsky, 1984; Zahn-Waxler et al., 2002).

Families' Demographic Resources

In exploring the GRRs, research studies have also demonstrated the possible role of the family's demographic resources and characteristics. For instance, Ristkari et al. (2008) reported that low levels of parental education level, death and serious illness of parents, and parental divorce contributed to lower levels of SOC among young men. Thus, higher levels of parents' education (Feldt et al., 2005), higher economic status (Geckova et al., 2010), and living with both parents (Ayo-Yusuf et al., 2009) contributed to higher level of SOC. Additionally, in accordance with the salutogenic framework assumptions on the GRRs (Antonovsky, 1979, 1987; Horsburgh & Ferguson, 2012), studies exploring families' demographic resources have also shown the role of familial economic wealth as a general resistance resource that increases individuals' opportunities to have SOC-promoting experiences (García-Moya et al., 2012).

Family Climate Factors

Several studies have highlighted the influential role of families' climate factors in SOC development across the lifespan. For example, in a study of elementary school children, Sharabi et al. (2011) emphasized the possible role of family cohesion, one of two dimensions in Olson's (1986) Circumplex Model of family climate, on children's SOC. Findings revealed that children in cohesive families reported higher levels of SOC compared to children within noncohesive families.

Family climate factors have been found to contribute during the adolescent period as well. For instance, data from García-Moya and her colleagues (García-Moya et al., 2012) demonstrated the role of family context as an important scenario in adolescents' SOC. This study yielded that among the family variables, the following had a significant individual influence on SOC during adolescence, of which the most important family dimensions were affection, ease of communication, and parental knowledge of their adolescents' life, such as their friends and leisure time activities. This study also demonstrated the contribution of the quality of relationships between the parents to adolescents' level of SOC. Similar results reported by Marsh et al. (2007) indicated the negative effect of parental high level of conflict in predicting levels of SOC in middle school youngsters. Furthermore, in an additional study on adolescents, Garcia-Moya et al. (2014) reported that the quality of the relationships between parents and their children was the most influential factor in explaining adolescent SOC.

The importance of the family environment on the development of SOC was similarly demonstrated in Silventoinen and colleagues' study (Silventoinen et al., 2014). The longitudinal study aimed to analyze genetic and environmental factors and their interaction affecting SOC among a large set of Finnish twins during young adulthood and during their home environment in childhood. The underlining assumption was based on evidence showing a strong genetic component behind psychological traits, such as personality and social attitudes (Bouchard & McGue, 2003). The study's results emphasized the significance of a supportive childhood home on the development of a strong SOC in early adulthood. Genetic differences between individuals explained a third to one-half of the variation of SOC, especially in supportive family environments. Children who grew up in supportive family climates and experienced fewer emotional tensions with their parents demonstrated more genetic and less environmental variation in SOC in adulthood than children who were raised in emotionally less favorable family climates.

Data from research on families from at-risk populations also emphasized the role of family factors in explaining variation in SOC. The following review focuses first on families with special needs. For example, among families with children with Autism Spectrum Disorder (ASD), the severity of the disorders and their typically developing siblings' resources influenced the latter's SOC. Additionally, this study also demonstrated that among the group with high severity ASD symptoms, a greater number of positive coping strategies buffered the typically developing siblings' SOC (Smith et al., 2015). Significant coping strategies that were strongly associated with higher SOC included engaging in demanding activities, ventilating feelings, avoiding problems, and solving family problems. The strongest positive correlation was engaging in demanding activities, whereas ventilating feelings had a negative correlation suggesting that typically developing siblings who did not get angry or complain had lower SOC scores.

Other findings related to ASD compared the levels of SOC in parents of children with autism and parents of typically developing children and also examined the association between SOC levels and coping strategies. Pisula and Kossakowska (2010) found that parents raising children with ASD had a lower level of SOC compared to parents raising children with more typical development. The SOC level of parents of children with ASD was positively correlated to seeking social support and self-controlling and negatively correlated with accepting responsibility and positive reappraisal. In the group of parents of children with ASD, positive correlations between distancing and total SOC, comprehensibility, and meaningfulness were revealed. The latter was perceived to indicate that having high levels of SOC orientation coincided with cognitive distancing from problems. These findings confirmed previous findings (Olsson & Hwang, 2008) that parents of children with ASD had lower levels of SOC than parents of typically developing children and emphasized that the high level of stress related to the demands associated with raising a child with ASD had a negative effect on parental SOC (Mak et al., 2007).

Moreover, Pisula and Kossakowska (2010) considered additional potential factors of lower SOC among parents of children with ASD. In line with Antonovsky's (1987) suggestion that SOC develops in childhood and early adolescence, they proposed that levels of the SOC may fluctuate with life's circumstances. Thus, challenging life experiences such as raising a child with ASD may affect the level of parental SOC.

Furthermore, in reviewing vulnerable life phases, such as prenatal and postpartum periods, Finnbogadottir and Perrson (2019) demonstrated the association between lower levels of SOC and a higher risk of depression among expectant fathers.

Reviewing at-risk families revealed several types of families, among which were those coping with traumatic life experiences, such as the Holocaust. Fossion et al. (2015) examined the consequences of extreme family functioning on resilience, SOC, anxiety, and depression. Results demonstrated that the children of Holocaust survivors' family types were more often damaged than in the general population. Growing in a damaged family impeded the development of coping strategies and enhanced the existence of depressive and anxiety disorders. In line with Fossion and colleagues' study (Fossion et al., 2014) on SOC and resilience in cases of multiple traumas, SOC was predicted to mediate between extreme families and the emergence of depressive and anxiety disorders. The recent study (Fossion et al., 2015) confirmed, in a group of children of Holocaust survivors, that which was observed among Holocaust survivors: SOC mediated between family types and depressive and anxiety disorders.

Similarly, Zeidner and Aharoni-David (2014) found indirect effects of SOC in the relationship between memory traces of specific traumatic experiences of Holocaust survivors and adaptive outcomes. They concluded that the horrors of the Holocaust recruited the survivors' inner strengths and coping resources, which in turn contributed to the development of a stronger sense of meaning and coherence, improving a better sense of mental health.

Finally, caring for a close relative in the home requires stress management. In a Swedish study, informal caregivers (n = 32) were interviewed about the generalized resistance resources and deficits they used for managing stress (Wennerberg et al., 2016, 2018). Caring in this context has been understood as a life phase, here referred to Caregivinghood, living in a dyad, and characterized by several domains (Wennerberg et al., 2019). In the caregiver domain, "Being someone significant in my own eyes" unites the essence of having access to GRRs stemming from oneself and "Being 'blessed' with a co-operative co-worker" that of having access to GRRs stemming from the care recipient. This may be the core in an orientation to life, which creates positive life experiences since it enables caregivers to find a "fit" between the possible and desired when resolving challenges (Wennerberg et al., 2016). "Experiencing personal deficiencies," when stemming from themselves and "struggling with an uncooperative co-worker," when stemming from their care recipients were found to be experiences of specific and generalized resistance deficits (Wennerberg et al., 2018).

Generalized Resistance Resources: The Community Level

School Setting

Studies of school settings focused attention on the effect of the school setting features on SOC and its contribution as a mediating factor. Throughout the school years, students are faced with an array of increasingly difficult challenges related to their academic functioning. For instance, a study of the Norwegian education system (Natvig et al., 2006) explored elementary through junior high school children focusing on age and gender comparisons of school-related stress and resources and their relations to the SOC construct. The sample consisted of 4116 school children aged 11, 13, and 15 years old. This study revealed that SOC was related to school-related characteristics, such as feeling pressured by schoolwork, social support from peers, and expectations. Sex and age variables played a significant role indicating that among the group of girls, the association between SOC and school-related characteristics was stronger among the youngest group.

In an attempt to explore the influence of school-related characteristics among youngsters with special needs, studies emphasized the prolonged academic challenges emerging from neurodevelopmental disabilities. As suggested by previous studies, these youngsters' difficulties at school remain a continuous source for increased stress, endless day-to-day struggling with age-appropriate academic roles, and with social and emotional challenges that in turn may contribute to their lower SOC (Idan, 2010; Idan & Margalit, 2014; Lackaye & Margalit, 2006).

As demonstrated by Idan's (2010) study, high levels of SOC were related to high levels of autonomy/competence, measured by a subscale of the Basic Psychological Needs instrument. In general, this construct refers to the individual's natural, innate, and constructive tendencies to develop a unified self. This tendency toward integration is characterized as involving autonomy, tending toward inner organization, self-regulation and homonymy, and tending toward integration of oneself with others. Healthy development involves the complementary functioning of these two aspects (Deci & Ryan, 2008). These inner resources, innate psychological needs, are the bases for integrating the differentiation of goal contents and regulatory processes. Should the needs—competence, autonomy, and relatedness—be satisfied, individuals will develop and function in healthy and optimal ways (Deci & Ryan, 2000).

Idan's (2010) findings showed that the highest levels of SOC and autonomy/competence were reported by females with SLD in a specialized high school compared to typically developing females and females with SLD from regular school classes. The highest levels of SOC and autonomy/competence among adolescent males were reported by typically developing males. This parallelism between females with SLD in a specialized high school and typically developing males, and more interestingly, the females' high scores in levels of SOC and autonomy/competence may be explained by the females' belief that they had more control over their lives. Consequently, these females with SLD from the specialized school were better able to predict their internal and external environments, whether they be positively inclined or not. An additional explanation may lie in the possible role of the classification following diagnosis as SLD in self-evaluation, which in turn may contribute to the level of SOC.

Consequently, as suggested by Idan (2010), girls who had never received such a diagnosis lacked this so-called protection, and bad grades may have been evidence that they were not smart enough to do well in school. On the other hand, boys who were diagnosed in the past with learning disabilities demonstrated declining levels of perceived intelligence regardless of their academic achievement. This suggests that boys may be more concerned with impersonal labeling removed from the classroom setting.

A prominent school-related feature is the role of the teacher as an extrafamilial significant other. An illustration of this, in a study focusing on the perception of teachers as a secure base among children with reading difficulties, Al-Yagon and Margalit (2006) revealed that children's reading difficulties affected their lower level of SOC. Children's perceptions of the teacher as a source of secure base were significantly related to high levels of SOC, emphasizing the possible protective role of extrafamilial figures who provide care and support in times of need.

The above review of school-related characteristics reveals the scarcity of studies is apparent and calls for further exploration, examining in depth the variables that were presented in addition to a variety of other school-related features that may shed light on the school community.

Community Feature

In an attempt to shift from the personal to the collective SOC, based on the understanding that an individual is part of a community, studies have explored possible features of communities that may contribute to collective SOC. Sense of community coherence (Peled et al., 2013) consists of the identical three components of the individual's SOC concept. Comprehensibility refers to the sense of predictability and security felt by the members of a community and the extent to which the community is comprehensible; manageability refers to the ability of the community to assist its members in times of need; and meaningfulness refers to the ability of the members of the community to express themselves in order to feel a higher level of satisfaction and interest within the community. Studies on community ecology revealed its role in predicting SOC development. Being a member of a minority group predicted lower SOC than being a member of a majority group (Braun-Lewensohn & Sagy, 2011a, 2011b). Additionally, social support (Marsh et al., 2007) and neighborhood or community cohesion (García-Moya et al., 2013; Marsh et al., 2007; Peled et al., 2013) were contributing factors in the development of a strong SOC.

In this context of community features, prior studies have also investigated communities that cope with high and extreme levels of stress, such as political violence and war. For example, studies focusing on SOC and political violence revealed SOC as a mediator between exposure to missile attacks and stress-related reactions among adolescents (Braun-Lewensohn et al., 2011) and as a mediator between attitudes toward war and peace within the Israeli–Palestinian conflict and anxiety reactions among adolescents living in a conflictual area (Braun-Lewensohn et al., 2015). In both studies, strong SOC was related to higher resiliency and lower levels of stress-related reactions. In line with the assumption that peaceful ideas were correlated to stronger SOC (Pham et al., 2010), outcomes from the study of Braun-Lewensohn et al.' (2015) suggested that adolescents who supported resolution of the Palestinian–Israeli conflict in peaceful ways had a stronger SOC and were less anxious. In contrast, those who supported more violent conflicts and war did not reveal this relationship. SOC acted as mediator between peace and war attitudes and anxiety solely for peaceful attitudes.

In the context of anxiety-inducing events, natural hazards have also been a source of testing the endurance and resilience of communities. In a study on human resilience in coastal ecosystems following disaster, Matin and Taylor (2015) demonstrated that people with higher education and secure livelihoods have significantly higher resilience scores—including SOC—than those with a lower educational level and insecure livelihoods.

Conclusions and Directions for Further Research and Interventions

Together, the surveyed research studies emphasized the need for continued in-depth exploration of the possible role of different GRR-RDs for understanding individuals' SOC in different developmental phases across the lifespan, as well as through the individual, family, and community ecological levels. Furthermore, based on the expansion to community SOC, such in-depth exploration regarding the GRR-RDs is required. Moreover, in examining the impact of GRR-RDs on individuals' and communities' levels of SOC, it seems important to reconsider the possible role of several factors as follows:

A. *Reciprocal Relationship Between GRR-RDs and SOC*

As mentioned above, the salutogenic theoretical framework proposed that over the lifespan, individuals may develop high levels of SOC through successful applications of GRR-RDs. At the same time, this theoretical framework also assumed a reciprocal and dynamic relationship between SOC and GRR-RDs. Consequently, whereas GRR-RDs may contribute to an individual's and community's levels of SOC, an individual's and community's levels of SOC may, in turn, contribute to mobilizing GRRs for enhancing the ability of stress management (Antonovsky, 1987; Sagy & Dotan, 2001). However, only few research studies reviewed in the present chapter examined this assumption on the reciprocal relationships between these two variables (e.g., Volanen et al., 2004), calling for future investigation regarding the possible bidirectionality of these interrelationships.

B. *Individuals' Differential Susceptibility to Environment Effects*

Previous studies have underscored that individuals may vary in their responsivity to the qualities of their environments, including their childrearing experiences (see Pluess & Belsky, 2011, for a review). These assumptions are generally framed in diathesis-stress or "dual risk" terms, proposing that some individuals tend to be more vulnerable due to their biological/neurological and or behavioral characteristics (i.e., "stress" or "risk 1") to the adverse effects of negative experiences and environmental qualities (i.e., "diathesis" or "risk 2") (Belsky et al., 2007; Belsky & Pluess, 2009; Trentacosta et al., 2008), whereas others may be relatively resilient. Findings from such studies have also pinpointed that individuals may vary not only in the degree to which they are vulnerable to the negative effects of adverse experiences but also, more generally, in their "developmental plasticity" (Boyce & Ellis, 2005). Accordingly, this hypothesis, which was termed the "biological sensitivity to context" (Boyce & Ellis, 2005), or "differential susceptibility hypothesis" (Belsky, 2005), assumes that individuals may vary in their susceptibility to both adverse and beneficial effects of childrearing influences.

Overall, studies analyzing the susceptibility factors that may contribute to individual children's differential susceptibility emphasized the possible role of three categories of variables, such as genetic factors (e.g., short allele of the serotonin transporter linked polymorphic region, 5-HITTLPR), physiological factors (e.g., cortisol reactivity), and behavioral factors (e.g., negative emotionality) (see Pluess & Belsky, 2011 for a review). Such findings call for comprehensive additional exploration regarding individuals' variations in genetic, biological, and behavioral sensitivities, which may predict their susceptibility not only to the adverse effects of GRR-RDs but also to beneficial effects of such factors. Such differential susceptibility has rarely been examined among communities, calling for future comprehensive investigation.

C. *Flexibility Versus Stability*

The current review raises an important question regarding the flexibility versus stability of SOC across the lifespan. Antonovsky (1987) hypothesized that SOC develops during childhood and stabilizes during the early adulthood stage. In contrast, other research proposed SOCs changes over an entire lifetime (e.g., Nilsson et al., 2003; Nilsson et al., 2010). These findings raise several important issues regarding the longitudinal fluctuations as well as stability versus flexibility in individual SOC across the different development phases.

D. *Hedonia, Eudaimonia, and Meaning in Life Perspectives*

In exploring the impact of GRR-RDs on individuals' levels of SOC, further studies may do well to consider exploring the possible role of three additional individual-level orientations—eudaimonia, hedonia (e.g., Huta & Waterman, 2014; Ryan & Deci, 2001; Ryff & Singer, 2008; Steger et al., 2008), and meaning in life (e.g., Costin & Vignoles, 2019; George & Park, 2016; Martela & Steger, 2016; Ryff, 1989). Briefly, eudaimonia is defined as striving to use and develop the best in oneself, in ways that are congruent with one's values and authentic self, including striving for excellence, meaning, acting with virtue, and having concerns beyond the self and beyond the immediate moment (e.g., Huta, 2012). Hedonia is defined as striving to experience pleasure, enjoyment, and comfort, whether through physical- or emotional-cognitive means (Huta & Ryan, 2010). The third concept—meaning in life—has been defined as comprising three distinct subconstructs: comprehension, purpose, and mattering (e.g., George & Park, 2016; Heintzelman & King, 2014; Martela & Steger, 2016; Steger, 2012). As argued by Martela and Steger (2016), *meaning in life* partially coincides with the eudaimonia concept as well as with the SOC concept. Much has been learned in recent years regarding these concepts and their association with a variety of well-being measures (e.g., George & Park, 2016; Huta & Waterman, 2014). However, the possible association with the SOC, as well as the possible role of concepts such as GRR-RDs, has not been sufficiently explored and calls for further investigation.

Selected GRR-RDs

Conceptual matters merit words of caution regarding the possible role of GRR-RDs in understanding individuals' levels of SOC. Since the GRR-RDs reviewed in the current chapter are only few of the possible individual, familial, and community factors, additional resources should be considered. Such resources may include the individual's self-regulation and executive functioning abilities, parental monitoring levels, and parental anxiety, as well as school climate and collective versus individual approach.

Furthermore, such resources may also include GRR-RDs that develop early in life (i.e., neonatal period and birth). As suggested by prior studies (Bauer et al., 2019; Hansson et al., 2008; Silventoinen et al., 2014), neuro-hormonal, epigenetic factors, exposure to risk conditions (e.g., maternal stressors and toxic substances), can set pathways for future well-being. However, such resources have been rarely examined within the SOC framework, calling for additional exploration.

Clinical and Interventional Implications

Acknowledging the importance of SOC as a factor contributing to effective coping with challenges and stressors and well-being, several intervention programs were developed in order to enhance SOC. These interventions highlight the factors that develop SOC throughout the lifespan and emphasize the flexibility of the construct and its potential influences (Janik & Kroger, 2007; Kahonen et al., 2012; Mayer & Boness, 2011; Pallasch & Hameyer, 2008). The following provides examples of interventions promoting SOC in different contexts.

Within the school setting, Mayer and Boness (2011) proposed a didactic model (the team ombuds model) which aimed at promoting SOC and transcultural competencies in educational contexts. Based on studies demonstrating that teachers perceived educational approaches such as concepts of intercultural communication as enriching and stimulating, strengthening self-consciousness, self-worth, and SOC (Pallasch & Hameyer, 2008), the model aimed at promoting GRRs of learners and teachers as well as at ameliorating comprehensibility, manageability, and meaningfulness. It was based on a vertical hierarchy of interacting social units in which learners created teams that were the basis of the educational process. The students who were in a position of trust worked closely with the teachers in resolving conflicts or improving interaction between the students and their teachers. This led to an increase in team competence and individual performance, which decreased feelings of anxiety, dissatisfaction, and uncertainty (Janik & Kroger, 2007). Thus, the learning input was acquired during teamwork (comprehensibility), teamwork was promoted (manageability), and students learned how to learn and set priorities according to their interests (meaningfulness).

Within an occupational context, Kahonen et al. (2012) reported on two group interventions (psychodramatic and analytic) promoting SOC in an occupational healthcare context. The psychodrama method was based on socio- and psychodramatic techniques, such as drawing, music, and writing, and muscle relaxation and exercises using the imagination. The analytic method (Foulkes & Anthony, 1990) was based on free-flowing discussions in order to provide the participants with (1) a sense of security and belonging on the collective level, creating an atmosphere that enables expression of personal feelings; (2) an ability to discuss the feelings awakened by the group on a projective level; and (3) an awareness of one's inner world and its development in the complex relationship between past and present on the transference level. The action-based psychodrama group showed a higher increase in SOC than the dialog-based analytic group, while the improvement in the latter group was significant during the 6-month follow-up. The study concluded that due to its effectiveness, group intervention should be considered an important strategy alongside improvement in the organizational climate and second, that it was possible to enhance SOC by a relatively short group intervention among employees suffering burnout symptoms.

References

Ainsworth, M. D., & Wittig, B. A. (1969). Attachment and exploratory behavior of one-year-olds in a strange situation. In B. M. Foss (Ed.), *Determinants of infant behavior* (Vol. 4, pp. 113–136). Methuen.

Allen, J. P. (2008). The attachment system in adolescence. In J. Cassidy & P. R. Shaver (Eds.), *Handbook of attachment: Theory, research, and clinical applications* (pp. 419–435). Guilford Press.

Al-Yagon, M. (2008). Maternal personal resources and children's socioemotional and behavioral adjustment. *Child Psychiatry and Human Development, 30*, 283–298.

Al-Yagon, M. (2010). Maternal emotional resources and socioemotional well-being of children with and without learning disabilities. *Family Relations, 59*, 152–169.

Al-Yagon, M. (2011). Fathers' emotional resources and children's socioemotional and behavioral adjustment among children with learning disabilities. *Journal of Child and Family Studies, 20*, 569–584.

Al-Yagon, M. (2014a). Child-mother and child-father attachment security: Security: Links to internalizing adjustment among children with learning disabilities. *Child Psychiatry and Human Development, 45*, 119–131.

Al-Yagon, M. (2014b). Fathers and mothers of children with learning disabilities: Links between emotional and coping resources. *Learning Disability Quarterly, 38*(2), 112–128. https://doi.org/10.1177/0731948713520556

Al-Yagon, M., & Margalit, M. (2006). Loneliness, SOC, and perception of teachers as a secure base among children with reading difficulties. *European Journal of Special Needs Education, 21*(1), 21–37.

Antonovsky, A. (1979). *Health, stress and coping*. Jossey-Bass.

Antonovsky, A. (1987). *Unraveling the mystery of health*. Jossey-Bass.

Antonovsky, A. (1991). The structural resources of salutogenic strengths. In C. L. Cooper & R. Payne (Eds.), *Personality and stress: Individual differences in the stress process*. Wiley.

Antonovsky, H., & Sagy, S. (1986). The development of a sense of coherence and its impact on responses to stress situations. *Journal of Social Psychology, 126*, 213–225.

Arteche, A., & Murray, L. (2011). Maternal affective disorder and children's representation of their families. *Journal of Child and Family Studies, 20*, 822–832.

Ayo-Yusuf, O. A., Reddy, P. S., & Van Den Borne, B. W. (2009). Longitudinal association of adolescents' sense of coherence with tooth-brushing using an integrated behaviour change model. *Community Dentistry and Oral Epidemiology, 37*(1), 68–77.

Bauer, G. F., Roy, M., Bakibinga, P., Contu, P., Downe, S., Eriksson, M., … Canal, D. J. (2019). Future directions for the concept of salutogenesis: A position article. *Health Promotion International*. https://doi.org/10.1093/heapro/daz057

Belsky, J. (1984). The determinants of parenting: A process model. *Child Development, 55*, 83–96.

Belsky, J. (2005). Differential susceptibility to rearing influences: An evolutionary hypothesis and some evidence. In B. Ellis & D. B. Jorklund (Eds.), *Origins of the social mind: Evolutionary psychology and child development* (pp. 130–163). Guildford.

Belsky, J., Bakermans-Kranenburg, M. J., & van Ijzendoorn, M. H. (2007). For better and for worse: Differential susceptibility to environmental influences. *Current Directions in Psychological Science, 16*, 300–304.

Belsky, J., & Barends, N. (2002). Personality and parenting. In M. H. Bornstein (Ed.), *Handbook of parenting* (Vol. 3, 2nd ed., pp. 415–438). Lawrence Erlbaum.

Belsky, J., & Pluess, M. (2009). The nature (and nurture?) of plasticity in early human development. *Perspectives on Psychological Science, 4*, 345–351.

Belsky, J., & Pluess, M. (2012). Differential susceptibility to long-term effects of quality of child care on externalizing behavior in adolescence? *International Journal of Behavioral Development, 36*(1), 2–10.

Bernier, A., & Matte-Gagne, C. (2011). More bridges: Investigating the relevance of self-report and interview measures of adults' attachment for marital and caregiving relationships. *International Journal of Behavioral Development, 35*, 307–316.

Bouchard, T. J., & McGue, M. (2003). Genetic and environmental influences on human psychological differences. *Journal of Neurobiology, 54*(1), 4–45.

Bowen, G. L., Richman, J. M., Brewster, A., & Bowen, N. (1998). Sense of school coherence, perceptions of danger at school, and teacher support among youth at risk of school failure. *Child and Adolescent Social Work Journal, 15*, 273–286.

Bowlby, J. (1973). *Attachment and loss: Anxiety, anger, and separation*. Basic Books.

Bowlby, J. (1982). *Attachment and loss: Attachment*. Basic Books. (Original work published 1969).

Boyce, W. T., & Ellis, B. J. (2005). Biological sensitivity to context: An evolutionary-developmental theory of the origins and functions of stress reactivity. *Development and Psychopathology, 17*, 271–301.

Braun-Lewensohn, O., Abu-Kaf, S., & Sagy, S. (2015). Attitudes towards war and peace and their relations with anxiety reactions among adolescents living in a conflictual area. *Journal of Youth Studies, 18*(1), 68–69.

Braun-Lewensohn, O., & Sagy, S. (2011a). Salutogenesis and culture: Personal and community sense of coherence among adolescents belonging to three different cultural groups. *International Review of Psychiatry, 23*(6), 533–541.

Braun-Lewensohn, O., & Sagy, S. (2011b). Coping resources as explanatory factors of stress reactions during missile attacks: Comparing Jewish and Arab adolescents in Israel. *Community Mental Health Journal, 47*(3), 300–310.

Braun-Lewensohn, O., Sagy, S., & Roth, G. (2011). Adolescents under missile attacks: Sense of coherence as a mediator between exposure and stress related reactions. *Journal of Adolescence, 34*, 195–197.

Campbell, S. B. (2003). *Behavior problems in preschool children: Clinical and developmental issues*. Guilford Press.

Cassidy, J., & Shaver, P. R. (2008). *Handbook of attachment: Theory, research, and clinical applications* (2nd ed.). Guilford Press.

Cohen, O. (1997). On the origins of a sense of coherence: Sociodemographic characteristics, or narcissism as a personality trait. *Social Behavior and Personality, 25*(1), 49–58.

Cohen, S. (2004). Social relationships and health. *American Psychologist, 59*, 676–684.

Collins, N. L., & Ford, M. B. (2010). Responding to needs of others: The caregiving behavioral system in intimate relationships. *Journal of Social and Personal Relationships, 27*, 235–244.

Costin, V., & Vignoles, V. L. (2019). Meaning is about mattering: Evaluating coherence, purpose, and existential mattering as precursors of meaning in life judgments. *Journal of Personality and Social Psychology.* https://doi.org/10.1037/pspp0000225

Daoud, N., Polsky-Berger, A., Abu-Kaf, S., & Sagy, S. (2015). *Sense of coherence among women in polygamous and monogamous marriages*. Manuscript in preparation.

Deci, E. L., & Ryan, R. M. (2000). The what and why of goal pursuits: Human needs and the self-determination of behavior. *Psychological Inquiry, 2*(4), 227–268.

Deci, E. L., & Ryan, R. M. (2008). Facilitating optimal motivation and psychological well-being across life's domains. *Canadian Psychology, 49*(1), 14–23.

Evans, W. P., Marsh, S. C., & Weigel, D. J. (2010). Promoting adolescent sense of coherence: Testing models of risk, protection, and resiliency. *Journal of Community and Applied Social Psychology, 20*, 30–43.

Feldt, T., Kokko, K., Kinnunen, U., & Pulkkinen, L. (2005). The role of family background, school success, and career orientation in the development of sense of coherence. *European Psychologist, 10*, 298–308.

Finnbogadottir, H., & Perrson, E. K. (2019). Lifestyle factors, self-reported health and sense of coherence among fathers/partners in relation to risk for depression and anxiety in early pregnancy. *Scandinavian Journal of Caring Sciences, 33*, 436–445.

Florian, V., Mikulincer, M., & Bucholtz, I. (1995). Effects of adult attachment style on the perception and search for social support. *Journal of Psychology, 129*, 665–676.

Fossion, P., Leys, C., Kempenaers, C., Braun, S., Verbanck, P., & Linkowski, P. (2014). Psychological and social-demographic data contributing to the resilience of Holocaust survivors. *Journal of Psychology, 148*(6), 641–657.

Fossion, P., Leys, C., Vandeleur, C., Kempenaers, C., Braun, S., Verbanck, P., et al. (2015). Transgenerational transmission of trauma in families of Holocaust survivors: He consequences of extreme family functioning on resilience, sense of coherence, anxiety and depression. *Journal of Affective Disorders, 171*, 48–53.

Foulkes, S. H., & Anthony, E. J. (1990). *Group psychotherapy*. Karnac.

García-Moya, I., Moreno, C., & Jiménez-Iglesias, A. (2013). Understanding the joint effects of family and other developmental contexts on the sense of coherence (SOC): A person-focused analysis using the Classification Tree. *Journal of Adolescence, 36*, 913–923.

Garcia-Moya, I., Moreno, C., & Rivera, F. (2014). Obtaining a hierarchy of contextual factors in shaping the SOC of male and female adolescents. *Journal of Happiness Studies, 15*, 1267–1287.

García-Moya, I., Rivera, F., Moreno, C., Lindström, B., & Jiménez-Iglesias, A. (2012). Analysis of the importance of family in the development of sense of coherence during adolescence. *Scandinavian Journal of Public Health, 40*, 333–339.

Geckova, A. M., Tavel, P., van Dijk, J., Abel, T., & Reijneveld, S. (2010). Factors associated with educational aspirations among adolescents: Cues to counteract socioeconomic differences? *BMC Public Health, 10*(1), 154.

George, L. S., & Park, C. L. (2016). Meaning in life as comprehension, purpose, and mattering: Toward integration and new research questions. *Review of General Psychology, 20*, 205–220.

Goodman, S. H., & Gotlib, I. H. (2002). *Children of depressed parents*. American Psychological Association.

Grossmann, K. E., Grossmann, K., & Waters, E. (2006). *Attachment from infancy to adulthood*. Guilford Press.

Hansson, K., Cederblad, M., Lichtenstein, P., Reiss, D., Pedersen, N., Belderhiser, J., et al. (2008). Individual resiliency factors from a genetic perspective: Results from a twin study. *Family Process, 47*(4), 537–555.

Heintzelman, S., & King, L. (2014). Life is pretty meaningful. *American Psychologist. 69*, 561–574.

Horsburgh, M. E., & Ferguson, A. L. (2012). Salutogenesis: Origins of health and sense of coherence. In V. H. Rice (Ed.), *Handbook of stress, coping, and health: Implications for nursing research, theory, and practice* (2nd ed., pp. 180–198). Sage Publications.

Huta, V. (2012). Linking peoples' pursuit of eudaimonia and hedonia with characteristics of their parents: Parenting styles, verbally endorsed values, and role modeling. *Journal of Happiness Studies, 13*, 47–61.

Huta, V., & Ryan, R. M. (2010). Pursuing pleasure or virtue: The differential and overlapping well-being benefits of hedonic and eudaimonic motives. *Journal of Happiness Studies, 11*, 735–762.

Huta, V., & Waterman, A. S. (2014). Eudaimonia and its distinction from hedonia: Developing a classification and terminology for understanding conceptual and operational definitions. *Journal of Happiness Studies, 15*, 1425–1456.

Idan, O. (2010). *Socio-emotional self-perceptions and family climate among students with learning disabilities in inclusive classes, typically achieving students from the same classes and students with severe learning disabilities in a special school and their hopeful thinking*. Thesis submitted for the degree "Doctor of Philosophy", Joan and Jaime Constantiner School of Education, Tel Aviv University.

Idan, O., & Margalit, M. (2014). Socio-emotional self-perceptions, family climate, and hopeful thinking among students with learning disabilities and typically achieving students from the same classes. *Journal of Learning Disabilities, 47*(2), 136–152.

Janik, S., & Kroger, J. (2007). *Das team-Ombuds-Modell*. Unpublished research paper.

Kahonen, K., Naatanen, P., Tolvanen, A., & Salmela-Aro, K. (2012). Development of sense of coherence during two group interventions. *Scandinavian Journal of Psychology, 53*, 523–527.

Lackaye, T., & Margalit, M. (2006). Comparisons of achievement, effort and self perceptions among students with learning disabilities and their peers from different achievement groups. *Journal of Learning Disabilities, 39*, 432–446.

Mak, W. W. S., Ho, A. H. Y., & Law, R. W. (2007). Sense of coherence, parenting attitudes and stress among mothers of children with autism in Hong Kong. *Journal of Applied Research in Intellectual Disabilities, 20*, 157–167.

Marsh, S. C., Clinkinbeard, S. S., Thomas, R. M., & Evans, W. P. (2007). Risk and protective factors predictive of sense of coherence during adolescence. *Journal of Health Psychology, 12*, 281–284.

Martela, F., & Steger, M. F. (2016). The three meanings of meaning in life: Distinguishing coherence, purpose, and significance. *The Journal of Positive Psychology, 11*, 531–545.

Matin, N., & Taylor, R. (2015). Emergence of human resilience in coastal ecosystmes under environmental change. *Ecology and Society, 20*(2), 43–52.

Mayer, C.-H., & Boness, C. (2011). Interventions to promoting sense of coherence and transcultural competences in educational contexts. *International Review of Psychiatry, 23*(6), 516–524.

Mikulincer, M., & Shaver, P. R. (2004). Security-based self-representations in adulthood: Contents and processes. In W. S. Rholes & J. A. Simpson (Eds.), *Adult attachment: Theory, research, and clinical implications* (pp. 159–195). Guilford Press.

Mikulincer, M., & Shaver, P. R. (2005). Mental representations of attachment security: Theoretical foundation for a positive social psychology. In M. W. Baldwin (Ed.), *Interpersonal cognition* (pp. 233–266). Guilford Press.

Mikulincer, M., & Shaver, P. R. (2007). *Attachment in adulthood: Structure, dynamics, and change*. Guilford Press.

Nash, J. K. (2002). Neighborhood effects on sense of school coherence and educational behavior in students at risk of school failure. *Children and Schools, 24*, 73–89.

Natvig, G. K., Hanestad, B. R., & Samdal, O. (2006). The role of the student: Salutogenic or pathogenic? *International Journal of Nursing Practice, 12*, 280–287.

Nilsson, B., Holmgren, L., Stegmayr, B., & Westman, G. (2003). Sense of coherence—Stability over time and relation to health, disease, and psychosocial changes in a general population. *Scandinavian Journal of Public Health, 31*, 297–304.

Nilsson, K. W., Leppert, J., Simonsson, B., & Starrin, B. (2010). Sense of coherence and psychological well-being: Improvement with age. *Journal of Epidemiol Community Health, 64*, 347–352.

Olson, D. H. (1986). Circumplex model VII: Validation studies and FACES III. *Family Process, 26*, 337–351.

Olsson, M. B., & Hwang, C. P. (2008). Socioeconomic and psychological variables as risk and protective factors for parental well-being in families of children with intellectual disabilities. *Journal of Intellectual Disability Research, 52*(12), 1102–1113.

Pallasch, W., & Hameyer, U. (2008). Lerncoaching: Coaching to improve learning. In *Theoretical basics and practical examples*. Juventa (German).

Peled, D., Sagy, S., & Braun-Lewensohn, O. (2013). Community perception as coping resource among adolescents living under rockets fire: A salutogenic approach. *Journal of Community Positive Practices, 4*, 681–702.

Pham, P. N., Vinck, P., & Weinstein, H. M. (2010). Human rights, transitional justice, public health and social reconstruction. *Social Science & Medicine, 70*(1), 98–105.

Pisula, E., & Kossakowska, Z. (2010). Sense of coherence and coping with stress among mothers and fathers of children with autism. *Journal of Autism Development Disorder, 40*, 1485–1494.

Pluess, M., & Belsky, J. (2011). Prenatal programming of postnatal plasticity. *Development and Psychopathology, 23*, 29–38.

Read, S., Aunola, K., Feldt, T., Leinonen, R., & Ruoppila, I. (2005). The relationship between generalized resistance resources, sense of coherence, and health among Finnish people aged 65–69. *European Psychologist, 10*, 244–253.

Ristkari, T., Sourander, A., Rønning, J. A., Nikolakaros, G., & Helenius, H. (2008). Life events, self-reported psychopathology and sense of coherence among young men-a population-based study. *Nordic Journal of Psychiatry, 62*, 464–471.

Ryan, R. M., & Deci, E. L. (2001). On happiness and human potentials: A review of research on hedonic and edaimonic well-being. *Annual Review of Psychology, 52*, 141–166.

Ryff, C. D. (1989). Happiness is everything, or is it? Explorations on the meaning of psychological well-being. *Journal of Personality and Social Psychology, 57*, 1069–1081.

Ryff, C. D., & Singer, B. H. (2008). Know thyself and become what you are: A eudaimonic approach to psychological well-being. *Journal of Happiness Studies, 9*, 13–39.

Sagy, S., & Antonovsky, H. (1996). Structural sources of the sense of coherence: Two life stories of Holocaust survivors in Israel. *Israel Journal of Medical Sciences, 32*(3–4), 200–205.

Sagy, S., & Antonovsky, H. (2000). The development of the sense of coherence: A retrospective study of early life experiences in the family. *International Journal of Aging and Human Development, 51*, 155.

Sagy, S., & Dotan, N. (2001). Coping resources of maltreated children in the family: A salutogenic approach. *Child Abuse & Neglect, 25*, 1463–1480.

Schnyder, U., Büchi, S., Sensky, T., & Klaghofer, R. (2000). Antonovsky's sense of coherence: Trait or state? *Psychotherapy and Psychosomatics, 69*, 296–302.

Seiffge-Krenke, I., & Beyers, W. (2005). Coping trajectories from adolescence to young adulthood: Links to attachment state of mind. *Journal of Research on Adolescence, 15*, 561–582.

Sharabi, A., Levi, U., & Margalit, M. (2011). Children's loneliness, sense of coherence, family climate and hope: Developmental risk and protective factors. *The Journal of Psychology, 146*(1–2), 61–83.

Silventoinen, K., Volanen, S.-M., Vuoksimaa, E., Rose, R. J., Suominen, S., & Kaprio, J. (2014). A supportive family environment in childhood enhances the level and heritability of sense of coherence in early childhood. *Social Psychiatry and Psychiatric Epidemiology, 49*(12), 1951–1960.

Smith, L. O., Elder, J. H., Storch, E. A., & Rowe, M. A. (2015). Predictors of sense of coherence in typically developing adolescent siblings of individuals with autism spectrum disorder. *Journal of Intellectual Disability Research, 59*(1), 26–38.

Solcova, I., Kebza, V., Kodl, M., & Kernova, V. (2017). Public health crisis in war and conflict – Health security in aggregate. *Central European Journal of Public Health, 25*(3), 222–227.

Srensen, T., Klungsyr, O., Kleiner, R., & Klepp, O. M. (2011). Social support and sense of coherence: Independent, shared and interaction relationships with life stress and mental health. *International Journal of Mental Health Promotion, 13*, 27–44.

Steger, M. F., Kashdan, T. B., & Oishi, S. (2008). Being good by doing good: Daily eudaimonic activity and well-being. *Journal of Research in Personality, 42*, 22–42.

Steger, M. F. (2012). Experiencing meaning in life: Optimal functioning at the nexus of well-being, psychopathology, and spirituality. In P. T. P. Wong (Ed.), *The human quest for meaning: Theories, research, and applications* (pp. 165–184). Routledge/Taylor & Francis Group.

Trentacosta, C. J., Hyde, L. W., Shaw, D. S., Dishion, T. J., Gardner, F., & Wilson, M. (2008). The relations among cumulative risk, parenting, and behavior problems during early childhood. *Journal of Child Psychology and Psychiatry, 49*, 1211–1219.

Wennerberg, M. M. T., Eriksson, M., Danielson, E., & Lundgren, S. M. (2016). Unravelling Swedish informal caregivers' Generalised Resistance Resources. *Scandinavian Journal of Caring Sciences, 30*, 602–613.

Wennerberg, M. M. T., Eriksson, M., Lundgren, S. M., & Danielson, E. (2018). Unravelling Swedish informal caregivers'. *Generalised Resistance Deficits, 32*, 186–196.

Wennerberg, M. M. T., Lundgren, S. M., Eriksson, M., & Danielson, E. (2019). Me and You in Caregivinghood – Dyadic resistance resources and deficits out of the informal caregiver's perspective. *Aging and Mental Health, 23*(8), 1041–1048.

Volanen, S. M., Lahelma, E., Silventoinen, K., & Suominen, S. (2004). Factors contributing to sense of coherence among men and women. *European Journal of Public Health, 14*, 322–330.

Waters, E., & Cummings, E. (2000). A secure base from which to explore close relationships. *Child Development, 71*, 164–172.

Weismann, U., & Hannoch, H.-J. (2011). Salutogenic perspectives on health maintenance: The role of resistance resources and meaningfulness. *Geropsychology, 24*(3), 127–135.

Ying, Y.-W., Lee, P. A., & Tsai, J. L. (2007). Attachment, sense of coherence, and mental health among Chinese American college students: Variation by migration status. *International Journal of Intercultural Relations, 31*, 531–544.

Zahn-Waxler, C., Duggal, S., & Gruber, R. (2002). Parental psychopathology. In M. H. Bornstein (Ed.), *Handbook of parenting* (Vol. 4, 2nd ed., pp. 295–327). Lawrence Erlbaum.

Zeidner, M., & Aharoni-David, E. (2014). Memories of Holocaust related traumatic experiences, sense of coherence, and survivors' subjective well-being in late life: Some puzzling findings. *Anxiety, Stress, & Coping, 28*(3), 254–271. https://doi.org/10.1080/10615806.2014.954244

13

Salutogenic Model of Health: Conceptual and Concrete Differences

Maurice B. Mittelmark, Marguerite Daniel, and Helga B. Urke

Introduction

This chapter discusses conceptual and concrete differences between generalized and specific resistance resources in the salutogenic model of health. How generalized resistance resources (GRRs) and specific resistance resources (SRRs) are developed differ, with implications for health promotion practice.

To summarize, the main idea is that GRRs arise from the cultural, social, and environmental conditions of living and early childhood rearing and socialization experiences, in addition to idiosyncratic factors and chance (Lamprecht & Sack, 2003; Lindström & Eriksson, 2005). SRRs, on the other hand, are optimized by societal action in which health promotion has a contributing role, for example, the provision of supportive social and physical environments.

The Salutogenic Model of Health Logic

Antonovsky (1987) called for research to develop scientific knowledge about strengthening the sense of coherence. This could be done by building on the resistance resources (RR) that are the properties of individuals, groups, and even situations. GRRs facilitate coping with stressors and strengthen the sense of coherence. Confronting the question of how a strong sense of coherence translates into better health, Antonovsky proposed that "a strong SoC […] allows one to 'reach out,' in any given situation, and apply the resources appropriate to that stressor" (Antonovsky, 1996, p. 15).

The highly simplified salutogenic model of health logic is

$$\text{RR} \rightarrow \uparrow \text{SOC} \rightarrow \uparrow \text{use of RR} \rightarrow \uparrow \text{HEALTH}$$

GRRs and SRRs will be formally defined later, but for now, GRRs are resources that have wide-ranging utility (one's social network, for example). In contrast, SRRs have situation-specific utility (e.g. an emergency phone number to reach the police). Antonovsky felt it was

> …imperative to focus on developing a fuller understanding of those generalized resistance resources that can be applied to meet all demands (Antonovsky, 1972, p. 541), while

> … [SRRs] are often useful in particular situations of tension. A certain drug, telephone lifelines of suicide prevention agencies… can be of great help in coping with particular stressors. But these are all too often matters of chance or luck, as well as being helpful only in particular situations…[and] … it is the GRR that determines the extent to which specific resistance resources are available to us (Antonovsky, 1979, p. 98–99).

This goes a great way toward explaining why Antonovsky's attention was mostly on the left side of this more detailed salutogenic model of health diagram:

$$\text{GRR} \rightarrow \uparrow \text{SOC} \rightarrow \uparrow \text{use of GRR} \\ \& \uparrow \text{use of SRR} \rightarrow \uparrow \text{HEALTH}$$

A more realistic depiction would be a systems-like diagram with double-headed arrows connecting everything to everything. The simplification above is useful for the present purpose, which is to elucidate the GRR/SRR distinction.

SRRs need not always be "matters of chance or luck". Indeed, it is an essential aspect of health promotion to replace chance and luck with fair and dependable availability of SRRs that support health. One of the highest priorities of health promotion is providing supportive environments for health (WHO, 2009). Supportive environments include both GRRs and SRRs, but as suggested in the salutogenic model of health logic above, they have distinctions.

Most of the space in this chapter is devoted to discussing the nature of SRRs and health promotion's role in their

M. B. Mittelmark (✉) · M. Daniel · H. B. Urke
Department of Health Promotion and Development, Faculty of Psychology, University of Bergen, Bergen, Norway
e-mail: maurice.mittelmark@uib.no

nurturance. However, some space is given to a brief overview of the nature of GRRs, to help illuminate distinctions, similarities, and interrelationships between GRRs and SRRs. The reader interested in a full exposition of GRRs is referred to Chap. 12 in this handbook and to chapter 4 in Antonovsky's *Health, Stress and Coping* Antonovsky (1979).

Antonovsky (1979, P. 99) defined a GRR as "any characteristic of the person, the group, or the environment that can facilitate effective tension management". He was quite clear that GRRs and SRRs are not exchangeable concepts: "…it is the GRR that determines the extent to which specific resistance resources are available to us… being literate or being rich… opens the way to exploitation of many specific resistance resources…" (Antonovsky, 1979, pp. 99–100). A perhaps more precise formulation is that when confronted with a particular stressor, a strong sense of coherence enhances one's ability to recognize and activate the most appropriate SRR from those that may be available.

Antonovsky (1979, pp. 103–119) discussed GRRs that operate through physical and biochemical mechanisms (e.g. immune function) that enable the acquisition of SRRs (as money may do), that are intrapersonal (e.g. with ego identity, intelligence, and coping), that are social (interpersonal ties and social embeddedness), and that are cultural (guiding as to how stressors should be encountered). GRRs play two important roles in coping: they help determine the strength of the sense of coherence, *and* they enable the use of specific resistance resources.

Specific Resistance Resources

Neither Antonovsky nor the few others who have written about SRRs have shown much interest in the GRR/SRR differentiation. For example, in Antonovsky's (1979) extremely detailed depiction of the salutogenic model of health (ibid, pp. 184–185), a strong sense of coherence is shown as mobilizing GRRs and SRRs, with no clear differentiation of the two. Both types of resistance resources are posited to have roles in avoiding stressors, in the definition of stimuli and non-stressors, and in overcoming stressors. Antonovsky hardly mentioned SRRs in his *Unraveling the Mystery of Health*, and he did not dwell on the distinction between GRRs and SRRs:

> What the person with the strong SoC does is … [choose] from the repertoire of generalized and specific resistance resources at his or her disposal… (Antonovsky, 1987, p. 138).

Others seem to agree that the GRR/SRR distinction is not particularly important. Poppius (2007) wrote about choosing "from the repertoire of generalized and specific resistance resources […] in what seems to be the most appropriate combination". Nene (2006) noted that the sense of coherence is influenced by GRRs and SRRs and makes no differentiation between them. Sullivan (2006) does make a differentiation, stating that nursing is a GRR while the nurse providing help with a particular problem is an SRR. Yet, Sullivan does not develop that distinction in terms of the role of sense of coherence. Haldeman and Peters (1988) intended to measure SRRs in a study to identify the combination of SRRs and tension that would best predict stress. They operationalized SRRs as satisfaction with family life and family finances, frequency of interactions with friends and relatives, and community resources used. These measures are distant from the concept of SRRs as distinguished from GRRs, even if the number of community resources is measured. SRRs are particular resources used in encounters with particular stressors, as in Antonovsky's example of using a suicide hotline by a suicidal person. Reininghaus et al. (2007) noted the distinction between GRRs and SRRs, in a study of the stress connected to assault on psychiatric nurses, and then rejected the distinction by creating a measure of "stress resistance resources" composed of self-esteem (a GRR), self-confidence (a GRR), received clinical supervision (an SRR), and staff support services (an SRR). Taylor (2004) differentiated GRRs and SRRs in her literature review of salutogenesis as a framework for child protection, but characterized both, without differentiation, as helping people to structure life experiences to reinforce the sense of coherence.

These citations are not "cherry-picked", highly selected counter-examples from an extensive literature in which GRRs and SRRs are discussed: they are all the instances in which SRRs received explicit attention in a reasonably thorough literature search.

Why do SRRs receive so little attention? One answer is that following Antonovsky's lead, there has been all-consuming attention to GRRs and the sense of coherence (Eriksson & Lindström, 2005) and its relationship to health and well-being (Eriksson & Lindström, 2006, 2007). Even if Antonovsky wished health promotion to focus on the sense of coherence as the dependent variable, most researchers have focussed on it as the independent variable. While this could be assumed to drive interest in SRRs as mediators in the sense of coherence/health relationship, such interest is not manifest. On the contrary, there has been little interest in the question of what *mediates* the connection between the sense of coherence and health, despite Antonovsky's postulation that a strong sense of coherence allows one, in any given situation, to apply the appropriate GRR and/or SRR (Antonovsky, 1979).

One additional, critical point needs to be made to clarify why SRRs have received little attention in salutogenic research and why this should be rectified. As already noted, Antonovsky viewed SRRs as all too often matters of chance or luck. In the mid-1990s, he observed that health promotion had not:

> ...confronted the question of the creation of the appropriate social conditions which underlie or facilitate health-promotive behaviors, for example adequate day care facilities and access to health care, not to speak of incomes adequate for decent nutrition and housing. (Antonovsky, 1996, p. 12)

Put in contemporary terms, Antonovsky referred to social determinants of health (e.g. the GRR "income") and supportive social environments (e.g. the SRR "daycare facilities"). Examined closely, what may be a GRR from one person's perspective may be an SRR from another person's perspective. For example, a child daycare facility is an SRR for the parents, and hopefully, a source of GRRs for the child. In contrast, an eldercare facility is an SRR for the resident *and* an SRR for relatives that need professional care assistance.

Antonovsky's criticism of health promotion for not confronting social conditions was perhaps valid for the approach to health promotion that dominated in Europe and the USA in the 1970s and 1980s, concerned mostly with individuals' responsibility for their health and calling for individuals to abandon their risk behaviour to prevent chronic diseases.

However, health promotion has evolved. The 1986 Ottawa Charter for Health Promotion acknowledged individuals' responsibility but emphasized the importance of social determinants of health and creating supportive environments (Eriksson & Lindström, 2008; Kickbusch, 2003). In recent decades, health promotion moved from an almost myopic concern with individuals' health-related lifestyles to a balanced concern with processes for empowering individuals and communities to control their health. In good part, this is accomplished by creating environments supportive of health, or "appropriate social conditions" in Antonovsky's words. Health promotion's concern with appropriate social conditions has taken two forms. One is an overarching emphasis on reducing social inequities in health by a fairer distribution of social resources (Marmot et al., 2008). The other is the health promotion "settings" approach, in which schools, workplaces, and whole communities are considered as locales for health promotion, expanding from the traditional locus of health care in doctors' offices, health clinics, and hospitals (Dooris et al., 2007; Poland et al., 2009). Does health promotion's settings approach mean that it has engaged the SRR concept or the GRR concept? A nuanced answer depends in part on a precise definition of specific resistance resources.

Definition of Specific Resistance Resources

A useful definition of SRRs must distinguish them from GRRs. Bengt Lindström is famous for his illustrated lectures on salutogenesis. A cartoon figure travels across the chalkboard, in the river of life, encountering stressors, trials, and tribulations, equipped with a knapsack stuffed with GRRs acquired during a lifetime (Fig. 13.1). The main point is that the GRRs are already available to be engaged as needed as one encounters various situations creating tension. In concert

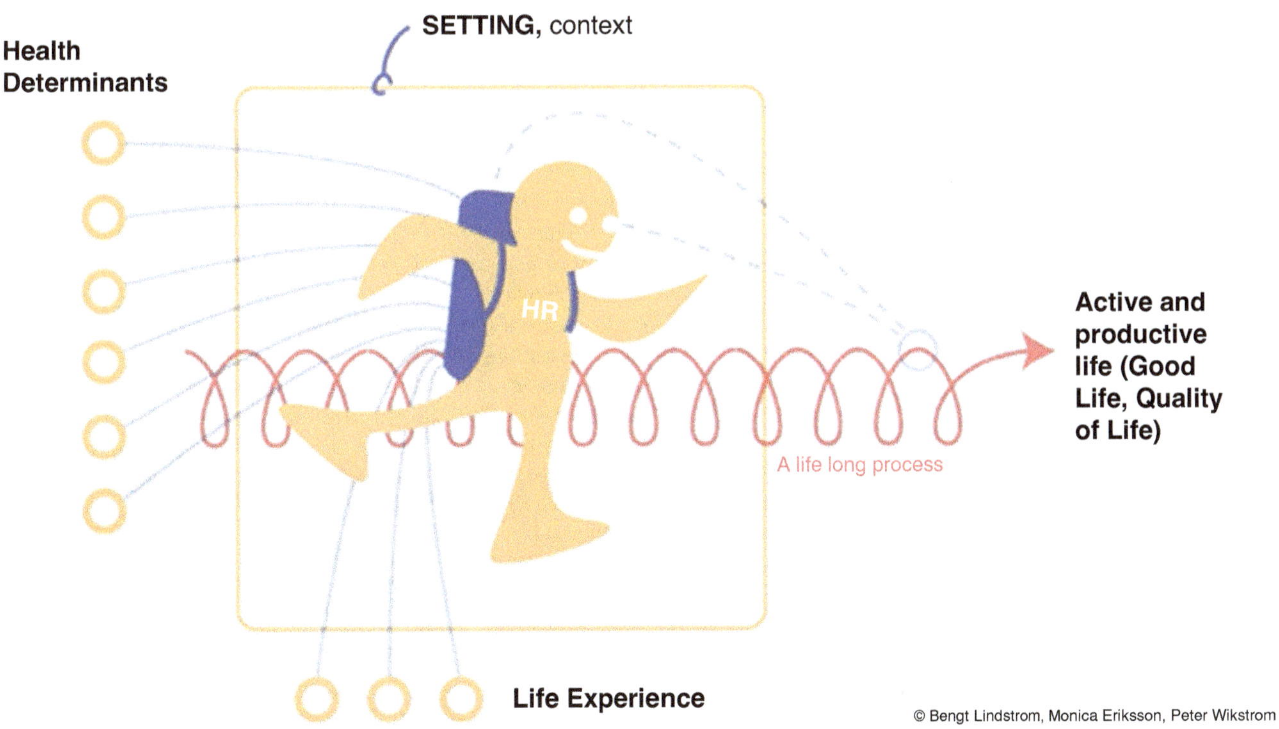

Fig. 13.1 Generalized resistance resources in the knapsack. (© Bengt Lindström, Monica Eriksson, Peder Wikström. All Rights Reserved)

with this metaphor, we conceptualize SRRs as available in the river, picked up and used as needed in specific encounters with stressors, and not necessarily placed in the knapsack afterwards. The relationship between GRRs and SRRs is that via the sense of coherence, GRRs enable one to recognize, pick up, and use SRRs in ways that keep tension from turning into debilitating stress, assuming useful SRRs are available.

A brief example: Having access to and understanding the empowering potential of the Internet is a GRR. The availability of information about your present worrying symptoms on Wikipedia is an SRR. That you have access to, and proactively search for, read, critically evaluate, and use the Wiki's information exemplifies the salutogenic model of health logic:

(a) GRR → ↑ use of SRR → ↑ HEALTH
(b) INTERNET → ↑ SPECIFIC WIKI → ↑ HEALTH

This is, of course, an oversimplification. For example, while the Internet has undoubtedly contributed to an enhanced sense of coherence for many people, it is but one of many GRRs having an equal or more significant influence on the sense of coherence. The diagram's point is not to depict the salutogenic model of health in detail but to show how GRRs and SRRs are substantially different. Of course, health promotion interventions might focus on both—increasing people's unfettered access to the Internet and their skill in using it (enhanced GRR) *and* making websites that address various specific health issues that are of salience when particular nasty symptoms pop up (enhanced SRR).

A formal definition of SRRs is shown in Fig. 13.2, using Facet Theory's sentence mapping approach (Borg & Shye, 1995; Canter, 2012). Antonovsky (1979) used the same approach to define key concepts, including health on the ease/dis-ease continuum (ibid, p. 65), GRRs (ibid, p. 103), and the sense of coherence (Antonovsky, 1987, p. 77). The elements in the three arrays of the mapping sentence definition are not meant to be exhaustive but rather are illustrative.

SRRs are instrumentalities whose meanings are defined in terms of the particular stressors they are invoked to manage.

A GRR is a generality, and an SRR is a particularity.

Usually, SRRs are not invoked unless tension is perceived to threaten to convert to debilitating stress, which many tensions do not. The salutogenic model of health is concerned with ubiquitous tensions that *can* convert to health-threatening levels of stress. Antonovsky (1979, pp. 89–90) listed these:

> …accidents and the survivors; the untoward experiences of others in our social networks; the horrors of history in which we are involved; intrapsychic, unconscious conflicts and anxieties; the fear of aggression, mutilation and destruction; the events of history brought into our living rooms; the changes of the narrower world in which we live, phase-specific psychosocial crises; other normative life crises—role entries and exits; inadequate socialization, underload, and overload; the inherent conflicts in all social relations; and the gap between culturally inculcated goals and socially structured means.

A useful examination of the differences between GRRs and SRRs should be undertaken with this understanding of psychosocial stressors in mind. At extremes—surviving a plane crash, taking an exam—stressors are stressors from the start or tensions that simply remain tensions.

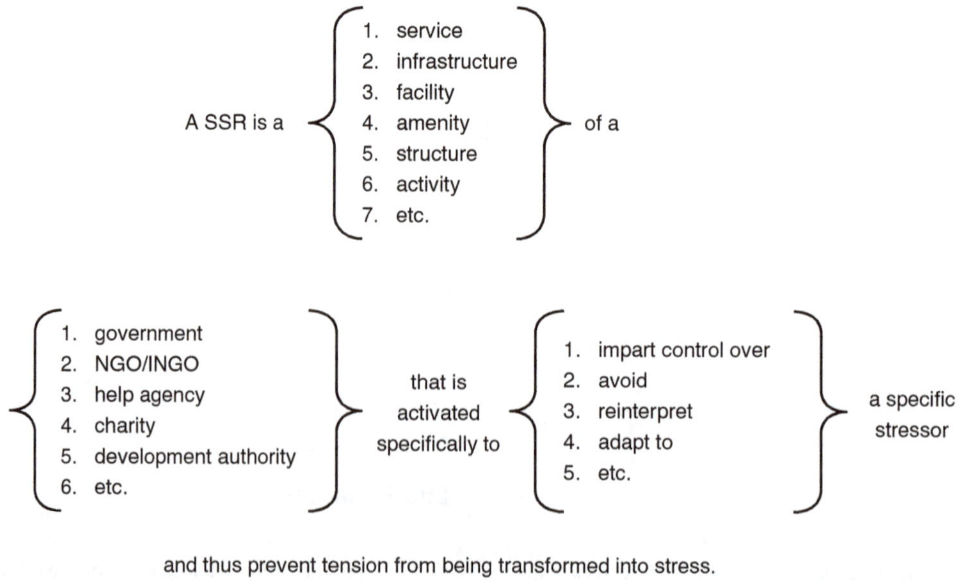

Fig. 13.2 Mapping sentence definition of specific resistance resources. (Reproduced with permission from Mittelmark et al. (2017))

Examples of Specific Resistance Resources

Health-Promoting Schools in Norway

Virtually all adolescents attending school are stressed by the demands of maturation, peer relations, teachers' demands, home and community conditions, and so on. In this cauldron of tension, schools in Norway (and in many other countries) have implemented *Health Promoting Schools* programmes which aim to support educational goals by attending to the health and well-being of all who inhabit the school milieu; students, teachers, administrators, parents, and neighbourhoods (Langford et al., 2015; Tjomsland et al., 2009; Wold & Mittelmark, 2018). The health-promoting school strives to meet these goals:

- Promote the health and well-being of students.
- Enhance the learning outcomes of students.
- Uphold social justice and equity concepts.
- Provide a safe and supportive environment.
- Promote student participation and empowerment.
- Link health and education issues and systems.
- Address the health and well-being issues of all school staff.
- Collaborate with parents and the local community.
- Integrate health into the school's ongoing activities, curriculum, and assessment standards.
- Set realistic goals built on accurate data and sound scientific evidence.
- Seek continuous improvement through ongoing monitoring and evaluation.

Thus, the health-promoting school aims to be a powerful GRR for the youth, the staff, the parents, and the surrounding community. The Norwegian school is also a repository of, or a portal to, some SRRs, offered through the school nursing service (Moen & Skundberg-Kletthagen, 2018) and other student-support services. Examples include support for pregnant students to help keep them in school, special education teachers and facilities equipped to help students with learning disabilities, and referral to community child protection services in cases of need.

These SRRs are present in or around the school, but they are not particularly salient to the adolescents that do not need them, and therefore do not use them. The school as a GRR helps contribute in a general way to strengthen the sense of coherence of many pupils, and a strong sense of coherence facilitates the uptake/use of particular SRRs when the need should arise. Let us consider two students. Jack has a typical day, experiencing "normal" strain and hassles, but nothing out of the ordinary happens. SRRs abound, but this student makes use of none of them; they are not salient. On the same day, Jill discovers she is pregnant, and her sense of coherence is high enough that she does not panic and sink into depression. Instead, she contacts the pregnancy support programme, which she knows about and trusts because of other pupils' good experiences. The pregnancy support programme is an SRR for this student, offering highly salient services at this inflection point in her life.

There is a vexing equity dimension to this. If SRRs are more readily available to those with lots of GRRs (e.g. money), SRRs might contribute to a widened equity gap. Equality in access to SRRs depends on a reasonably fair distribution of GRRs, so health promotion needs to focus on both types.

Child Health in the Andean Highlands in Peru

Perhaps the most apparent SRRs are social services established to provide targeted assistance to groups living in conditions that impart severe vulnerability (Mittelmark, 2021). A prime example was documented in research in a remote and low-income district in the Andean highlands in Peru (Urke et al., 2013). The field researcher (Urke) interviewed mothers with local reputations for providing good childcare. All the mothers participated in a Peruvian NGO-run social and health programme. The interviewer did not mention the NGO programme—a clear example of a social services SRR—to avoid prompting. The respondents explicitly referred to it and attributed improved health-related knowledge and skills to the NGO interventions that included education about nutritious meal preparation, childcare skills, and sanitation practices. This project also illuminated the close relation between GRRs and SRRs. There was some evidence that the women with more GRRs (such as money and social support in the home and the community) benefited more from the NGO's activities than did the women with fewer GRRs.

Support Services for Orphaned Children and Adolescents in Botswana

Another example of NGO-as-SRR is described in research from Botswana (Thamuku & Daniel, 2012). In collaboration with the Botswana Department of Social Services, the Botswanan NGO People and Nature Trust developed a programme called Ark for Children to provide support services for orphaned children and adolescents. They employ culturally appropriate interventions to strengthen orphans and build them into cohesive groups of age-mates who support each other. *Ark for Children* organizes 16-day retreats for up to 40 adolescent orphans from the same village. The retreats harken to historical *Setswana* initiation rites and link with cultural traditions recognized by the members of the adolescents' community. The adolescents are followed up in a 3-year support programme. This is an illuminating example of an SRR (*Ark for Children*) that builds GRRs (social cohesion and supportive ties).

Sexual Orientation and Gender-Identity Support Services in the USA

Identity-based adversity begins early in life, affecting the availability and development of GRRs. Young people's experience of sexual orientation prejudice is exemplified in many cases by bullying, harassment, rejection, social isolation, and internalization of negative attitudes and beliefs. Gender-identity adversity is framed by stigma arising from societal norms and biases (Horn, 2019). While sexual preference-related adversity is typically an emergent feature in adolescence and young adulthood, gender-role tension may have roots in earliest childhood behaviour. Little boys are encouraged to dress, think, and act like boys "should" and little girls to act like girls, with norms varying according to their culture. Boys holding hands beyond young childhood is not gender-consistent in many cultures but is normative in other cultures. This points out that salutogenesis' relevance to identity-based adversity, tension, and coping is complex, rooted in culture and impacting one's early life experience, the acquisition of GRRs, the availability and use of SRRs, and therefore the development of the SOC.

In this chapter on the nature of SRRs, we turn aside momentarily, noting that the experience of and developing resilience to gender-related prejudice may be a GRR. In their research with young adults in the USA, Schmitz and Tyler's (2018) respondents explained it in ways like this: *"[My lesbian identity] opens up a lot more doors… I think that [it] opens up opportunities for friendship because you like to confide in people that have similar situations, so I think it builds stronger relationships"*.

Now narrowing the discussion to SRRs, we focus on just one dimension of salutogenesis and gender-based identity: the tension, stress, and coping-enabling SRRs of young persons with lesbian, gay, bisexual, transgender, and queer (LGBTQ[1]) identities. In coping research with lesbian, gay, and bisexual (LGB) American Latino and non-Latino young adults, Toomey et al. (2018) examined the use of three types of coping strategies: engagement of SRRs, alternatives-seeking strategies (e.g. finding new friends), and cognitive strategies (e.g. imagining a better future). Regarding SRRs, respondents reported employing a closely knit constellation of coping behaviours, including getting involved in LGBT groups and organizations, looking for services for LGBT youth, and looking for information on LGBT issues.

Similar findings are reported by Asakura (2016), whose LGBTQ respondents reported coping by engaging in collective action, by participating in safe social spaces like gay-straight alliances, and by accessing social services from organizations that welcome gender and sexual diversity among youth. Likewise, Schmitz and Tyler (2018) observed the importance of institutional support in LGBT coping. As one college student expressed it, "[the campus] is very open and accepting… there are plenty of resources on campus, specifically for LGBT students".

Non-institutional SRRs in Caregiving Dyads in Sweden

Figure 13.2 may convey an impression that SRRs are exclusively facilities and organizations whose mission is to provide specific types of assistance to people with particular needs. Yet, the definition does embrace the concept of SRRs in the private sphere ("activities", listed sixth in the first facet of the definition). This has been well described in a Swedish programme of research with caregiving dyads in which care was provided to persons aged 65+ (Wennerberg et al., 2016). Caregivers' overall feelings of competence in being a caregiver—a GRR in the researchers' analysis—were bolstered by caregiver SRRs such as having enough physical strength to provide physically demanding care activities (e.g. lifting) and having the professional/technical knowledge required for managing complex medication regimes. In these caregiving dyads, having children and grandchildren functioned as an SRR, a shared experience that was a mutual pleasure to the dyad (Wennerberg et al., 2019). A mutual understanding of the caregiving situation and good dyad communication skills was also revealed as an important SRR (ibid). For dyads in assisted living facilities, the facility—an SRR—enabled caregivers to gain/regain personal SRRs that had been problematic in their homes (SRR deficits). Examples cited by respondents included shopping facilities in the living complex, elevators, and apartments that were disability adapted (Eriksson et al., 2017).

The Swedish studies cited above also report findings regarding general and specific resources deficits (GRDs and SRDs) (Wennerberg et al., 2019). A discussion of GRDs and SRDs is beyond this chapter's scope. Still, it is in place to mention that the general-specific differentiation also pertains to negative life experiences, unsuccessful tension management, and a weakened sense of coherence. A caregiver's loss of a well-functioning partner is simultaneously a GRD—the

[1] Some of the acronyms used below vary from this form, following the usages of the various authors cited.

fading quality and equality of a mutually caring and sharing relationship—and an SRD as in the care receiver's reduced ability to reciprocate care (ibid).

Conclusion

This chapter's aim has been modest, to illuminate a part of the salutogenic model of health that seems to be overlooked—SRRs have as much or more relevance to health promotion practice as do GRRs. By drawing attention to SRRs, one also draws attention to what should be a core aim of health promotion: to ensure that the availability of the right SRR at the right time is not all too often a matter of "chance or luck", as Antonovsky worried.

References

Antonovsky, A. (1972). Breakdown. A needed fourth step in the conceptual armamentarium of modern medicine. *Social Science and Medicine, 6*, 537–544.

Antonovsky, A. (1979). *Health, stress and coping*. Jossey-Bass.

Antonovsky, A. (1987). *Unraveling the mystery of health—How people manage stress and stay well*. Jossey-Bass.

Antonovsky, A. (1996). The salutogenic model as a theory to guide health promotion. *Health Promotion International, 11*(1), 11–18.

Asakura, K. (2016). Paving pathways through the pain: A grounded theory of resilience among lesbian, gay, bisexual, trans and queer youth. *Journal of Research on Adolescence, 27*(3), 521–536.

Borg, I., & Shye, S. (1995). *Facet theory: Form and content*. Sage.

Canter, D. (Ed.). (2012). *Facet theory: Approaches to social research*. Springer.

Dooris, M., Poland, B., Kolbe, L., De Leeuw, E., McCall, D. S., & Wharf-Higgins, J. (2007). Healthy settings. In D. V. McQueen & C. M. Jones (Eds.), *Global perspectives on health promotion effectiveness* (pp. 327–352). Springer.

Eriksson, M., & Lindström, B. (2005). Validity of Antonovsky's sense of coherence scale: A systematic review. *Journal of Epidemiology and Community Health, 59*(6), 460–466.

Eriksson, M., & Lindström, B. (2006). Antonovsky's sense of coherence scale and the relation with health: A systematic review. *Journal of Epidemiology and Community Health, 60*(5), 376–381.

Eriksson, M., & Lindström, B. (2007). Antonovsky's sense of coherence scale and its relation with quality of life: A systematic review. *Journal of Epidemiology and Community Health, 61*(11), 938–944.

Eriksson, M., & Lindström, B. (2008). A salutogenic interpretation of the Ottawa Charter. *Health Promotion International, 23*(2), 190–199.

Eriksson, M., Wennerberg, M. M. T., Lundgren, S. M., & Danielson, E. (2017). "Self-employed" in caregiving hood: The contribution of Swedish informal caregivers' environmental and contextual resistance resources and deficits. *Societies, 7*(3), 19. https://doi.org/10.3390/soc7030019

Haldeman, V. A., & Peters, J. M. (1988). Using resistance resources to reduce stress: A study of rural Nevadans. *Journal of Family and Economic Issues, 9*(4), 357–366.

Horn, S. S. (2019). Sexual orientation and gender identity-based prejudice. *Child Development Perspectives, 13*(1), 21–27.

Kickbusch, I. (2003). The contribution of the World Health Organization to a new public health and health promotion. *American Journal of Public Health, 93*(3), 383–388.

Lamprecht, F., & Sack, M. (2003). Vulnerability and salutogenesis in health and disease. *Public Health Reviews, 31*(1), 7–21.

Langford, R., Bonell, C., Jones, H., Pouliou, T., Murphy, S., Waters, E., ... Campbell, R. (2015). The World Health Organization's Health Promoting Schools framework: A Cochrane systematic review and meta-analysis. *BMC Public Health, 15*(1), 130.

Lindström, B., & Eriksson, M. (2005). Salutogenesis. *Journal of Epidemiology and Community Health, 59*(6), 440–442.

Marmot, M., Friel, S., Bell, R., Houweling, T. A., Taylor, S., & Commission on Social Determinants of Health. (2008). Closing the gap in a generation: Health equity through action on the social determinants of health. *The Lancet, 372*(9650), 1661–1669.

Mittelmark, M. B. (2021). Resilience in the salutogenic model of health. In M. Ungar (Ed.), *Multisystemic resilience: Adaptation and transformation in changing*. Springer.

Mittelmark, M. B., Bull, T., Daniel, M., & Urke, H. (2017). Specific resistance resources in the salutogenic model of health. In M. B. Mittelmark, S. Sagy, M. Eriksson, G. Bauer, J. M. Pelikan, B. Lindström, & G. A. Espnes (Eds.), *The handbook of salutogenesis*. Springer International Publishing.

Moen, Ø. L., & Skundberg-Kletthagen, H. (2018). Public health nurses' experience, involvement and attitude concerning mental health issues in a school setting. *Nordic Journal of Nursing Research, 38*(2), 61–67.

Nene, N. (2006). *Compassion fatigue and the sense of coherence in caregivers working with sexually abused children in Soweto*. Doctoral dissertation, University of the Witwatersrand, Johannesburg.

Poland, B., Krupa, G., & McCall, D. (2009). Settings for health promotion: An analytic framework to guide intervention design and implementation. *Health Promotion Practice, 10*(4), 505–516.

Poppius, E. S. K. O. (2007). *The sense of coherence and health. The effects of the sense of coherence on risk of coronary heart disease, cancer, injuries and all-cause mortality*. Tampereen yliopisto.

Reininghaus, U., Craig, T., Gournay, K., Hopkinson, P., & Carson, J. (2007). The high secure psychiatric hospitals' nursing staff stress survey 3: Identifying stress resistance resources in the stress process of physical assault. *Personality and Individual Differences, 42*(3), 397–408.

Schmitz, R. M., & Tyler, K. A. (2018). 'Life has actually become more clear': An examination of resilience among LGBTQ young adults. *Sexualities, 22*(4), 710–733.

Sullivan, G. C. (2006). Evaluating Antonovsky's Salutogenic Model for its adaptability to nursing. *Journal of Advanced Nursing, 14*(4), 336–342.

Taylor, J. S. (2004). Salutogenesis as a framework for child protection: Literature review. *Journal of Advanced Nursing, 45*(6), 633–643.

Thamuku, M., & Daniel, M. (2012). The use of rites of passage in strengthening the psychosocial well-being of orphaned children in Botswana. *African Journal of AIDS Research, 11*(3), 215–224.

Tjomsland, H. E., Iversen, A. C., & Wold, B. (2009). The Norwegian network of health promoting schools: A three-year follow-up study of teacher motivation, participation and perceived outcomes. *Scandinavian Journal of Educational Research, 53*(1), 89–102.

Toomey, R. B., Ryan, C., Diaz, R. M., & Russell, S. T. (2018). Coping with sexual orientation-minority stress. *Journal of Homosexuality, 65*(4), 484–500.

Urke, H. B., Bull, T., & Mittelmark, M. B. (2013). Child diet and healthy growth in the context of rural poverty in the Peruvian Andes: What influences primary caregivers' opportunities and choices? *Global Health Promotion, 20*(3), 5–13.

Wennerberg, M. M. T., Eriksson, M., Danielson, E., & Lundgren, S. M. (2016). Unravelling Swedish caregivers' generalized resistance resources. *Scandinavian Journal of Caring Sciences, 30*, 602–613.

Wennerberg, M. M. T., Lundgren, S. M., Eriksson, M., & Danielson, E. (2019). Me and you in caregivinghood – Dyadic resistance resources and deficits out of the informal caregiver's perspective. *Aging & Mental Health, 23*(8), 1041–1048.

Wold, B., & Mittelmark, M. B. (2018). Health-promotion research over three decades: The social-ecological model and challenges in implementation of interventions. *Scandinavian Journal of Public Health, 46*(20_suppl), 20–26.

World Health Organization. (2009). *Milestones in health promotion. Statements from global conferences*. WHO Press, World Health Organization.

Part III

Life Course and Sense of Coherence (SOC)

14

Importance of SOC in the Life Course

Claudia Meier Magistretti

Introduction

Antonovsky understood the sense of coherence (SOC) as the outcome of learning processes that begin at the time of birth, or even earlier. To create a strong SOC, these processes should provide challenges that are perceived as consistent, that allow participation, and are characterised by an underload–overload balance. Initially, Antonovsky considered the SOC to be relatively stable after early adulthood, with only minor fluctuations occurring after that. Later, he clarified that stability of the SOC pertains mainly for adults with a strong SOC, since "the person who has, in early adulthood, crystallised a strong SOC, [has] the ability to bring into play the generalised resistance resources available to him or her" (Antonovsky, 1987, p. 121).

Antonovsky assumed that early childhood is a critical period to create a strong SOC. He conceptualised the infant as an active subject that can interact in ways that produce stable, consistent response interactions (Antonovsky, 1987, p. 94). These actions occur very early, according to Antonovsky, immediately after birth.

Relating to Bowlby's attachment theory, he developed the idea that a strong sense of comprehensibility is fostered early in life by the consistent experience of parents' and other caregivers' responsiveness and sensitivity. Still, Antonovsky criticised the imperative for parents to be always consistent and responsive, stating that real life is far more complex. Perfectly responsive parents do not exist, because multiple tasks and demanding environments are the reality for all. On the contrary, "natural" frustrations are necessary to create a sense of comprehensibility. When the infant learns that objects and satisfactions can disappear and reappear, he or she learns about the continuity (and to a certain extent the predictability) of social interactions.

C. Meier Magistretti (✉)
Centre for Health Promotion and Participation, Lucerne University of Applied Sciences and Arts, Lucerne, Switzerland
e-mail: claudia.meiermagistretti@hslu.ch

Manageability is, according to Antonovsky, built by experiences of load balance fostered by parents that respect their child's abilities at different stages of development. Using the example of forced toilet training in toddlers, Antonovsky describes how overloading demands are created when the biological and psychological realities of the child are not sufficiently recognised. Consequently, the development of the sense of manageability can be disturbed or hindered by inappropriate expectations of a child's caregivers. In Antonovsky's thinking, load balance is achieved when a demand corresponds to the child's development state, in the sense that it is somehow "reasonable" and when it is subjected to the child's choice.

The sense of meaningfulness develops by participation in decision-making, which in early childhood occurs when the infant experiences that his or her actions produce the desired reaction in the adult. "To the extent that desired outcome is contingent on the infant and child's action", Antonovsky stated, "it can reasonably be said that early on there is participation in decision making" (Antonovsky, 1985, p. 97). The sense of meaningfulness in the early stage of life is fostered by the infant's experience of being able to pressure the environment to act and thereby comprehend that she or he *matters* to the parents or other caregivers.

In adolescence, the SOC is potentially volatile, and the basis that has been laid in childhood for a strong the SOC may become upset. This stage of life is characterised by transitions and a constant balancing of a fragile identity between "not anymore" and "not yet". Antonovsky related the development of the SOC to Erik Erikson's main developmental tasks that adolescents have to face in all cultures:

- First, they are challenged to develop a personality within a social reality that they have to understand.
- Second, they have to "get their act together" to acquire a "vitalising sense of reality" (Erikson, 1950, p. 89).
- Third, they need growing experience mastering challenges.

The sense of comprehensibility is reinforced by the growing ability of the adolescent to develop a sense of reality. The experience of mastering challenges nurtures the sense of manageability. The sense of meaningfulness is supported by a "vitalising" way to deal with reality. Still, Antonovsky appreciated that adolescence is a fragile period of life, needing adult guidance.

Adulthood is perceived as a period of life where roles and GRRs are decisive for the development of the SOC and for shaping identity. Antonovsky assumed that in the first decade of adulthood, an individual tends to put together the new roles he or she assumes at work, in partnership, in creating a family, and in society. While some of these new roles may weaken the individual's SOC, others may strengthen it. The SOC is assumed to remain somewhat volatile in this period of life. Antonovsky supposed (but gave indications of not being entirely convinced) that at the end of the second decade, individuals have sorted out or accepted the different areas of life, and "one has attained a given location on the SOC continuum" (Antonovsky, 1987, p. 119).

Following Antonovsky's passing in 1994, Lindström and Eriksson (2010) defined the development of the SOC as a *lifelong learning* process. Analysing SOC levels in different age groups in longitudinal studies, they observed the SOC's tendency to strengthen with age (Lindström & Eriksson, 2010). The strengthening of the SOC over the lifespan is—neglecting some fluctuations—continuous, consistent over different measurement scales (SOC-13, the SOC-29), steady, and moderate.

Nevertheless, we know little about how the development of a stronger SOC occurs. Only recently, Maas and colleagues (2017) investigated mechanisms strengthening the SOC in adults. They found that systematic, coherent experiences in everyday life might play a crucial role in building a strong SOC.

Significant life events may cause fluctuations in the SOC. Becoming a parent, for example, is posited to be s a critical life experience that may alter one's SOC (Lindström et al., 2017). From the perspective of anthropological pedagogics, we can hypothesise that the SOC, as any other learning outcome, could benefit from sensitive phases of development. These have been studied in children as a developmental phase of specific readiness to learn, which enables a person to acquire specific skills and characteristics relatively effortlessly (e.g. Montessori, 1995). Further investigation of the SOC as a lifelong learning process may reveal critical points throughout life when the SOC is particularly prone to change.

As the preceding discussion shows, the development of the SOC is understood as a lifelong learning process. Among the important questions about this process are as follows:

- What are the crucial factors that contribute to build, enhance, and strengthen the SOC during the life course?
- Is the role of the SOC in coping stable during the life course, or does it have different functions at different life stages? For example, does the SOC open one to new GRRs at the beginning and facilitate access to GRRs later in life?
- Can salutogenic interventions strengthen the SOC during various phases in the lifespan?

The chapters in this part of the Handbook tackle all three of these questions with varying emphasis at different periods of life.

Childhood and Families

Chapter 15 on salutogenesis and the sense of coherence in families and children deals with the contributions of children's environments to the adjustment of children with typical development and the development of children with special needs. The chapter starts with a short description of childhood development. Orly Idan and colleagues report on their comprehensive literature review covering 20 years of research and 44 studies from 15 countries, including children from infants and toddlers through preschool to school-aged children up to 12 years of age. The construction and use of the children's SOC scale and methodological considerations are discussed. Also in focus is the influence of the SOC on various health outcomes, and children's emotional, social, and cognitive development (both in children with regular development and in children facing challenging life circumstances, health-related adversity, and special needs).

The chapter concludes that the SOC plays a significant protective role at school and emphasises the crucial role of teachers' ability to engage with children in responsive and caring relationships. For families with children with special needs, the SOC is demonstrated to be a significant protective factor related to coping and hopeful thinking, as well as to parental adjustment and effective coping outcomes. The chapter also provides examples of programs to foster the SOC in young children, by promoting play and reinforcing self-worth in the first years of school.

Adolescence

In Chap. 16 by Braun-Lewensohn and colleagues, the focus is on salutogenesis and the sense of coherence during the adolescent years. The authors' approach is itself salutogenic, in the sense that they develop their arguments in line with a positive youth development perspective. Adolescents are appreciated as individuals eager to explore the world, to acquire competence, and to struggle with challenges and difficulties, rather than as a vulnerable group in need of risk prevention, cure, and treatment for maladaptive tendencies.

Still, the literature is replete with studies of the authors' review of more than 30 studies in 16 countries shows a significant role of the SOC for physical and mental health, health behaviour, social adaption, and academic or professional success of adolescents. This is demonstrated for the individual the SOC (in several studies measured by specific adolescent the SOC scales) and hypothesised for family and community the SOC. In adolescence, the SOC is a predictor for physical health and the use of medication in consequence.

The studies reviewed in this chapter confirm that a strong SOC is associated with reduced stress, and decreased internalising/externalising of problems. Related to health behaviours, adolescents with stronger SOC report a more healthy lifestyle as well as a better quality of life and well-being. The authors report on studies observing that a strong SOC in adolescence is associated with higher levels of physical activity and exercise, less tobacco and alcohol use, and healthier eating habits.

Factors strengthening the SOC in adolescence are discussed, with an emphasis on the child's socio-ecological context, such as open family communication, child-centred parenting, and parents' knowledge regarding their children's activities. The authors also discuss how social support and neighbourhood and community cohesion may play a positive role in the development of a strong SOC in adolescence.

Transitions in Adulthood

Salutogenic research with adults has focused on their roles in workplaces, families, communities, and caregiving institutions. Researchers have tended to neglect the lifetime and developmental perspective of adult age. This might reflect a general view of the adult as a performing, not as a developing individual. It might be, as well, a consequence of methodological difficulties in describing transitions at various points of life in biographies that may deviate from a formerly "normal" life course, becoming more and more diverse.

Nevertheless, lifespan developmental psychology of the past two decades provides an understanding of adulthood as a series of interrelated transitions (Sugarman, 2001). Transition periods have been shown to play a crucial role in one's adaption to life stressors, and the development of physical and mental health throughout the life course.

In Chap. 17, Claudia Meier Magistretti and Beat Reichlin treat the topic of the transition from adolescence to adulthood and focus on young adults facing difficulties during this transition. Young adults not in education, employment, or training (NEETs) emerged only recently as an interest in public health and health promotion debate. Although estimates of the number of NEETS vary, the problem seems to be global and growing. This has stimulated the International Labour Organisation to talk in terms of "a generation at risk". Yet, the many programs that try to support NEETs fail to reach them and guide them successfully into work, housing, and social participation.

The authors consider why current initiatives to assist NEETs do not produce sustainable effects. "Helping" systems regard NEETs as patients, cases, or not yet enabled adults and thereby fail to meet their needs as well as their potential. Confronting the limits of current approaches, the authors emphasise the need for a salutogenic orientation in research and practice with NEETs. To provide guidance and inspiration in this direction, the authors describe new and promising NEET initiatives. These initiatives are characterised by having a genuine health orientation, NEET participation, the centrality of learning processes, and flexible, adaptive models of individual and social development in combination with enhanced employment, education, training, and entrepreneurship opportunities.

In Chap. 18, Ottomar Bahrs and colleagues focus on the transition from middle to late adulthood. The questions of when and how past transitions affect subsequent aging are discussed. While middle age was long considered undramatic, the authors state that it is increasingly gaining profile. They focus on a phase typically observed in the sixth decade of life, characterised by the initiation of the transition to deprofessionalisation and change of responsibilities within the family when crisis and chronic situations can lead to the need for help from health professionals.

Bahrs and colleagues deliberate on how a dialogue between middle-aged adults and professionals can contribute positively to the naming, modification, design, and further development of health goals, linking physiological and unconscious processes to the theory of salutogenesis.

Notably, the authors frame illness processes from the perspective of salutogenic resources, also discussing the *benefits* of crises experienced in middle adulthood.

I hope the authors' novel ideas about a salutogenic perspective on life in middle adulthood will inspire researchers and practitioners to a more innovative approach to this large segment of society.

Older Age

In Chap. 19, Maria Koelen and Monica Eriksson consider the meanings of the concepts of healthy aging, aging well, salutogenic aging, and reciprocity between the SOC and aging processes. They discuss how the community can provide resources to strengthen older adults' SOC, perceived well-being, and quality of life. Quoting "It's not how old we are; it's how we are old", the authors illuminate critical differences in understanding healthy aging by professionals, researchers, and older people themselves.

While professionals tend to focus on negatively phrased topics (e.g. disability, disease, loneliness), older people emphasise a supportive social environment, the ability to use resources, to manage restrictions, and to make one's own decisions. As the authors clarify, evidence on the potential for enhanced health at older age points clearly to these factors: participation in social networks, contact with family and friends, and engagement in leisure and social activities. Since many of the prerequisites to strengthen general resistance resources (GRRs), specific resistance resources (SRRs), and the SOC are provided by or mediated through the community, the authors emphasise the role of intergenerational and age-friendly communities in providing supportive neighbourhood environments, social cohesion, and adequate transportation facilities for older people, and support for their ability to continue living in their own homes.

Enhancing the Sense of Coherence along the Life Span

Chapter 20, by Eva Langeland and colleagues, is titled *Effectiveness of interventions to enhance the sense of coherence in the life course: a summary of the empirical evidence.* It provides an overview of the effectiveness of programs and interventions that aim to strengthen the SOC throughout the lifespan. The authors report on more than 40 studies investigating the effectiveness of interventions to strengthen the SOC. They structure and summarise findings for young people, employed and unemployed adults, health professionals, people with disabilities, people with psychosomatic and mental health problems, people with physical problems, hospital patients, and older people. Even though most studies are limited to short-term pre-test and post-test study designs, a few studies have investigated the effects of intervention for longer follow-up periods of up to several months, and even more than 1 year.

The authors classified interventions on the extent of their salutogenic orientation, defining criteria for salutogenic interventions based on Antonovsky's theory and current research. They found that the effective interventions aiming at strengthening the SOC might have three qualities: they facilitate access and use of GRRs and SRRs, they foster active participation, and they understand SOC development as a learning process. The authors conclude that more intervention studies are needed, with (a) a more robust grounding in salutogenesis principles, (b) larger sample sizes, (c) longer follow-up periods, and (d) stronger research designs. Overall, the chapter indicates that it is possible to improve the SOC throughout the whole life course and that health promotion professionals' work to enhance the SOC should embrace a person-centred, resource-oriented approach.

Knowledge, Gaps, and Perspectives

In closing, we return to the three questions posed at the start of this chapter:

- What are the crucial factors that contribute to build, enhance, and strengthen the SOC during the life course?
- Is the role of the SOC in coping stable during the life course, or does it have different functions at different life stages? For example, does the SOC open one to new GRRs at the beginning and facilitate access to GRRs later in life?
- Can salutogenic interventions strengthen the SOC during various phases in the lifespan?

Addressing the first question on crucial factors that contribute to a strong SOC in the various phases of the life course, the authors of these chapters are unanimous about the significance of a strong linkage between the development of the SOC and the availability and use of GRRs. Even though GRRs change during a lifespan, the family, the social circle, and the community environment are crucial to the development of a strong SOC from early life to old age. At all life stages, the SOC is the product of the *interaction* of an individual and the environment—of the SOC, GRRs, and SRRs.

Therefore, the enrichment, attainability, and accessibility of resources are crucial to strengthening the SOC. This conclusion, based on mounting evidence presented in these chapters, is supportive of Antonovsky's contention that the most significant potential for strengthening the SOC lies in the availability and use of resistance resources.

Yet, as he regretfully noted, fostering resistance resources in a significant way depends on "radical change in the institutional, social, and cultural settings that shape people's life experiences" (Antonovsky, 1987, p. 124). Those levels of social life are rarely subjects of health research and not a primary focus of the chapters discussed here. However, this subject is taken up in other parts of this Handbook, most notably in Chap. 24 on the application of salutogenesis in politics and policy-making.

The answer to the second question is that we lack sufficient evidence to comment decisively about the stability of the SOC during the life course and its functions at different ages. There is a striking lack of research on healthy adults and little research on weak SOC and how to strengthen it. Questions of how a strong SOC is created in children are partly answered, but we do not know how a strong SOC is created and maintained in adulthood, and we do not know how stable positive changes in people's SOC are over the lifetime. This gap might be due to the view of the adult as a performer of different roles, rather than as an individual in development. Therefore, salutogenic research investigates adults mainly as employees, parents, patients, caregivers, or inhabitants of cities or communities.

The third question, on how to strengthen the SOC, can be answered to a degree. It seems the SOC can be influenced at any age and in many life situations, as Chap. 20 on salutogenic interventions discusses. Antonovsky suggested that lasting SOC strength is obtained when interventions enable people to perceive coherent life experiences, when they learn how to nourish their sense of comprehensibility, meaningfulness, and manageability.

References

Antonovsky, A. (1985). The life cycle, mental health and the sense of coherence. *Israel Journal of Psychiatry & Related Sciences, 22*(4), 273–280.

Antonovsky, A. (1987). *Unraveling the mystery of health: How people manage stress and stay well.* Jossey-Bass.

Erikson, E. (1950). Growth and crises of the healthy personality. *Psychological Issues, 1*, 50–100.

Lindström, B., Berg, M., Meier Magistretti, C., Perez-Botella, M., & Downe, S. (2017). The salutogenic approach to maternity care - from theory to practice and research. In Sinclair et al. (Eds.), *New thinking on improving maternity care*. Pinter & Martin Ltd.

Lindström, B., & Eriksson, M. (2010). *The Hitchhiker's guide to salutogenesis: Salutogenic pathways to health promotion*. Helsinki.

Maass, R., Lindstrom, B., & Lillefjell, M. (2017). Neighborhood-resources for the development of a strong the SOC and the importance of understanding why and how resources work: A grounded theory approach. *BMC Public Health, 17*(1), 704.

Montessori, M. (1995). *The absorbent mind.* Henry Holt & Co.

Sugarman, L. (2001). *Lifespan development. Frameworks, accounts, and strategies* (2nd ed.). Psychology Press.

15

SOC and Salutogenesis: A Study of Families and Childhood

Orly Idan, Orna Braun-Lewensohn, Bengt Lindström, and Malka Margalit

Introduction

Infancy and early childhood are distinct developmental periods in which young children differ significantly from older children, adolescents, and adults in terms of cognitive skills, language and communication, self-regulation, and socioemotional functioning (Mowder et al., 2009). The science of early childhood development demonstrates that the foundations for sound mental health are built early in life, as early experiences shape the architecture of the developing brain (Miller & Kinsbourne, 2012). These important experiences include children's relationships with parents, caregivers, relatives, teachers, and peers, which play a critical role in shaping social, emotional, and cognitive development. Recent research indicates that early intervention can have a positive impact on the trajectory of common emotional or behavioral problems as well as on outcomes for children with adversities and disorders (National Scientific Council on the Developing Child, 2012). Adverse experiences early in life, particularly for vulnerable children, have been shown to predict the emergence of later physical and mental health problems (Edwards et al., 2003). Although mental health challenges for young children share many biological and behavioral characteristics with those of older children and adults, several aspects differentiate early childhood from later developmental stages. First, emotional health for young children is very strongly influenced by their environment and the nature of their relationships and the support or risks these relationships confer. Therefore, it is essential to examine the quality of the children's environments and relationships to tap the risks for adversaries and the protective factors that may assist in promoting mental and physical health. Second, cognitive, social, and emotional characteristics are all intertwined within the architecture of the brain, and these capacities vary at different developmental stages. Children understand, manage, think, feel, and talk about their experiences differently at different ages. These developmental differences are important to understanding the behavioral and emotional risks and protective factors involved. Finally, in early childhood, it can be challenging to distinguish temporary deviations in behavior from persistent problems, or typical differences in maturation from developmental delays (Rubin et al., 2006).

From birth, children develop their abilities to experience and express a diverse range of emotions, as well as their capacity to cope with and manage different feelings (Thompson & Lagattuta, 2006). The development of these capabilities occurs at the same time as a wide range of highly visible skills in mobility, cognition, and communication (Thompson, 2001). The foundations of social competence that are developed in the first 5 years are linked to emotional well-being and affect a child's ability to functionally adapt in school later on and form promoting relationships during adolescence and adulthood (Cassidy & Shaver, 1999). Therefore, it is important to address children's affective and cognitive aspects. Failure to address difficulties in the socioemotional domain may result in missed opportunities for interventions at critical periods (National Scientific Council on the Developing Child, 2004).

The emotional experiences of newborns and young infants occur for the most while interacting with their caregivers.

O. Idan (✉)
School of Psychology, Interdisciplinary Center (IDC), Herzliya, Israel
e-mail: oidan@idc.ac.il

O. Braun-Lewensohn
Conflict Management and Resolution Program, Ben-Gurion University of the Negev, Beer Sheva, Israel

B. Lindström
NTNU Center for Health Promotion Research, Norwegian University of Science and Technology, Trondheim, Norway
e-mail: bengtblind@hotmail.com

M. Margalit
Tel Aviv University, and Peres Academic Center, Rehovot, Israel

Associations between positive emotions and the availability of responsive caregivers are strengthened during infancy in both behavior and brain architecture (Cassidy, 1994). Toddlers and preschool children depend on their emerging capacities to interpret their personal experiences and understand what others are doing and thinking, as well as to interpret the distinctions between different responses to them. By the end of the preschool years, children who have acquired emotional regulation skills can use their awareness of their own and others' feelings to interact daily (Thompson & Lagattuta, 2006). Studies on preschool children have shown how the interrelated development of emotion and cognition relies on the emergence, maturation, and interconnection of complex neural circuits in multiple areas of the brain (Davidson et al., 2002). A large-scale study examining a biopsychosocial model of risk and resilience on behavior at preadolescence indicated the importance of biological and psychosocial factors, including the SOC, on resilient outcomes and preadolescents' mental health (Agnafors et al., 2017).

Thus, the emotional development of young children is correlated to the characteristics of the environments in which they live, including their families, school, and community (Reid et al., 2002). A Children's Sense of Coherence Scale (CSOC) based on the three components of the SOC construct was developed (Margalit & Efrati, 1995).

Children's Sense of Coherence Scale

The Children's Sense of Coherence Scale (CSOC) (Margalit & Efrati, 1995) is an adaptation of the Antonovsky Orientation to Life (Sense of Coherence—SOC) Scale (Antonovsky, 1987). In line with the sense of coherence construct and the adults' scale, a children's version (CSOC) was developed, field-tested, and revised several times at the Special Education Laboratory in Tel-Aviv University.

Due to the children's young age and reservations regarding the ability of children to comprehend the construct and scale, it was decided to develop a scale that would meet the unique characteristics of the target population. The scale was developed in collaboration with Aaron and Helen Antonovsky. The scale included distractors relating to the children's lives and activities. The CSOC's wording, the order of words, examples, and distracters were examined to ensure the comprehension of young children and the inclusion of age-appropriate content. Since its development, several new versions have been used, such as for junior high school students, omitting the distracter items, for example, "I'm interested in lots of things" and "I'm interested in lots of things in my class" (for school-based research, or "at home"—for family-based research). In general, distractors were coherent with culture.

The children's scale was tested on children of age 5 to adolescents. Comprehension was examined using unstructured interviews; a series of retests verified stability. Conceptually, the items were derived from SOC-29 and the three components of the SOC. This consisted of 16 primary items and 3 filler items on a four-point Likert scale (the range was reduced to 4 from "never" (1) to "always" (4)). Scores ranged from 16 to 64, with items describing the children's feeling of confidence in their world, as expressed in their sense of comprehensibility—understanding their environment (i.e., "I feel that I don't know what to do in class"); sense of manageability—feelings of control, and confidence that when help is needed, it will be available (i.e., "when I want something, I'm sure I'll get it"); and meaningfulness interest in investing efforts in different tasks (i.e., "I'm interested in lots of things") (Alpha = 0.72). Similar to the SOC scoring procedures, a high score reflected a high level of CSOC.

Studies using the CSOC explored children's personal and contextual resources and their ability to perceive family, social, and educational environments as structured and meaningful realities. The following section presents studies that used CSOC.

Studies on SOC During Childhood

A systematic search for studies on children and SOC between the years 2000 and 2019 in online databases (PsychoInfo, Ebsco, Proquest, APApsycnet, SocioFile, SAGE, Web of Science, and PubMed) using keywords (sense of coherence, salutogenesis, children, and family) and Boolean operators, presented 44 studies from 15 countries. Table 15.1 summarizes the studies.

Two major foci emerged from the review of the studies: Children's SOC within the family, school, peer group, and community environments and CSOC as a predictor of children's health and health behavior. The studies relating to CSOC and different contextual environments may be divided into three age groups/developmental stages: the preschool age stage, the elementary school-age stage, and a prolonged stage from infant to adolescence/adulthood focusing on families of children with special needs.

SOC and the Child's Environments: Family, School, Peers, and Community

The salutogenic paradigm focuses on promoting growth and adjustment. The following research deals with the contributions of children's environments: families, friends, and school systems, to the adjustment of children with typical development and children with special needs. The resilience

Table 15.1 Studies (2000–2019) on SOC during childhood

Author	Year	Place	Population	Variables	Results
1. Agnafors et al.	2017	Sweden	889 children and mothers from a birth cohort	Maternal symptoms of depression, psychological risk, children's experiences of life events, genetic polymorphisms, child temperament, social functioning, maternal sense of coherence	The l/l genotype of the serotonin-transporter-linked polymorphic region was associated with lower internalizing scores, but not mainly related to the level of adversity. An easy temperament was associated with resilience for children exposed to high adversity. Social functioning was found to be promotive independent of the risk level
2. Al-Yagon	2003	Israel	145 mother–child dyads of 5–6.5-year-old kindergartners with/without mild developmental delays	Children: developmental delay status, temperament, gender, loneliness, SOC, friendship nomination, attachment security style; mother's SOC, family cohesion and adaptability	Child's SOC demonstrated that the attachment pattern mediator variable significantly explained 15% of the variance among children with developmental delays. Children with secure attachment reported higher levels of SOC than children with insecure attachment
3. Al-Yagon	2007	Israel	110 mother–child dyads of 8–11-year-old schoolchildren with/without LD	Children: LD and non-LD group, gender, loneliness, SOC, attachment security style, hope; mothers: coping, affect, experience in close relationships, child behavior	Mothers' low use of avoidant coping strategies and less avoidance in close relationships with significant others were found to moderate the effect of children's disabilities on children's levels of loneliness, hope, and secure attachment
4. Al-Yagon	2008	Israel	58 mother–child dyads of 8–11-year-old schoolchildren	Children: loneliness, SOC, mother-rated behavior; mothers: SOC, attachment style, loneliness	Maternal SOC significantly contributed to all child socioemotional adjustment measures and attachment scores
5. Al-Yagon	2010	Israel	205 mother–child dyads of 8–12-year-old schoolchildren with/without LD	Children: LD and non-LD group, gender, SOC, attachment security style, hope, effort; mothers: experiences in close relationships, affect, child behavior	Children's adjustment and SOC mediated associations between maternal emotional resources and children's well-adjusted functioning. The significantly lower SOC among children with LD emphasized this coping resource
6. Al-Yagon	2011	Israel	205 father–child dyads of 8–12-year-old schoolchildren with/without LD	Children: LD and non-LD group, gender, SOC, loneliness, attachment security style, hope, effort; fathers: coping, SOC, child behavior	The mediating role of CSOC emerged for both groups in the association between fathers' resources and children's well-adjusted functioning. The significantly lower SOC among children with LD emphasized this coping resource
7. Al-Yagon	2012	Israel	312 8–12-year-old schoolchildren with/without LD and their parents	Children: LD and non-LD group, gender, SOC, loneliness, attachment security style, hope; parents: child behavior	Children who felt securely attached to both parents reported a higher global orientation or enduring tendency to see the world as comprehensible, manageable, and meaningful than children who felt securely attached to only one parent or neither parent. In contrast, children who exhibited insecure attachment to both parents appeared to be the most vulnerable in forming coping resources

(continued)

Table 15.1 (continued)

Author	Year	Place	Population	Variables	Results
8. Al-Yagon	2014	Israel	107 children with LD and 98 children with typical development ages 8–12 years	Children's attachment with father and mother, loneliness, SOC, hope, effort, internalizing behavior syndrome	Results indicated the unique and complementary roles played by children's attachment with the father and with the mother for explaining children's internalizing socioemotional variables. The LD group's heightened vulnerability to insecure attachment relationships with significant others was revealed
9. Al-Yagon	2015	Israel	107 parent couples with LD children and 98 couples with typically developing children, ages 8–12 years	Parents' low anxious/avoidance attachment, low/high negative affect, active/avoidant coping, SOC	Results revealed the contribution of fathers' high attachment anxiety to their greater use of active coping strategies; a lower effect of avoidant attachment than anxious attachment in discriminating between individuals' coping strategies was found; higher levels of positive affect significantly contributed to parents' higher SOC level for groups of fathers and mothers of children with LD
10. Al-Yagon and Cinamon	2008	Israel	96 mother–child dyads of 8–12-year-old schoolchildren with/without LD	Children: LD and non-LD group, gender, attachment security style; mothers: experiences in close relationships, affect, work–family relations, SOC, family cohesion, and adaptability	Higher maternal perceptions of the world as comprehensible, manageable, and meaningful contributed significantly to children's secure attachment and level of connection, closeness, and involvement between the family members
11. Al-Yagon and Margalit	2006	Israel	266 third graders with/without reading difficulties	Loneliness, SOC, children's appraisal of the teacher as a secure base	Children's perception of their teacher as their secure base correlated significantly with higher levels of SOC and lower levels of loneliness
12. Al-Yagon and Mikulincer	2004	Israel	196 8–11-year-old schoolchildren with/without LD; 23 homeroom teachers	Children: LD and non-LD group, gender, loneliness, SOC, attachment security style; teachers: ratings of children's academic functioning	Secure attachment classification correlated significantly with higher levels of SOC and lower levels of loneliness
13. Berntsson and Gustafsson	2000	Sweden	1163 7–12-year-old schoolchildren	Psychosomatic complaints, mental stability, family activities, parents' health status, gender, parents' social class, education, income, ethnicity, employment, and family structure	Predictors of psychosomatic complaints were mother's health, child's mental stability, contacts with peers, long-term illness, and via other factors, parents' SOC, social competence, and school satisfaction
14. Bonanato et al.	2009	Brazil	546 mother–child dyads of 5-year-old preschool children	Mothers' SOC, oral health status, social class	Mothers with lower levels of SOC were more likely to have children with decayed teeth or filled teeth regardless of the child's social class and gender
15. Dabrowska	2003	Poland	77 parents of children with cerebral palsy (CP) and 62 parents of typically developing children	Coping, stress, SOC	Parents of children with cerebral palsy, reporting higher levels of SOC, less often used avoidance, wishful thinking, and resignation as coping strategies than parents reporting lower levels of SOC

Author	Year	Place	Population	Variables	Results
16. Dabrowska	2008	Poland	128 fathers of children with and without developmental disabilities	SOC, coping	Fathers of children with developmental disabilities reported lower levels of SOC more frequently and used strategies of avoidance compared to fathers with higher levels of SOC that used confrontation more frequently and positive reappraisal and problem-solving behavior
17. Efrati-Virtzer and Margalit	2009	Israel	337 schoolchildren grades 3–6 with/without behavior difficulties (BD); 47 teachers	Children: SOC, loneliness, peer nominations; teachers: hyperactive behavior, aggressive behavior, academic achievements	Teachers evaluated students with BD as achieving lower academic grades and displaying higher levels of hyperactive behavior and aggression. Children with BD were less accepted by their peers, reported lower levels of SOC and higher levels of loneliness. Students who were rated by their teachers as revealing higher levels of hyperactive and aggressive behavior experienced lower levels of personal coherence
18. Einav et al.	2012	Israel	111 mother–child dyads of infants ages 3–24 months with developmental delays	SOC, family cohesion and adaptability, coping, hope	Mothers with high levels of SOC and with high coping strategies felt more hopeful. In families characterized by flexibility and open to changes, mothers reported higher levels of coping that contributed to their hope measure. Family cohesion was interrelated with mothers' SOC, but not directly related to coping or hope. Cohesion was related to hope only indirectly, mediated through mothers' SOC
19. Eli et al.	2016	Sweden	565 mothers of 4-year olds	SOC, maternal and child characteristics, pressuring or restrictive feeding practices	Child gender, age, and BMI were not associated with SOC. Lower SOC was associated with controlling practices and with concern about child weight and eating
20. Feldman et al.	2018	Israel	1719 fifth and sixth graders from 29 schools	SOC, hopeful thinking, loneliness, family cohesion, effort, success in school	The results support the distinctive contribution of family cohesion and the mediating roles of sense of coherence and hope (as protective factors) as well as loneliness (as a risk factor) in predicting students' school effort
21. Forinder et al.	2005	Sweden	52 patients ages 9–22 years (at least 3 years following stem cell transplant (SCT))	Late effects in each of eight predefined problem categories, patient activity, SOC, quality of life	SOC scores for younger children (ages 9–12 years) showed that the SCT group was on par with that of both the norm groups and other chronically ill children. The mean value for the younger children in the SCT group was on par with that of the norm group
22. Groholt et al.	2003	The five Nordic countries	9524 2–17-year-old children of which 35% were co-responders (with their parents), 2% children	Parental SOC, parental health, marital status, education, socioeconomic status, income, child chronic health condition, child gender	Compared to the higher social classes, low levels of SOC were more common in the lower classes. The association of child health with parental SOC was found to be disability-specific (diabetes, epilepsy, psychiatric problems)

(continued)

Table 15.1 (continued)

Author	Year	Place	Population	Variables	Results
23. Hedov et al.	2002	Sweden	207 parents of children (ages 3.5–7 years) with down's syndrome (DS), 237 parents of healthy children	Parents' groups, SOC, parental self-perceived stress, frequency of gainful employment, amount of time spent on child care	Mean SOC scores of the parents of children with DS did not differ from those of the control group. Parents from both groups who experienced lower stress in parenthood had a stronger SOC
24. Hintermair	2004	Germany	235 mothers of children ages 1–13 years with hearing impairments	SOC, stress, life satisfaction, social support, age, gender, education, means of communication with children	Mothers with a stronger SOC had an advantage in coping with the experience of raising a deaf and hard of hearing child over mothers with lower SOC scores. SOC was of greater importance than experienced social support
25. Honkinen et al.	2005	Finland	1231 12-year-old schoolchildren	Profession of parents, gender, SOC, physical activity, weight, academic achievements, social support, class climate, psychosomatic symptoms	SOC and variables of social support were found significantly associated with perceived health. Physical exercise and SOC were associated with perceived health and father's occupation, and low SOC was found to be independently associated with relatively poor health
26. Jellesma et al.	2006	Netherlands	153 8–13-year-old schoolchildren at three levels of somatic complaints	Groups: Low somatic complaints, many somatic complaints, clinical group; happiness, anger, fear, sadness, depressiveness, emotion awareness, SOC	The clinical group and the children with many somatic complaints reported more negative moods on the anger, sadness, and fear scale, more difficulty differentiating emotions, and a lower SOC
27. Kan et al.	2015	Japan	1497 men and 1764 women from the Stratification, Health, Income, & Neighborhood Study (J-HINE)	Mastery, SOC, childhood SES, self-related health, psychological distress	Mastery and SOC significantly and independently mediated the association between childhood SES and current health in the total sample after adjusting for age, gender, and respondent education, regardless of the type of SES or health outcome indicators. SOC significantly mediated the association between parents' education and current health only among women, and it mediated the association between perceived childhood SES and current health only among men
28. Krause	2011	Germany	226 5–10-year-old schoolchildren; longitudinal	Health promotion by self-worth reinforcement program, SOC, feeling of self-worth, sense of belonging	Developing sense of coherence in promoting mental health in schoolchildren was perceived fundamental and most effective in the early years of childhood, requiring training of professionals within the school
29. Liberman et al.	2013	Israel	50 5–6-year-old schoolchildren with/without developmental coordination disorder	Gender, mother education, family income, place of living, movement, children's partaking (completed by parents for ages 4–6.5), performance skills, SOC, hope, effort	Levels of SOC, hope, and effort in children with DCD were lower than their typically developing peers. The explanatory variables (SOC, hope and effort, motor skills, and processing skills) did not predict either the diversity or the frequency measures of participation

30. Londal	2010	Norway	36 8–9-year-old children participating in an after-school program; 4 months, qualitative	Play, SOC	Play in the ASP had considerable potential for promoting the children's SOC. Most of the children in the study experienced their world as comprehensible, manageable, and meaningful. Negative thoughts and feelings were reduced during bodily play. Play offered particularly strong opportunities for the children themselves to shape outcomes and interact with children
31. Mak et al.	2006	Hong Kong	157 mothers of children with autism (ages 1–28)	Severity of autistic symptoms, SOC, parenting attitudes, parenting stress, age, education, marital status, income	Mothers with a higher level of SOC reported less stress than those with a lower level. SOC had a moderating effect on the association between symptom severity and parenting stress
32. Margalit et al.	2006	Israel	80 mothers of children ages 2–39 months exhibiting delayed development	SOC, family cohesion and adaptability, mood, coping, parenting stress	Mothers from noncohesive families with lower SOC experienced higher levels of stress than mothers from cohesive families with higher SOC. Mothers from noncohesive families with lower SOC experienced lower levels of positive mood than mothers from cohesive families with high SOC
33. Most et al.	2000	Israel	98 5–6.4-year-old preschool children with/without risk for developing LD	Groups (at risk and not at risk), gender, phonological awareness skills, loneliness, SOC, peer acceptance	Children at risk scored lower on phonological awareness, loneliness, SOC, peer acceptance. The largest group of children at risk had the lowest levels of SOC and phonological awareness skills
34. Nammontri et al.	2013	Thailand	257 10–12-year-old schoolchildren; 133 intervention group	Clinical variables, oral health-related quality of life, SOC, oral health beliefs	Greater SOC predicted positive health beliefs and fewer symptoms. Intervention provided evidence that SOC influences oral health-related quality of life
35. Natvig et al.	2006	Norway	4116 schoolchildren age 11, 13, and 15 years.	Age, gender, SOC, supportive school climate, learning conditions, school-related stress	In analyses of all resources and stress factors, the strongest and most adverse associations with the SOC were seen with feeling pressured by schoolwork. Among girls, this association was strongest for the youngest group. School-related factors represent both resource and stress factors of importance for the SOC
36. Neves et al.	2019	Brazil	769 5-year-old preschoolers from public and private schools	Parental/caregiver SOC, SES, untreated dental caries,	The prevalence of clinical consequences of untreated dental caries was low in the present sample and was associated with socio-demographic factors (type of preschool, caregiver's age, and the number of children in the family) and SOC
37. Oelofsen and Richardson	2006	United Kingdom	104 fathers and mothers of preschool children (average age 43.8 months) with/without developmental disabilities	Family structure, parental age, socioeconomic classification, child gender, child age, SOC, parenting stress, parental health status, parental social support	Parents of children with DD reported parenting stress within the clinical range, weaker SOC, and poorer health than parents of children without DD. Mothers of children with DD reported poorer health, higher levels of parenting stress, and weaker SOC than their partners

(continued)

Table 15.1 (continued)

Author	Year	Place	Population	Variables	Results
38. Olsson and Hwang	2002	Sweden	429 fathers and mothers of children ages 0–16 years with/without intellectual disability	Parental group, SOC, depression	Parents of children with ID who reported low levels of SOC were more depressed than control parents with low levels of SOC. No relation was found between the age of the child and SOC levels in parents of children with ID
39. Pisula and Kossakowska	2010	Poland	45 couples of parents to children ages 3–7 years with/without autism	Parental gender, education, employment, time spent caring for the child, SOC, ways of coping	Parents of children with autism had lower total SOC, meaningfulness, and manageability, compared with controls, and used escape avoidance coping more often. SOC level was positively associated with seeking social support and self-controlling and negatively with accepting responsibility and positive reappraisal
40. Ray et al.	2009	Finland	772 parent–child dyads of 10–11-year-old schoolchildren	Children: meal patterns, food frequency intake; parents: SOC, eating patterns	A weaker parental SOC was associated with children's irregular meal patterns, more frequent intake of energy-rich foods, and less frequent intake of nutrient-rich foods
41. Sharabi et al.	2012	Israel	287 10–11.6-year-old schoolchildren	Loneliness, SOC, hope, effort, family cohesion, and adaptability	Four family profiles were identified: Children in the two cohesive families' clusters reported the lowest levels of loneliness and the highest levels of personal strengths. Children within noncohesive family clusters reported the highest levels of loneliness and the lowest levels of SOC
42. Sivberg	2002		37 families, 66 parents of children with and without autism	Coping, coping behavior, strain, SOC	Parents of children with autism reported low levels of SOC. Lower levels of coping were associated with higher levels of strain on the family system, and the level of strain on the family system was higher in the families with a child with an autism spectrum disorders (ASD)
43. Svavarsdottir et al.	2005	Iceland	76 American families (75 mothers and 62 fathers) and 103 Icelandic families (103 mothers and 74 fathers)	Family adaptation, family hardiness, SOC, caregiving demands, family demands, severity of illness	SOC and family hardiness predicted family adaptation. Icelandic mothers perceived their family's adaptation more favorably than American mothers. Regarding fathers, family demands predicted adaptation. SOC moderated the effect of family demands on adaptation for both parents
44. Torsheim et al.	2001	Norway	1592 grade 6, 1534 grade 8, 1605 grade 10 children	Health complaints/symptoms, school-related stress, SOC	Age group comparisons revealed that the association between SOC and stress weakened with age. Association between SOC and health complaints grew stronger

approach defines assumptions about the critical predictors of the full potential of children to learn and to thrive in diverse settings regardless of personal and environmental challenges and risk factors (Damon, 2004). A major role of resilient research is to identify the complex transactions and processes among internal and external (risk and protective) factors that affect children's resilience and sense of coherence (Margalit, 2003).

Sense of coherence at the preschool age stage Children of various ages, with a strong sense of coherence, may perceive their day-to-day experiences as comprehensible and manageable. To compare the sense of coherence of typically developing preschool children with preschool children having special needs, studies have examined children and their parents in various social contexts (Al-Yagon, 2003; Margalit, 1998; Most et al., 2000). In a sample of 187 preschool children ages 4.9–6.3 years, children who were identified as at risk for developing learning disabilities (LD), even before they were formally diagnosed and labeled, had a weaker sense of coherence, had fewer friends, and were less accepted by their peers. The sense of coherence assessment revealed the children's heterogeneity, and even among the group of typically developing children, a small subgroup could be defined with a very low sense of coherence and many social challenges. Also, in line with the salutogenic paradigm, special attention was given to a small subgroup of children within the group of children at risk whose sense of coherence was high. The relatively small extreme groups may add to the understanding of the development of coherence from early developmental stages (Margalit, 1998).

The children with a risk for developing learning disabilities received tutoring on an individual and small group basis during school time by the special education teachers. The focus was on language enrichment and basic learning skills. The sense of coherence of a subgroup of these preschool children (N = 67) was tested. Significant differences were noted in the comparisons between the sense of coherence scores at the beginning of the intervention and at the mid-year evaluation. However, no significant differences were found between mid-year and the end of the year. The correlations between the first and the second assessments of children's sense of coherence were significant (0.34) and between the second and the third assessments (0.32) as well. It can be concluded that at this age, there was some level of flexibility in the children's sense of coherence. Remedial training on delayed academic, language, and cognitive functioning was related to an increased sense of coherence and a narrowing of the gap with the typically developing group (Margalit, 1998).

Language difficulties and social-emotional challenges are often considered as two separate risk factors at the preschool age stage. A study of preschool children explored the relations between children's sense of coherence, loneliness, and phonological awareness. Phonological awareness consists of language skills such as awareness of the structure of sounds in words and sentences. Research reports that they predict reading acquisition (Most et al., 2000). The study examined the phonological awareness skills, loneliness, sense of coherence, and peer acceptance among 98 children ages 5.0–6.4 years. Children at risk had lower achievements as a group on the phonological awareness measures, reported weaker CSOC, viewed themselves as lonelier, and were less accepted by their peers.

Family ecology is comprised of parental, familial, and environmental characteristics that may affect the capacity of the family to provide optimal care (Greenberg et al., 1993). Olson (2000) identified cohesion and adaptability as two major parameters for evaluating the functioning of a family. Cohesion refers to the extent of connection, closeness, and involvement between the family members. Adaptability reflects the family's capability to change as an adaptation to developmental and external pressures (Olson, 1986, 2000). A family system has been considered balanced when it demonstrates moderate scores on these two dimensions. In a study examining SOC, attachment security style, loneliness, and temperament of 145 children ages 5–6.5 years with and without developmental delays, and their mothers' SOC and family cohesion and adaptability, children having a secure attachment to their mothers reported a stronger SOC than children having an insecure attachment (Al-Yagon, 2003).

In summary, the studies on preschool children identified SOC as an important protective factor that differentiated children with typical development and high-risk children, even before their formal assessment and measurable academic challenges.

Sense of coherence at the elementary school-age stage The transfer to elementary schools expands the variability of the factors that affect and are affected by the children's sense of coherence. Children's academic success, social competence, and coping capabilities contribute to their well-being and adjustment during that period, while academic, social, and behavior difficulties may be considered risk factors. Interactions with teachers and peers have a profound impact on children's life quality. Multiple studies examined the relations between children's sense of coherence and their family; their perceptions of teachers' support, peer friendships, and their overall school experience, revealing the complex and multivariate interactions at the elementary school-age stage (Al-Yagon, 2007, 2008, 2010, 2011, 2012; Al-Yagon & Cinamon, 2008; Al-Yagon & Margalit, 2006; Al-Yagon & Mikulincer, 2004; Efrati-Virtzer & Margalit, 2009; Liberman et al., 2013; Sharabi et al., 2012).

To further clarify the role of teachers in understanding children's sense of coherence, the attachment conceptualization (that was developed for children–mothers' relations) was adapted to schools' relationships. Children's perceptions of the teachers as a secure base were examined, and the results revealed that secure attachment patterns expressed in the development of close relationships with teachers predicted children's SOC and loneliness (Al-Yagon & Margalit, 2006; Al-Yagon & Mikulincer, 2004). Children, who felt that their teachers were more available to them and more accepting, reported a stronger SOC and less feelings of loneliness.

In another study (Efrati-Virtzer & Margalit, 2009), the characteristics of children with behavior difficulties were examined (behavior difficulties included verbal and physical aggression toward children and objects). The age range of these children was 9–12 years, and they were compared with children with no adjustment problems from the same classes. Results revealed that the behavior difficulties contributed to the explanation of social and academic functioning and were linked to social difficulties—in terms of lower peer acceptance and increased rejection by children in their classes, as well as to lower academic achievement. Children with disruptive behavior also reported weaker levels of CSOC. Those children with stronger CSOC revealed emotional self-regulation and participated in fewer behavior conflicts at school. It is not clear whether a weaker SOC was the outcome of the multiple academic, social, and behavior difficulties or predicted them. Students with a weaker SOC were less accepted by their peers and rated as more rejected by them.

The study of social relations at school provided additional validation to the complexity of the interacting variables. The most common approach for identifying a child's status in class is done by asking the children to state the names of their best friends (and those that they do not like) as measures of social acceptance and rejection. The construct of reciprocal positive nomination (mutual friendship) attracted increased research attention since it provided information on mutual perceptions, reflecting the interpersonal attraction and liking where within a pair of children, each one selected the other as a friend (Yugar & Shapiro, 2001). If the positive mutual nomination was an important indicator in reflecting friendship and explaining decreased alienation experience in schools, the reciprocal negative nomination (mutual selection within a dyad of children of the least liked child in the class) extended the understanding of the increased experience of social isolation, identified enemies in classes and enhanced feelings of social exclusion and loneliness. It is not surprising that they were related to a weaker SOC (Efrati-Virtzer & Margalit, 2009).

Research on elementary schoolchildren with and without developmental delays and their families identified SOC as playing a significant protective role during the first year at school. In a study on 50 schoolchildren ages 5–6 years with and without developmental coordination disorder (DCD), levels of CSOC, hope, and effort in children with DCD were lower than their typically developing peers. Significant correlations were found between CSOC to the children's involvement in daily activities in a variety of environments. The CSOC was related to the children's independence and enjoyment from participation in age-appropriate social and leisure activities (Liberman et al., 2013).

The Relations Between Children's SOC and Families' Characteristics

Several studies have shown that maternal coping resources moderated the effect of children's learning disabilities on secure attachment, levels of loneliness, feelings of hope, and future expectations. The degree to which the learning disability affected the children's socioemotional academic competence and social interrelations was related to the type of coping their mothers employed and their reliance on social support (Al-Yagon, 2007, 2008, 2010, 2011, 2012, 2014, 2015; Al-Yagon & Cinamon, 2008): Maternal SOC significantly enhanced the child's socioemotional adjustment measures and attachment scores (Al-Yagon, 2008); children's adjustment and SOC mediated associations between maternal emotional resources and children's well-adjusted functioning. The significantly weaker SOC among children with learning disabilities (LD) emphasized this coping resource (Al-Yagon, 2010); studies also recognized the significance of children's relations not only with mothers but also with fathers. The mediating role of CSOC emerged for children with and without learning disabilities in the association between fathers' resources and children's well-adjusted functioning (Al-Yagon, 2011); children who felt securely attached to both parents reported a higher global orientation or enduring tendency to see the world as comprehensible, manageable, and meaningful than children who felt securely attached to only one parent or neither parent. In examining the differences in the role of attachment with fathers and mothers, Al-Yagon (2014) reported that in the model modified for elementary schoolchildren with severe learning disabilities (SLD), a higher number of significant paths emerged between child–mother attachment relationships and internalizing measures than for child–father attachment. Data also showed that attachment with fathers contributed mainly to children's coping resources (i.e., SOC, hope, and effort), whereas attachment with mothers contributed to a broader range of internalizing adjustment measures including not only SOC but also self-reported loneliness and parent-rated internalizing problems. In investigating the coping resources of parents of children with LD and children with typical development, Al-Yagon (2015) highlighted the potential role of parents' affect. Specifically, higher levels of positive affect significantly contributed to parents' stronger SOC for fathers and mothers of children with LD. However, greater negative affect contributed to greater utilization of active and avoidance coping strategist only for mothers of children with LD. Furthermore, children who exhibited insecure attachment to both parents appeared to be the most vulnerable in forming coping resources (Al-Yagon, 2012; Al-Yagon & Cinamon, 2008).

Parents comprise only in part family cohesion. In a study on 287 schoolchildren ages 10–12 years, four family profiles were identified: children in the cohesive families' clusters reported the lowest levels of loneliness and the strongest levels of CSOC, whereas children within noncohesive family clusters reported the highest levels of loneliness and the weakest levels of CSOC (Sharabi et al., 2012). Additionally, the degree of cohesion within families was found to predict effort investment and success in school. Feldman et al. (2018) revealed that family cohesion and the mediating roles of SOC and hope (protective factors), as well as loneliness (risk factor), contributed significantly in predicting school effort among elementary school pupils.

In conclusion, during elementary school, children acquired basic learning skills, established positive and negative relations with teachers and peers, and their functioning predicted their life quality, as well as presenting special academic and behavior challenges. At this age stage, SOC was shown to provide a unique and relatively stable index of children's social and emotional adjustment and well-being. The entrance to high schools and the adolescence age stage not only provided extended opportunities but also revealed continued difficulties and new challenges. A study of the Norwegian education system explored elementary through junior high schoolchildren focusing on age and gender comparisons concerning school-related stress and resources and their relations to the SOC construct. The sample consisted of 4116 schoolchildren ages 11, 13, and 15 years. SOC was related to feeling pressured by schoolwork, social support from peers, and expectations. Among girls, this association was strongest for the youngest group. School-related factors were shown to represent both resource and stress factors related to the SOC (Natvig et al., 2006).

From infancy to adolescence/adulthood: Families of children with special needs Children with special needs are considered a source of distress to their families. Their increased levels of stress reflect their emotional reactions to the unexpected and challenging reality of having children with developmental disabilities and behavior challenges. The fathers' and mothers' SOC reflects the impacts of the prolonged stress but at the same time reveals their parental resources that may be conceptualized as resources that serve as protective factors (Margalit, 1994).

Research on infants and preschool children with developmental delays and their families (Einav et al., 2012; Hedov et al., 2002; Margalit et al., 2006; Oelofsen & Richardson, 2006; Pisula & Kossakowska, 2010) identified the parents' SOC as meaningful for the development of their children. In a study of 111 mother–child dyads of infants ages 3–24 months with developmental delays, mothers with strong levels of SOC and with high coping strategies felt more hopeful. The family cohesion (the mothers' perceptions that their family members were close to one another and provided support when needed) was interrelated with mothers' SOC. Cohesion was related to hopeful thinking only indirectly, mediated through mothers' SOC. Only for mothers who reported strong levels of SOC was the family support meaningful in the prediction of hopeful thinking (Einav et al., 2012).

Mothers from noncohesive families with weaker SOC experienced higher levels of stress than mothers from cohesive families with stronger SOC in a study examining SOC, family cohesion and adaptability, mood, coping, and parenting stress of 80 mothers of children ages 2–39 months exhibiting delayed development. Furthermore, mothers from noncohesive families with weaker SOC experienced lower levels of positive mood than mothers from cohesive families with a strong SOC (Margalit et al., 2006). Oelofsen and Richardson (2006), studying fathers and mothers of preschool children with developmental disabilities (DD), found that parents of children with DD reported parenting stress within the clinical range, weaker SOC, and poor health than the comparison group—parents of children without DD. The study's results focused the attention on the mothers who, as the major caregiving parent, experienced more stress than the fathers and reported more health problems, and weaker SOC than the fathers.

Studies focusing on parents to children with special needs emphasized the significance of SOC with parenting stress: parents of children with cerebral palsy, reporting a stronger SOC, less often used avoidance, wishful thinking, and resignation as coping strategies than parents reporting a weaker SOC (Dabrowska, 2003); parents of children with Down's syndrome as well as the comparison group had a stronger SOC when their stress level was lower (Hedov et al., 2002); and fathers of children with developmental disabilities reported a weaker SOC more frequently and used strategies of avoidance compared to fathers with a stronger SOC that used confrontation more frequently and positive reappraisal and problem-solving behavior (Dabrowska, 2008).

In a study on parents of children with autism, the parents reported a weaker SOC than the comparison group and used avoidance coping more often. Among parents of children with autism, the SOC level was positively associated with seeking social support and self-controlling and negatively with accepting responsibility and positive appraisal. The results demonstrated that the frequency of using accepting responsibility strategy increased with decreasing levels of SOC among the parents. This may suggest that one of the consequences of low SOC may be a self-blame tendency for the occurrence of stressful situations related to parenting a child with special needs (Pisula & Kossakowska, 2010). This confirms earlier findings of a weaker SOC among parents of children with autism (Olsson & Hwang, 2002; Sivberg, 2002).

Several studies explored SOC in families of children with developmental disorders from birth to adolescence (ages 1–13, 0–16 years) and/or adulthood (ages 1–28 years). Hintermair (2004) studied 235 mothers of children ages 1–13 years with hearing impairments and found that mothers with stronger SOC had an advantage in coping with the experience of raising a deaf and hard of hearing child over mothers with weaker SOC scores. SOC was of greater importance than experienced social support. Similarly, Olsson and Hwang (2002) studied 429 fathers and mothers of children from birth to 16 years of age with and without intellectual disability (ID). They found that parents of children with ID who reported low levels of SOC were more depressed than control parents with low levels of SOC. No relation was found between the age of the child and the levels of SOC in parents of children with ID. In a study of children, adolescents, and young adults with autism, Mak et al. (2007) reported that mothers with a strong SOC reported less stress than those with a weak SOC. SOC had a moderating effect on the association between symptom severity and parenting stress.

In summary, the studies on families of children with special needs identified SOC as a significant protective factor related to effective coping and hopeful thinking that differentiated between families of children with typical development and families of children with special needs. Understanding the relationship between SOC and coping among parents of children with special needs provides insight into the mechanisms involved in parental adjustment and effective coping outcomes.

SOC as Predictor of Health and Health Behavior

In the past decade, research has shown the relationship between social factors, health, and disease, focusing attention on salutogenic models, concentrating on personal control. This trend followed former studies that revealed that persons with a strong SOC tended to manage stress better, whereas persons with a weak SOC tended to be more sensitive to health challenges and illness (Lundberg & Nystrom, 1994). Recent multiple pieces of research on SOC and health have identified SOC as a predictor of health and health behavior (Berntsson & Gustafsson, 2000; Bonanato et al., 2009; Forinder et al., 2005; Groholt et al., 2003; Honkinen et al., 2005; Jellesma et al., 2006; Kan et al., 2015; Krause, 2011; Løndal, 2010; Nammontri et al., 2013; Ray et al., 2009; Torsheim et al., 2001).

Studies examined the determinants of psychosomatic complaints in children. They found that the predictors of psychosomatic complaints were the mother's health, child's mental stability, contacts with peers, long-term illness, and, via other factors, parents' SOC, social competence, and school satisfaction (Berntsson & Gustafsson, 2000). Furthermore, in an attempt to understand the relationship between poor perceived health during childhood and an individual's well-being throughout life, 1231 12-year-old schoolchildren in Finland were studied. SOC and variables of social support were found significantly associated with perceived health. Physical exercise and SOC were associated with perceived health and father's occupation, and weak SOC was found to be independently associated with relatively poor health (Honkinen et al., 2005). Kan et al. (2015) demonstrated the mediating role of SOC on the association between childhood economic status and health in the community adult population of Japan. SOC significantly mediated the association between parents' education and current health among women and mediated between perceived childhood socio economic status (SES) and current health among men.

Studies focusing on the relation of somatic complaints and emotional functioning of children pinpointed attention to the existence of emotional problems in children who reported somatic complaints. Jellesma et al. (2006) studied 153 schoolchildren ages 8–13 years at three levels of somatic complaints (few, many, and clinical). The results showed that the clinical group and the children with many somatic complaints reported more negative moods on the anger, sadness, and fear scale, more difficulty differentiating emotions, and a weaker SOC than the group with fewer complaints. Torsheim et al. (2001) studied 1592 sixth-grade children, 1534 eighth-grade children, and 1605 tenth-grade children in an attempt to tap the role of SOC and school-related stress as predictors of health complaints. Age group comparisons revealed that the association between SOC and stress grew weaker with age, whereas the direct association between SOC and health complaints grew stronger. Fifty-two patients aged 9–22 years, who had stem cell transplant at least 3 years before the study, participated in a study of health and quality of life. The scores obtained on SOC for younger children (ages 9–12 years) showed that children in the SCT group have a SOC level equal to that of both the norm groups and other chronically ill children. The mean value for the younger children in the SCT group was in line with that of the norm group of children age 9 (Forinder et al., 2005).

Parents' SOC and Children's Health

The parents' role in predicting their children's health and health behavior was examined based on the salutogenic model. The relation between parental SOC and child health was explored in a large-scale study (Groholt et al., 2003) in the five Nordic countries, which included 9524 children ages 2–17 years, of which 35% co-responded with their parents due to their young age. Compared to the higher social classes, low levels of SOC were more common in the lower socio-economic classes. The association of child chronic health complaints with weak parental SOC was found to be disability-specific (diabetes, epilepsy, and psychiatric problems). Parents of children with diabetes, epilepsy, or psychiatric problems had 2–5 higher odds of having weak SOC compared to parents of children without a specific diagnosis.

Ray et al. (2009) studied 772 parent–child dyads of 10- to 11-year-old schoolchildren to find the relationship between food intake and parents' SOC. Weaker parental SOC was associated with children's irregular meal patterns, more frequent intake of energy-rich foods, and less frequent intake of nutrient-rich foods. Eli et al. (2016) found that mothers who had a stronger SOC were less likely to engage in pressuring or restrictive feeding practices. Resilience to stress reduced counterproductive practices, even in the presence of concern about the child's weight.

In another study, mothers with weaker levels of SOC were more likely to have children with decayed teeth or filled teeth regardless of the child's social class and gender (Bonanato et al., 2009). In contrast, the prevalence of clinical consequences of neglected dental caries was low among children attending public and private preschools in Brazil. It was associated with stronger levels of parental/caregiver SOC (Neves et al., 2019).

In a study identifying the predictors of adaptation and assessing potential moderating effects of parents' sense of coherence and family hardiness on the relationship of severity of illness of a child with asthma, SOC and family hardiness predicted family adaptation. Icelandic mothers perceived their family's adaptation more favorably than American mothers. Regarding the fathers, family demands predicted adaptation. SOC moderated the effect of family demands on adaptation for both parents (Svavarsdottir et al., 2005).

Intervention programs promoting children's health In addition to identifying SOC as a significant protective factor related to effective coping, the contribution of the salutogenic paradigm in explaining successful coping with stressors and health promotion has guided the development of intervention programs promoting health and health behavior. The following studies are examples of such intervention programs involving children and their families.

An intervention program based on the salutogenic model promoting oral health resulted in improved oral health. The intervention provided evidence that SOC influenced the oral health-related quality of life (Nammontri et al., 2013). Positive health beliefs and a stronger SOC were found to predict positive health beliefs and fewer symptoms. An additional intervention program focused on promoting play in an after-school program (ASP) had considerable potential of promoting the children's SOC. Most of the children in the study experienced their world as comprehensible, manageable, and meaningful. Negative thoughts and feelings were reduced during play. Play offered particularly strong opportunities for the children themselves to shape outcomes and interact with children, promoting their SOC (Løndal, 2010).

In another intervention program that aimed to promote health resources in children, 226 schoolchildren ages 5–10 years participated in a longitudinal self-worth reinforcement program. The results showed that developing SOC as a part of promoting mental health in schoolchildren is most effective during the early years of childhood. This finding emphasized the need to train professionals within the school (Krause, 2011).

Conclusions and Future Research Directions

The results of the surveyed studies support the conceptualization of the SOC construct as an important personal resource that develops during childhood. Stresses and challenges are a part of children's lives. However, most children who have a strong SOC can transform their potential resources into actuality, thereby promoting well-being. Children and adolescents with a strong SOC may have a good comprehension of most of their contextual conditions, situational demands, and personal experiences. They may feel relatively in control of their lives and may consider most of their tasks and participation in age-appropriate activities as meaningful, significant, and worth of investing the effort. When they face a stressful situation, they can select the appropriate strategies to cope effectively with the stressors. Thus, acquiring a wide range of coping strategies, alongside an emphasis on collaborative activities, developing social partnerships that respect different voices and self-reliance, may enhance the youngsters' resilience and motivation to invest effort to reach their preferred goals (Margalit, 1998). Consistency, a special cognitive challenge for children, may strengthen comprehensibility; an overload–underload balance, a special risk for children who struggle with school demands, may affect manageability; and the participation in socially valued decision-making may strengthen meaningfulness (Margalit, 2008).

The results of these studies have clear educational implications for school systems at various age groups in terms of prevention and intervention planning. The early manifestations of the developing SOC, as a personal resource, and the results that indicate that stresses and difficulties are disclosed in weaker levels of SOC, call for early awareness and empowering programs within educational systems. In addition, the results that show the impact of effective intervention not only on better academic functioning but also on friendship development and significant growth incoherence justify focused attempts on early intervention before SOC is structured and stabilized. The studies demonstrated the importance of early comprehensive intervention, as well as the significant value of preventive measures through sensitizing teachers not only to meet crises and difficulties but also especially to provide attentive support to the children's experiences. Preventive programs that empower children's abilities to integrate their thinking and learning skills with the abilities to regulate their feelings (emotion regulation) and actions (behavioral competence) promote growth, effort, and motivation (Idan & Margalit, 2011). School-based intervention programs and teachers' training promoting salutogenic approaches in class are required, alongside family-based interventions and parents' training, to promote salutogenic approaches in the home.

In the reviewed studies, children with typical development and children with developmental disabilities, learning disabilities, and various additional adjustment challenges were included. Most children who reported higher levels of loneliness also experienced a weak sense of coherence. In several studies, the weak sense of coherence was related to children's current distress, as well as to early expressions of adjustment difficulties and family climate. Mothers' sense of coherence was found as an important personal resource that enabled successful attachment relations and was related to children's sense of coherence (Al-Yagon & Mikulincer, 2004). Special attention was provided to groups of children with developmental or contextual challenges that reported levels of sense of coherence compatible with their typically developing peers. Thus, the awareness of the fact that difficulties never appeared in isolation, encouraged the multidimensional prevention and intervention approaches that treated not only academic or behavior challenges, but supported the whole child who had been developing satisfactory social relations while struggling with difficulties, to support coping and celebrate success and competencies. The salutogenic paradigm provides a structure to this planning, by emphasizing comprehensibility (explaining and clarifying the goals and the procedures), manageability (teaching the required skills to reach these goals), and meaningfulness (enhancing motivation and involvement in the effort).

Research presented in this review demonstrated the importance of the salutogenic approach in developmental research of children and adolescents and its potential for educational planning. The studies emphasized the interacting role of academic demands and social challenges with the SOC, clarifying the dynamic interactions between academic and socioemotional factors and children's readiness to treat their difficulties as challenges worthy of effort investment. These findings emphasized the major role of resilience approaches, considering SOC as a predictor in explaining well-being and adjustment, and calling for the future development of comprehensive educational intervention programs (Idan & Margalit, 2011).

To benefit schools and children from the salutogenic approach, two future research directions are needed. First, there is a need for longitudinal studies that will document changes and stabilities in the development of CSOC. Through longitudinal studies, we can clarify the interactions between the stabilization and the flexibility of children's SOC within different contextual conditions. Second, research calls for cross-cultural comparisons of the sense of coherence development. There is a need for a coordinated international collaboration for longitudinal research to explore the interactions of SOC between cultures, families, schools, communities, and children's different growth paths.

References

Agnafors, S., Svedin, C., Oreland, L., Bladh, M., Comasco, E., & Sydsjö, G. (2017). A biopsychosocial approach to risk and resilience on behavior in children followed from birth to age 12. *Child Psychiatry & Human Development. 48*, 584–596.

Al-Yagon, M. (2003). Children at-risk for developing learning disorders: Multiple perspectives. *Journal of Learning Disabilities, 36*(4), 318–335.

Al-Yagon, M. (2007). Socioemotional and behavioral adjustment among school-age children with learning disabilities: The moderating role of maternal personal resources. *The Journal of Special Education, 40*(4), 205–217.

Al-Yagon, M. (2008). Maternal personal resources and children's socio-emotional and behavioral adjustment. *Child Psychiatry & Human Development, 30*, 283–298.

Al-Yagon, M. (2010). Maternal emotional resources and socio-emotional well-being of children with and without learning disabilities. *Family Relations, 59*, 152–169.

Al-Yagon, M. (2011). Fathers' coping resources and children's socio-emotional adjustment among children with learning disabilities. *Journal of Learning Disabilities, 44*(6), 491–507.

Al-Yagon, M. (2012). Subtypes of attachment security in school-age children with learning disabilities. *Learning Disability Quarterly, 35*(3), 170–183.

Al-Yagon, M. (2014). Child-mother and child-father attachment security: Links to internalizing adjustment among children with learning disabilities. *Child Psychiatry and Human Development, 45*, 119–131.

Al-Yagon, M. (2015). Father and mothers of children with learning disabilities: Links between emotional and coping resources. *Learning Disability Quarterly, 38*(2), 112–128.

Al-Yagon, M., & Cinamon, G. R. (2008). Work-family relations among mothers of children with learning disorders. *European Journal of Special Needs Education, 23*, 91–107.

Al-Yagon, M., & Margalit, M. (2006). Loneliness, sense of coherence, and perception of teachers as a secure base among children with reading difficulties. *European Journal of Special Needs Education, 21*(1), 21–37.

Al-Yagon, M., & Mikulincer, M. (2004). Socioemotional and academic adjustment among children with learning disorders: The mediational role of attachment-based factors. *The Journal of Special Education, 38*(2), 111–124.

Antonovsky, A. (1987). *Unraveling the mystery of health*. Jossey-Bass.

Berntsson, L. T., & Gustafsson, J.-E. (2000). Determinants of psychosomatic complaints in Swedish schoolchildren aged seven to twelve years. *Scandinavian Journal of Public Health, 28*, 283–293.

Bonanato, K., Palva, S. M., Pordeus, I. A., Ramos-Jorge, M. L., Barbabela, D., & Allison, P. J. (2009). Relationship between mothers' sense of coherence and oral health status of preschool children. *Caries Research, 43*, 103–109.

Cassidy, J. (1994). Emotion regulation: Influences of attachment relationships. In N. A. Fox (Ed.), *The development of emotion regulation and dysregulation: Biological and behavioral aspects* (*Monographs of the Society for Research in Child Development*) (Vol. 59(2–3, Serial No. 240), pp. 228–249).

Cassidy, J., & Shaver, P. R. (Eds.). (1999). *Handbook of attachment: Theory, research, and clinical applications* (pp. 89–111). Guilford.

Dabrowska, A. (2003). Sense of coherence in parents of children with cerebral palsy. *Psychiatria Polska, 41*(2), 189–201.

Dabrowska, A. (2008). Sense of coherence and coping with stress in fathers of children with developmental disabilities. *Polish Psychological Bulletin, 39*(1), 29–34.

Damon, W. (2004). What is positive youth development? *Annals of the American Academy of Political and Social Science, 591*, 13–30.

Davidson, R. J., Lewis, M., Alloy, L. B., Amaral, D. G., Bush, G., Cohen, J., et al. (2002). Neural and behavioral substrates of mood and mood regulation. *Biological Psychiatry, 52*(6), 478–502.

Edwards, V. J., Holden, G. W., Felitti, V. J., & Anda, R. F. (2003). Relationship between multiple forms of child maltreatment and adult mental health in community respondents: Results from the Adverse Childhood Experiences Study. *The American Journal of Psychiatry, 160*(8), 1453–1460.

Efrati-Virtzer, M., & Margalit, M. (2009). Students' behaviour difficulties, sense of coherence and adjustment at school: Risk and protective factors. *European Journal of Special Needs Education, 24*(1), 59–73.

Einav, M., Levi, U., & Margalit, M. (2012). Mothers' coping and hope in early intervention. *European Journal of Special Needs Education, 27*(3), 265–279.

Eli, K., Sorjonen, K., Mokoena, L., Pietrobelli, A., Flodmark, C.-E., Faith, M. S., & Nowicka, P. (2016). Associations between maternal sense of coherence and controlling feeding practices: The importance of resilience and support in families of preschoolers. *Appetite, 105*, 134–143.

Feldman, D. B., Einav, M., & Margalit, M. (2018). Does family cohesion predict children's effort? The mediating roles of sense of coherence, hope and loneliness. *The Journal of Psychology, 152*(5), 276–289.

Forinder, U., Löf, C., & Winiarski, J. (2005). Quality of life and health in children following allogeneic SCT. *Bone Marrow Transplantation, 36*(2), 171–176.

Greenberg, M. T., Speltz, L., & DeKlyan, M. (1993). The role of attachment in the early development of disruptive behavior problems. *Development and Psychopathology, 5*, 191–213.

Groholt, E.-K., Stigum, H., Nordhagen, R., & Kohler, L. (2003). Is parental sense of coherence associated with child health? *European Journal of Public Health, 13*, 195–201.

Hedov, G., Anneren, G., & Wikblad, K. (2002). Swedish parents of children with Down's syndrome. *Scandinavian Journal of Caring Science, 16*, 424–430.

Hintermair, M. (2004). Sense of coherence: A relevant resource in the coping process of others of deaf and hard of hearing children? *Journal of Deaf Studies and Deaf Education, 9*(1), 15–26.

Honkinen, P.-L. K., Suominen, S. B., Valimaa, R. S., Helenius, H. Y., & Rautava, P. T. (2005). Factors associated with perceived health among 12-year-old school children. *Scandinavian Journal of Public Health, 33*, 35–41.

Idan, O., & Margalit, M. (2011). The salutogenic orientation: Children's sense of coherence and hopeful thinking in education of children and adolescents. *TEME*, Special Issue, *24*(4), 5–18.

Jellesma, F. C., Rieffe, C., Terwogt, M. M., & Kneepkens, C. M. F. (2006). Somatic complaints and health care use in children: Mood, emotion awareness and sense of coherence. *Social Science & Medicine, 63*, 2640–2648.

Kan, C., Kawakami, N., & Umeda, M. (2015). Mediating role of psychological resources on the association between childhood socioeconomic status and current health in the community adult population of Japan. *International Journal of Behavior Medicine, 22*, 764–774.

Krause, C. (2011). Developing sense of coherence in educational contexts: Making progress in promoting mental health in children. *International Review of Psychiatry, 23*(6), 525–532.

Liberman, L., Ratzon, N., & Bart, O. (2013). The profile of performance skills and emotional factors in the context of participation among young children with Developmental Coordination Disorder. *Research in Developmental Disabilities, 34*(1), 87–94.

Løndal, K. (2010). Children's lived experience and their sense of coherence: Bodily play in a Norwegian after-school program. *Child Care in Practice, 16*(4), 391–407.

Lundberg, P., & Nystrom, F. H. (1994). Sense of coherence, social structure, and health. *European Journal of Public Health, 4*, 252–257.

Mak, W. W. S., Ho, A. H. Y., & Kaw, R. W. (2007). Sense of coherence, parenting attitudes ad stress among mothers of children with autism in Hong Kong. *Journal of Intellectual Disability Research, 20*, 157–167.

Margalit, M. (1994). *Loneliness among children with special needs: Theory, research, coping, and intervention*. Springer.

Margalit, M. (1998). Loneliness and coherence among preschool children with learning disabilities. *Journal of Learning Disabilities, 31*(2), 173–180.

Margalit, M. (2003). Resilience model among individuals with learning disabilities (LD): Proximal and distal influences. *Learning Disabilities Research & Practice, 18*(2), 82–86.

Margalit, M. (2008). *The salutogenic paradigm in education: Promoting well-being of children and their families*. Paper presented at the International Seminar on Salutogenesis, Helsinki.

Margalit, M., Al-Yagon, M., & Kleitman, T. (2006). Family subtyping and early intervention. *Journal of Policy and Practice in Intellectual Disabilities, 3*(1), 33–41.

Margalit, M., & Efrati, M. (1995). Loneliness, coherence, and companionship among children with learning disorders. *Educational Psychology, 16*(1), 69–79.

Miller, J. G., & Kinsbourne, M. (2012). Culture and neuroscience in developmental psychology: Contributions and challenges. *Child Development Perspectives, 6*(1), 35–41.

Most, T., Al-Yagon, M., Tur-Kaspa, H., & Margalit, M. (2000). Phonological awareness, peer nominations, and social competence among preschool children at risk for developing learning disabilities. *International Journal of Disability, Development & Education, 47*(1), 89–105.

Mowder, B. A., Rubinson, F., & Yasik, A. E. (2009). Current status and future directions. In B. A. Mowder, F. Rubinson, & A. E. Yasik (Eds.), *Evidence based practice in infant and early childhood psychology* (pp. 703–715). Wiley.

Nammontri, O., Robinson, P. G., & Baker, S. R. (2013). Enhancing oral health via sense of coherence: A cluster randomized trial. *Journal of Dentistry Research, 92*(1), 26–31.

National Scientific Council on the Developing Child. (2004). *Children's emotional development is built into the architecture of their brains*. (Working paper 2). Retrieved from Center on the Developing Child website http://www.developingchild.harvard.edu

National Scientific Council on the Developing Child. (2012). *Establishing a level foundation for life: Mental health begins in early childhood.* (Working paper 6). Retrieved from Center on the Developing Child website http://www.developingchild.harvard.edu

Natvig, G. K., Hanestad, B. R., & Samdal, O. (2006). The role of the student: Salutogenic or pathogenic? *International Journal of Nursing Practice, 12*(5), 280–287.

Neves, E. T. B., Perazzo, M. F., Gomes, M. C., Ribeiro, I. L. A., Paiva, S. M., & Granville-Garcia, A. F. (2019). Association between sense of coherence and untreated dental caries in preschoolers: a cross-sectional study. *International Dental Journal, 69*, 141–149.

Oelofsen, N., & Richardson, P. (2006). Sense of coherence and parenting stress in mothers and fathers of preschool children with developmental disability. *Journal of Intellectual & Developmental Disability, 31*(1), 1–12.

Olson, D. H. (1986). Circumplex model VII: Validation studies and FACES III. *Family Process, 26*, 337–351.

Olson, D. H. (2000). Circumplex model of marital and family systems. *Journal of Family Therapy, 22*, 144–167.

Olsson, M. B., & Hwang, C. P. (2002). Sense of coherence in parents of children with different developmental disabilities. *Journal of Intellectual Disability Research, 46*(7), 548–559.

Pisula, E., & Kossakowska, Z. (2010). Sense of coherence and coping with stress among mothers and fathers of children with autism. *Journal of Autism & Developmental Disorders, 40*, 1485–1494.

Ray, C., Suominen, S., & Roos, E. (2009). The role of parent's sense of coherence in irregular meal pattern and food intake pattern of children aged 10–11 in Finland. *The Journal of Epidemiology and Community Health, 63*(12), 1005–1009.

Reid, J. B., Patterson, G. R., & Snyder, J. (2002). *Antisocial behavior in children and adolescents: A developmental analysis and model for intervention.* American Psychological Association.

Rubin, K., Bukowski, W., & Parker, J. (2006). Peer interactions, relationships, and groups. In W. Damon & R. M. Lerner (Eds.), *Handbook of child psychology* (Vol. 3: Social, emotional, and personality development. (N. Eisenberg, Vol. Ed.), 6th ed., pp. 571–645). Wiley.

Sharabi, A., Levi, U., & Margalit, M. (2012). Children's loneliness, sense of coherence, family climate and hope: Developmental risk and protective factors. *The Journal of Psychology, 146*(1–2), 61–83.

Sivberg, B. (2002). Family system and coping behaviors. *Autism, 6*(4), 397–409.

Svavarsdottir, E. K., Rayens, M. K., & McCubbin, M. (2005). Predictors of adaptation in Icelandic and American families of young children with chronic asthma. *Family & Community Health, 28*(4), 338–350.

Thompson, R. A. (2001). Development in the first years of life. *The Future of Children, 11*(1), 20–33.

Thompson, R. A., & Lagattuta, K. (2006). Feeling and understanding: Early emotional development. In K. McCartney & D. Phillips (Eds.), *The Blackwell handbook of early childhood development* (pp. 317–337). Blackwell.

Torsheim, T., Aaroe, L. E., & Wold, B. (2001). Sense of coherence and school related stress as predictors of subjective health complaints in early adolescence: Interactive, indirect or direct relationships? *Social Science & Medicine, 53*, 603–614.

Yugar, J. M., & Shapiro, E. S. (2001). Elementary children's school friendship: A comparison of peer assessment methodologies. *School Psychology Review, 30*(4), 568.

16

Adolescence, Salutogenesis and SOC

Orna Braun-Lewensohn, Orly Idan, Bengt Lindström, and Malka Margalit

The Developmental Stage of Adolescence

Adolescence is a period of growth and development between childhood and adulthood. This developmental period involves new demands on the individual. A major task of this period is moving toward independence from dependency on the family; therefore, peers become a crucial socialization circle for the adolescent (Romeo, 2013; Spear, 2013). During this period, several physiological and cognitive changes occur as young people confront developmental tasks and challenges. During the last decade, there has been a marked increase in neurobiological research on cognitive, emotional, and behavioral changes, and development during adolescence. These studies have found that cognitively, adolescents, as well as adults, can suppress responses when no emotional information is provided (Tottenham et al., 2011). However, it is the avoidance of social cues during challenging situations in which adolescents have a difficulty to make a proper and rational response (Casey & Caudle, 2013). Thus, it seems that tension between regulation of behavior and sensitivity to positive environmental cues makes the response of the individual during the period of adolescence more complex (Somerville et al., 2011).

The adolescent, at the very best, can only have gained a tentative strong SOC, which may be useful for a short-range prediction about coping with stressors and health status (Antonovsky, 1987, p. 107).

O. Braun-Lewensohn (✉)
Conflict Management & Resolution Program, Ben-Gurion University of the Negev, Beer Sheva, Israel
e-mail: ornabl@bgu.ac.il

O. Idan
School of Psychology, Interdisciplinary Center (IDC), Herzliya, Israel

B. Lindström
NTNU Center for Health Promotion Research, Norwegian University of Science and Technology, Trondheim, Norway
e-mail: bengtblind@hotmail.com

M. Margalit
Tel Aviv University, Peres Academic Center, Rehovot, Israel

In line with the positive youth development perspectives (Damon, 2004), there is a growing recognition of the individuals who are eager to explore the world, to acquire competence, and to struggle with challenges and difficulties. This approach focuses on productive activities rather than on trying to cure and treat maladaptive tendencies. The agenda is to maximize the potential of the individual and to reduce the potential of hazardous, destructive, and antisocial behaviors (Lerner & Benson, 2003). The period of adolescence is a particularly important developmental stage since social, emotional, and cognitive processes are involved in attempts to navigate increasingly complex relationships (Blakemore & Mills, 2014). Indeed, it is during these years that abstract thinking and cognitive processing develop along with enhanced moral reasoning and judgment. These positive processes enable the adolescent to explore the world, gain competences, and contribute to the world surrounding him/her (Damon, 2004). As children age, their coping repertoire expands and shifts from primarily external, behavior-oriented to more internal, cognitively based strategies (Aldwin et al., 1994).

The advanced forms of reflection, such as the ability to consider things in hypothetical and abstract terms, and the ability to monitor one's cognitive activity during the process of thinking, enable adolescents to see from the perspective of other persons, to plan, to anticipate the future consequences of an action, and to offer alternative explanations of events. Cognitive mastery is, therefore, an important contribution to young people's ability to manage or regulate their feelings and to control their emotions and/or avoid being overwhelmed by them (Garnefski et al., 2001). These abilities also have the potential to influence the emotional–motivational and behavioral components of sense of coherence (SOC). It is during these years, as young people move from one experience of using specific coping resources to another, that different resources can be reviewed and crystalized.

In the following section, we present adjustments to the SOC questionnaire and discuss a variety of ways that researchers have approached the study of salutogenesis and adolescence.

Studies of SOC During Adolescence

Our literature search used Ebsco, PsycInfo, PubMed, SocioFile, and GoogleScholar, and we searched the sites of the publishers Sage, Springer, and Wiley. We looked at the last decade from 2014 to 2019 and included the search words: adolecs*, youth, sense of coherence, and salutogenesis. We came up with more than 30 articles and research from 16 countries in Europe, the Middle East, Australia, and the United States. Table 16.1 summarizes these studies.

The following themes emerged from the identified studies.

Table 16.1 Studies of SOC during adolescence

Author	Year	Place	Population	Variables	Results
1. Abu-Kaf et al.	2017	Israel	Jewish and Bedouin adolescents, aged 14–18, during a period of escalated political violence	SOC, hope, anxiety, anger	Bedouin Arab adolescents reported lower levels of SOC and higher levels of hope and anger, compared to Jewish adolescents. SOC contributed significantly to the reduction of state anxiety only among the Jewish adolescents
2. Abu-Kaf & Braun-Lewensohn	2019	Israel	Bedouin Arab adolescents, 14–18 years old, during three periods of escalated political violence	SOC, hope, anxiety, anger, psychological distress	Over time, SOC was found to be a significant predictor of those stress reactions, whereas the association between hope components and stress reactions weakened over time
3. Al-Said et al.	2018	Israel	Bedouin adolescents, 13–18 years old, from recognized and unrecognized villages; some had experienced home demolitions	SOC, emotional reactions	Stress reactions were strongest among adolescents from unrecognized villages with demolitions. Personal SOC was related to fewer emotional reactions among the adolescents from recognized villages. Among adolescents from unrecognized villages, especially adolescents living in an unrecognized village with demolitions, a stronger SOC was linked to stronger emotional reactions
4. Aitcheson et al.	2017	Gaza	11th–12th grade Palestinians in refugee camps	Depression, anxiety, coping skills, self-regulation, optimism, parenting style, family sense of coherence, national identity, ethnic identity	Adolescents with stronger national identity, stronger family SOC, greater self-regulation, and more optimism reported less severe depressive and anxious symptoms. Age, optimism, family SOC, ethnic identity, self-regulation, and coping skills were all significant predictors of resilience
5. Barni & Danioni	2016	Italy	Italian adolescents between 14 and 19 years old	Values, SOC	Adolescents' conservative and self-transcendent values were the most important predictors of their SOC. The greater the importance placed on conservatism and self-transcendence, the stronger the confidence in the perception that problems to be faced are clear, manageable, and worthy of commitment and engagement
6. Braun-Lewensohn et al.	2015	Israel	Jewish and Arab adolescents aged 14–19	SOC, community SOC, participation in extra-curricular activities, exposure to violence	Jewish adolescents reported significantly stronger SOC and community SOC. They participated more in extra-curricular activities and were more exposed to and victimized by violence. While SOC was an asset among both groups, participation in extra-curricular activities was an asset only for the Arab youth

Table 16.1 (continued)

Author	Year	Place	Population	Variables	Results
7. Braun-Lewensohn	2016	Israel	16–18 year olds during a social protest	Values, SOC, social responsibility, civic efficacy, hope	Values and SOC explained civic engagement, while only universal and collective in-group values and civic engagement directly explained citizens' efficacy
8. Braun-Lewensohn et al.	2017	Israel	Secular Jewish, religious Jewish and Bedouin Arab adolescents aged 12–18	SOC, hope	Religious Jews reported the strongest SOC and Bedouin Arabs reported the strongest hope. In both Jewish groups, significant correlations were found between the expectation component and/or global hope and SOC. However, no links were found between global hope or its components or dimensions and SOC among the Bedouin Arab group
9. Braun-Lewensohn et al.	2018	Israel	Bedouin Arab adolescents, 14–18 years old, in 2010 and 2015	SOC, anxiety, anger	In the 2010 sample, unlike in many stable Western societies, the stronger the SOC, the more severe the stress reactions. However, in 2015, the results resembled those reported in Western cultural settings and the stronger the SOC, the fewer symptoms of stress were reported
10. Braun-Lewensohn & Al-Said	2018	Greece	Syrian refugee adolescents aged 13–18	Exposure to war, appraisal of danger, receiving aid, SOC, wishes and expectations, internalizing and externalizing problems	Boys, younger adolescents, and those who had more recently arrived in the refugee camp reported stronger SOC. The amount of time spent in the refugee camp, gender, exposure to war situations, and appraisal of danger all contributed to the explained variance in the different psychological problems. However, SOC mediated the relationships between all of the sociodemographic and situational variables and the examined psychological problems
11. Carneiro et al.	2017	Brazil	29 adolescents with MPS and 29 adolescents without MPS, and their mothers	SOC, MPS	The SOC of the mothers of adolescents with MPS was associated with the adolescents' experiences with dental caries. Improving mothers' SOC should contribute to a better quality of life for their children
12. da Costa et al.	2017	Brazil	12–15 years	SOC, self-perceived dental aesthetics, Dental Aesthetic Index	SOC was associated with self-perceived dental aesthetics. Among the adolescents with no need for orthodontic treatment, those with a low SOC perceived their dental aesthetics more negatively than those with high levels of SOC; SOC being higher in the younger
13. Elfassi et al.	2016	Israel	8th–11th grade from three communities	Community SOC, involvement in risk behaviors	Community SOC is a significant protective factor that could be related to reduced involvement in risk behaviors
14. El-Shahawy et al.	2015	USA, California	Adolescents attending high school	SOC, smoking behavior, smoking expectations	SOC was correlated with baseline cigarette smoking and next-year smoking expectation. SOC did not predict change in cigarette smoking or change in next-year smoking

(continued)

Table 16.1 (continued)

Author	Year	Place	Population	Variables	Results
15. Evans & Davis	2018	USA, Nevada	30 American Indian (AI) youth 14–18 years old	SOC, psychological problems, historical loss	Higher levels of SOC predicted fewer historical trauma-related symptoms. SOC may enhance AI youth's sense of belonging by countering the effects of thwarted belongingness
16. Garcia-Moya et al.	2014	Spain	Spanish adolescents	Bullying victimization, physical and psychological symptoms, SOC	Weak-SOC adolescents were significantly more likely to be bullied. In addition, among weak-SOC adolescents, there was a significant association between having been bullied and physical and psychological symptoms. In contrast, among strong-SOC adolescents, having been bullied was not significantly associated with increased physical complaints and its effects on psychological complaints seemed to be weaker
17. Huss et al.	2018	Israel	14- to 16-year-old Bedouin youth	Drawing on coping resources	The findings reveal and concretize a mismatch between SOC among these youth and the predominant Western understanding of coping in terms of meanings, manageability, and comprehensibility of coping methods
18. Jakobsson	2014	Sweden	15- to 18-year-old Swedish adolescents	Participation in a sport club, SOC, and its components	The teenagers found sports fun and meaningfulness because they experienced learning and development. They found competition challenging, and they enjoyed the involvement and engagement with others
19. Kalagy et al.	2017	Israel	Ultra-Orthodox and national religious adolescents aged 14–18.	Attitudes toward the military operation, Attitudes toward the Israeli–Palestinian conflict, SOC, anxiety, anger	SOC was positively related to more wars Hawkish attitudes among the national religious group. SOC was negatively related to peaceful resolution Dovish attitudes among the ultra-Orthodox adolescents. In both groups, SOC was negatively related to anxiety
20. Krok	2015	Poland	Older adolescents, 16–20 years old	SOC, optimism, subjective and psychological well-being	Direct and indirect effects of SOC on subjective and psychological well-being measures were found, suggesting that optimism served as a partial mediator. SOC should not be interpreted as an autonomous resource contributing to a favorable development of late adolescents' well-being, but as a factor that works in connection with dispositional optimism
21. Lage et al.	2017	Brazil	Adolescents	SOC, oral clinical examinations	Higher mother's SOC and adolescent's SOC were protective factors against dental caries among the adolescents
22. Latzer et al.	2019	Israel	Boys in grades 8–12	SOC, body shape, eating attitudes, eating disorder	SOC was negatively correlated with developing an eating disorder
23. Lindblom et al.	2017	Sweden	14- to 21-year- olds in pre-criminal and early criminal phases	Criminal Thinking Styles (PICTS), SOC	Cognitive intervention shows promise for reducing criminal thinking patterns and increasing SOC, which may have beneficial effects on the behavior of young offenders

Table 16.1 (continued)

Author	Year	Place	Population	Variables	Results
24. Moksnes et al.	2014	Norway	Adolescents, 13–18 years old	Stress, SOC, emotional symptoms	Girls scored higher than boys in terms of stress related to peer pressure, home life, school performance, school/leisure conflict, and emotional symptoms. Conversely, boys reported higher SOC than girls. SOC was strongly and inversely associated with emotional symptoms, especially anxiety among girls. SOC also moderated the association between stress related to peer pressure and depressive symptoms among both genders
25. Moksnes & Haugan	2015	Norway	Adolescents, 13–18 years old	SOC, life satisfaction, stress	Boys reported higher scores for SOC and life satisfaction, whereas girls scored higher than boys in most of the stressor domains. There was a significantly strong and positive association between SOC and life satisfaction, independent of age, and each individual stressor
26. Moksnes & Lazarewicz	2016	Norway	Adolescents, 13–18 years old		Adolescents aged 13–14 years had significantly higher SOC scores than those aged 15–16. A significant positive association was found between self-esteem and SOC when controlling for sex, age, stress, subjective health complaints, and subjective health. Neither sex nor age moderated the relationship between self-esteem and SOC
27. Rizou et al.	2017	Greece	Children, 10–18 years old, with epilepsy	Disease characteristics, perception of the illness, psychological distress, sleep problems, somatic complaints	A brief self-regulation-based intervention may have beneficial effects for children and adolescents suffering from epilepsy, through improvements in coherence, psychological distress, and sleep problems
28. Shreuder et al.	2014	Netherland	Adolescents and young adults, 17–22 years old	Semi-structured interviews to elicit their experiences from a salutogenic perspective	Analysis revealed that several on the youth care farm worked well for the youngsters and contributed to their personal development and to their SOC: the feeling that the world is or can be meaningful, comprehensible, and manageable, associated with positive outcomes in endeavors linked to improving health and well-being
29. Smith et al.	2015	USA	Adolescents aged 11–18 with a sibling diagnosed with autism	Coping orientation, relationships, SOC, psychological problems	The stress of autism spectrum disorder (ASD) severity and adjustment resources are related among typically developing (TD) adolescents who have an autistic sibling. There was a strong relationship between TD sibling adjustment and SOC. A greater number of positive coping strategies buffered TD sibling coherence levels when ASD severity scores were high
30. Super et al.	2018	Netherland	Vulnerable youth, 12–23 years old	Behavior, school performance, subjective health and well-being, self-regulation skills, SOC, sports participation	Sports participation was positively related to pro-social behavior, subjective health, well-being, and SOC

(continued)

Table 16.1 (continued)

Author	Year	Place	Population	Variables	Results
31. Ustinavičienė et al.	2018	Lithuania	Adolescents aged 13–18	Amount of time spent playing computer games, types of games, SOC	Boys and girls aged 13–15 with a weak SOC were significantly more likely to play action or combat computer games for 5 or more hours per day, in comparison to the respondents who had a strong SOC
32. Vilija & Romualdas	2014	Lithuania	8th graders	Posttraumatic stress (PTS) symptoms, daily consumption of unhealthy foods, physical inactivity, smoking, SOC	All lifetime traumatic events were associated with PTS symptoms, as well as were consumption of unhealthy foods. SOC weakened the strength of those associations
33. Wadsby et al.	2014	Sweden	High-school students	Parental bonding, psychiatric symptoms, SOC	SOC was higher among teens with alternating residences and teens living with both parents, but it was lower among those living with a single parent
34. Wang et al.	2014	Australia	Adolescents with heart disease, 12–20 years old	Quality of life, adolescents' knowledge of their cardiac condition, anxiety, depression, perceived social support, Life Orientation, SOC	Health-related quality of life was found to be positively correlated with low levels of anxiety and depression, a good understanding of their cardiac condition, feelings of optimism, adequate social support, and a strong SOC
35. Würtz et al.	2015	Denmark	7th and 8th graders	Use of over-the-counter painkillers, pain, well-being, friends, SOC	Girls with a weak SOC (the lowest first quartile) had a significantly increased risk of receiving unemployment benefits, social assistance and disability benefits, compared with girls with a strong SOC. For boys, only minor protective and non-significant differences were found
36. Xu et al.	2019	China	Middle- and high-school students	Socioeconomic status, maternal care and control, SOC, depression	Socioeconomic status, maternal care, and adolescent SOC were positively related to each other and negatively related to adolescent depressive symptoms. Socioeconomic status was associated with adolescent depressive symptoms indirectly through maternal care separately, as well as through maternal care and adolescent SOC sequentially

Adaptations of the SOC Questionnaires

Based on the original SOC questionnaire (Antonovsky, 1983), several researchers have examined the adaptability of the questionnaire to adolescent populations. For example, *the adolescent sense of coherence scale* (Antonovsky & Sagy, 1986) was adjusted to fit adolescents' characteristics, that is, development of self-identity, orientation to one's self society, confusion, unpredictable changes, close emotional ties with parents for the development of open communication, stability of the community, etc. Several items were removed from the original 29-item scale, and others were rephrased to make sure that adolescents understand the items (Antonovsky & Sagy, 1986), ending up with the final version of 13 items which is considered as a single factor and not the three separate components—meaningfulness, comprehensibility, and manageability (Hagquist & Andrich, 2004). Many studies have used this scale, and reliability proved to be very good ($\alpha \approx 0.80$). Another approach to the adaptation of the scale to the adolescence developmental stage was based on the use of the child version (CSOC) without the examples and distractors for younger children. The description of the CSOC can be found in the chapter on children (Margalit & Efrati, 1996). The adolescence adaptation from the CSOC consisted of 16 items (e.g., "When I want something I'm sure I'll get it"; "When I need help there is someone around to help me"), on a five-point Likert-type scale ranging from 1 (never) to 5 (always). A Cronbach's alpha of 0.78 was obtained (Levi et al., 2014).

The SOC Construct During Adolescence

The stability question regarding SOC accompanied this construct since the beginning of research about it. Antonovsky and Sagy (1986) argued that SOC should be strengthening during adolescence and stabilized toward the end of this developmental period. However, studies that addressed the issue of age and the stability of SOC revealed inconsistencies (Apers et al., 2013; Ayo-Yusuf et al., 2008; Garcia-Moya et al., 2013a, b, c, d; Kristensson & Öhlund, 2005; Moksnes et al., 2012). Indeed, Eriksson and Lindström (2007) stated that SOC is likely to vary during adolescence due to developmental changes, transitions, and challenges. While some researchers did not find differences among various age groups (Honkinen et al., 2008) and claimed the existence of SOC stability during adolescence (Kröninger-Jungaberle & Grevenstein, 2013), others focused on the variability between groups of adolescents between younger and older adolescents (Garcia-Moya et al., 2013a, b, c, d) as well as between groups with strong versus weak scores of SOC. The group with a weaker SOC reported more variability in its SOC scores (Buddeberg-Fischer et al., 2001).

Moreover, during periods of political violence, studies have shed light on the impacts of fragile periods and documented a drop in SOC levels during acute stress situations. However, once the acuteness is over, the SOC gains back its strengths (Braun-Lewensohn et al., 2013). Nevertheless, when adolescents face chronic states of stress, such as longitudinal missile attacks, the deterioration of the SOC remained stable over time (Braun-Lewensohn & Sagy, 2010).

Other *demographic characteristics,* apart from age, have significant roles in the determination of the SOC levels. Gender differences were examined, and many studies showed that the SOC scores of boys were higher than the scores of girls (Apers et al., 2013; Dorri et al., 2010; Evans et al., 2010; Kristensson & Öhlund, 2005; Moksnes et al., 2011, 2012; Nio, 2010). Also, socioeconomic status plays an important role in the SOC prediction. Thus, higher levels of parents' education (Feldt et al., 2005; Geckova et al., 2010; Ristkari et al., 2009), higher economic status (Geckova et al., 2010), and living with two parents (Ayo-Yusuf et al., 2009) have been important indicators of stronger SOC. Lastly, membership in a minority group in different cultures around the world predicted weaker SOC scores than those of majority groups (Braun-Lewensohn, 2014; Braun-Lewensohn & Sagy, 2011a, b; Glanz et al., 2005).

SOC, Health, Mental Health, and Psychosocial Behavior

Examining the various studies, we found that the relations of health, mental health, and psychosocial behaviors with SOC were explored. More specifically, researchers investigated the SOC as a predictor of health outcomes, mental health, and diverse health-promoting behaviors during adolescence.

Several studies examined the relations between the SOC and general health (Eriksson & Lindström, 2006; Nilsson et al., 2003). Stronger SOC was related to better-perceived health, while weaker SOC was related to medication use. Moreover, SOC was negatively related to reported health problems (Blom et al., 2010; Garcia-Moya et al., 2013a, b, c, d; Geckova et al., 2010; Honkinen et al., 2005; Koushede & Holstein, 2009; Mattila et al., 2011; Modin et al., 2011; Moksnes et al., 2011; Myrin & Lagerström, 2006).

Other examinations related to health focused on groups with specific health problems. For example, surprisingly, adolescents with heart problems were found to have a stronger SOC compared to healthy adolescents. These results were explained by the fact that youngsters with such chronic disease have learned to cope with their problem, which increased their manageability, besides having existential implications that increased their meaningfulness. Moreover, a supportive home environment experienced by these adolescents emphasizes specific life events as being more comprehensible, manageable, and meaningful; hence, nurtured feelings of SOC (Luyckx et al., 2012). More expected results were found for adolescents with epilepsy where a weaker SOC was found in the long run, reflecting the experience of losing control during seizures and difficulty in assessing when to expect the next seizure. Following this line, those adolescents with no seizures had a stronger SOC (Gauffin et al., 2010).

Mental health has been the focus of numerous studies that examined diverse outcomes. Stress-related outcomes such as anxiety, anger, depression, psychological distress, and other emotional and internalizing or externalizing problems were examined in the context of political violence (Braun-Lewensohn & Sagy, 2010, 2011a, b; Sagy & Braun-Lewensohn, 2009) and with regard to challenging and extreme life events such as child abuse (Gustafsson et al., 2010) or juvenile delinquency (Koposov et al., 2003). However, adolescents were also examined during regular daily life with "normal" life stressors, such as academic, school, or peer pressure as well as family conflicts (Moksnes et al., 2012, 2013; Nielsen & Hansson, 2007; Ristkari et al., 2009; Simonsson et al., 2008). All these studies confirm that the SOC can be considered a resilience factor. It can be concluded that a strong SOC predicts reduced stress and decreased internalizing or/and externalizing problems.

Moreover, examining the relationships of SOC with *psychosocial behaviors* even strengthens the consideration of SOC as a resilient factor. Accordingly, results of various studies showed that adolescents with stronger SOC reported a healthier lifestyle, a better quality of life, and well-being (Honkinen et al., 2009; Neuner et al., 2011). The healthy lifestyle is related, on the one hand, to physical activities and exercises (Bronikowski, 2010) and, on the other hand, to smoking habits, alcohol abuse (Garcia-Moya et al., 2013a, b, c, d, 2013a; Myrin & Lagerström, 2006; Nielsen & Hansson, 2007), and eating habits (Myrin & Lagerström, 2006). Similarly, the relations between SOC and oral behavior (e.g., toothbrush habits) were reported. Stronger SOC was linked to lower gingivitis, more willingness to change toothbrush habits, and especially increased tooth brushing (e.g., Ayo-Yusuf et al., 2008, 2009; Dorri et al., 2010).

Ecological Contexts: Family, School, Peers, and Community

Ecological contexts (Bronfenbrenner, 1977, 1979; Bronfenbrenner & Morris, 2006) extend the consideration from a focus on the personal level to awareness and sensitization to contextual characteristics and systemic consideration such as the families, schools, and communities. Several family-related factors were examined in relation to the SOC. For example, open family communication (Garcia-Moya et al., 2013a, b, c, d; Marsh et al., 2007), focused parenting style (Garcia-Moya et al., 2013a, b, c, d), and parents' knowledge regarding their children activities (Garcia-Moya et al., 2013a, b, c, d) were considered positive contributors to the development of a strong SOC. In addition, child-centered parenting during adolescence (examined within a longitudinal paradigm) predicted a stronger SOC at adulthood (Feldt et al., 2005).

In addition to examining family contexts and factors which could enhance or reduce personal SOC, few studies also related to family sense of coherence as another source to rely on when facing difficulties and/or stressful situations. Likewise the personal SOC, it was found that also family SOC is a resilient factor, and adolescents with stronger family SOC reported reduced stress (Sagy & Braun-Lewensohn, 2009; Sagy & Dotan, 2001).

Another important ecological system is *school*. While the family dimension produced mainly studies that pinpointed attention at the contribution of family characteristics to the development of SOC, studies of schools focused attention on outcomes, examining the adolescents' achievement and adjustment, and their relationship to SOC as a mediation factor. Within the educational systems, a stronger SOC predicted high grades and enhanced academic motivation and success. Lower stress levels were also reported as related to stronger SOC (Honkinen et al., 2005; Kristensson & Öhlund, 2005; Lackaye & Margalit, 2006). Moreover, stronger SOC was linked to social competence (Mattila et al., 2011; Moksnes et al., 2011).

The school system provides a unique opportunity to look at particular populations with regard to SOC. Adolescents with learning disabilities are an additional example of the importance of the SOC (Idan & Margalit, 2014; Lackaye & Margalit, 2006). These youngsters are identified by their chronic academic challenges emerging from neurodevelopmental difficulties. Their difficulties at school systems remain a continuous source for increased stress, endless day-to-day struggling with age-appropriate academic roles, and with social and emotional consequences. Indeed their sources of stress are not dramatic, but their lasting impact is expressed in weaker SOC. Studies placed the SOC as a mediator of hopeful thinking, predicting adjustment and effort investment in school. The adolescents' systems, such as families, schools, and communities, may further clarify the important role of the SOC and the factors that predict its development.

The focus on *peer relations and community atmosphere* produced studies that explored these factors as predictors of SOC development. An additional group of studies explored SOC as a collective construct contributing to the mental health of adolescents. Exploring SOC as a dependent variable, it seems that social support (Marsh et al., 2007), neighborhood or community cohesion (Garcia-Moya et al., 2013a, b, c, d; Marsh et al., 2007; Peled et al., 2013), and success in school (Garcia-Moya et al., 2013a, b, c, d) are all constructive in the development of strong SOC.

To expand the measurement of the SOC from the personal to the collective level, the *sense of community coherence* instrument was developed, which includes the components of comprehensibility, manageability, and meaningfulness (Braun-Lewensohn, 2014; Braun-Lewensohn & Sagy, 2011b; Peled et al., 2013). *Comprehensibility* refers to the sense of predictability, safety, and security felt by members of the community and the extent to which that community is understandable. A community's *manageability* expresses its ability to assist its members, via treatment providers and group programs, among others, in times of crisis and distress. Lastly, the higher the level of *meaningfulness* among the members of a community, the abler they are to express themselves, and the higher the likelihood that they will feel satisfied with and challenged and interested by what the community has to offer them (Braun-Lewensohn & Sagy, 2011b). Recent studies showed that indeed the sense of community coherence is another source of support for coping during adolescence when facing acute or chronic types of stress, especially among collectivist cultures (Braun-Lewensohn, 2014; Braun-Lewensohn & Sagy, 2011b; Peled et al., 2013).

Conclusions, Implications, and Directions for Future Research

This chapter focused on the sense of coherence and salutogenesis during the developmental period of adolescence. While in many ways, adolescents appear to function similarly to adults, numerous cognitive, biological, and behavioral processes are formed and shaped on the path to maturity and normative adulthood.

A recent review on salutogenesis and the concept of SOC examined the influence of different factors such as gender and age as well as different developmental contexts (family, school, peers, and neighborhood) on the development of SOC (Rivera et al., 2013). In our current review, we extended conceptualization and research results regarding SOC during this important developmental period of adolescence within a different orientation. Mainly, we addressed how the SOC questionnaire was adopted to fit adolescent populations, as well as the clarifying ways how SOC is linked to different health, mental health, and psychosocial behaviors in different ecological contexts. We can conclude that the review of studies from around the world in the last decade demonstrated that personal and systemic (i.e., family and community) SOC are important resources for coping with a wide variety of stressful situations. The survey of the studies shows that the SOC may be considered as a protective factor for adolescents in different cultures. During adolescence, the SOC may contribute to moderating and mediating stress experiences and may also play a protective role, similar to that of the mature adult SOC.

The educational and community implications of the current consideration of the SOC as a critical resource call for the sensitizing educators and community workers to the importance of the salutogenic construct. Future empowering programs should be guided by this construct, leading to the development of prevention/inoculation to stress planning as well as programs promoting positive psychosocial and healthy behaviors and academic success.

Our review raises several directions for future research in the field of salutogenesis and the sense of coherence during adolescence. Despite developments, there are still some issues that require attention. This includes the role of family coherence as a protective factor for health and mental health, for success in school, and psychosocial behaviors that determine their relationships and their attitudes toward each other. Moreover, non-western cultural groups were less studied in this context. When studied, some questions regarding the universality of the concept of SOC were raised (Braun-Lewensohn & Sagy, 2011a). Thus, it seems important to examine this issue further. We should focus on the meanings of sense of coherence in such cultures as well as the understanding of the questionnaire and the implication of SOC in such societies.

References

Abu-Kaf, S., & Braun-Lewensohn, O. (2019). Coping resources and stress reactions among Bedouin Arab adolescents during three military operations. *Psychiatry Research, 273*, 559–566.

Abu-Kaf, S., Braun-Lewensohn, O., & Kalagy, T. (2017). Youth in the midst of escalated political violence: Sense of coherence and hope among Jewish and Bedouin Arab adolescents. *Child and Adolescent Psychiatry and Mental Health, 11*(1), 42.

Aitcheson, R. J., Abu-Bader, S. H., Howell, M. K., Khalil, D., & Elbedour, S. (2017). Resilience in Palestinian adolescents living in Gaza. *Psychological Trauma Theory Research Practice and Policy, 9*(1), 36.

Aldwin, C. M., Levenson, M. R., & Spiro, A. (1994). Vulnerability and resilience to combat exposure: Can stress have lifelong effects? *Psychology and Aging, 9*(1), 34.

Al-Said, H., Braun-Lewensohn, O., & Sagy, S. (2018). Sense of coherence, hope, and home demolition are differentially associated with anger and anxiety among Bedouin Arab adolescents in recognized and unrecognized villages. *Anxiety, Stress, and Coping, 31*(4), 475–485.

Antonovsky, A. (1983). The sense of coherence: Development of a research instrument. WS Schwartz Research Center for Behavioral Medicine, Tel Aviv University, Newsletter and Research Reports 1:1–11.

Antonovsky, A. (1987). *Unraveling the mystery of health: How people manage stress and stay well*. Jossey-Bass.

Antonovsky, H., & Sagy, S. (1986). The development of a sense of coherence and its impact on responses to stress situations. *The Journal of Social Psychology, 126*(2), 213–226.

Apers, S., Moons, P., Goossens, E., Luyckx, K., Gewillig, M., Bogaerts, K., & Budts, W. (2013). Sense of coherence and perceived physical health explain the better quality of life in adolescents with congenital heart disease. *European Journal of Cardiovascular Nursing, 12*(5), 475–483.

Ayo-Yusuf, O. A., Reddy, P. S., & Van Den Borne, B. W. (2008). Adolescents' sense of coherence and smoking as longitudinal predictors of self-reported gingivitis. *Journal of Clinical Periodontology, 35*(11), 931–937.

Ayo-Yusuf, O. A., Reddy, P. S., & Van Den Borne, B. W. (2009). Longitudinal association of adolescents' sense of coherence with toothbrushing using an integrated behaviour change model. *Community Dentistry and Oral Epidemiology, 37*(1), 68–77.

Barni, D., & Danioni, F. (2016). Adolescents' basic personal values and sense of coherence. *Personality and Individual Differences, 102*, 46–50.

Blakemore, S.-J., & Mills, K. L. (2014). Is adolescence a sensitive period for sociocultural processing? *Annual Review of Psychology, 65*(1). https://doi.org/10.1146/annurev-psych-010213-115202

Blom, E. C. H., Serlachius, E., Larsson, J. O., Theorell, T., & Ingvar, M. (2010). Low sense of coherence (SOC) is a mirror of general anxiety and persistent depressive symptoms in adolescent girls – A cross-sectional study of a clinical and a non-clinical cohort. *Health and Quality of Life Outcomes, 8*(1), 58.

Braun-Lewensohn, O. (2014). Coping resources and stress reactions among three cultural groups one year after a natural disaster. *Clinical Social Work Journal, 42*(4), 366–374.

Braun-Lewensohn, O. (2016). Sense of coherence, values, youth involvement, civic efficacy and hope: Adolescents during social protest. *Social Indicators Research, 128*(2), 661–673.

Braun-Lewensohn, O., Abu-Kaf, S., & Kalagy, T. (2017). Are 'sense of coherence' and 'hope' related constructs? Examining these concepts in three cultural groups in Israel. *The Israel Journal of Psychiatry and Related Sciences, 54*(2), 17–24.

Braun-Lewensohn, O., & Al-Said, H. (2018). Syrian adolescent refugees: How do they cope during their stay in refugee camps? *Frontiers in Psychology, 9*. https://doi.org/10.3389/fpsyg.2018.01258

Braun-Lewensohn, O., Alziadneh, S., & Eisha, H. (2015). Coping resources and extra-curricular activity as explanatory factors of exposure to violence: Comparing Jewish and Arab youth in Israel. *The Journal of Primary Prevention, 36*(3), 167–176. https://doi.org/10.1007/s10935-015-0385-4

Braun-Lewensohn, O., Huss, E., Al-Said, H., & Ganayeim, H. (2018). Bedouin adolescents: Are their coping resources stable over time? In K. A. Moore & P. Buchwald (Eds.), *Stress and anxiety. Theories and realities* (pp. 97–105). Logos.

Braun-Lewensohn, O., & Sagy, S. (2010). Sense of coherence, hope and values among adolescents under missile attacks: A longitudinal study. *International Journal of Children's Spirituality, 15*(3), 247–260.

Braun-Lewensohn, O., & Sagy, S. (2011a). Coping resources as explanatory factors of stress reactions during missile attacks: Comparing Jewish and Arab adolescents in Israel. *Community Mental Health Journal, 47*(3), 300–310.

Braun-Lewensohn, O., & Sagy, S. (2011b). Salutogenesis and culture: Personal and community sense of coherence among adolescents belonging to three different cultural groups. *International Review of Psychiatry, 23*(6), 533–541.

Braun-Lewensohn, O., Sagy, S., & Roth, G. (2011). Coping strategies as mediators of the relationship between sense of coherence and stress reactions: Israeli adolescents under missile attacks. *Anxiety, Stress, and Coping, 24*(3), 327–341.

Braun-Lewensohn, O., Sagy, S., Sabato, H., & Galili, R. (2013). Sense of coherence and sense of community as coping resources of religious adolescents before and after the disengagement from the Gaza Strip. *The Israel Journal of Psychiatry and Related Sciences, 50*(2), 110–117.

Bronfenbrenner, U. (1977). Toward an experimental ecology of human development. *The American Psychologist, 32*(7), 513.

Bronfenbrenner, U. (1979). *The ecology of human development*. Harvard University Press.

Bronfenbrenner, U., & Morris, P. A. (2006). The bioecological model of human development. In R. M. L. W. Damon (Ed.), *Handbook of child psychology* (Theoretical models of human development) (Vol. 1, 6th ed., pp. 793–828). Wiley.

Bronikowski, M. (2010). Is sense of coherence needed to keep youth physically active? *Medicina Dello Sport; Rivista di Fisiopatologia Dello Sport, 63*(4), 465–483.

Buddeberg-Fischer, B., Klaghofer, R., & Schnyder, U. (2001). Sense of coherence in adolescents. *Sozial- und Präventivmedizin, 46*(6), 404–410.

Carneiro, N. C., Duda Deps, T., Campos França, E., Ribeiro Valadares, E., Almeida Pordeus, I., & Borges-Oliveira, A. C. (2017). Oral health of children and adolescents with mucopolysaccharidosis and mother's sense of coherence. *Special Care in Dentistry, 37*(5), 223–229.

Casey, B. J., & Caudle, K. (2013). The teenage brain: Self-control. *Current Directions in Psychological Science, 22*(2), 82–87.

da Costa, A. C., Rodrigues, F. S., da Fonte, P. P., Rosenblatt, A., Innes, N. P. T., & Heimer, M. V. (2017). Influence of sense of coherence on adolescents' self-perceived dental aesthetics: A cross-sectional study. *BMC Oral Health, 17*(1), 117.

Damon, W. (2004). What is positive youth development? *The Annals of the American Academy of Political and Social Science, 591*(1), 13–24.

Dorri, M., Sheiham, A., Hardy, R., & Watt, R. (2010). The relationship between sense of coherence and toothbrushing behaviours in Iranian adolescents in Mashhad. *Journal of Clinical Periodontology, 37*(1), 46–52.

Elfassi, Y., Braun-Lewensohn, O., Krumer-Nevo, M., & Sagy, S. (2016). Community sense of coherence among adolescents as related to their involvement in risk behaviors. *Journal of Community Psychology, 44*(1), 22–37.

El-Shahawy, O., Sun, P., Tsai, J. Y. K., Rohrbach, L. A., & Sussman, S. (2015). Sense of coherence and tobacco use myths among adolescents as predictors of at-risk youth cigarette use. *Substance Use & Misuse, 50*(1), 8–14.

Evans, W., & Davis, B. (2018). Exploring the relationship between sense of coherence and historical trauma among American Indian youth. *American Indian and Alaska Native Mental Health Research (online), 25*(3), 1–25.

Evans, W. P., Marsh, S. C., & Weigel, D. J. (2010). Promoting adolescent sense of coherence: Testing models of risk, protection, and resiliency. *Journal of Community and Applied Social Psychology, 20*(1), 30–43.

Eriksson, M., & Lindström, B. (2006). Antonovsky's sense of coherence scale and the relation with health: A systematic review. *Journal of Epidemiology and Community Health, 60*(5), 376–381.

Eriksson, M., & Lindström, B. (2007). Antonovsky's sense of coherence scale and its relation with quality of life: A systematic review. *Journal of Epidemiology and Community Health, 61*(11), 938–944.

Feldt, T., Kokko, K., Kinnunen, U., & Pulkkinen, L. (2005). The role of family background, school success, and career orientation in the development of sense of coherence. *European Psychologist, 10*(4), 298–308.

García-Moya, I., Jiménez-Iglesias, A., & Moreno, C. (2013a). Sense of coherence and substance use in Spanish adolescents. Does the effect of SOC depend on patterns of substance use in their peer group? *Adicciones, 25*(2), 109.

García-Moya, I., Moreno, C., & Jiménez-Iglesias, A. (2013b). Understanding the joint effects of family and other developmental contexts on the sense of coherence (SOC): A person-focused analysis using the classification tree. *Journal of Adolescence, 36*(5), 913–923.

García-Moya, I., Moreno, C., & Braun-Lewensohn, O. (2013c). Neighbourhood perceptions and sense of coherence in adolescence. *The Journal of Primary Prevention, 34*(5), 371–379.

García-Moya, I., Rivera, F., & Moreno, C. (2013d). School context and health in adolescence: The role of sense of coherence. *Scandinavian Journal of Psychology, 54*(3), 243–249.

García-Moya, I., Suominen, S., & Moreno, C. (2014). Bullying victimization prevalence and its effects on psychosomatic complaints: Can sense of coherence make a difference? *The Journal of School Health, 84*(10), 646–653.

Garnefski, N., Kraaij, V., & Spinhoven, P. (2001). Negative life events, cognitive emotion regulation and emotional problems. *Personality and Individual Differences, 30*(8), 1311–1327.

Gauffin, H., Landtblom, A. M., & Räty, L. (2010). Self-esteem and sense of coherence in young people with uncomplicated epilepsy: A 5-year follow-up. *Epilepsy & Behavior, 17*(4), 520–524.

Geckova, A. M., Tavel, P., van Dijk, J., Abel, T., & Reijneveld, S. (2010). Factors associated with educational aspirations among adolescents: Cues to counteract socioeconomic differences. *BMC Public Health, 10*(1), 154.

Glanz, K., Maskarinec, G., & Carlin, L. (2005). Ethnicity, sense of coherence, and tobacco use among adolescents. *Annals of Behavioral Medicine, 29*(3), 192–199.

Gustafsson, P. E., Nelson, N., & Gustafsson, P. A. (2010). Diurnal cortisol levels, psychiatric symptoms and sense of coherence in abused adolescents. *Nordic Journal of Psychiatry, 64*(1), 27–31.

Hagquist, C., & Andrich, D. (2004). Is the sense of coherence-instrument applicable on adolescents? A latent trait analysis using Rasch-modelling. *Personality and Individual Differences, 36*(4), 955–968.

Honkinen, P. L., Aromaa, M., Suominen, S., Rautava, P., Sourander, A., Helenius, H., & Sillanpää, M. (2009). Early childhood psychological problems predict a poor sense of coherence in adolescents: A 15-year follow-up study. *Journal of Health Psychology, 14*(4), 587–600.

Honkinen, P. L., Suominen, S., Helenius, H., Aromaa, M., Rautava, P., Sourander, A., & Sillanpää, M. (2008). Stability of the sense of coherence in adolescence. *International Journal of Adolescent Medicine and Health, 20*, 85–91.

Honkinen, P. L. K., Suominen, S. B., Välimaa, R. S., Helenius, H. Y., & Rautava, P. T. (2005). Factors associated with perceived health among 12-year-old school children. Relevance of physical exercise and sense of coherence. *Scandinavian Journal of Public Health, 33*(1), 35–41.

Huss, E., Braun-Lewensohn, O., & Ganaim, H. (2018). Using arts-based research to overcome the mismatch between Western and Indigenous forms of coping of Bedouin youth. *International Journal of Psychology, 53*(S2), 64–71.

Idan, O., & Margalit, M. (2014). Socioemotional self-perceptions, family climate, and hopeful thinking among students with learning disabilities and typically achieving students from the same classes. *Journal of Learning Disabilities, 47*(2), 136–152.

Jakobsson, B. (2014). What makes teenagers continue? A salutogenic approach to understanding youth participation in Swedish club sports. *Physical Education and Sport Pedagogy, 19*(3), 239–252.

Kalagy, T., Braun-Lewensohn, O., & Abu-Kaf, S. (2017). Youth from fundamentalist societies: What are their attitudes towards war and peace and their relations with anxiety reactions? *Journal of Religion and Health, 56*(3), 1064–1080. https://doi.org/10.1007/s10943-017-0358-4

Koposov, R. A., Ruchkin, V. V., & Eisemann, M. (2003). Sense of coherence: A mediator between violence exposure and psychopathology in Russian juvenile delinquents. *The Journal of Nervous and Mental Disease, 191*(10), 638–644.

Koushede, V., & Holstein, B. E. (2009). Sense of coherence and medicine use for headache among adolescents. *The Journal of Adolescent Health, 45*(2), 149–155.

Kristensson, P., & Öhlund, L. S. (2005). Swedish upper secondary school pupils' sense of coherence, coping resources and aggressiveness in relation to educational track and performance. *Scandinavian Journal of Caring Sciences, 19*(1), 77–84.

Krok, D. (2015). Religiousness, spirituality, and coping with stress among late adolescents: A meaning-making perspective. *Journal of Adolescence, 45*, 196–203.

Kröninger-Jungaberle, H., & Grevenstein, D. (2013). Development of salutogenetic factors in mental health – Antonovsky's sense of coherence and Bandura's self-efficacy related to Derogatis' symptom check list (SCL-90-R). *Health and Quality of Life Outcomes, 11*(1), 80.

Lackaye, T. D., & Margalit, M. (2006). Comparisons of achievement, effort, and self-perceptions among students with learning disabilities and their peers from different achievement groups. *Journal of Learning Disabilities, 39*(5), 432–446.

Lage, C. F., Fulgencio, L. B., Corrêa-Faria, P., Serra-Negra, J. M., Paiva, S. M., & Pordeus, I. A. (2017). Association between dental caries experience and sense of coherence among adolescents and mothers. *International Journal of Paediatric Dentistry, 27*(5), 412–419.

Latzer, Y., Weinberger-Litman, S. L., Spivak-Lavi, Z., & Tzischinsky, O. (2019). Disordered eating pathology and body image among adolescent girls in Israel: The role of sense of coherence. *Community Mental Health Journal, 55*(7), 1246–1252.

Lerner, R. M., & Benson, P. I. (2003). *Developmental assets and asset-building communities: Implications for research, policy, and practice*. Kluwer Academic/Plenum.

Levi, U., Einav, M., Ziv, O., Raskind, I., & Margalit, M. (2014). Academic expectation and actual achievement: The roles of hope and effort. *European Journal of Psychology of Education, 29*(3), 367–386.

Lindblom, S., Eriksson, L., & Hiltunen, A. J. (2017). Evaluation of the cognitive intervention programme 'A New Direction' targeting young offenders in Sweden. *Journal of Scandinavian Studies in Criminology and Crime Prevention, 18*(2), 176–190.

Luyckx, K., Missotten, L., Goossens, E., & Moons, P. (2012). Individual and contextual determinants of quality of life in adolescents with congenital heart disease. *The Journal of Adolescent Health, 51*(2), 122–128.

Margalit, M., & Efrati, M. (1996). Loneliness, coherence and companionship among children with learning disorders. *Educational Psychologist, 16*(1), 69–79.

Marsh, S. C., Clinkinbeard, S. S., Thomas, R. M., & Evans, W. P. (2007). Risk and protective factors predictive of sense of coherence during adolescence. *Journal of Health Psychology, 12*(2), 281–284.

Mattila, M. L., Rautava, P., Honkinen, P. L., et al. (2011). Sense of coherence and health behaviour in adolescence. *Acta Paediatrica, 100*(12), 1590–1595.

Modin, B., Östberg, V., Toivanen, S., & Sundell, K. (2011). Psychosocial working conditions, school sense of coherence and subjective health complaints. A multilevel analysis of ninth-grade pupils in the Stockholm area. *Journal of Adolescence, 34*(1), 129–139.

Moksnes, U. K., Espnes, G. A., & Haugan, G. (2013). Stress, sense of coherence, and emotional symptoms in adolescents. *Psychology & Health, 29*(1), 32–49.

Moksnes, U. K., Espnes, G. A., & Haugan, G. (2014). Stress, sense of coherence and emotional symptoms in adolescents. *Psychology & Health, 29*(1), 32–49.

Moksnes, U. K., Espnes, G. A., & Lillefjell, M. (2012). Sense of coherence and emotional health in adolescents. *Journal of Adolescence, 35*(2), 433–441.

Moksnes, U. K., & Haugan, G. (2015). Stressor experience negatively affects life satisfaction in adolescents: The positive role of sense of coherence. *Quality of Life Research, 24*(10), 2473–2481.

Moksnes, U. K., & Lazarewicz, M. (2016). The association between self-esteem and sense of coherence in adolescents aged 13–18 years—The role of sex and age differences. *Personality and Individual Differences, 90*, 150–154.

Moksnes, U. K., Rannestad, T., Byrne, D. G., & Espnes, G. A. (2011). The association between stress, sense of coherence and subjective health complaints in adolescents: Sense of coherence as a potential moderator. *Stress and Health, 27*(3), e157–e165.

Myrin, B., & Lagerström, M. (2006). Sense of coherence and psychosocial factors among adolescents. *Acta Paediatrica, 97*(6), 805–811.

Neuner, B., Busch, M. A., Singer, S., Moons, P., Wellmann, J., Bauer, U., & Hense, H. W. (2011). Sense of coherence as a predictor of quality of life in adolescents with congenital heart defects: A register-based 1-year follow-up study. *Journal of Developmental and Behavioral Pediatrics, 32*(4), 316–327.

Nielsen, A. M., & Hansson, K. (2007). Associations between adolescents' health, stress and sense of coherence. *Stress and Health, 23*(5), 331–341.

Nilsson, B., Holmgren, L., Stegmayr, B., & Westman, G. (2003). Sense of coherence-stability over time and relation to health, disease, and psycho-social changes in a general population: A longitudinal study. *Scandinavian Journal of Public Health, 31*(4), 297–304.

Nio, K. (2010). Sense of coherence in adolescents with congenital cardiac disease. *Cardiology in the Young, 20*(5), 538.

Peled, D., Sagy, S., & Braun-Lewensohn, O. (2013). Community perception as coping resource among adolescents living under rocket fire: A salutogenic approach. *Journal of Community Positive Practices, 4*, 681–702.

Ristkari, T., Sourander, A., Rønning, J. A., et al. (2009). Childhood psychopathology and sense of coherence at age 18: Findings from the Finnish from a boy to a man study. *Social Psychiatry and Psychiatric Epidemiology, 44*(12), 1097–1105.

Rivera, F., García-Moya, I., Moreno, C., & Ramos, P. (2013). Developmental contexts and sense of coherence in adolescence: A systematic review. *Journal of Health Psychology, 18*(6), 800–812. https://doi.org/10.1177/1359105312455077

Rizou, I., De Gucht, V., Papavasiliou, A., & Maes, S. (2017). Evaluation of a self-regulation based psycho-educational pilot intervention targeting children and adolescents with epilepsy in Greece. *Seizure, 50*, 137–143.

Romeo, R. D. (2013). The teenage brain: The stress response and the adolescent brain. *Current Directions in Psychological Science, 22*, 140–145.

Sagy, S., & Braun-Lewensohn, O. (2009). Adolescents under rocket fire: When are coping resources significant in reducing emotional distress? *Global Health Promotion, 16*(4), 5–15.

Sagy, S., & Dotan, N. (2001). Coping resources of maltreated children in the family: A salutogenic approach. *Child Abuse & Neglect, 25*(11), 1463–1480.

Schreuder, E., Rijnders, M., Vaandrager, L., Hassink, J., Enders-Slegers, M. J., & Kennedy, L. (2014). Exploring salutogenic mechanisms of an outdoor experiential learning programme on youth care farms in the Netherlands: Untapped potential? *International Journal of Adolescence and Youth, 19*(2), 139–152.

Simonsson, B., Nilsson, K. W., Leppert, J., & Diwan, V. K. (2008). Psychosomatic complaints and sense of coherence among adolescents in a county in Sweden: A cross-sectional school survey. *BioPsychoSocial Medicine, 2*(4), 8.

Smith, L. O., Elder, J. H., Storch, E. A., & Rowe, M. A. (2015). Predictors of sense of coherence in typically developing adolescent siblings of individuals with autism spectrum disorder. *Journal of Intellectual Disability Research, 59*(1), 26–38.

Somerville, L. H., Hare, T., & Casey, B. J. (2011). Frontostriatal maturation predicts cognitive control failure to appetitive cues in adolescents. *Journal of Cognitive Neuroscience, 23*(9), 2123–2134.

Spear, L. (2013). The teenage brain: Adolescents and alcohol. *Current Directions in Psychological Science, 22*, 152–157.

Super, S., Verkooijen, K., & Koelen, M. (2018). The role of community sports coaches in creating optimal social conditions for life skill development and transferability–a salutogenic perspective. *Sport, Education and Society, 23*(2), 173–185.

Tottenham, N., Hare, T. A., & Casey, B. J. (2011). Behavioral assessment of emotion discrimination, emotion regulation, and cognitive control in childhood, adolescence, and adulthood. *Frontiers in Psychology, 2*, 39. https://doi.org/10.3389/fpsyg.2011.00039

Ustinavičienė, R., Škėmienė, L., Lukšienė, D., Radišauskas, R., Kalinienė, G., & Vasilavičius, P. (2018). Association between computer game type, playing time and sense of coherence in Lithuanian adolescents. *Central European Journal of Public Health, 26*(3), 209–214.

Vilija, M., & Romualdas, M. (2014). Unhealthy food in relation to posttraumatic stress symptoms among adolescents. *Appetite, 74*, 86–91.

Wadsby, M., Priebe, G., & Svedin, C. G. (2014). Adolescents with alternating residence after parental divorce: A comparison with adolescents living with both parents or with a single parent. *Journal of Child Custody, 11*(3), 202–215.

Wang, Q., Hay, M., Clarke, D., & Menahem, S. (2014). Associations between knowledge of disease, depression and anxiety, social support, sense of coherence and optimism with health-related quality of life in an ambulatory sample of adolescents with heart disease. *Cardiology in the Young, 24*(1), 126–133.

Würtz, E. T., Fonager, K., & Mortensen, J. T. (2015). Association between sense of coherence in adolescence and social benefits later in life: A 12-year follow-up study. *BMJ Open, 5*(1), e006489.

Xu, F., Cui, W., Xing, T., & Parkinson, M. (2019). Family socioeconomic status and adolescent depressive symptoms in a Chinese low- and middle-income sample: The indirect effects of maternal care and adolescent sense of coherence. *Frontiers in Psychology, 10*, 819.

17

NEET Youth, Salutogenesis and SOC

Claudia Meier Magistretti and Beat Reichlin

Introduction

Young adults not in education, employment, or training (NEETs) emerged as an interest of public debate in the 1990s (Hussmanns et al., 1990). The debate was taken up by the fields of health promotion and public health in the mid-2000s. NEETs, also referred to as "disconnected youth", have since been a priority topic in policymaking (Levitan, 2005) and research (Patel et al., 2007).

In the years following the banking crisis of 2008, unemployment levels rose, and youth unemployment rates were substantially higher than those for adults (Robertson, 2018). The numbers of young people not in education, employment, or training remained stable even in those countries where employment rates increased remarkably (Carcillo et al., 2015; Wilson & Bivand, 2014). However, a decline in the numbers of NEETs due to economic improvement had been expected in the following years (Fernandes & Gabe, 2009). Additionally, the share of well-educated youth among NEETs was rising (Carcillo et al., 2015) as well as the proportion of rural NEETs among young adults (Simões, 2018). In accordance, data from Eurostat (2020) reveal disparities within countries and show higher rates of NEETs in rural than in urban contexts, especially in southern and eastern European countries (Eurostat, 2020). These developments indicate that disconnectedness in young adults is not exclusively due to an economic crisis in general.

The global estimates of numbers of NEETs vary widely since indicators of NEET and age groups included in the group of "young adults" differ markedly among available studies and between disciplines (Fernandes & Gabe, 2009) and countries (Elder, 2015). For example, NEET young adults have been defined, ranging from 15 to 30 years of age. The Organisation for Economic Co-operation and Development (OECD) defines two groups of young NEETs, one from 15 to 19 and a second from 20 to 24 years. Referring to the second age group of young adults ages 20 to 24 years, estimates for NEETs in different countries vary for men from 5.1% (Czech Republic) to 28.6% (Italy) and women from 4.4% (Switzerland) to 44.4% (Turkey) of the total number of young people in the corresponding age group (OECD, 2021). The US Social Science Research Council (Measure of America) estimated NEETs' rates as 12% of the general population in the same age group (OECD, 2018; Burd-Sharp & Lewis, 2017). The European Commission counts 4.6 million young people in NEET situations all over Europe, yet again considering a different range of ages (15–24 years). Using this calculation, 20.4% of the young people ages 14–25 years throughout Europe are unemployed, not in education and not in training (European Commission, 2016). However, the prevalence differs substantially among European regions. Rates of NEET status in 20- to 24-year-olds are much lower (approximately 8.5–11%) in central and northern European countries compared to southern European countries with rates of 23% (examples of Spain and Greece, OECD, 2021). The pattern in all regions shows that women are more affected than men worldwide—even in regions with low numbers of young adults in a NEET situation (Fig. 17.1).

The problem of young people not in education, employment, or training represents a global concern (McGorry, 2019). Studies, reports, and position papers cover a wide range of countries with various economic backgrounds all over the world. They reach from Scandinavia (Bania et al., 2019; Stea et al., 2019) to Mexico (Gutiérrez-García et al., 2018) and Australia (Rodwell et al., 2018), from Japan (Genda, 2007) to Europe (European Commission, 2016) and South Africa (Hallstein Holte et al., 2018). They cover the United Kingdom (Goldman-Mellor et al., 2016), Senegal (Cabral, 2018), and the United States (Carcillo et al., 2015), as well as South Korea (Noh & Lee, 2017) Austria (Tamesberger &

C. Meier Magistretti (✉)
Centre for Health Promotion and Participation, Lucerne University of Applied Sciences and Arts, Lucerne, Switzerland
e-mail: claudia.meiermagistretti@hslu.ch

B. Reichlin
Centre for Health Promotion and Participation, Lucerne University of Applied Sciences and Arts, Lucerne, Switzerland

Centre of Child and Adults Protection, Lucerne University of Applied Sciences and Arts, Lucerne, Switzerland

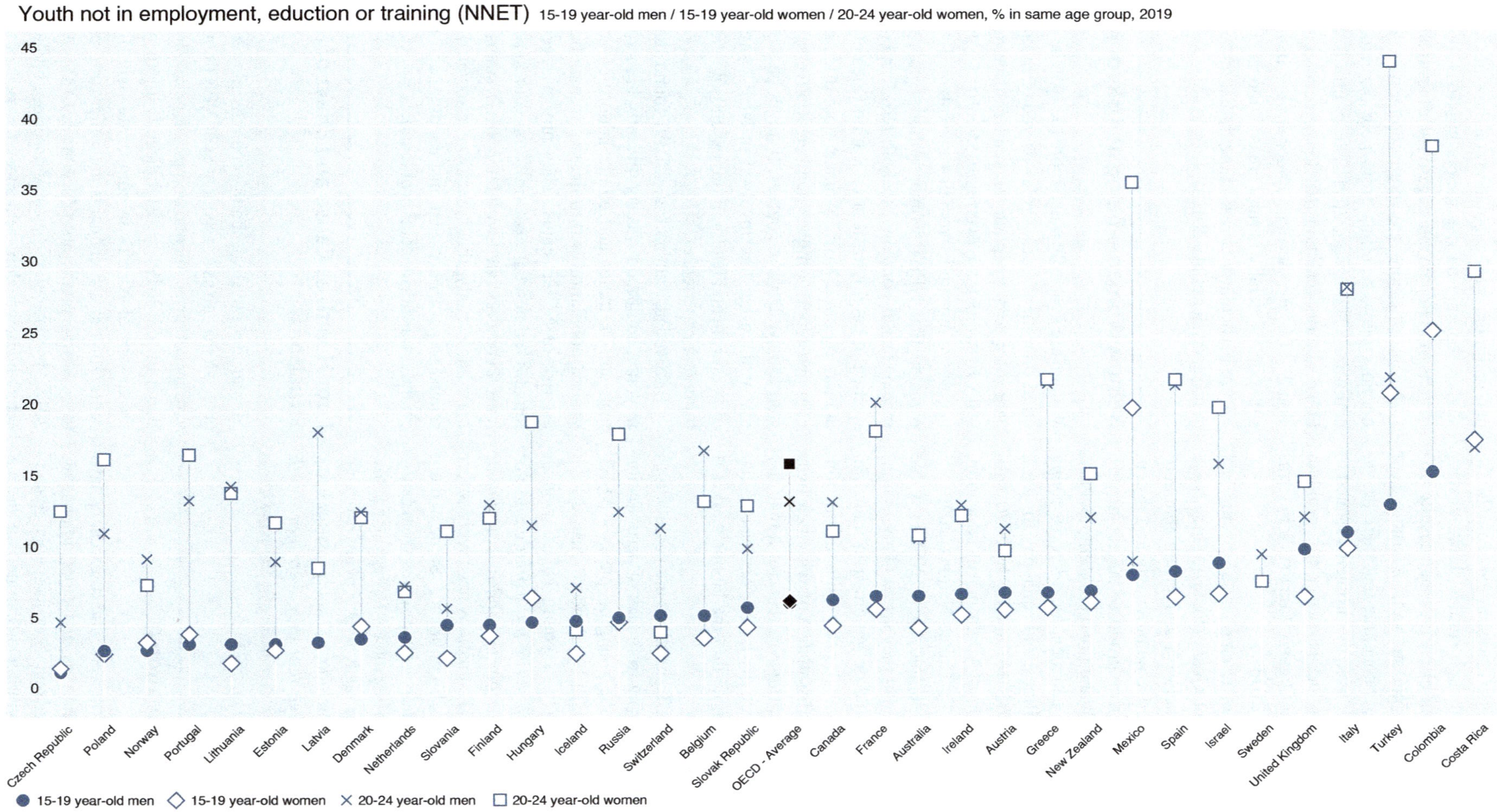

Fig. 17.1 `Youth not in education, employment, or training (NEET) (indicator), 20–24-year-olds / 20–24-year-old men / 20–24-year-old women, % in same age group. (Reprinted with permission from OECD (2021))

Johann Bacher, 2014), and Switzerland (Baggio et al., 2015), among other countries. Even though studies show substantial differences in the definition of NEETs and despite differences in the economic situations and welfare structures of the various countries, all authors conclude that there are no valuable and functioning solutions to the problems related to NEET (Bania et al., 2019). The persistence of this problem has led the International Labour Organisation to talk in terms of "a generation at risk" (ILO, 2013).

The urgency of the problem is emphasised by the UN 2015 Sustainable Development Goals (SDGs). Goal No 8 aims to "promote sustained, inclusive and sustainable economic growth, full and productive employment, and decent work for all". Within this goal, two proposed targets identify youth: (i) by 2030, achieve full and productive employment and decent work for all women and men, *including for young people* and persons with disabilities, and equal pay for work of equal value (United Nations, 2016), and (ii) by 2020, substantially reduce the proportion of youth not in education, employment, or training (NEET) (United Nations, 2020).

Despite being deprived of employment, NEETs value work as much as other youths, and they are as likely as non-NEETs to think that work would be important in their life. Therefore, the lack of a job has an impact on life satisfaction. NEETs report higher levels of dissatisfaction with their lives compared to non-NEETs. This suggests that, for a majority of youth, unemployment or inactivity is not a choice and that they would be willing to integrate into the labour market if they could (OECD, 2016).

On an individual level, NEET situations are perceived as a burden and a source of suffering from lack of participation and life perspective: Most of the young people in a NEET situation did not become NEETs by choice (Chen, 2011). In a Japanese qualitative study, a young NEET woman framed this in clear words: *"If you're not working and not in school or training, it will be boring, and it is no fun at all"* (Chen, 2011, p. 36). NEET situations negatively affect young adults' self-esteem and self-confidence. Some of them stated that it was difficult to defend themselves from being exploited. They felt they had to be grateful for having a job at all, and therefore they had to be ready to accept any working conditions. As Chen (2011) concludes, *"Their previous work experiences led them to believe that they were not worth much and that their choices for succeeding in the workforce were limited"* (Chen, 2011, p.41).

Risk Factors and Risk Situations

Since the banking crisis, policymakers, and researchers have increasingly focused on the analyses of factors influencing NEET. Studies have concentrated mainly on individual characteristics such as gender and migration background on the one hand and macro-level social factors such as economic growth and minimum-wage regulations on the other hand. In general, studies focusing on risk factors in NEET situations and the deficits of young people negatively affected are predominant.

NEET situations are more common in lower socioeconomic groups, resulting from poor participation in formal education (Thompson, 2011; Duckworth & Schoon, 2012). Other authors maintain that lower educational and professional skills are the main underpinning factors of a NEET situation, especially in rural areas (Simões, 2018). Care leavers are particularly at risk in the transition to adult independence (Akister et al., 2010).

Being a Woman—Being at Risk for NEET

Women are generally much more likely to be in a NEET situation than men. Caring roles as young mothers or in other care roles do not explain the gender difference, and the reason why women are overrepresented in the group of disconnected young adults remains unexplained. A recent study revealed that NEET women suffered poorer physical and mental health compared to both NEET men and same-age women in employment or education (Stea et al., 2019). The authors reported NEET women more often endure physical pain and report a higher number of adverse experiences as well as have fewer resources. It might be worth considering that women become involved in NEET situations because of poorer mental health, more psychosomatic disorders, and traumatic experiences.

In Sweden, Bania et al. (2019) found that NEET status in young adulthood was significantly higher among females than among males and ethnic minorities compared to the general population, with minority women bearing the highest risk of NEET status. They further specify that among females, adolescent peer problems and hyperactivity problems were associated with later NEET status. In contrast, in male adolescents, this status was associated with problems related to poor peer relations, conduct, and physical health (mainly musculoskeletal problems).

Poor Health as Cause and Effect of NEET Situations

Mental and physical health problems play a crucial role as antecedents and as consequences of NEET conditions. Across various countries, mental and physical health problems (e.g., Bania et al., 2019) are significantly more prevalent in the pre-history of NEETs in comparison with their non-NEET peers. In contrast, cannabis and other drug use do not seem to be strong predictors (Zuccotti & O'Reilly 2019; Cabral, 2018). In particular, the early onset of childhood mental and behavioural problems enhances the risk of a NEET status (Rodwell et al., 2018). A Canadian research group showed that NEET status was thrice as prevalent in young adults with psychotic developments as in the peer population (Iyer et al., 2018). In line with this finding, O'Dea et al. (2014) found a high proportion of NEETs among mental help-seekers. Compared to their peers in education, training, or work, they were more likely to be male and to have a history of criminal charges and/or economic hardship. They also showed a more advanced stage of mental illness with symptoms of poor mental health (risky cannabis use, higher levels of depression, poorer social functioning and greater disability). Even minor mental problems may increase the risk of NEET status. A study based on census data in the US describes three main groups of NEETs: young mothers and young carers, young adults with disabilities or health problems, and young people (mainly young men) who do not have any overt disadvantage, but who cannot find a way to enter the labour market (Fernandes and Gabe, 2009). A randomised study in Greece showed increasing symptoms of anxiety and depression in young people between 15 and 24 years of age the longer the duration of NEET situations (more than one year) and the older the young person (Basta Maria Basta et al., 2019). Other authors emphasise the heterogeneity of the NEETs as well as their multiple and various burdens of poverty, mental illness, social deprivation, low education, and low self-esteem that are a reinforcing determinant of a NEET situation (Stea et al., 2019; Carcillo et al., 2015). Baggio et al. (2015) therefore conclude from their study on causal paths analysis that NEET status is a consequence of mental health and thereby induced substance use is a way of self-medication rather than a cause. According to Basta Maria Basta et al. (2019), studies from countries with significantly different economic and cultural backgrounds, such as Australia, the United Kingdom, Mexico, Japan, Sweden, and Switzerland, that explored associations between NEET status, mental health, and substance use confirm these associations between NEET status, mood disorders, suicidal behaviours, depressive symptoms, and substance use.

Other authors question the prominent role of mental health problems in the genesis of NEET situations: Gutiérrez-García et al. (2018) conducted a representative, prospective, longitudinal 8-year cohort study in Mexico City with 1000 adolescents aged 12–17 years in wave 1 and 19–26 years at the second point of measurement. They found no marked differences between young people in NEET situations and their working or studying peers of the same age group. The authors conclude: *"NEET youth were not that different from their peers...The greatest differences between NEET youth and all their peer groups were their increased risks of incident suicidal behaviour"* (Gutiérrez-García et al., 2017).

A third perspective relates to NEET situations due to mental problems in young adults to general societal developments. Robertson (2018) assumes that underlying societal circumstances may further hamper the transition to adulthood. He states that the pathways from adolescence to adulthood are prolonged, more complicated, and more individual in general: Those who manage well find a broader range of opportunities and those who do not face NEET situations very often have health problems. Robertson (2019) states that health-risk factors facing young people increase due to the trend towards a prolonged and complicated period of transition from youth to independent adulthood. During this transition period, unemployment is likely and has the potential to increase stress, mental health issues, use of drugs, promiscuity, eating disorders, and self-harm. Stewards and colleagues confirmed this observation in a British study, where NEETs were significantly more likely than non-NEETs to be smokers, not to participate in sport, and have an unhealthy BMI (Stewart et al., 2017).

NEET status itself causes health-damaging effects. A meta-synthesis shows evidence that young people are especially vulnerable to health problems when unemployed or working in precarious conditions (Vancea & Utzet, 2016). Bruckner et al. (2010) confirm that levels of demand for youth mental health services are related to levels of unemployment. Japanese researchers show that young people whose expected returns from working are low tend to refrain from working and seeking jobs (Genda, 2007). This is particularly true for young women, the less educated, and the long-term jobless. Young people seem to resign at an early age with unforeseeable and presumed catastrophic long-term consequences for their lives, their health, and their changes to participate in society.

Programs and Projects to Resolve an Unresolved Global Problem

In parallel to the growing scientific interest, an equally growing number of policies, projects, and initiatives have evolved that aim at integrating and educating the young NEET adults by supported education, supported employment, supported housing, and other means of social welfare. The results of these efforts are discouraging (Strandh et al., 2015). Even though a small number of studies show that individual job placement is useful in helping young adults to attain employment (Bond et al., 2016), two persisting problems remain unresolved. First, most young adults who are not in employment stay out of the reach of these measures or they fail to complete programs within the predefined (and economically guaranteed) time. Secondly, most of the labour policy programs are tailored for and successful with men, but not (equally) effective for women (Bacher et al., 2017).

Very few scientific evaluations of the various existing programs are available. The retrievable evaluations consist of short-term evaluations of effectiveness or customer satisfaction. No studies on long-term effects of supported education or supported employment on the specific group of young adults in NEET situations could be located. These findings correspond to statements by several authors (e.g., Robertson, 2018) describing a lack of strong evidence for the effectiveness of back-to-work programs. Accordingly, in a previous literature review, Lakey et al. (2001) revealed a near absence of evidence for the health effects of labour market programs for NEET young people.

In Taiwan, a 4- to 10-month program named "Flying young"was offered nationwide to young people in a NEET situation (Chen, 2011). Although the program was targeted at this group, was tailored to this group locally, and participants were offered monetary compensation that allowed them to make a living, the retention rate was low. Of the participants, 59% did not complete the program. Those who finished had little to say about the job skills they had learned in the program. They considered the program to be of low practical help to participants. It did not increase their chances of employment, but it provided social and emotional support and helped them feel better about themselves (Chen, 2011). These findings are in line with the results of Swiss authors who conclude that the broad and heterogeneous projects in the field of supported education and supported employment for young adults widely lack evidence of effectiveness (Sabatella & Wyl, 2017). A large variety of offers and programs of assessed quality and adequate length (24-month duration on average) did result in a meagre success rate. For example, 8% of participants completed an apprenticeship (Sabatella & Wyl, 2017). Moreover, the contribution of the programs to the success is much lower than the two main determinants for successful integration: neither was related to professional support but rather to an individual's motivation and their parents' or their informal network and relationships to employers (Sabatella & Wyl, 2017).

From a policy point of view, Bacher et al. (2017) conclude that there is no "one-size-fits-all" solution for reducing the number of young people in NEET situations. Group-specific aspects related to age, migration, and gender should be considered in order not to leave behind young women and migrants. The most promising structural intervention, according to the authors, consists of an active labour market policy (Bacher et al., 2017).

Young people with psychological problems have even lower chances of finding access to the labour market due to stigmatisation and self-stigmatisation of psychological and psychiatric problems (O'Dea et al., 2016). However, there is no association between a change in depression and a change in NEET status in the same study on young adults with depression. The authors conclude that psychiatric and other services need to address functional outcomes and re-engagement with education and employment in addition to symptom reduction. Re-employment improves the health of formerly unemployed adults in general (Rueda et al., 2012) (Bjarnason & Sigurdardottir, 2003): The best health outcomes result when full-time employment and role satisfaction are achieved.

The social risks influencing the likelihood of NEET status are multi-dimensional, so interventions that focus on one risk factor are likely to be inadequate (Duckworth & Schoon, 2012). Overall, the conclusion might be Shore and Tosun's (2017): "One of the main reasons for this failure is that the proposed activities do not match NEETs' needs".

A Salutogenic Perspective on NEET Situations

Given the failure of support initiatives for young adults in NEET conditions, this field needs new and different approaches as well as new questions. It is crucial to understand who these young people in NEET situations are, what they need, and how they could receive appropriate support in improving their quality of life and their life perspectives, with or without becoming educated, employed, and trained. To date, such a comprehensive approach to the NEET situation is lacking; it is necessary to develop an approach that incorporates the experiences and visions of these youth, their relations with formal and informal systems, as well as their cultural and economic condition (Simões & Drumonde, 2016). Salutogenesis may offer a framework towards a new understanding, a comprehensive approach, and a different way of handling the problem. It focuses on resources and capabilities instead of risks, deficits, and predefined "normality". We, therefore, attempt to illuminate the situation of NEETs from the perspective of salutogenic theory and research by advancing a new approach to learning and research with NEETs and with their non-NEET peers. In this section, we present some first results of a current research program and conclude with future policies and practices.

We conducted literature research on the Web of Science to retrieve publications that link the topic of NEETs to salutogenesis. We limited the publications years to 2006 to 2019 and used the keywords salutogenesis, sense of coherence, SOC combined with NEET, disconnected youth, and other terms. We could not find any study that did explicitly link salutogenesis or SOC to NEET situations or disconnected young adults. Therefore, we recurred to publications that throw light on related topics, such as research on SOC and unemployment in general.

We know from studies conducted with unemployed populations that Sense of Coherence (SOC) is a strong predictor for positive outcomes in terms of re-employment: SOC is an important personal resource that enhances the chances of re-entering the labour market after unemployment (Vastamäki et al., 2011), independent of educational level, age, gender, and duration of unemployment. The SOC of adolescents may affect their stress and coping in much the same way as is seen in adults (Eriksson & Lindström, 2005), young people are especially vulnerable to health problems when unemployed or working under precarious conditions. This is mainly true for their higher risk of mental health disorders, health-risk behaviour, poor quality of life, and occupational injuries (Vancea & Utzet, 2017). Again, SOC is a crucial buffer when coping with unemployment and marginalisation in the early years of adult life. Starrin et al. (2001) found that in unemployed young adults who were exposed to a greater degree of financial hardship as well as to more shaming experiences, the mean SOC score was much lower compared to young unemployed men and women who were not victims of financial deprivation and shaming experiences.

Consequently, we assume that strengthening SOC in NEET situations is a feasible approach to support young adults. Dealing openly with experiences of shame, providing minimal basic incomes and housing may be the first important psychological and material resistance resources in this process. Additionally, a salutogenic approach may be more attractive and motivating for affected youth than the current paradigms that ask them to fit into defined programs and life plans defined by educators, experts, and rehabilitation systems.

A 3-Year Peer-to-Peer Study to Understand Young Adults in NEET Situations

We assume that a salutogenic perspective on young people in NEET situations will reveal new approaches to urgently needed solutions. According to Antonovsky and following his example, we must ask new questions. These questions should shift from the deficit-oriented approach in the literature and include the central concepts of the theory of salutogenesis. What are the resources of these young adults? How do they build their SOC? How do their resources, coping, and coherence fit with the support systems they find in their societies? These questions were addressed in a 3-year study of 76 NEETs in the German-speaking part of Switzerland. The study was based on three assumptions:

- We need to ask new questions.
- We need to use new research methods.
- We need to work with researchers in the same age group as the NEETs.

It is difficult and costly to reach NEETs (Stea et al., 2019), and it is difficult to gain the confidence of these young adults who have mostly had various adverse experiences with the social-care system (Genda, 2007). We, therefore, worked with students of the social work department at a Swiss university, assuming that each of them would know a friend, colleague, or relative in a NEET condition. To allow the young researchers to ask new questions, we excluded questions regarding the causes and history of the NEET situation, and we chose a process-oriented design, following the method of rhizomatic learning and research by Deleuze and Guattari (1988). Rhizomatic research attempts to overcome hierarchical and binary thinking that traditionally leads to a top-down process in scientific approaches that generate hypotheses, methods, and results. In contrast, a rhizome, according to Deleuze and Guattari (1988), is an "image of thought", analogous to the botanical rhizome, which is a stem of plants that sends out roots and shoots from its nodes. In other words, the ontological thinking by Deleuze and Guattari (1988) can be understood by analogy with these rhizomes in nature. The underpinning concept of rhizome ontology is that material and semiotic entities have the same ontological status, that is, both material entities and discursive statements are "real" in an identical way. Deleuze and Guattari (1988) do talk about assemblages of entities as active, creative affected and affecting processes that define and limit themselves and each other, as rhizomes of plants do in nature. Deleuzian ontology (and in consequence rhizome research) is based on the assumption that reality is made up of discursive statements and material entities, both of which are active, mutually affecting, and affecting the world. Therefore, this research methodology and design shifts from a deductive and hierarchical conceptualisation towards a process of interacting with the question of interest. In this process, the research question, the researchers, and reality affect influence and change each other mutually. This ontology has a broad impact on research and learning, as some of the fundamental principles of rhizome research demonstrate (Clarke & Parsons, 2013). Box 17.1 describes the basic principles.

Box 17.1 Principles and Methods of Rhizomatic Research

Nomadism: Rhizome researchers are «nomadic» in the sense that they transcend the current state of knowledge and allow them themselves to be led by the research question and the research process. They might change along the process of moving from place to place, idea to idea, and concept to concept. Nomadism demands an openness to interrelationships even if these interrelationships present places and concepts that are not traditionally linked.

Assemblages: An assemblage consists of heterogeneous components and forces that form a unity by working together as a whole to produce or create a temporary entity. The components of an assemblage have traditionally been considered separate. Rhizome research deliberately sees things, processes, and people as equally important elements co-creating assemblages. Therefore, researchers link seemingly unconnected aspects (for example, architectural, technological, emotional, and discursive aspects)—into assemblages and they consider elements that seem less likely to provide research insights rather than dismissing them as being irrelevant.

Deterritorialisation: Rhizome researchers develop sensitivities to elements/people that are not part of the status quo.

Affect: In rhizome research, emotions (affects) are not considered to be confounders that have to be controlled or at least reflected. Emotions like interest, fear, compassion, etc. *are means of gaining knowledge and insight. They co-create and co-direct the research process that ideally will allow the research project to control itself.*

The students learned these principles at the beginning of the course in a challenging process. They found themselves in a very open situation and soon recognised the parallels to the situation of their peers in NEET conditions. They had to find their way into a completely new and uncertain process, make efforts without ensured success, and did not know whom and how to ask for help. These students left the "secure ground" of professionals "knowing" solutions for problems, and they accessed the topic of NEETs with a humbler and more open attitude of learning.

The overarching aim of the study was to understand the inner and outer world of young adults in NEET situations. Within this frame, students were free to choose their specific research questions, which they then studied together in two phases of fieldwork, each 2 weeks long. In between the fieldwork periods, they gathered all together in a 1-day marketplace workshop, where each group's study was discussed with other students, tutors, teachers, and an artist. The marketplace served as a reflection on the ongoing research process and as a support to further orient and specify the research questions for the second period of fieldwork.

Research questions varied broadly: How do NEETs with a psychiatric diagnosis and those without view their lives? How much or how little do NEETs accept their reality of living and themselves? Where do young adults in NEET situations find resources for their everyday struggle? Why are they in a NEET situation? What are their dreams and their visions of life? (cf. Box 17.2). The results are presented in the following section.

Box 17.2 Research Questions and Methodology

The research methods used by students were predominantly qualitative approaches focusing on interviews of different types. Guideline-based, narrative, and biographical interviews were conducted. In some cases, the storytelling method or (photograph) diaries were also used, since some of the young adults in NEET situations were often able to express themselves better with this method. Some of the student's groups choose to explore and contrast two perspectives: the one of the young adults in NEET-situations and the ones of the results professionals of their help systems. They conducted a first field work with young adults, discussed the results and generated questions for the second phase of field work, where they interviewed social workers, psychiatrists, youth workers, working educators, family nurses, and other professionals. The latter presented the experiences of young adults in comparison with an expert view and gathered information on the type of cooperation between professionals. The 22 groups dealt with a wide variety of questions, which allows the results presented to be used to form different categories and summarise complexes of questions:

The study groups that explored the experiences of young adults pursued the following questions:

- *How do those affected experience working with help systems?*
- *What kinds of plans and visions do those affected have?*
- *What is important in the area of housing?*
- *What was supportive in the socialisation process?*
- *What do those affected do in their free time?*
- *How do those affected experience their everyday life?*
- *What kind of support do affected people want?*

Study groups dealing with institutional support systems attempted to answer the following summarising sets of questions:

- *What form can inter-institutional cooperation between the support systems take?*
- *Which accesses to support systems are open to affected persons?*
- *What options are available to those not recognised as disabled by the social security system?*

Study groups that focused on the closest personal environment dealt with the following questions:

- *How do relatives experience their everyday life with those affected?*
- *What support do relatives want?*

A total of 116 interviews were conducted, of which 76 were with affected persons, 7 with relatives, 25 with professionals, and 6 with young adults who formerly were in NEET situations that they ended by successfully integrating into work or education.

Tutors accompanied the students during two research phases of 2 days each, and they received support in the evaluation of their results by targeted feedback. It quickly became apparent that a significant challenge was to establish contact with young adults in NEET conditions. The second field phase built on the evaluation of the first phase. Often this led to a revised question and also to more precise interest in knowledge. The implementation of the principles and methods of rhizomatic research was a continuous learning process requiring reflection by all participants. Altogether 80 students participated in the course over the three terms of investigation that extended over 3 years.

Generalised and Specific Resistance Resources of Young Adults in NEET Situations

The prerequisites for the sense of coherence (SOC) are general resistance resources (GRRs), conceptualised as any physical, material, cognitive, emotional, attitudinal, interpersonal, social, or macro-sociocultural characteristics of an individual to cope with a wide variety of stressors (Lindström & Eriksson, 2010). Specific resistance resources (SRRs) are individualised, dependent on the person's particular context, and used during certain circumstances (Antonovsky, 1987; Mittelmark et al., 2017). In terms of young adults in NEET situations, GRRs are resources that generally allow access to societal roles and participation, for example, education, social belonging, and societal and political participation. SRRs are those specifically needed to overcome the hardship of NEET situations and their negative consequences on health, for example, integration programs, social assistance, and psychiatric or psychotherapeutic treatment. The results are presented alongside the generalised and specific resistance resources.

In the 3 years of rhizomatic research, both young adults and the professionals who supported them were interviewed. The patterns of their narratives show remarkable differences,

Table 17.1 Contrasting the perceptions of young adults and professionals

General Resistance Resources (GRR)	Young adults' perception of GRR	Professionals' perception of GRR
Employment	Very important	Important
Time	Very important	Important
Stigma	Important	Important+
Housing	Very important	Somehow important
Personal development and identity	Very important	Somehow important
Coping skills	Very important	Somehow important
Visions and perspectives	Important	Not relevant
Leisure	Important	Not relevant
Peers and friends	Important	Not relevant

which might explain why the variety of assistance available does not reach the young adults in the NEET situation. There seems to be a misfit of concepts, attitudes, and expectations between the two systems of help-seekers and professionals. Of the nine key resources of well-being that young adults emphasise, only three were fully shared by the representatives of the helper system, three were mentioned but defined differently, and three of the young adult's key issues were perceived as irrelevant (Table 17.1).

Both young adults in NEET situations and social workers in the helper system consider work and employment as a key issue and central goal. Young adults' difficulties in finding employment on the first job market were confirmed by social workers who stated that there were too few employers ready to hire young adults with psychological and/or social difficulties or handicaps. Employers often perceived the available programs of supported training, supported education, or supported employment as too bureaucratic and too complicated. At the same time, the young adults found them as too demanding, difficult, and stressful. In Switzerland, programs for youth in NEET situations that focus on education, training, and employment are either funded by municipalities or by national insurance systems. Both demand defined steps of success within fixed time limits, which means that if predefined objectives are not achieved within the required time, support is discontinued and young adults find themselves back in the NEET situation. Support systems are fragmented, and in the majority of cases, continuity between different support systems is not provided. In consequence, the young adults themselves should seek and find consecutive programs. This proves to be an excessive demand for many since they struggle with feelings of shame and low self-esteem. A common consequence is a nomadic journey of attempts, failures, disruptures, and new attempts that may last 5, 8, or more years (Mögling et al., 2015).

Accordingly, time was mentioned as an important issue by both young adults and social workers. They talked about the time young people lose finding relevant information about support systems, the time they lose trying to overcome failures, and the time they wait for replies or authorisations from the helper system, communities, or health insurance. Once they are in a support system, young adults feel themselves being under constant time pressure to shape their personal and psychological development in a way to follow the demands and time limits of educational and welfare systems.

The young NEET adults' perception of illness, diagnosis, and stigma corresponded with the view of professionals in the support systems, which reveals the important impact and correlation of psychiatric diagnosis, mental problems, and stigmatisation. As the young adults stated in the interviews, a psychiatric diagnosis can be both a support and a burden for them. Some find it helpful to have an explanation for their suffering; others reinforce their already existing self-deprecation. The researchers observed that diagnoses received before adolescence shape individuals' self much more strongly than diagnoses made in early adulthood. In surprising contrast, a psychiatric illness, by itself, was viewed positively. The young adults in our study emphasised that mental health problems can be a reason to engage in a process of critical self-analysis and a starting point for personal growth: "People without mental health problems can easily go through life without reflecting on who they are". For a process of personal reflection and growth, young adults in this study consider it important to have access to a value-free, non-judgmental environment, be this nature, animals, sports, music, a theatre group, or something else. Only when they start to compare themselves with others (or with people on social media), do they start to doubt their lives and themselves. There, a vicious circle may start where low self-esteem and self-stigmatisation weaken the process of becoming healthy as well as achieving social and professional participation.

Communicating the diagnosis remains difficult due to employers' contradictory attitudes: They want to be informed of a job applicant's psychiatric problems, but employers also think they would not employ the applicant if they knew of a psychiatric diagnosis (Baer et al., 2017). The young adult's experiences described in the interviews mirror this contradiction. To receive support, they must communicate the psychiatric diagnosis, but consequently, they experience, "employers don't feel confident about your abilities, and you feel like a burden to them. And you're perceived as your diagnosis only; you're not perceived as a person. This makes you feel unhopeful".

A second group of resources concerns housing as well as psychological and coping resources. Housing, "to have a place of your own where you feel secure and are free to live your life", as one of the young adults framed it, is considered important by professionals and young adults alike. Views diverge, however, about the way housing should be provided. Young adults consider housing as a basic resource. *"Housing means intimacy. My home gives me security and is a place in which I can determine what happens"*. From there, they can start to find training, participate in professional education, and find employment. They are also convinced that having their place to live in would help them to become more independent and gain self-esteem: *"If I feel at ease at home and can live the way I want, I'm fine and I can use my energy for the next task"*.

The support system instead follows an opposing logic: As long as young adults do not earn their living, as long as they have not completed their professional education, and as long they have not learned to manage a household, they are better in sheltered housing, where social workers and social pedagogues take care of them. Consequently, situations perceived as humiliating by young adults in NEET situations persist: *"My apartment is one the region pays for. It bothers me when the social worker comes into the house unannounced and does what he wants, whether I am at home or not. I have no privacy for myself and my family in this apartment – he even looks in the fridge"*.

The support system offers sheltered or accompanied housing in institutions that generally are not conceptualised for young adults in NEET situations. As a result, they found themselves in institutions for people with handicaps or patients with severe psychiatric disorders—a situation they found depressing.

For professionals, one's place to live is a reward, but for these young adults, it is a prerequisite to building up an independent life. "Housing First" projects in the US, Canada, and recently Europe, especially Finland, may well prove the young adults right. In most existing welfare models, individuals should graduate through a social rehabilitation process to earn their housing. The housing first principle suggests a paradigm shift. Instead of an ultimate goal, housing is considered a first step, a basis, and a precondition to start and succeed in the social recovery process. Results of recent randomised controlled trials (RCTs) show better outcomes in housing first programs than in the traditional educational models for quality of life, mental health, social inclusion, and other parameters (Aubry et al., 2019). Some social workers in our study did not acknowledge the young adult's wish for independent housing. One stated: *"They need to consume, to have everything, iPhone, computer; brand-name clothing is huge today. I think those are more important for the young than having an apartment of their own"*.

Attitudes towards psychological and coping resources also differ between young adults and social workers. Individual biographies of young adults in NEET situations show an almost unbreakable will to succeed, to achieve, and to survive. Five to ten attempts at integration, education, or training were frequent among the young adults in the interviews. *"You need persistence and a strong will to survive"*, one of them stated. This contrasts with the beliefs of professionals. They don't emphasize persistence but the capability to sacrifice, to adapt to given circumstances.

Similarly, the concept of identity is perceived differently by professionals and young adults. The young adults interviewed said that all they asked and wished for was to be accepted and appreciated the way they are. It was the strong conviction of all interviewees that they are—presumably special—but full human beings, with identities of their own. In contrast, the professionals demonstrated the conviction that these young adults would stay in a state of "not yet", still searching for themselves and still in the process to become and to build up a personal identity. These contrasting perceptions are not explicitly exchanged or expressed in routine interactions between the partners involved. Nevertheless, such a stark contrast can hinder a genuine and functional working alliance.

The third group of general resistance resources was composed of those aspects of life quality that were not perceived and were therefore not addressed by supporting systems and professionals. However, they were of crucial importance to young adults in NEET situations. One of the most prominent findings was that young adults were surprised to be asked about their aims and visions in life. They said that their visions had never been a topic of interest for professionals of the helping systems. In line with these NEET adults' statements, some representatives of the support system affirmed they never ask about visions, since the young adults might be overstrained by this question (because they are not able to reflect on and express themselves). The visions of their future the young adults described were modest but still far away from their current living situations. They dreamed of having a place to work, becoming an appreciated member of the community/society, doing something meaningful, and having a family—if possible outside the city and in the countryside. Stable relationships were a constant wish since most of the young adults interviewed looked back on a life full of interrupted relationships within the family, but also with peers and the various professionals of support systems they had known, worked with, and then lost. Money was not the main issue: They wanted to be economically self-supporting, and they aimed at living a simple life in which they had enough money not to suffer from a deficiency.

Support systems for young adults in NEET situations are mainly directed at education, employment, and training that are usually rather difficult to achieve. In our interviews, young adults emphasised the important role of leisure activities. They are considered to be an opportunity for positive experiences, a source of self-esteem, and a relatively easily accessible resource since professional background or education usually are not requested to take part in sports or groups of creative, social, or other leisure activities. In leisure groups, social background or position are less important than shared interests and activities. Some leisure groups are aware of this and actively involve people in difficult living situations. Social workers stated that leisure time is not important. In their views, hobby and leisure activities are a later priority of learning—a successful integration into working life comes first. Social welfare professionals could but rarely do support leisure initiatives of young adults in NEET conditions, predominantly for economic reasons. These opinions contrast with the view of the young adults who feel that it is easier for them to find access to leisure groups than to professional or educational systems. The importance young people in NEET situations attribute to leisure activities in this peer-to-peer study contrast with research (OECD, 2016) that found NEETs are less likely than non-NEET youth to think that leisure time is very important for their life. The different findings may be due to differing research questions and methods as well as to the fact that most participants in our sample suffered from slight or moderate mental problems. For them, leisure groups were a gate for social contact and participation, since stigmatisation is less prominent, access is easier, especially when peers accompany young NEETs.

Peers compose the third GRR in the group of NEETs' resources neglected by professionals but considered important by the young adults in our interviews. Some of them have lost former friends due to mental problems, the NEET status, and the stigmatisation of both. They were living a rather lonely life but claimed to have "many friends", who on closer inspection turned out to be friends on Facebook, Instagram, or Twitter with whom they have no personal contact in real life. Still, young adults consider these friends very important and spend a significant amount of time with them on social media. Others could keep friendships with former friends who are not in a NEET situation and reported they receive support from them, but also "a situation of equality and belonging without any power gap". Ideally, friends support or can cope with the specific vulnerability the young NEET adults show, as one NEET adult describes his peer group: "*Everyone knows about my illness and my problems. I don't have to pretend, and I can be sad and calm. Even when I feel very bad, I can always be there and do not have to be involved. But I can take part in fun evenings without having to do anything or to pretend. This helps me a lot. We care for each other. We have agreed on a sign language: When I raise my hand, they all know that I don't want to talk now*".

A third group of the young adults in our sample found new friends during previous treatments in psychiatric hospitals or detoxification clinics with whom they kept contact after the treatments. These friends were considered emotional resources and people to talk with about problems, but since most of them are in NEET situations as well, they were not of practical support. In contrast, social workers and other professionals either ignore peers, regard them as a private matter, or have a more negative perspective of NEETs' peers, fearing their harmful influence. In any case, friends and peers were not involved in integrative, therapeutic, or supportive treatment nor did professionals in this sample provide support in developing a private social network.

To conclude, young adults in NEET situations and the professionals who support them share a common view, but with differing understandings, of the GRRs regarding work, education, housing, psychological and coping capabilities, and the insight that de-stigmatisation of NEET situations are needed. Professionals ignore or are unaware of the resources that might be crucial to strengthen the SOC of young adults. Closing this gap in the perception of support systems may help to empower young adults to more easily access and use both GRRs and SRRs.

Specific Resistance Resources (SRRs) and the Support System

The support system can be viewed as the organ to facilitate the access to or to provide specific resistance resources that are needed in NEET situations to access the GRRs described above. An inconsistency between the high number of available supporting programs and the persistent stability of the number of young adults in NEET situations calls for an explanation. To discover the reasons for this inconsistency, a group of questions in our study addressed the young adults' perception of the helper system.

In Switzerland, young adults in NEET situations who have access to the support system are usually accompanied by an average of five different institutions (Baer et al., 2015). Institutions and their representatives lack time and resources, so they rarely coordinate with each other or actively involve their clients. This results in a lack of cooperation among professionals and requires young adults to spend a substantial amount of time and energy keeping appointments, which gives them the impression they are being "administered". They described their situation by asking a question: "Are we all puppets?" This lack of coordination often results in young adults being buffeted about on their journey among the different support systems because of bureaucratic and legal requirements. Since the institutions, not the young adult, lead the process, dealing with access to protected personal data needs time.

Moreover, every institution sticks to its profile, and tasks and transitions between support systems are often not provided. Sometimes, specific support is even lacking: One participant stated: *"I'm too sick for the primary labour market, but I am too strong for the second – what shall I do?"* Others stated that they think that each program might be useful and valuable, but that all lack flexibility and their criteria for admission, progress, and success are unduly restrictive.

In sum, the misfit between institutional support and individual needs may be due to a support system that functions within a financial, organisational logic that cannot respond to individual life circumstances and development processes. As our research shows, support by non-profit organizations was a crucial factor for NEETs who were able to overcome their situation. Private services could provide the support and time the young adults needed because of flexible economic standards. In contrast, most of the public support programs demand specific progress within a predefined time.

Inter-institutional coordination, in particular, appears to be poorly developed. For example, young adults in NEET situations perceive that there is too little communication among the experts involved; they also experience the individual processes offered by institutional helpers as closed systems. Moreover, when different institutions are connected, the number of professionals with whom a young adult speaks considerably increases. Finally, the highly specialised support systems make things even more difficult: Individual aspects of problems only are tackled, but the situation of the individual as a whole is not seen.

Discussion

Among the most striking results were those that expressed the individual needs, dreams, wishes, and future perspectives of the young adults in NEET situations. It was impressive to learn that what they wanted was normality. They defined this based on their needs (see also Table 17.1). In contrast, institutional support systems take a different approach. Their focus is on integration through work, and their priority is for NEETs to earn a living. The promotion of earning capacity is seen as the key. Support systems seem to not take into account the normal range of up to 6 years in differences in psychological and social development among children and adolescents. In line with other authors (Maguire, 2015), we consequently can assume that the problem of NEET situations in early adulthood is at least partly due to the misfit of offered support by organisations and the individual needs of development. Here, we will claim that the system could work much more effectively if the support system were able to understand the young adults and their situation in terms of the SOC and the GRRs.

The normative structure of support offers hinders young NEETs from accessing GRRs. The final question by the student interviewers addresses this: "Why are there no niche offers in the first labour market for NEETs?" A possible solution to this lack and dilemma may be to create new and adequate GRRs in a "third" labour market overlapping and bridging the first and the second ones. Recent initiatives in Portugal provide promising examples. In *Highlights of an untold story,* Simões (2018) described an initiative for rural NEETs. Cooperation among youth and social workers, farmers, and ecologists led to the development of a training and entrepreneur's program. It broke the former rule for NEETs to fit into pre-designed projects. It allowed them to work, be trained, and build up their business project within a flexible system of transition to the labour market in an eco-agriculture cooperative. The project, called *Terra nostra,* was based on an equality approach to talks, learning, and evolving. It thereby addressed important dimensions of the SOC: *comprehensibility* was tackled by learning and gradually understanding, *manageability* by developing a business with an income, and *meaningfulness* by planning a personal future. *Terra nostra* consisted of several offers for young adults in NEET situations that were multi-level, open, easily accessible, and flexible. The main elements of the program were as follows: Integration of young adults in NEET situations into an eco-agriculture social business.

- The launch of one's own small business, with the support of project partners.
- Linkage to local food production businesses where apprenticeships took place while the apprentices were mentored by *Terra nostra*.

Terra nostra take into account that many young adults in NEET situations look back on a history of educational failure or underachievement. It is based on individualised informal learning in contrast to the formal educational system that overemphasises labour market demands. This approach refuses traditional teacher-centred methodologies and rigid curricula and instead fosters informal learning techniques, allowing individuals to take the time they need to evolve. Learning sessions occur mostly in the field rather than in a traditional classroom environment. Direct observation, demonstration, peer mentoring, small-group problem-solving, and learning diaries are the primary teaching methods used in this bottom-up learning and teaching process, during which the youths' questions and contributions are the starting point for exploring training topics.

Terra nostra and the young adults together developed a system of after-learning transition to the labour market offering three pathways: the creation of an eco-agriculture social business, which could integrate some of the youths; entrepreneurship, for example, participants could create their own small business with the support of the project's partners; and integration into food production businesses where apprenticeships took place. This is also in contrast to traditional services that do not consider the young adults' expectations and predominantly offer counselling and training in narrowly defined work alternatives to low-skilled intensive labour (Carcillo et al., 2015; Tosun, 2017). The system offered flexibility in that youths could combine various solutions according to their personal needs (Simões, 2018).

The authors conclude that at all stages, projects should be organised as laboratories in which youth can understand, by themselves, the demands, the achievements, and the barriers to activities, with minimal (but significant) input from professionals. Together, self-determination and free experimentation are elements of an activation formula that becomes a sense of empowerment otherwise seldom experienced by NEETs (Simões & Drumonde, 2016).

From a salutogenic viewpoint, projects like *Terra nostra* reconstruct the distinction between SRR and GRR in the sense that they combine them in a new way. When we regard such projects in relation to our results from NEET and professional interviews, we observe that *Terra nostra* covers all but one GRR dimension (see Table 17.1). We propose three main qualities for suitable and effective Specific Resistance Ressources (SRRs). First, successful support should provide a particular experience of coherence for the NEETs. The experience of resources, not their availability, is crucial for strengthening SOC (Maass et al., 2017). Young adults who have the opportunity to learn according to their capabilities and within an encouraging and open process are much more likely to live positive experiences of resources than those who feel overwhelmed by long curricula of aims, objectives, and abilities they have to achieve within a predefined limit of time.

Second, professionals' attitudes towards young adults should be shaped by respect, equity, and trust in processes of growth, rather than based on systems of control and mistrust.

And third, young adults need challenging and demanding, but yet flexible and individualised pathways to achieve the societal autonomy they wish for. These pathways need supported transitions in between different support systems as well as the willingness of professionals to cooperate and invest in transprofessional and interdisciplinary networks.

In sum, support systems and young adults have so far agreed on the GRRs to be achieved, but support systems have not yet been able to design adequate, accessible, and attractive SRRs for young adults. *Terra nostra* is one example of how to create them. Others are strongly needed, not only for the benefit of young adults: "Greater cooperation between youths, social agents, and producers (not to mention political decision-makers) would result in a win-win situation: not only would youths and social organisations find alternatives for youth employment based on local opportunities, but producers could also use an additional channel to tackle the increasing labour force shortage" (Simões, 2018). Thereby, the NEET situation could become a collective challenge and would no longer be defined as an individual failure. Moreover, the thousands and thousands of young people in NEET situations around the globe would no longer be an overload for fragmented services but rather a valuable resource for society.

Support systems are thus challenged to understand the young adults in order to strengthen their SOC. This means understanding the inner reality of these young adults rather than attempting to fit them into economy-driven, rigid programs (Lindström & Eriksson, 2010; Meier Magistretti et al.,

2016, 2019). One of the key capacities in professionals that our study revealed to be positively associated with NEETs' successful transitions was to bear NEETs' insecurity and their periods of no apparent progress. We thus suggest that the professionals should commit themselves to acquire a more profound understanding instead of providing fast, predefined solutions. Another factor that strengthens SOC is the professionals' agility and flexibility in following their clients and challenging them with adequate and attractive tasks (Antonovsky, 1987).

Future Questions and Developments

Young adults in NEET conditions tend to preserve coherence and SOC by narrowing their radius of action. Alcohol and drug consumption, excessive online gaming, and other behaviours (that may even grow to become lifestyles) serve as a means to maintain or create a world that is understandable, manageable, and meaningful. In online games, for example, they understand their tasks, they can manage them, and the achievement of different levels provides motivation and a sense of meaningfulness. Focusing on gaming, the young adults can successfully fade out other sectors of life, for example, work and employment, that potentially weaken their SOC. Antonovsky (1987) stated that the boundaries people set about which parts of the world and life we consider of importance affect the SOC. He further assumed that the boundaries cannot be illimitably restricted but must include the person's inner feelings, the closest interpersonal relations, the main occupation, and the main existential themes. Hochwälder (2019), referring to Antonovsky, proposes a "measure of the boundaries, or in other words, a measure of which sectors of the world and life the person takes into consideration when assessing his or her SOC" (Hochwälder, 2019, S.4). Even though this measure is still lacking, the concept of boundaries is a useful heuristic for practical work with young adults in NEET situations. Assuming that current behaviours of these young people serve to maintain the four basic functions of SOC by narrowing their world, setting boundaries to sectors of life they do not threaten their experience of coherence. The task of professionals then might be to support young adults to widen their boundaries slowly. The example of terra nova shows this is possible. Other, more various and new initiatives are to be developed to create perspectives and sustainable quality of life for young adults in NEET situations.

Finally, new questions risen by students in the rhizomatic research program mentioned above should receive more attention, and difficulties now perceived as individual problems could be recognised as (also) societal ones. Basic questions of what is and who defines quality of life will arise.

References

Akister, J., Owens, M., & Goodyer, I. M. (2010). Leaving care and mental health: Outcomes for children in out-of-home care during the transition to adulthood. Health Research Policy and Systems, 8, 10. https://doi.org/10.1186/1478-4505-8-10.

Antonovsky, A. (1987). *Unraveling the mystery of health: How people manage stress and stay well.* Jossey-Bass.

Aubry, T., Bourque, J., Goering, P., Crouse, S., Veldhuizen, S., LeBlanc, S., Cherner, R., Bourque, P. E., Pakzad, S., & Bradshaw, C. (2019). A randomised controlled trial of the effectiveness of Housing First in a small Canadian City. *BMC Public Health, 19*(1154), 1–14. https://doi.org/10.1186/s12889-019-7492-8

Bacher, J., Koblbauer, C., Leitgöb, H. et al. Small differences matter: How regional distinctions in educational and labour market policy account for heterogeneity in NEET rates. Journal for Labour Market Research51, 4 (2017). https://doi.org/10.1186/s12651-017-0232-6.

Baer, N., Altwicker-Hámori, S., Juvalta, S., Frick, U & Rüesch, P. (2015). Report under the second multiannual research programme on invalidity and disability (in German). (FoP2-IV), Nr. 19/15. Bern: Bundesamt für Sozialversicherungen. Available: https://www.sciencedirect.com/science/article/pii/S1054139X14003863?via%3Dihub. Accessed June 2020.

Baer, N. Frick, U., Auerbach, S. & Basler, M. (2017). The daily madness. Swiss executives' perceptions of employees with psychological problems. Lucerne University, Lucerne (in German). https://www.hslu.ch/de-ch/soziale-arbeit/ueber-uns/institute/sozialmanagement-sozialpolitik-und-praevention/praevention-und-gesundheit/studie-der-taegliche-wahnsinn/. Accessed 22 May 2020.

Baggio, S., Iglesias, K., Deline, S., Studer, J., Henchoz, Y., Mohler-Kuo, M., & Gmel, G. (2015). Not in education, employment, or training status among young Swiss men. longitudinal associations with mental health and substance use. *Journal of Adolescent Health, 56*, 238–243. https://doi.org/10.1016/j.jadohealth.2014.09.006

Bania, E. V., Eckhoff, C., & Kvernmo, S. (2019). Not engaged in education, employment or training (NEET) in an Arctic sociocultural context: The NAAHS cohort study. *BMJ Open, 9*, e023705. https://doi.org/10.1136/bmjopen-2018-023705

Basta Maria Basta, M., Karakonstantis, S., Koutra, K., Dafermos, V., Papargiris, A., Drakaki, M., Tzagkarakis, S., Vgontzas, A., Simos, P., & Papadakis, N. (2019). NEET status among young Greeks: Association with mental health and substance use. *Journal of Affective Disorder, 253*, 210–217.

Bjarnason, T., Sigurdardottir, T. J. (2003). Psychological distress during unemployment and beyond: Social support and material deprivation among youth in six northern European countries. p. 973985. https://doi.org/10.1016/S0277-9536(02)00109-0

Bond, G. R., Drake, R. E., & Campbell, K. (2016). Effectiveness of individual placement and support supported employment for young adults. *Early Intervention in Psychiatry, 10*(4), 300–307. https://doi.org/10.1111/eip.12175

Bruckner, T. A., Snowden, L., Subbaraman, M. S., Brown, T. T. (2010). Economic antecedents of Medicaid-financed mental health services among youths in California. p. 490. https://doi.org/10.2753/IMH0020-7411390204

Burd-Sharp, S. & Lewis, K. (2017). Promising gains, persisting gaps. Youth disconnection rates for states, metro areas, rural and urban areas, and counties as well as by gender and race/ethnicity. Measure of America of the Social Science research council. Available: http://measureofamerica.org/youth-disconnection-2017/

Cabral, F. J. (2018). Key drivers of NEET phenomenon among youth people in Senegal. *Economics Bulletin, 38*(1), 248–261.

Carcillo, S., Fernandez, R., Könis, S. & Minea, A. (2015). NEET youth in the aftermath of the crisis: challenges and policies, OECD social, employment and migration working papers, No. 164, OECD Publishing, Paris, https://doi.org/10.1787/5js6363503f6-en.

Chen, Y. W. (2011). Once a NEET always a NEET? Experiences of employment and unemployment among youth in a job training programme in Taiwan. *International Journal of Social Welfare, John Wiley & Sons, 20*(1), 33–42. https://ideas.repec.org/a/wly/injsow/v20y2011i1p33-42.html

Clarke, B., & Parsons, J. (2013). Becoming rhizome researchers. *Reconceptualising Educational Research Methodology, 4*(1), 35–43.

Deleuze, G., & Guattari, F. (1988). *A thousand plateaus*. Athlone.

Duckworth, K., & Schoon, I. (2012). Beating the odds: Exploring the impact of social risk on young people's school-to-work transitions during recession in the UK. *National Institute Economic Review, 222*, R38–R51.

Elder, S. (2015). *What does NEET mean and why is the concept so easily misinterpreted? Work4Youth publication series, techn Geneva*. Employment Policy Department, International Labour Office, http://www.ilo.org/employment/areas/youth-employment/work-for-youth/publications/technical-briefs/WCMS_343153/lang--en/index.htm.

Eriksson, M., & Lindström, B. (2005). Validity of Antonovsky's sense of coherence scale: A systematic review. *Journal of Epidemiology and Community Health, 59*, 460–466. https://doi.org/10.1136/jech.2003.018085

European Commission. (2016). *Youth unemployment by sex, age and educational attainment level*. Eurostat. http://appsso.eurostat.ec.europa.eu/nui/submitViewTableAction.d

Eurostat (2020). Statistics ond young people neither in employment nor in education or training. Available: https://ec.europa.eu/eurostat/statistics-explained/index.php/Statistics_on_young_people_neither_in_employment_nor_in_education_or_training. Accessed August 2020.

Fernandes, A. L., & Gabe, T. (2009). *Disconnected youth: A look at 16- to 24-year olds who are not working or in school*. Congressional Research Service. https://digital.library.unt.edu/ark:/67531/metadc700799/

Genda, Y. (2007). Jobless youths and the NEET problem in Japan. *Social Science Japan Journal, 10*(1), 23–40. https://doi.org/10.1093/ssjj/jym029

Goldman-Mellor, S., Caspi, A., Arseneault, L., Ajala, N., Ambler, A., Danese, A., et al. (2016). Committed to work but vulnerable: Self-perceptions and mental health in NEET 18-year olds from a contemporary British cohort. *Journal of Child Psychology and Psychiatry, 57*, 196–203.

Gutiérrez-García, R. A., Benjet, C., Borges, G., Méndez Ríos, E., & Medina-Mora, M. E. (2018). Emerging adults not in education, employment or training (NEET): Socio-demo-graphic characteristics, mental health and reasons for being NEET. *BMC Public Health, 18*, 1201.

Gutiérrez-García, R. A., Benjet, C., Borges, G., et al. (2017). NEET adolescents grown up: Eight-year longitudinal follow-up of education, employment and mental health from adolescence to early adulthood in Mexico City. *European Child & Adolescent Psychiatry, 26*, 1459. https://doi.org/10.1007/s00787-017-1004-0

Hallstein Holte, B., Swart, I., & Hiilamo, H. (2018). The NEET concept in comparative youth research: The Nordic countries and South Africa. *Journal of Youth Studies, 22*(2), 256–272. https://doi.org/10.1080/13676261.2018.149640

Hochwälder, J. (2019). *Sense of coherence: Notes on some challenges for future research* (pp. 1–8). Psychological Reports. https://doi.org/10.1177/2158244019846687

Hussmanns, R., Mehran, F., & Verma, V. (1990). *Surveys of economically active population, employment, unemployment and underemployment: An ILO manual on concepts and methods*. Geneva.

International Labour Organisation (ILO). (2013). *Global employment trends for youth 2013; a generation at risk*. ILO.

Iyer, S., Mustafa, S., Gariépy, G., et al. (2018). A NEET distinction: Youths not in employment, education or training follow different pathways to illness and care in psychosis. *Social Psychiatry and Psychiatric Epidemiology, 53*, 1401–1411. https://doi.org/10.1007/s00127-018-1565-3

Lakey, J., Mukherjee, A., White, M. (2001). London Policy Studies Institute [Google Scholar]).

Levitan, M. (2005). *Out of school, out of work . . . Out of luck? New York City's disconnected youth*. Community Service Society.

Lindström, B., & Eriksson, M. (2010). *The Hitchhiker's guide to Salutogenesis*. Helsingfors.

Maass, R., Lindstrom, B., & Lillefjell, M. (2017). Neighborhood-resources for the development of a strong SOC and the importance of understanding why and how resources work: A grounded theory approach. *BMC Public Health, 17*(1), 704. https://doi.org/10.1186/s12889-017-4705-x

Maguire, S. (2015). NEET, unemployed, inactive or unknown – Why does it matter? *Educational Research, 57*(2), 121–132. https://doi.org/10.1080/00131881.2015.1030850

McGorry, P. (2019). Building the momentum and blueprint for reform in youth mental health. *Lancet, 6*(6), 459–461. https://doi.org/10.1016/S2215-0366(19)30050-1

Meier Magistretti, C., Downe, S., Lindstrøm, B., Berg, M., & Tritten-Schwarz, K. (2016). Setting the stage for health: Salutogenesis in midwifery professional knowledge in three European countries. *International Journal of Qualitative Studies on Health and Wellbeing, 11*(1), 33155.

Meier Magistretti, C., Topalidou, A., & Meinecke, F. (2019). The sense for coherence – Approaching a new concept in salutogenic theory. (in German). In C. Meier Magistretti et al. (Eds.), *Salutogenese kennen und verstehen* (pp. 119–134). Hogrefe.

Mittelmark, M. B., Sagy, S., Eriksson, M., Bauer, G., Pelikan, J. M., Lindström, B., & Arild Espnes, G. (2017). *The handbook of Salutogenesis*. Springer.

Mögling, M., Tillmann, F., & Reissig, B. (2015). *Disconnected young adults and challenges for youth welfare. A study by the German Youth Institute under the authority of the Vodafone Foundation. (in German)*. Düsseldorf. Available: https://www.stiftungen.org/uploads/tx_leonhardtdyncontent/downloads/Entkoppelt-vom-System.pdf (accessed May 2020)

Noh, H., & Lee, B. J. (2017). Risk factors of NEET (Not in Employment, Education or Training) in South Korea: An empirical study using panel data. *Asia Pacific Journal of Social Work and Development, 27*, 1. https://doi.org/10.1080/02185385.2017.1289860

O'Dea, B., Glozier, N., Purcell, R., et al. (2014). A cross-sectional exploration of the clinical characteristics of disengaged (NEET) young people in primary mental healthcare. *BMJ Open, 4*, e006378. https://doi.org/10.1136/bmjopen-2014-006378

O'Dea, B., Lee, R. S. C., McGorry, P. D., et al. (2016). A prospective cohort study of depression course, functional disability, and NEET status in help-seeking young adults. *Social Psychiatry and Psychiatric Epidemiology, 51*, 1395–1404. https://doi.org/10.1007/s00127-016-1272-x

OECD. (2016). The NEET challenge: What can be done for jobless and disengaged youth? *Society at a glance*. OECD Social Indicators. p. 13–68. https://doi.org/10.1787/9789264261488-en

OECD. (2018). Education at a glance. Education at a Glance. https://doi.org/10.1787/19991487.

OECD. (2021). "Youth not in employment, education or training (NEET)" (indicator), https://doi.org/10.1787/72d1033a-en. Accessed on 15 March 2021.

Patel, V., Fisher, A. J., Hetrick, S., & McGorry, P. (2007). Mental health of young people: A global public-health challenge. *Lancet, 369*, 1302–1313. https://doi.org/10.1016/S0140-6736(07)60368-7

Robertson, P. J. (2018). Developing career capabilities in "NEET" young people: Experiences of participants in the Prince's trust team program. *British Journal of Guidance & Counselling, 46*(6), 752–764. https://doi.org/10.1080/03069885.2018.1434130

Robertson, P. J. (2019). The casualties of transition: The health impact of NEET status and some approaches to managing it. *British Journal of Guidance & Counselling, 47*(3), 390–402. https://doi.org/10.1080/03069885.2018.1455168

Rodwell, L., Romaniuk, H., Nilsen, W., Carlin, J., Lee, K., & Patton, G. (2018). Adolescent mental health and behavioural predictors of being NEET: A prospective study of young adults not in employment, education, or training. *Psychological Medicine, 48*(5), 861–871. https://doi.org/10.1017/S0033291717002434

Rueda, S., Chambers, L., Wilson, M., Mustard, C., Rourke, S. B., Bayoumi, A. (2012). Association of returning to work with better health in working-aged adults: A systematic review. 541556. https://doi.org/10.2105/AJPH.2011.300401

Sabatella, F. & Wyl, A. (2017). Supported education in Switzerland. Sustaining young people in the transistion to working life. (in German). ZHAW Zürcher Hochschule für Angewandte Wissenschaften. https://doi.org/10.21256/zhaw-1315.

Shore, J. & Tosun, J. (2017). Assessing youth labour market services: Young people's perceptions and evaluations of service delivery in Germany. Public Policy and Administration. https://doi.org/10.1177/0952076717722192.

Simões, F. (2018). How to involve rural NEET youths in agriculture? Highlights of an untold story. *Community Development, 49*(5), 556–573. https://doi.org/10.1080/15575330.2018.1531899

Simões, F., & Drumonde, R. (2016). Os desafios da reconversão profesional de jovens nas atividades do setor primário: O caso do projeto Terra Nostra (The challenges of youths' professional reskilling in the primary sector: The case of the project Our Land). In G. Rocha, R. Gonçalves, & P. D. Medeiros (Eds.), *Juventude(s): Novas realidades, novos olhares (Youth: New realities, new approaches)* (pp. 103–122). Húmus.

Starrin, B., Jönsson, K., & Rantakeisu, U. (2001). Sense of coherence during unemployment. *International Journal of Social Welfare, 10*, 107–116. https://doi.org/10.1111/1468-2397.0016

Stea, T. H., Abildsnes, E., Strandheim, A., & Haugland, S. H. (2019). Do young people who are not in education, employment or training (NEET) have more health problems than their peers? A cross-sectional study among Norwegian adolescents. *Norsk Epidemiologi, 28*(1–2), 89–95. https://doi.org/10.5324/nje.v28i1-2.3055

Stewart, C. H., Berry, P., Przulj, D., et al. (2017). Cancer-related health behaviours of young people not in education, employment or training ('NEET'): A cross-sectional study. *BMC Cancer, 17*, 165. https://doi.org/10.1186/s12885-017-3157-0

Strandh, M., Nilsson, K., Nordlund, M., & Hammarström, A. (2015). Do open youth unemployment and youth programs leave the same mental health scars?--evidence from a Swedish 27-year cohort study. *BMC Public Health, 15*, 1151. https://doi.org/10.1186/s12889-015-2496-5

Tamesberger, D., & Johann Bacher, J. (2014). NEET youth in Austria: A typology including socio-demography, labour market behaviour and permanence. *Journal of Youth Studies, 17*(9), 1239–1259. https://doi.org/10.1080/13676261.2014.901492

Thompson, R. (2011). Individualisation and social exclusion: The case of young people not in education, employment or training. *Oxford Review of Education, 37*(6), 785–802. https://doi.org/10.1080/03054985.2011.636507

Tosun, J. (2017). Promoting youth employment through multi-organisational governance. *Public Money and Management, 37*(1), 39–46. https://doi.org/10.1080/09540962.2016.1249230

United Nations. (2016). SDG, Goal 8, Concept notes. https://unstats.un.org/sdgs/files/metadata-compilation/metadata-goal-8.pdf. Accessed on 16 Mar 2021.

United Nations. (2020). SDG, Goal 8, Concept notes: Promote sustained, inclusive and sustainable economic growth, full and productive employment and decent work for all, Target 8.6: By 2020, substantially reduce the proportion of youth not in employment, education or training. https://unstats.un.org/sdgs/metadata/files/Metadata-08-06-01.pdf. Accessed on 16 Mar 2021.

Vancea, M., & Utzet, M. (2016). How unemployment and precarious employment affect the health of young people: A scoping study on social determinants. *Scandinavian Journal of Public Health, 45*(1), 73–84. https://doi.org/10.1177/1403494816679555

Vancea, M., & Utzet, M. (2017). How unemployment and precarious employment affect the health of young people: A scoping study on social determinants. *Scandinavian Journal of Public Health, 45*(1), 73–84. https://doi.org/10.1177/1403494816679555

Vastamäki, J., Paul, K. I., & Moser, K. (2011). How stable is sense of coherence? Changes following an intervention for unemployed individuals. *Scandinavian Journal of Psychology, 50*, 161–171.

Wilson, T., & Bivand, P. (2014). *Equitable full employment: A jobs recovery for all (touchstone extra pamphlet)*. Trades Union Congress.

Zuccotti, C. V., & O'Reilly, J. (2019). Ethnicity, gender and household effects on becoming NEET: An intersectional analysis. *Work, Employment and Society, 33*(3), 351–373. https://doi.org/10.1177/0950017017738945

18

Middle Adulthood, Salutogenesis and SOC

Ottomar Bahrs, Felix Deymann, and Karl-Heinz Henze

Introduction

The life course can be understood as a dynamic learning process that is socially pre-structured in the sense of electoral opportunities but is experienced and lived individually (Erikson, 1980). This is how life phases with expected developmental tasks and corresponding risk-resource profiles can be described – culturally differently structured. Besides, critical – usually unexpected – life events must be taken into account, which in turn present specific challenges and require flexible coping strategies. The formation of personal and social identity (Goffman, 1975) is thus a continuous challenge of 'making yourself who you are' (Sartre, 1964, p. 1977–1979, translated by the authors) and which is also expressed in the formation of the SOC (Antonovsky, 1987; Ventegodt et al., 2003).

For a long time, the late middle age has been considered an undramatic phase of life, but it is increasingly beginning to acquire its particular profile (Perrig-Chiello & Perren, 2005; Perrig-Chiello et al., 2008). We focus here on a phase typically observable in the sixth decade of life, which can be described as the initiation of the transition to devocationalization and a change in family responsibilities. It is thus an approach towards balancing and future orientation, looking for a coherent life.

Crises, whatever their causes, as well as long-standing problems, can lead to a need for help from health professionals who can provide support in defining individual health objectives and in developing ways to achieve them according to the situation, the person and the problem. The often implicit personal life goals must be taken into account.

This chapter uses a case study to illustrate how general practitioners can contribute by using a specific framework for encounters (*review dialogue*) to the naming, modification, design and development of health goals. Further, we want to illustrate how this kind of encounter can promote the use and formation of salutogenic resources, and how this relates to the life situation and life history of persons in chronic conditions. We focus on the challenges of the sixth decade of life – here, especially the care and support of parents as the continuing effect of developmental tasks. From this perspective, for example, the tasks of developing autonomy and detaching oneself from the parental home, which is typically on the agenda in earlier phases of life, become relevant again in a modified form. The meaning of the tasks at hand is shown employing a biographical reconstruction and gives an idea of the interweaving of coexisting constellations in the family context (cf. Oevermann, 2000). This chapter underlines, based on the specific transitional situation in the sixth decade of life, that life tasks need to be emphasized and taken into account for the joint negotiation of health goals.

We illustrate that individual health goals, such as those discussed in the context of long-term care by family doctors and agreed upon by the patient and the doctor, are the more likely to be achieved the more closely they correspond to the implicit life tasks (Bahrs & Henze, 2019). It requires a relationship based on understanding and mutual acceptance, in which the interlocutors can meet as subjects and take into account their particular contextual conditions. The dialogue aims at enabling the person seeking help to find individual solutions, extends the concept of shared decision-making (Elwyn et al., 2012), which is usually related to the agreed-upon treatment plans, by the definition of the underlying problems and thus becomes an action-guiding philosophy. We show that this participatory approach helps to strengthen the sense of meaningfulness, and thus the SOC as a whole (Antonovsky, 1987).

O. Bahrs (✉)
University of Düsseldorf, Düsseldorf, Germany

Umbrella Organization Salutogenesis, Göttingen, Germany
e-mail: obahrs@dachverband-salutogenese.de

F. Deymann
University of Göttingen, Göttingen, Germany

K.-H. Henze
Lou Andreas-Salomé Institut for Psychoanalysis and Psychotherapy, Göttingen, Germany

The chapter illustrates this process with a case study based on a series of four detailed family doctor-patient interviews (review dialogues) and a subsequent narrative interview lasting three hours. By systematically relating narrated life, experienced life and lived life to one another, we depict the process of forming resources and identity and illustrate its structuring function for the formation of relationships. It becomes clear that there is an inherent healing potential in the narration itself (Rosenthal, 1995; Nünning & Nünning, 2019).

First, we outline specific features of the sixth decade of life with a particular focus on gender aspects. Further, we outline the selected theoretical aspects regarding our case study. We deal with the life course as a contradictory unit of socialization and individuation, which is mentally processed in the form of a biography. The life course is organized along with life phases and life tasks, the mastering of which is challenging and involves learning processes. These can be crisis-like, but it is precisely phases of transition that offer the chance to mature. The development of ego-identity and the relationship between identity and SOC are lifelong processes (Lindström & Eriksson, 2010).

Late Middle Age: Time for Stocktaking

Preliminary note: the cited empirical results do not always refer precisely to the sixth decade of life. In the study by Lademann and Kolip (2005), for example, a broader age group between 45 and 65 years is considered. In their comparative study, Perrig and Höpflinger (2001) refer, amongst other things, to the age group of 50- to 55-year-olds.

Particularities of the Sixth Decade of Life

The life span between the 50th and 60th year of life is less clearly organized as a specific life phase than some earlier and later stages of life (Perrig-Chiello & Perren, 2005). In this decade, the confrontation with illness, dying and death occurs more frequently, for example, through reports from the environment, illness or death of a family member. Concerning parents, the probability of care and nursing tasks increases (Höpflinger & Perrig-Chiello, n.d.). Increasingly, physical limitations are becoming apparent, for example, at the level of sports or more general physical activities.

There are several specific health changes in the late middle age group, for example, the prevalence of many chronic diseases - such as skeletal and cariovascular diseases and cancer - are increasing (Lademann & Kolip, 2005). Possible functional limitations also evoke a changed body life. This requires repeated repositioning of the attitude towards the body. It should be noted that the body is involved in perception and communication and can be the object of observation and evaluation of one's perception and the perception of others. As the performer of the self, it also has a recursive effect on the self through its performance (Corbin & Strauss, 1988, 2004, p. 70–86). According to Foucault, the body is produced through discursive practices. It is socially and culturally constructed. For example, scientific disciplines provide patterns of thinking or interpretation, which then become part of everyday knowledge and have an impact on action. This mediated knowledge influences how the body is spoken about in our society. Discourses are thus inseparably connected with power (Gugutzer, 2002, 2004). Since the body is also a significant factor in the self-value representation of the individual, constant identity work is required.

In the sixth decade of life, children will usually move out or have already left the parental home. The parents have to focus more strongly on themselves or the couple's relationship again and, if necessary, realigning oneself. Reasons for change often result from crisis-like events such as separation, divorce and loss of a loved one. In other areas of life, too, there is a stocktaking of the goals of life that are strived for, achieved and not achieved. The life priorities and plans of the past will become at the latest now a virulent and partly emotionally occupied topic. An example from two psychotherapeutic consultations – conducted by one of the authors – illustrate this:

> Mrs. A., 55 years old: 'Now in the menopause, I have a growing feeling of physical insecurity, sometimes I sit there and have stomach aches, become thin-skinned and more vulnerable. Sometimes I feel guilty because of the breakdown of the relationship with my parents. My son is an adult, sometimes I think I should have done more for him, but I know it's over. Certain doors close.'

Here begins a reflexive and affective process of coming to terms with the situation, which – perhaps through mourning – is an essential prerequisite for moving from passively resigned accepting of what happened to an integrative perspective or inner balance and experience of self-efficacy. Perhaps the result will be a similar insight as with Mrs. B.:

> Mrs. B., 57 years old: 'My marriage is deadlocked, nothing more will happen. I was depressed often and for a long time, wondering how it came about. Then the thought came up: "What do I want to experience anymore?" So the thought came to me, "When one door closes, another opens." I began to reorient myself professionally.'

Against the background of increasing life expectancy, new challenges, fields of activity and responsibilities may arise, combined with the recognition that stable limits of previous life may be shifted. It can even be experienced as enriching and enjoyable to face new challenges. For example, grandchildren may enrich life towards the end of the decade.

Significant social and cultural dimensions influence the specific life situation or the design of life plans. These include, for example, growing income disparities, such as the level of education or access to education (Perrig-Chiello & Höpflinger, 2001, p. 106).

Gender

Gender has a biological and social dimension, which is interrelated in the broadest sense. 'Gender' refers to sex in the sense of cultural, social or societal construction. It is expressed, for example, in the role of the sexes or gender identity. Gender construction affects social interactions and attributions from the beginning of the life course, and therefore gender-specific differences result in the respective phases of life.

Concerning the sex differences described in the following, it should be noted that other variables have a causal, moderating and differentiating effect, especially influences of socioeconomic status (education, occupation, income). Life situation, attitudes to health and the resulting behaviour diverge for gender groups (Backes, 1998; Backes & Wolfinger, 2009).

Women, in particular, have to integrate family tasks and gainful employment and have more discontinuous career paths compared to men. Moreover, women are more likely to have jobs 'with less room for manoeuvre and autonomy' and are paid less for comparable work than men (Lademann & Kolip, 2005, p. 81).

Looking at the sixth decade of those born between 1950 and 1959 on the basis of the German Ageing Survey (1996 to 2017), women are somewhat more satisfied with their lives than men during this phase. Satisfaction is highest at the beginning of the sixth decade and then decreases (Vogel et al., 2019, p. 14–15).

The drug consumption of women is comparatively higher, whereby hormone therapy playing a particularly relevant role during and after menopause. According to Lademann and Kolip (2005), its appropriateness must be questioned and partly interpreted as an indication of a tendency to medicalization.

Women are usually responsible for family health and more often make use of screening examinations and medical assistance (Robert Koch Institute, 2014; Beutel et al., 2019). Compared to men, affective disorders, anxiety disorders and somatoform disorders are more frequently diagnosed in women of the sixth decade of life. The most frequent cause of death in women is breast cancer (Lademann & Kolip, 2005, p. 63–64).

Care work is unequally distributed between the sexes. In addition to caring for grandchildren, care activities include, in particular, the support and care of relatives. Concerning the cohort of those born between 1950 and 1959, there is a probability of care and nursing tasks of 23% for women and 16% for men (Vogel et al., 2009, p. 29).

The data of a representative telephone survey by the Robert Koch Institute (Wetzstein et al., 2015) confirm and complete the picture. According to these data, although the share of men providing nursing care is increasing, private home care is predominantly provided by women (Wetzstein et al., 2015, p. 3). The study does not make any specific statements for the sixth decade of life, but tendencies become apparent that are equally relevant for this age group. In general, about two-thirds of the carers across all age groups are women, and one third are men. As the extent of care increases, the share of women in the care of relatives increases (Wetzstein et al., 2015, p. 8). Nurses with a high level of care receive less social support than non-nurses, and the health status of carers is worse than that of non-carers.

The German Institute for Economic Research (DIW) has determined the importance of informal care in Germany for the years 2001 to 2012 and states that employed caregivers are more satisfied than non-employed caregivers, the satisfaction of caregivers is significantly lower compared to people who do not provide care and the general life satisfaction decreases with increasing care provision (Geyer & Schulz, 2014, p. 299–300). Conversely generally applies: prerequisites for greater life satisfaction are 'good health resources and a low level of stressors such as chronic anxiety, social isolation and problems with the immediate family' (Perrig-Chiello & Hutchison, 2010, p. 204).

The least willingness to care is found amongst people with high social status (Wetzstein et al., 2015, p. 8). Presumably, in contrast to families with a lower social status, they have more options at their disposal, such as the financed delegation of care tasks to third parties.

Care work, therefore, has many possible implications, such as restricted or (temporarily) abandoned employment, limited prevention opportunities, increased psychosocial burdens and limited options for realizing interests, needs and requirements. However, this probably does not concern care activities per se. Depending on the relationship with the person being cared for, work can also strengthen the SOC with meaningful and enriching experiences, experiences of satisfaction.

Men's life expectancy is shorter than that of women. In 2012, men in the age group between 50 and 60 had a mortality risk that was at least 1.7–1.8 times higher. The mortality of unmarried men is higher than that of married men, that is, partnership or marriage, and family can act as protective resources or health-promoting context. Concerning diseases of the circulatory system, especially coronary heart disease (age group 45–65 years), there is a 2.9-fold excess mortality rate compared to women. Lung tumours, external causes (e.g. injuries, accidents) and diseases of the digestive and respiratory systems are comparatively more frequent causes of death in men (Lademann & Kolip, 2005, p. 16; Robert Koch Institute, 2014). In a gender comparison, men display more frequent tobacco consumption, overweight and more inadequate nutritional behaviour. Health-endangering alcohol consumption is also higher amongst working men than amongst inactive men (Lademann & Kolip, 2005, p. 41; Robert Koch Institute, 2014). Compared to women, men are more likely to have jobs with higher physical stress (Lademann & Kolip, 2005, p. 81).

It is interesting to note that men's health awareness is much more developed than their health behaviour (Faltermaier, 2004). The development of health awareness may be counteracted by traditional concepts of self and masculinity that support 'risky' health behaviour, and corresponds to 'masculinity concepts'. If one pursues this aspect further and assumes that the definition of male identity continues to be strongly influenced by the professional role, then it should be noted that in the sixth decade, the forthcoming retirement with the expected loss of significance, status and relationships will cast its shadow. Often there are no alternative concepts to this. Instead, a mental and affective confrontation with the upcoming life changes is fended off.

The Biography as a Learning Process

The development of a human being can be understood as a contradictory unity of forming him/her into a member of society (socialization) and shaping his/her unique characteristics (individuation). In his concept of existential psychoanalysis, Sartre starts from a double birth of man, which he calls constitution (Sartre, 1977-1979, Vol. 1) and personalization (Sartre, 1977-1979, Vol. 2 and 3). On the one hand, man as a biological and social being finds himself in a world of social facts. Thus, body, history and environment determine a priori the chances for the social place that a person will be able to occupy and constitute a part of the social body: 'The meaning of life comes to the living person through the human society that sustains him and through the parents who engender him' (Sartre, 1981, p. 134). On the other hand, the social body reproduces and transforms itself through the social practice of the members of society who, through their designs, make themselves into individuals and thus, to a certain extent, occupy self-defined places. 'To live is to produce meanings' (Sartre, 1981, p. 15).

Sartre – similar to Antonovsky regarding the SOC (Antonovsky, 1987) – assumes an autopoietic process. In every situation, man is confronted with a pre-structured world with various (thought and) action possibilities, which he cannot use simultaneously. He has to make choices (with always incomplete information), and thus at the same time invents the basic structure of his life project. Man first sets the values that define him. Nevertheless, the choice as a project in a self-structured world is, in turn, conditional. 'The basic behaviours are only accepted if they exist first' (Sartre, 1977-1979, Vol. 1, p. 53, translated by the authors). The constitution, as a meaningful body, is first conveyed in baby care. Although in this form of interaction, the actors refer particularly clearly to each other as 'whole people', the 'basic choice' as the attitude towards oneself and the world always concerns the psychosomatic unit and therefore has an affective structure. It indicates that 'hidden core(s) in which the experienced body and the sense mix' (Sartre, 1977-1979, Vol. 1, p. 56, translated by the authors).

Biography denotes 'the subjective construction or coherence formation of lived life'; it is the result of a 'conferring of meaning and significance' or 'the active performance of the subject through which the past is reorganized in the face of the present and the future' (Marotzki, 1990, p. 77). By their biography, which is continuously being newly constructed or changed, individuals simultaneously construct, reflect and develop drafts for action about the future perspective of life.

The biography is also 'the place where the individual processes of reflection and learning are synchronized' (Maier-Gutheil, 2015, p. 15). 'From a process perspective, experiences of everyday life, as well as crises, form potential triggers for learning activities' (Maier-Gutheil, 2015, p. 11), which can relate to attitudes, patterns of interpretation, experiences, self-awareness and resources. This happens in the most diverse learning contexts, such as family and relatives, leisure activities, job, sport, cultural and social gatherings and in contacts with professional helper systems, such as in the family-doctor relationship.

Life Stages and Life Tasks

Any age phase can be understood as a product of cultural representations, social constructions, social institutionalizations and structural principles as well as biological mechanisms. An order takes place through the life course, which is characterized by distinctive transitions and phases of life. In Kohli's sense, it is a system of rules built up over time (van Dyk, 2015, p. 48). As an example, the family life cycle is briefly sketched out here in line with Hegemann et al. (2000). It comprises key stages such as 'birth', 'early childhood', 'schooling', 'adolescence', 'early adult life with entry into the world of work, a transition to starting a family', 'bringing up children', 'midlife crisis with reassessments and reorientations', 'ageing', 'exit from working life', 'old age', 'very old age' and 'dying and death'.

With the increasing pluralization of life worlds, modernization and differentiation in postmodern societies, however, life courses are less structurally framed; there is a growing diversity of role patterns and individual design options (Eikelpasch & Rademacher, 2004, p. 59; Bauman, 2001; Gilleard & Higgs, 2019). Despite the growing flexibility of life courses, specific developmental tasks and challenges must be mastered in each of these phases against the background of corresponding risk and resource profiles. Therein, the here and now is not conceivable without the experienced past and the anticipated future.

The transitions or transitional periods between the respective phases are partly characterized by normative crises, which can be accompanied by severe challenges and instabilities. Transitions are 'life events that require coping with discontinuities on several levels, accelerate processes, stimulate intensified learning, and are perceived as significant biographical experiences of change in identity development' (Griebel & Niesel, 2011, p. 37–38).

Learning in Crises: Continuity and Break

The transitions between development phases, life stages or life spans (Baltes, 1987) are associated with numerous new requirements. This refers to challenges such as integrating new roles and dealing with changing life contexts and self and identity issues (e.g. family changes and entry into or termination of working life) (Griebel & Niesel, 2011, p. 37–38). It requires an intensified and accelerated learning process. Whilst anticipated grand-parenthood represents, for example, a positively experienced transition (Perrig-Chiello & Perren, 2005, p. 178), tasks arising with the parents' need for care or accompanying the dying mother/father are very stressful or ambivalent (Perrig-Chiello & Höpflinger, 2001, p. 106).

Crisis events beyond transitions can, of course, occur at any time and within any phase of life. The reasons can be strokes of fate, such as the loss of essential caregivers or the occurrence of severe illness or misfortune at work, break-up of relationships and much more. Even seemingly processed previous life experiences, conflicts and crises can then become virulent again, and existing certainties and an inner sense of security can dissolve. On an individual level, initial denial tendencies and affects such as grief, fears, helplessness, excessive demands, stagnation, helplessness and hopelessness, as well as body-related complaints, can occur. At the same time, in the sense of a learning process, the crisis opens up an opportunity for developmental steps by acceptance (e.g. of limits to the controllability of life; Lindström & Eriksson, 2010, p. 13) balancing and reflexive processing of the past life, the here and now and the view of the presumed future. The balancing does not only refer to supposedly missed chances and failures but also to experiences that represent abilities or growth potentials, where one experienced satisfaction or pride. Ideally, the image of a realm of possibilities can emerge, combined with an experience of one's potentials (and limitations) as well as emerging needs and desires: Do I now want to change something in and about the previous life model? If so, what? How could I start to realize this?

Identity, SOC and Life Cycle

According to Antonovsky (1979, p. 110), ego-identity plays a central role in the field of generalized resistance resources. Ego-identity can be understood concerning the subject as an inner, interactive and constant process of everyday identity work. It is regulative that makes it possible to experience oneself as 'the same' in different social situations, and it is constantly re-established in interaction with other subjects. However, it is also a (self-)attribution that can be recognized by third parties, through which the person remains recognizable as identical in different situations (and is thus reliable). For this, several competencies must be acquired, including the ability to fill the contradictions of life with meaning and to synthesize them. This development is interactive and takes place against the background of societal, social and cultural conditions (Bohleber, 1997; Höfer, 2006; Keupp, 1997; Keupp et al., 2006; Krappmann, 1975, 1997).

An important question is how the relationship between ego-identity development and the SOC could look like. Höfer (2006) has attempted to analyse this. Before we describe her considerations, the SOC will be outlined in short.

In the salutogenic model, the sense of coherence (SOC) is of central importance. According to Antonovsky, it is composed of three dimensions, comprehensibility, manageability and meaningfulness, and it is a general and profound life orientation. It is a 'dispositional orientation rather than a response to a specific situation' (Antonovsky, 1987, p. 75). The SOC represents 'the extent to which one has a pervasive enduring though dynamic feeling of confidence that (1) the stimuli deriving from one's internal and external environments in the course of living are structured, predictable and explicable (2) the resources are available to one to meet the demands posed by these stimuli; and (3) these demands are challenges, worthy of investment and engagement' (Antonovsky, 1987, p. 19). The SOC is developing based on life experiences such as 'experiences of consistency, participation in decisions and a balance between demands and resources' (Faltermaier, 2006, p. 190; Antonovsky, 1987). In contrast to Antonovsky's early, but later modified, hypothesis, the SOC seems to have developmental potential beyond the age of 30 and is even expected to increase in the further course of life (Lindström & Eriksson, 2010, p. 23–25). In this respect, the SOC represents a dynamic process not only in childhood and youth but also in later life cycles.

Höfer (2006) conceptualizes 'identity as a source of the feeling of coherence' (2006, p. 57). It represents a 'reflexive frame of reference' within which the individual deals with his or her own life, for example, and attempts to 'develop coherent passages of internal and external demands' (Höfer, 2006, p. 60). SOC is formed on evaluations of how everyday demands are dealt with and expresses, as Antonovsky (1979) puts it, the relationship to the world (Höfer, 2006, p. 62). In Höfer's view, the SOC is the result of many successful identity-shaping experiences. The better the subject succeeds in creating 'links in his projects and experiences the project designs as subjectively coherent and authentic, the stronger the SOC will be' (Höfer, 2006, p. 63). One may assume that there will also be a positive feedback effect from the SOC on the feeling of identity.

Salutogenesis as Relationship-Related Health Development and Learning Process

The development of identity and the SOC takes rise within the framework of processes of interaction and social exchange (Antonovsky, 1987, p. 92–94). These processes last a whole lifetime and are never completed (Lindström & Eriksson, 2010). How this connection is formed is specific to the individual, and it is expressed in one's relationship to the world as a whole, in one's relationship to others and in relation to oneself (especially one's body). This specific style can also be expressed in health and illness behaviour as well as in the formation of symptoms, insofar as these are understood as part of a communicative process and can be attributed as active contributions (Sartre, 1977-1979; Weizsäcker, 1956; Uexküll, 2004).

Although the formation of health is designed as a result of self-regulation, professional support is required in special cases. In the fields of care, counselling, therapy and (family) practice, the relationship between the (two) actors is also of central importance. If the person seeking help feels taken seriously and appreciated as a person when interacting with a professional contact person, he/she can also experience him/herself and his/her relationships in a new way. He/she learns to make use of previously unknown resources and can subsequently test and stabilize the development potential in everyday life.

The long-term care of (healthy and) sick people requires a hermeneutic case understanding, taking somatic, psychosocial, sociocultural and ecological aspects into consideration. Hermeneutic case understanding is 'a specific professional activity, which is patient-centered, context-related, biographical and within a joint interpretive community (inclusion of the patient's concept of illness) and has a case-specific individual result' (Bahrs, 2012, p. 356).

Striving for a trusting, cooperative and open relationship includes, for example: establishing a stable work alliance, continuous cooperation, active listening, trying to understand the patients and their (family) life situation as well as an orientation towards his resources and strengths (cf. Honermann et al., 1999). A fundamental acceptance of the patients as experts of themselves promotes all three components of the help-seeking person's SOC.

Case Study: 'I Have Lost Sight of My Goal'

If you ask people about the most important thing in their lives, many will say: 'Health.' On closer listening, it quickly becomes apparent that the respective meaning of health is individual (Matthiessen, 2010; Sturmberg et al., 2019).

What is called and desired as 'health' is by no means arbitrary. We are all born into a particular, historically grown cultural and social environment so that this framework already shapes many of our perceptions and feelings in everyday life and social relationships. Against this background, we learn to interpret our own physically mediated experiences, to perceive signs of well-being and discomfort in ourselves and others and to differentiate more and more between ideas of desirable 'health' and 'illness'. What we consider to be 'healthy' and 'ill' is thus also an expression and result of a social learning experience (Payer, 1993; Faltermaier, 2009; Helmich et al., 1991) and relates to social developmental tasks faced by the individual (Buddeberg, 2003).

In this learning process, there are always situations in which the participants have different views on whether or not a behaviour or condition should be assessed as 'sick' or 'healthy'. According to this, 'health' is not an inherent fixed characteristic of the person, but rather the result of negotiations taking place in interpersonal relationships (Balint, 1957). Health is (also) between people, and thus social 'treatment' is also required to contribute to social recovery (Weizsäcker, 1930).

The development of the SOC is mediated through social relations and social interaction. Every human being has developmental potentials (GRR) from birth and learns to use these potentials (or is hindered in doing so) through interaction with the social environment (Antonovsky, 1987). The development of the SOC is, therefore, a lifelong process in which the primary caregivers (family) play a central role, which is later supplemented and/or temporarily replaced by other supporting persons in the social environment (family, friends, colleagues) and professional helpers. They can promote the further development of the SOC, especially in accompanying transitional crises. But to bring about sustainable change, it is necessary to expand the opportunities for influencing the shaping of one's own living conditions. A vital catalyst can be the family doctor, who plays the role of an 'elective relative' for many people.

Family doctors are often the first point of contact for health issues, and they often treat family members and people from social neighbourhoods over a long time. Therefore, patients and doctors usually assume that they know each other well and act following their respective needs. Admittedly, essential aspects – especially psychosocial aspects – regularly remain unaddressed. The patient and the doctor attribute to each other – often unnoticed by both – that the other person does not want to discuss this or is unable to do so – likewise an 'agreement in misunderstanding' (Brucks et al., 1998, p. 43). Thus, it is not discussed what health means for the patient and if or how it is worthwhile for him/her to be healthy or to become healthy again (Bahrs & Matthiessen, 2007). The treatment thus becomes a routine act, which is carried out like a ritual (Balint, 1975).

The long-term care of chronically ill people is a significant challenge for the doctor-patient relationship. This challenge pertains, at least implicitly, to all relevant areas of the life of the patient and his or her social and family network. As a rule, long-term care includes spontaneous treatment related to an acute problem on the one hand and regular, quasi-ritualized checks concerning diagnosed chronic diseases with an already established treatment regime on the other. However, there is no 'natural point in time' to reflect on the various aspects together to enable comprehensive treatment; a conversation setting is required that is free from acute pressure to act and well-established routines. The instrument of review dialogue (RD) offers the opportunity to leave the routines, to assess the significance of already known facts and to gain new insights into relevant life contexts and so to win a comprehensive understanding of the patient in terms of an 'overall diagnosis' (Balint, 1957).

The review dialogue was developed in a model project (Bahrs & Matthiessen, 2007, Bahrs, 2011a; Rojatz et al. in Chap. 38 in this book). In the trial phase, general practitioners specifically invited some patients with chronic illnesses outside of the usual consultation hours for a 20- to 30-minute conversation to develop jointly an understanding of the overall situation. Furthermore, the aim was to find out one or two health goals relevant to the patients and to develop jointly an individual treatment plan tailored to these goals. The development was regularly reviewed in three further meetings in the following year; successes were acknowledged and, if necessary, the goals were modified, or new ways of achieving them were looked for (Bahrs, 2011b).

The following example is based on four consecutive videotaped review dialogues and additional information from a three-hour biographical interview with the patient. The review dialogues (Table 18.1) took place in 2012/2013

Table 18.1 Health goals and their development over time (Bahrs et al., 2017)

Review dialogue	I (June 2012)	II (October 2012)	III (January 2013)	IV (July 2013)
Symptoms	Back pain, visual disturbances	Complaints without organic findings	Feeling for own body lost	Visual disturbances, tensions
Topics	Care for the father, emotional support for the mother	Father has been diagnosed with incurable cancer	Organization of palliative care for father and emotional support for mother	Father has died → supporting the mother, mourning
Agreed health goals	1. Less pain in movement	'Total package' (feel better and more relaxed in the body, less pain, become aware of one's capabilities)	1. Improve fitness	1. Improve fitness and movement
	2. Improve vision		2. Be aware of one's capabilities	2. Decrease stress
Success concerning the achievement of health goals		Less pain; visual problems remain unchanged	Improved mobility, aid is organized	Death of the father, self-care is hardly possible
Developmental task	Respect the autonomy of both (parents and oneself), pledge support	Acknowledge limitations, accept help	Prepare to say goodbye, secure aid and take care of oneself	Mourning, prepare for new projects
GP's significant intervention/flash	'You have an enormous sense of duty. You could have said: "Mum, you know what, you move into sheltered living and see who's taking care of you!" Of course, you can't do that. When I hear you talk about your backaches, I think, 'This woman has a heavy load to bear"'	'A health goal can be to ensure that you are doing well and that you make good decisions. That you don't unpack everything and you don't say, "'Okay, next job, next job, next job." Instead, you take a closer look at your own limitations'	'You're a family of caring women'	'Whenever you want to move forward and develop, there is something physical, that stops you. And then you stay with your mother'
Metaphor	'My mother follows me like a shadow'	'I'm afraid not to come back again'	'I feel totally let down'	'My vision is blurred, and I don't want to have to live with that anymore'

within the framework of the BALANCE project (Bahrs et al., 2015, 2017).

Dr. Angela Mead[1] is 50 years old and has been a general practitioner for 12 years. Since then, she has known her patient Mrs. Pamela Smith, 58 years old, an engineer by profession, having been a housewife for about 20 years and now working as a freelance archery trainer. She is married to Mr. John Smith, a 62-year-old hard-working academic who appears to be in good health and is described as a 'centre of tranquillity'. Pamela Smith visits her doctor about once a month, often because of back pain. Dr. Mead also treats Mrs. Smith's parents Mary and Martin Philipp. Both live, albeit in their apartment, in the same house as Mrs. Smith. The 87-year-old Martin Philipp has been suffering from type I diabetes for many years, which he has managed well with the support of his wife. In the meantime, dementia has developed, the need for care has grown and 82-year-old Mary Philipp now also needs the help of her daughter, Pamela Smith. Dr. Mead knows the other family members – the two sons Gerald and Thomas, who are already studying, and the husband Johann Smith – from sporadic encounters.

A Brief Characterization of the Encounters

Review Dialogue I: Problem outline: current situation, challenges and development task

In the first review dialogue, Mrs. Smith complains of back pain and visual disturbances, which massively restrict her mobility and frighten her. She comments on her situation, which is dominated by caring for her mother and father. Since early childhood, she was significantly influenced by her mother's panic attacks: '*My mother is like a shadow*'. Although Dr. Mead knows and treats the entire family, the mother-daughter constellation has never been an issue of the consultations with the family doctor. The general practitioner learns that Mrs. Smith's main development task is one of attaining autonomy and not the support of her parents. Although both actors are aware of this fundamental problem, this is not reflected in their prioritization of the two primary health objectives. These relate instead to the physical complaints, which usually would be treated by specialists (orthopaedist/physiotherapist, ophthalmologist).

Review Dialogue II: The body is taking part in the communication: the need for self-protection and defining one's own health goals

Medical examinations in the following three months do not show any organic findings for Pamela's complaints. But Mrs. Smith reports a reduction in her back pain resulting from physiotherapy, but an increase in new problems for which no physical or organic cause can be found. She narrates on the diagnosis of an incurable carcinoma in her father and her lack of care for herself. Her mother does not understand the situation and Mrs. Smith is left alone regarding the organization of her father's care. Instantly, Dr. Mead suggests that the already agreed health goals (less pain in movement and improved vision) should be supplemented to include the importance of self-awareness and empowerment ('total package'). She supports Pamela Smith's insight that it is crucial to perceive and recognize one's limitations and to allow help. Pamela Smith's homework is to pay attention to her strengths.

Review Dialogue III: Farewell, mourning, setting limits, relief and hope for new beginnings

Mrs. Smith seems to progress. Having organized outpatient palliative care for her father, emotional support for her mother and body therapy (acupuncture) for herself, she has become physically more mobile again. She acknowledges the painful reality and prepares for the imminent farewell to her father's death. Because of the experienced help, she can imagine a further development of the mother-daughter relationship, which releases both of them from their mutual dependence. Nevertheless, Pamela worries that her mother might be overwhelmed by the care of the dying father. The mother cannot yet come to terms with the situation and believes – following a family-mediated ethical imperative – that she has to cope with everything herself. Dr. Mead points out that in this *'family of caring women'* all women tend to overtax themselves. *'You are very close to it, aren't you?'* The doctor now directs attention to relaxation possibilities and lets Pamela find legitimate and necessary free space for herself with her artistic activities on the one hand and with indispositions on the other. Although it is difficult for her to attend and support her dying father, Mrs. Smith is optimistic regarding the future.

Review Dialogue IV: Being thrown back and ambivalence

However, the hope for structural change is deceptive. Mrs. Smith reports that on his deathbed, her father obliged her to look after her mother. Mary Philipp also loses her independence after her husband's death. Again, Pamela Smith suffers from tension, cardiac arrhythmia and visual problems without any apparent physical causes. Her father has passed on in the meantime, and her mother now needs her intensive support. Mrs. Smith is fundamentally concerned about her eye problems: *'My vision is blurred, and I don't want to have to live with that.'* Dr. Mead draws a line between Mrs. Smith's attempts to increase her independence, her increase in pain and physical symptoms and her remaining with her mother. Dr. Mead suggests seeking professional psychotherapeutic support, but Mrs. Smith rejects this idea and shows interest in further review dialogues with Dr. Mead.

[1]All names and other personal identifiers in the case study have been changed to protect privacy and confidentiality.

The pattern of the mother-daughter relationship, which has been established for more than 50 years, apparently cannot be abandoned. For all her resentment about her domestic situation, Pamela Smith seems to prefer the security of the ever-same to the uncertainties that come with a change.

Pamela Smith has developed remarkable self-help potentials and makes full use of these resources. With Qi Gong and dance, she uses body-oriented offers that promote mindfulness and enable social support in groups. She is active as an artist and is also successful in this. What all these activities have in common is that Pamela gets into a flow and creates a new reality for herself for a limited time, in which she can transcend the boundaries that are so obvious in everyday life.

However, she has to return to this everyday life again and again, and so she will probably continue to depend on the help of Dr. Mead.

Health Goals and Biographical Development Tasks in the Course of the Review Dialogues

As usual in primary care, the starting point of any treatment is the physical complaints presented by the patient. In the first review dialogue, Dr. Mead initially assumes difficulties in the current family situation as a background for Mrs. Smith's raw feeling of tension. However, Mrs. Smith sees her husband and her sons as havens of tranquillity. Problems and stress are connected to her family of origin.

Caring for elderly family members is a typical development task for Mrs. Smith's present life stage. Both the development task, in general, and Mrs. Smith's living situation, in particular, are well known to Dr. Mead. However, the doctor unexpectedly becomes aware of the interdependence between Mrs. Smith and her parents, a situation that has existed from her childhood to the present. Detachment from the mother remains a development task to be attained in the future. The phrase 'we are a double-pack' reveals the severance of her dependence and lack of respect ('flash', (Balint & Norell, 1975)). Further, Mrs. Smith missed a socially competent mother in her childhood and adolescence who would promote her self-development extensively. Therefore, she has only been able to attain her goals to a limited extent across the developmental phases, such as self-confidence and security, autonomy and detachment from early bonds.

The 'in-between' in this family are characterized in particular by anxiety, which characterizes the family atmosphere as a whole (GRD) and is expressed in different ways by several members of the family (family SOC; see Vossler, 2001, Braun-Lewensohn et al., 2017) (Table 18.2). The panic attacks of her mother are caused by traumatizing war experiences which seems to be a silenced taboo: *'The worst was actually that my mother did not confess it. It happened already when I was a child. Nobody could ever know that. Even we children did not know what was going on.'* (Review Dialogue I).

Mrs. Smith suffered from panic attacks during her studies, whilst her son, later on, develops similar symptoms from

Table 18.2 Diseases/illnesses across the life span

Development phase	Diagnosis according to the patient	Treatment	Important life data	Stressors	Expressive content
Childhood and youth (< 20)	Scoliosis	Gypsum bed and physiotherapy	Panic attacks of the mother	Structural overload in care, role reversal daughter/mother Back problems as 'birth defect' Back strengthening required	Structural lack of back support
Young adulthood (20–35)	Panic attacks; arrhythmias	Talk therapy	Strenuous studies; separation from a partner	Recognition through performance is no longer sufficient; insult (rejection by the partner and his family and thus simultaneously the separation from the family of origin fails ('heartache')	Fear of failure and loss of face
Middle adulthood (approx. 35–50)	Disc prolapse; sinusitis; fears of the oldest son	General practitioner, specialists; talk therapist	Birth of children; being no longer in work	Constitutional 'deficiency' and permanent overstrain are reflected in organic damage and massive crises	Body strike
Mature adulthood (from 50)	Iritis; disc prolapse; hip necrosis (or arthrosis?); sinusitis; mitral valve collapse	General practitioner, specialist; alternative therapy	The eldest son leaves home; the parents need care End-of-life care for father (cancer) and emotional support for mother	Accompanying the dying father (cancer) and emotional support for the mother. Extending and intensifying multiple physical complaints and impairment of perception (vision) and movement. Comprehensive insecurity (no physical feeling, goal lost)	Restriction of perception and movement

Modified following Bahrs et al. (2017)

time to time during school lessons. Both her son and herself improved through talk psychotherapy (SRR). Mrs. Smith's manifold physical complaints, however, are connected to her occurring fear, and the repeated investigations remain fruitless in the long term. Nevertheless, the investigation is effective in terms of short-term treatments, and Mrs. Smith feels fine. This intervention expands physical exclusion diagnostics: it is based on personal recognition and a biographical understanding (GRR).

Support has its limits where the predominance of the family task cannot be resolved by reflection. When the father on his deathbed commits Pamela Smith once again to taking care of her mother, the family force field is restaged, which Pamela Smith can hardly escape.

> *And my father then somehow did a tiny ceremony. (...) But he just said, 'I promise with all my heart and all my hand', but I don't know what? And then he shook hands with everyone. (...) He tried terribly hard. (...) But I actually thought that it was really important to let someone go. (...) He can't really only leave after we have said that we would take care of our mother and it would all be done, he doesn't need to worry (crying). (Biographical interview)*

The Body as Mediator

In the following, we assume that the body has a double function. It mediates between inner and outer demands and is the gateway to and part of the environment and the world around us. On the one hand, the body can be regarded as a thing amongst things, as a machine, so to speak, which controls itself according to describable rules. On the other hand, it can be seen as interpreting and expressing carrier of meaning, in which social rules are inscribed, manifested, expressed and reinvented. The self-regulation and impression/expression of the living body (Leib) are the result of a continuous learning process, with the SOC acting as its virtual coordination centre. This learning process is also expressed in the history of symptom formation. The reconstruction of the formation of symptoms in the context of life history is therefore also a key to understanding the world view (and thus to the development of the SOC).

The following description is hypothetical. We cannot describe in detail the relationship between biography, symptom formation and the development of coping mechanisms in the whole life course of Mrs. Smith. However, we have put information from the various documented conversations into a *mental order* that takes up the patient's self-interpretations, the doctor's interpretations and our reflections. This is intended to illustrate a *possible development* on a case-by-case basis.

Since the peculiarities of the sixth decade of life are based on the increase of meaning in the course of life and cannot be understood if one does not think of the preceding experiences, we follow the process as a whole.

In her childhood, Pamela experiences perception and interpretation of physical phenomena in the mirror of her environment. Thus, Pamela Smith's back problems are interpreted as a (congenital) malposition (scoliosis), which has to be 'straightened out' via plaster bed and physiotherapy. A retrospective alternative interpretation could be that the child, carrying a heavy load, has a hard time getting into an upright position from the beginning and needs continuous support.

In young adulthood, the body increasingly becomes a means of perception and expression, which is gradually and consciously acquired. Pamela Smith speaks about this time as having panic attacks, nervousness and heartache, which are associated with high-performance requirements in a male-dominated study and with an insulting separation from the life partner. She must become aware of the expressive content of the body's events in the therapeutic dialogue. Although she describes the conversations as helpful, she sees the central support above all in the helpful attitude of the (future) husband, that is, especially not in a *therapeutic* relationship.

In adulthood, following pregnancy and birth, back problems reappear, now in the area of the cervical spine and accompanied by temporary numbness in the face. Metaphorically speaking, fainting and loss of face could be associated with this – but any of the participants does not express such thoughts. The overwhelming effect, however, becomes practically tangible. What had been described as a structural weakness in childhood, but not perceived as suffering, now becomes painfully acute and calls urgently for treatment and a change of attitude. This is expressed in giving up one's job and changing roles. The underlying distress is not felt by Pamela but is delayed and communicated via her son's fears.

In late adulthood, the variety and intensity of the symptoms increase. In temporal connection with the increasing need for care of the parents, vision problems occur, which particularly frighten Pamela Smith, because she 'is a person who does it with her eyes' (Review Dialogue I). Due to a renewed herniated disc and hip problems, she is also severely impaired in her mobility. Heart rhythm disturbances and stomach problems direct attention inwards and Pamela Smith becomes a problem altogether: 'I am a terribly nervous shit' (Biographical interview). The complaints call for a rethinking of the family division of labour and the self-perceived mission. However, Pamela Smith cannot draw the obvious conclusions from this. At her father's deathbed, she is once again obliged to care for her family, so that her freedom of self-definition proves to be limited. The doctor raises the question whether 'whenever you want to go forward on your own, what physical stops you? And then you stay with your mother?' (Review Dialogue IV). Since real independence from her mother is not possible, Mrs. Smith is referred to a virtual reality (painting) in which she invents herself grandiosely and thus, in a way, exceeds the physical limits.

Using the example of back problems, we summarize the formation of the body and the attribution of meaning (Leder, 1990). The formation of symptoms is a simultaneous process of illness and recovery, as well as the emergence of resistance deficits and the development of resources. Back problems accompany Pamela Smith throughout her life. Diagnoses such as scoliosis or pelvic obliquity indicate structural problems (GRD) whose effects can at best be limited by physiotherapy (SRR). As an adult, Pamela Smith learns that dance and Taiji not only encourage movement (SRR) but are also fun and convivial (GRR). Her sister, a physiotherapist, emphasizes the success: 'I never thought you would get your back so straight again' (Biographical interview) (SRR→GRR→SOC). Increasingly, however, Pamela Smith has to accept that she can only influence the healing process to a limited extent (GRD) and that the muscles temporarily work against each other (SRD). This tension can be seen as an expression of a lack of fit between internal and external demands (Uexküll, 2004). The general practitioner states: 'The muscular system is the largest sensory organ of the body. All feelings, tension, external influences, and internal influences are also mediated via the muscle fibers.' Interpreting posture in a broader sense (SOC), the doctor advises a fundamental change of attitude (GRR). Pamela Smith looks for therapeutic support in the complementary medical field (acupuncture) (SRR) and benefits in particular from her self-chosen hobby, painting (SRR → GRR). 'When I paint, when I am somehow switched off, I am complete with myself. (...) I am then simply beamed away' (Biographical interview) (SRR → GRR → SOC).

The corporeal history includes the formation of the body as well as the development of resources. So, we would like to emphasize that Pamela Smith has considerable personal (resistance) resources (Antonovsky, 1987). She is ambitious and persistent as we can learn from her educational, professional and sports development. She is creative as well, expressing her point of view by painting, dancing, and her love for music. Having done Taiji exercise for 20 years, she is reflective and sensitive to her physical reactions.

In conclusion, she conceptualizes health and illness in a differentiated way. She organizes herself and gains support through her laity system (friends and colleagues) and professionals in her complementary and biomedical system. Additionally, she manages to apply the philosophy of the review dialogues, wondering what she has said: 'I cannot see the goal at archery.' Becoming aware of the underlying meaning of her wording, she concludes that she has to ask again: *'What are my life goals?'* (Review Dialogue IV).

Development of the SOC in the Life Course

Antonovsky regarded consistency, a good load balance and participation in shaping the outcome as crucial for the development of the SOC (Antonovsky, 1987, 92). In this perspective, we can imagine the development of the SOC in the case of Pamela Smith roughly as follows (see Table 18.3):

Table 18.3 Resource development across the life span

Development phase	Important life date	Symptom formation as an adaptive process	Generalized resistance resources (GRR)	Specific resistance resources (SRR)	SOC
Childhood and youth (< 20)	Growing up in a city in an industrial region; 5-year younger sister Secondary school and apprenticeship; panic attacks of the mother – parents war children	No information	Secondary school, apprenticeship, technical secondary school Younger sister starts studying directly at about the same time Finances: rather tight	Back gymnastics Technical secondary school	*Comprehensibility:* clear rules about role behaviour, but the background cannot be addressed (latently diffuse) *Manageability:* tends to be overburdening *Meaningfulness:* (relatively low) *Participation:* relatively little *Emotional closeness:* not with the mother, maybe with the father, possibly with the sister

(continued)

Table 18.3 (continued)

Development phase	Important life date	Symptom formation as an adaptive process	Generalized resistance resources (GRR)	Specific resistance resources (SRR)	SOC
Young adulthood (20–35)	Study and work in a male-dominated field of work; (humiliating) partner separation	Development of autonomy as a challenge and excessive demand; social limitation creates fear, which is physically felt and expressed as well as withdrawn from being addressed	Access to university on the second educational pathway, studying	Successful use of talk therapy The new partner is helpful	*Comprehensibility*: unclear; fails in interaction with a milieu foreign to her *Manageability:* enormous performance despite obstacles *Meaningfulness:* critical *Participation:* (follows the marked path) *Emotional closeness:* critical
Middle adulthood (approx. 35–50)	Birth of children; being no longer in work: change of roles/compromise (no 'male' career) Living with the parents	The shift of fear to the body and other family members – the experience of limits goes hand in hand with a stronger outward orientation	Stable partnership Financially well-off New resources through leisure time and help in the field of sports and alternative therapies	GP, specialists, individual talk therapist, family talk therapy, acupuncture, Taiji, dancing, music, archery, a gymnastics group	*Comprehensibility:* not prepared for the 'female' role, sister as an unattainable role model *Manageability:* takes a step back from the role of housewife and mother; creates a parallel network; uses professional helpers *Meaningfulness:* fragile *Participation:* unclear; has to look after parents again whilst starting a family *Emotional closeness:* yes, regarding the partner, but problems with the family of origin
Mature adulthood (from 50)	The eldest son leaves home; the parents need care End-of-life care for father (cancer) and emotional support for mother	Transformation crisis and reorientation	Stable partnership, financially well-off; regular contact to the sister Turns hobby into a profession (archery trainer); mediation training; access to various support systems; further training in artistic design, mediator training	GP: review dialogue; specialist; alternative therapy; can access various support systems (hospice association, group for dementia patients and relatives, palliative care doctors, hospice, Taiji, painting)	*Comprehensibility:* high, but she can hardly escape the operating rules *Manageability:* manages the terminal care successfully, organizes help (professional helpers, sister, friends, etc.). Body as mediator *Meaningfulness:* rather high *Participation:* She increasingly learns to organize her own space *Emotional closeness:* to husband (anchor); also to sons

- As a child, Pamela experiences herself as particularly crucial in terms of the support of the mother and receives recognition for her seemingly remarkable independence. She develops the necessary knowledge of rules and handling skills for this, which go far beyond what can be expected at her age. Since the mother's fears are taboo as a central theme, there is a systematic limit to comprehensibility that lies like a veil of uncertainty over everyday life. Accordingly, the experienced recognition is not based on actual participation (see Antonovsky, 1987, p. 92), but on the successful completion of a role. Reduced attention to self-care accompanies the development of care competencies.
- In young adulthood, some of these duties are transferred to the younger sister. Pamela 'pulls herself out' and seeks

recognition through successes in studies and work. Here she reaches the limits of her social skills and experiences rejections that centrally touch the sense of meaningfulness. In this crisis, she receives considerable support from her future husband (emotional bonds), but after her sister's departure, she once again becomes the primary contact person for her mother.
- With birth and motherhood, Pamela Smith gives up the possibility of a professional career. She now opens up new social contacts and areas of realization outside the family through sport and health education.
- In the sixth decade of her life, she can fall back on this extended network. She can assess the situation (comprehensibility) and organize help (manageability). Therefore, to others such as her doctor at the beginning of review dialogues, her resources appear strong. However, she has difficulties in accepting the help and follows a traditional family pattern ('caring women') (meaningfulness). One could, therefore, assume that her sense of meaningfulness temporarily decreases with increasing awareness of her overall situation.

In the course of her life, Pamela Smith succeeds in differentiating her strategy of 'pulling herself out' in a socially acceptable way and in strengthening her sense of meaningfulness: In her artistic activities, she was able to express her specific style. Her mentor acknowledged that Pamela had her own world and was an artist. Pamela felt this as a knighthood since she had not studied art. Pamela Smith proudly sums up: 'I have quite a few facets' (Biographical interview).

Discussion

Our considerations on the sixth decade of life are based on the situation in modern industrialized countries, where – with sometimes remarkable differences depending on social situation and cultural conditions – the average life expectancy is now over 80 years. Middle age is, therefore, less characterized by intervals related to years of life than by upcoming developmental tasks and is altogether a phase of transition in which a balance is being taken, and new orientations are possible.

An individual case cannot exhaust the variety of possible developmental trajectories. Still, it can illustrate a pattern that has heuristic value and contribute to the further development of research and practice. In the following, we discuss the relationship between the conceptual considerations presented at the beginning and our case study.

Double Birth: Constitution and Personalization

Pamela Schmidt not only has back problems as a constant companion, but she also lives them and redesigns herself and her environment accordingly. An active sportswoman, for example, becomes a coach who acknowledges her limitations and passes on her knowledge.

Special Features of the Sixth Decade of Life

Like many others, Pamela Smith's condition is becoming increasingly chronic – from a persistent illness to findings which, on closer examination, have a history that would have made an 'epicritic case evaluation' (Brucks et al., 1998, 43) worthwhile even in her 20s and 30s. Supporting and caring for the ageing parents are typical tasks of this phase of life, but in Pamela Smith's case, they are an explosive, ongoing issue. Thus, the question becomes virulent again with the care of the dying father: What is worth living for? In this situation, Pamela Smith can use the offer of the review dialogues (SRR) for a new orientation, strengthen her resources (GRR) and make her life more coherent, strengthening SOC.

Critical Life Events

The burdens associated with cancer, terminal care and the death of the father are dramatic. However, they are not entirely unexpected for Pamela Smith so that she can cope with them, partly with external help (SRR). The same applies to her own slipped disc. Her vision problems, on the other hand, are new, unexpected and throw her off track. The fact that she can *readjust her gaze*, so to speak, is a remarkable achievement and indicates a change that now allows her to define goals more strongly herself (GRR→SOC). The crisis becomes an opportunity.

Identity, SOC and Life Cycle

We interpret Pamela Smith's development as a (dis)continuous process of learning and competence development, in the course of which she has reoriented herself and yet remained recognizable. Although she repeatedly encounters limits, which are mainly due to the logic of interaction and the context of obligations in her family of origin, she is increasingly succeeding in opening up a new scope and becoming a person recognizable beyond the role-mediated action ('personalization'). Interestingly, the discrepancy between performance and autonomy becomes noticeable, so that her salutogenic resources seem to be decreasing despite the apparent development of competencies. We term this *flexibilization* (analogous to Antonovsky's reflections on the rigid SOC, Antonovsky, 1987, 24f), which is also expressed in increased attentiveness towards her own body.

Development of the SOC

For Pamela Smith, the development of the SOC is closely linked to health crises and upheavals. Illness and recovery are to be understood as temporary changes of location on the health-ease-disease continuum (Antonovsky, 1987). Phases of illness, although associated with limitations, can enable further development in the long term, so we propose to view the dynamic health-illness process as a whole, as 'the adaptation of the whole person to his entire past, to his present and to the visible forms of his future' (Sartre, 1981, p. 168).

Salutogenesis is both a biological and a social process (Sturmberg et al., 2019). Every human being is endowed with the capacity for self-regulation and yet, as a social being, cannot survive alone. The significant others enable, promote and limit the process of maturation, and thus salutogenesis takes place from the beginning as a bodily as well as a social process. If the abilities to cope with a situation are not sufficient (SRD) – for example, in case of chronic illness – professional support (SRR) may be necessary, ideally with a salutogenic orientation (Mittelmark et al., 2017).

Caring for patients with chronic conditions implicitly evokes the definition of life goals and the conduct of a healthy lifestyle. Treatment, life goals and lifestyle need to be aligned (Johnston et al., 2007). However, patients are often unaware of these interlinkages, and the general practitioner needs to create awareness around these issues and thereby provide the opportunity to reinvent their life history. Health and illness then cease to be real antagonisms (Antonovsky, 1987); they are strongly connected (Weizsäcker, 1956; Antonovsky, 1979, 1987) and part of the life process.

The presented person-centred care requires a new format of a conversation, empathy and time management (Coulter et al., 2013; Walseth et al., 2011; Derksen et al., 2017; Henselmans et al., 2015). We propose to perform review dialogues to apply this person-centredness. This case study shows the practical realizations of such professional interaction. This interaction needs to be designed as a process in which both conversation partners need to reinvent their roles as doctor and patient.

Doing this, both can experience that other ways of thinking and acting can be transferred. Ideally, in the sense of empowerment, this experience leads to lasting changes in behaviour and attitude patterns in everyday life and thus becomes a salutogenic resource (strengthening SOC). The experience with review dialogues shows that storytelling itself contributes to the development of health (Nünning & Nünning, 2019). Still, it also shows that repeated offers and opportunities for discussion and thus a certain continuity are needed. Primary care must be developed into a health-promoting setting (see Chap. 38 for a discussion of this issue).

According to our analysis, although the tasks Pamela Smith is facing become particularly urgent in the sixth decade of her life, they have been pending for some time. A resource-oriented offer of conversation – let's call this *development dialogue* – would, therefore, have made sense at an earlier point in time, starting, so to say, at another point of the health-ease-disease continuum.

The case study illustrates the limitations of medical interventions in doctor-patient interaction. Despite Pamela Smith's awareness and considerable personal resources, the patient does not succeed in becoming independent, due to her strong inner commitment towards her father and the experience of overwhelming social pressures.

Both, the patient and the general practitioner, sustain the established relationship pattern, and it might be assumed that Mrs. Smith will in the future continue to present somatic complaints to her general practitioner to recharge emotionally (Helmich et al., 1991). In the future, physical discomfort may continue to be a cause and expression of concern for Mrs. Smith, but in the knowledge of the possible professional help (SRR), and the experience of being able to rely on her family doctor (GRR), the visit can take place with less distress. The thought of the possible help may be occasionally enough (SOC), and the visits to the doctor may become less frequent. To prevent medicalization and somatic fixation, both actors will repeatedly be required to reject this invitation for constant repetition of their communication pattern and develop beyond it.

The case study underlines that the development of the SOC is a lifelong process and that change can be achieved even in (chronic) situations that appear to be frozen. It shows that such (health) crises indicate the need for change and can also be the beginning of change. It becomes clear that existing resources can be used for coping with them, of which those seeking help are often not even aware. It is evident that new potentials can be developed – and that for successful outcome support by 'obstetricians' with a 'sense for coherence' (Meier Magistretti et al., 2019) may be necessary. Given the current social organization of life courses, it is to be expected that such assessments and redrafts will become more frequent in the sixth decade of life. Still, given the pluralization of life plans, they are also possible in other stages of life. It, therefore, seems sensible to us to determine the individual need for support against the background of upcoming development tasks and long-term structuring life goals. As the health behaviour of women and men diverges, there are gender-specific resources and risk profiles to be considered.

References

Antonovsky, A. (1979). *Health, stress and coping*. Jossey-Bass.

Antonovsky, A. (1987). *Unravelling the mystery health – How people manage stress and stay healthy*. Jossey-Bass.

Backes, G. M. (1998). Individualisierung und Pluralisierung der Lebensverhältnisse: Familie und Alter im Kontext der Modernisierung. *Zeitschrift für Familienforschung, 2*, 5–29.

Backes, G. M., & Wolfinger, M. (2009). Frauen ab 50 – ´andere´ Chancen und Risiken des Alter(n)s? In B. Blättel-Mink & C. Kramer (Eds.), *Doing Aging – Weibliche Perspektiven des Älterwerdens* (pp. 93–104). Nomos.

Bahrs, O. (2011a). Fallverstehen in der hausärztlichen Langzeitversorgung. *Familiendynamik, 36*(2), 2–11.

Bahrs, O. (2011b). Der Bilanzierungsdialog – Eine Chance zur Förderung von Ressourcenorientierung in der Langzeitversorgung von Patienten mit chronischen Krankheiten. *GGW, 11*(4), 7–15.

Bahrs, O. (2012). Hermeneutisches Fallverständnis – Versuch einer Annäherung. *Z Allg Med, 88*, 355–361. https://doi.org/10.3238/zfa.2012.0355-0361

Bahrs, O., Heim, S., Löwenstein, F., & Henze, K. H. (2017). Review dialogues as an opportunity to develop life course specific health goals. *International Journal of Person Centered Medicine, 7*, 98–106.

Bahrs, O., & Henze, K. H. (2019). From shame to pride – Initiation of processes of De-stigmatisation in review dialogues. In C. Mayer & E. Vanderheiden (Eds.), *Transforming shame in culture and context: Practical applications and exercises for growth* (pp. 363–378). Springer.

Bahrs, O., Henze, K. H., Löwenstein, F., Abholz, H. H., Ilse, K., Wilm, S., Bureick, G., & Heim, S. (2015). Review dialogues as an opportunity to develop a person-related overall diagnosis. *International Journal of Person Centered Medicine, 5*, 112–119.

Bahrs, O., & Matthiessen, P. F. (Eds.). (2007). *Gesundheitsfördernde Praxen - Die Chancen einer salutogenetischen Orientierung in der hausärztlichen Praxis*. Hans Huber.

Balint, E., & Norell, J. S. (1975). *Fünf Minuten pro Patient. Eine Studie über die Interaktionen in der ärztlichen Allgemeinpraxis*. Suhrkamp.

Balint, M. (1957). *The doctor, the patient and his illness*. Tavistock.

Balint, M. (1975). *Das Wiederholungsrezept: Behandlung oder Diagnose?* Klett.

Bauman, Z. (2001). *The individualized society*. Polity Press.

Beutel, M. E., Brähler, E., & Tibubos, A. N. (2019). Gender und psychische Gesundheit. Bedeutung für die psychotherapeutische Praxis. In I. Moeslein-Teising, R. Schäfer, & R. Martin (Eds.), *Geschlechter-Spannungen* (pp. 54–65). Psychosozial Verlag.

Bohleber, W. (1997). Zur Bedeutung der neueren Säuglingsforschung für die psychoanalytische Theorie der Identität. In H. Keupp & R. Höfer (Eds.), *Identitätsarbeit heute. Klassische und aktuelle Perspektiven der Identitätsforschung* (pp. 93–119). Suhrkamp.

Braun-Lewensohn O, Idan O, Lindström B, Margalit M (2017) Salutogenesis: Sense of coherence in adolescence. In: Mittelmark MB, Sagy, S, Eriksson S, Bauer GF, Pelikan JM, Lindström B, Espnes GA (eds.) The handbook of Salutogenesis, Springer International Publishing, p 123–136.

Brucks, U., Wahl, W. B., & Schüffel, W. (1998). Die Bedingungen für Veränderungen erkennen: Salutogenese in der Praxis. In W. Schüffel, U. Brucks, R. Johnen, V. Köllner, F. Lamprecht, & U. Schnyder (Eds.), *Handbuch der Salutogenese* (pp. 37–53). Konzept und Praxis. Ullstein Medical.

Buddeberg, C. (Ed.). (2003). *Psychosocial medicine*. Springer.

Corbin, J. M., & Strauss, A. L. (1988). *Unending work and care: Managing chronic illness at home*. Jossey-Bass.

Corbin, J. M., & Strauss, A. L. (2004). *Weiterleben lernen. Verlauf und Bewältigung chronischer Krankheit* (2nd ed.). Hans Huber.

Coulter A, Roberts S, Dixon A. (2013). Delivering better services for people with long-term conditions: Building the house of care. The kings fund. http://www.kingsfund.org.uk/publications/delivering-better-services-people-long-term-conditions. Accessed 24 Apr 2017.

Derksen, F., Olde Hartman, T. C., Av, D., Plouvier, A., Bensing, J., & Lagro-Janssen, A. (2017). Consequences of the presence and absence of empathy during consultations in primary care: A focus group study with patients. *Patient Education and Counseling, 100*, 987–993.

Eikelpasch, R., & Rademacher, C. (2004). *Identität. transcript*. Verlag.

Elwyn, G., Frosch, D., Thomson, R., et al. (2012). Shared decision making: A model for clinical practice. *Journal of General Internal Medicine, 27*, 1361–1367. https://doi.org/10.1007/s11606-012-2077-6

Erikson, E. H. (1980). *Identity and the life cycle*. Norton.

Faltermaier, T. (2004). Männliche Identität und Gesundheit. Warum Gesundheit von Männern? In T. Altgeld (Ed.), *Männergesundheit. Neue Herausforderungen für Gesundheitsförderung und Prävention* (pp. 11–33). Weinheim.

Faltermaier, T. (2006). Die Salutogenese als Forschungsprogramm und Praxisperspektive. Anmerkungen zu Stand, Problemen und Entwicklungschancen. In H. Wydler, P. Kolip, & T. Abel (Eds.), *Salutogenese und Kohärenzgefühl. Grundlagen, Empirie und Praxis eines gesundheitswissenschaftlichen Konzepts* (3rd ed., pp. 185–196). Juventa.

Faltermaier, T. (2009). Gesundheit: Körperliche, psychische und soziale Dimensionen. In J. Bengel & M. Jerusalem (Eds.), *Handbuch der Gesundheitspsychologie und Medizinischen Psychologie* (pp. 46–57). Hogrefe.

Geyer, J., & Schulz, E. (2014). Who cares? Die Bedeutung der informellen Pflege durch Erwerbstätige in Deutschland. *DIW Wochenbericht, 14*, 294–303.

Gilleard, C., & Higgs, P. (2019). The individualization of ageing. In P. Naskali, J. Harbison, & S. Begum (Eds.), *New challenges to ageing in the rural north. International perspectives on aging, vol 22* (pp. 241–251). Springer. https://doi.org/10.1007/978-3-030-20603-1_15

Goffman, E. (1975). *Stigma. Über Techniken der Bewältigung beschädigter Identität*. Suhrkamp.

Griebel, W., & Niesel, R. (2011). *Übergänge verstehen und begleiten. Transitionen in der Bildungslaufbahn von Kindern*. Cornelsen.

Gugutzer, R. (2002). *Leib, Körper und Identität. Eine phänomenologisch-soziologische Untersuchung zur personalen Identität*. Westdeutscher Verlag.

Gugutzer, R. (2004). *Soziologie des Körpers*. transcript-Verlag.

Hegemann, T., Asen, E., & Tomson, P. (2000). *Familienmedizin für die Praxis*. Schattauer.

Helmich, P., Hesse, E., Köhle, K., Mattern, H. J., Pauli, P., Uexküll, T., & Wesiack, W. (1991). *Psychosoziale Kompetenz in der ärztlichen Primärversorgung*. Springer.

Henselmans, I., Heijmans, M., Rademakers, J., & Sv, D. (2015). Participation of chronic patients in medical consultations: patients' perceived efficacy, barriers and interest in support. *Health Expectations, 18*, 2375–2388.

Höfer, R. (2006). Kohärenzgefühl und Identitätsentwicklung. Überlegungen zur Verknüpfung salutogenetischer und identitätstheoretischer Konzepte. In H. Wydler, P. Kolip, & T. Abel (Eds.), *Salutogenese und Kohärenzgefühl. Grundlagen, Empirie und Praxis eines gesundheitswissenschaftlichen Konzepts* (3rd ed., pp. 57–69). Juventa.

Honermann, H., Müssen, P., Brinkmann, A., & Schiepek, G. (1999). *Ratinginventar lösungsorientierter Interventionen: Ein bildgebendes Verfahren zur Darstellung ressourcen- und lösungsorientierten Therapeutenverhaltens*. Vandenhoeck und Ruprecht.

Höpflinger F, Perrig-Chiello P. (n.d.) Mittleres Erwachsenenalter im gesellschaftlichen Wandel. Homepage Höpflinger, www.hoepflinger.com/fhtop/fhmidage1.html

Johnston, O., Kumar, S., Kendall, K., Peveler, R., Gabbay, J., & Kendrick, T. (2007). Qualitative study of depression management in primary care: GP and patient goals, and the value of listening. *The British Journal of General Practice, 57*, 872–879.

Keupp, H. (1997). Diskursarena Identität: Lernprozesse in der Identitätsforschung. In H. Keupp & R. Höfer (Eds.), *Identitätsarbeit heute. Klassische und aktuelle Perspektiven der Identitätsforschung* (pp. 11–39). Suhrkamp.

Keupp, H., Ahbe, T., Gmür, W., Höfer, R., Mitzscherlich, B., Kraus, W., & Straus, F. (2006). *Identitätskonstruktionen. Das Patchwork der Identitäten in der Spätmoderne* (3rd ed.). Reinbek bei Hamburg.

Krappmann, U. (1975). *Soziologische Dimensionen der Identität* (4th ed.). Klett-Cotta.

Krappmann, U. (1997). Die Identitätsproblematik nach Erikson aus einer interaktionistischen Sicht. In H. Keupp & R. Höfer (Eds.), *Identitätsarbeit heute; Klassische und aktuelle Perspektiven der Identitätsforschung* (pp. 66–92). Suhrkamp.

Lademann, J., & Kolip, P. (2005). In B. Deitermann, J. Bucksch, & M. Schwarze (Eds.), *Gesundheit von Frauen und Männern im mittleren Lebensalter*. Robert-Koch-Institut.

Leder, D. (1990). Clinical interpretation: The hermeneutics of medicine. *Theoretical Medicine, 11*, 9–24.

Lindström B, Eriksson M. (2010). The Hitchhiker's guide to Salutogenesis. Salutogenetic pathways to health promotion. Folkhälsan Research Centre, Health Promotion Research (eds.), Research Report, 2.

Maier-Gutheil, C. (2015). Lern- und Bildungsprozesse im Lebenslauf – Befunde empirischer Forschung und Perspektiven der Theorieentwicklung. Zeitschrift für Weiterbildungsforschung, Report 38:7–22. https://doi.org/10.1007/s40955-015-0008-y

Marotzki, W. (1990). *Entwurf einer strukturalen Bildungstheorie: biographietheoretische Auslegung von Bildungsprozessen in hochkomplexen Gesellschaften*. Weinheim.

Matthiessen, P. F. (2010). Paradigmenpluralität, Salutogenese und ärztliche Praxis. *Der Mensch – Zeitschrift für Salutogenese und anthropologische Medizin, 41*, 6–21.

Meier Magistretti, C., Topalidou, A., & Meinecke, F. (2019). Sense FOR Coherence – der Sinn FÜR Kohärenz: Annäherungen an ein mögliches Konzept. In C. Meier Magistretti, B. Lindström, & M. Eriksson (Eds.), *Salutogenese kennen und verstehen* (pp. 119–135). Hogrefe.

Mittelmark, M. B., Bull, T., Daniel, M., & Urke, H. (2017). Specific resistance resources in the Salutogenic model of health. In M. B. Mittelmark, S. Sagy, S. Eriksson, G. F. Bauer, J. M. Pelikan, B. Lindström, & G. A. Espnes (Eds.), *The handbook of Salutogenesis* (pp. 71–76). Springer International Publishing.

Nünning, V., & Nünning, A. (2019). How to stay healthy and Foster Well-being with narratives, or: Where narratology and Salutogenesis could meet. In J. Alber & G. Olson (Eds.), *How to do things with narrative – Cognitive and diachronic perspectives* (pp. 157–186). Walter de Gruyter.

Oevermann, U. (2000). *Die Methode der Fallrekonstruktion in der Grundlagenforschung sowie der klinischen und pädagogischen Praxis In: Kraimer, K (ed) Die Fallrekonstruktion – Sinnverstehen in der sozialwissenschaftlichen Forschung* (pp. 58–156). Suhrkamp.

Payer, L. (1993). *Andere Länder, andere Leiden: Ärzte und Patienten in England, Frankreich, den USA und hierzulande*. Campus.

Perrig-Chiello, P., & Höpflinger, F. (2001). *Zwischen den Generationen. Frauen und Männer im mittleren Lebensalter*. Seismo Verlag.

Perrig-Chiello, P., Höpflinger, F., & Suter, C. (2008). *Generationen – Strukturen und Beziehungen*. Generationenbericht Schweiz.

Perrig-Chiello, P., & Hutchison, S. (2010). Family caregivers of elderly persons. A differential perspective on stressors, Ressources and Well-Being. *The Journal of Gerontopsychology and Geriatric Psychiatry, 23*(4), 195–206.

Perrig-Chiello, P., & Perren, S. (2005). Biographical transitions from a midlife perspective. *Journal of Adult Development, 12*(4), 169–181. https://doi.org/10.1007/s10804-005-7085-x

Robert Koch Institut (Ed.). (2014). *Gesundheitliche Lage der Männer in Deutschland*. Beiträge zur Gesundheitsberichterstattung des Bundes.

Rosenthal, G. (1995). *Erlebte und erzählte Lebensgeschichte: Gestalt und Struktur biographischer Selbstbeschreibungen*. Campus.

Sartre, J.-P. (1964). *Marxismus und Existentialismus – Versuch einer Methodik*. Rowohlt.

Sartre, J-P. (1977-1979). Der Idiot der Familie. Rowohlt, Reinbek bei Hamburg, (Vol 1–5).

Sartre, J.-P. (1981). *The family idiot: Gustave Flaubert 1821–1857*. Vol. 1 (trans. Cosman, C.). University of Chicago Press.

Sturmberg, J. P., Picard, M., Aron, D. C., Bennett, J. M., Bircher, J., de Haven, M. J., Gijzel, S. M. W., Heng, H. H., Marcum, J. A., Martin, C. M., Miles, A., Peterson, C. L., Rohleder, N., Walker, C., Olde Rikkert, M. G. M., & Melis, R. J. F. (2019). Health and disease - emergent states resulting from adaptive social and biological network interactions. *Frontiers in Medicine, 6*, 59. https://doi.org/10.3389/fmed.2019.00059

Uexküll, T. (Ed.). (2004). *Psychosomatische Medizin* (4th ed.). Urban und Schwarzenberg.

Ventegodt, S., Andersen, N. J., & Merrick, J. (2003). The life Mission theory II. The structure of the life purpose and the Ego. *The Scientific World Journal, 3*, 1277–1285. https://doi.org/10.1100/tsw.2003.114

Vogel, C., Wettstein, M., & Tesch-Römer, C. (2019). Frauen und Männer in der zweiten Lebenshälfte – Älterwerden im sozialen Wandel. Bundesministerium für Familie, Senioren. In Frauen und Jugend (Ed.), *Frauen und Männer in der zweiten Lebenshälfte – Älterwerden im sozialen Wandel. Zentrale Befunde des Deutschen Alterssurveys (DEAS) 1996 bis 2017*. Bundesministerium für Familie, Senioren, Frauen und Jugend (BMFSFJ).

Vossler, A. (2001). Der Familien-Kohärenzsinn als kollektives Konzept: Das Ganze ist mehr als die Summe seiner Teile. *Zeitschrift für Gesundheitspsychologie, 9*, 112–122.

Walseth, L. T., Abildsnes, E., & Schei, E. (2011). Patients' experiences with lifestyle counselling in general practice: A qualitative study. *Scandinavian Journal of Primary Health Care, 29*, 99–103.

Weizsäcker, V. (1930). *Soziale Krankheit und soziale Gesundung*. Springer.

Weizsäcker, V. (1956). *Pathosophie*. Vandenhoeck und Ruprecht.

Wetzstein, M., Rommel, A., & Lange, C. (2015). Pflegende Angehörige - Deutschlands größter Pflegedienst. In Robert Koch-Institut Berlin (Ed.). GBE kompakt. https://doi.org/10.17886/RKI-GBE-2016-018

19

Elderly, Salutogenesis and SOC

Maria Koelen and Monica Eriksson

Introduction

Population ageing is a global trend. For example, in the EU-27 population, the share of the older population (65 and above) increased from 13.9% in 1991 to 19.7% in 2018 (Eurostat, 2018). It is expected that by 2060, the share of those 65 years and over will account for 29.5% of the EU-27 population (Eurostat, 2013). Moreover, we can observe a worldwide increase in very old people, aged 85 and over. The ageing of the population results from decreasing fertility rates, but also from increasing life expectancy rates and the progressive ageing of the ageing population itself. These latter trends are partially attributable to improved quality of nutrition, and advances in medicine, especially knowledge about diseases and their control, and to developments such as early detection of colorectal and breast cancer in screening programmes which increase the chances of survival. Improvements in housing, nutrition and sanitation standards have also contributed to improved life expectancy (Staehelin, 2005).

In middle- and high-income countries, years added to life are generally lived in good health. However, because more people live into old age and because chronic diseases – such as cancers, diabetes, heart disease, Alzheimer disease and related dementias – more frequently occur in the older population, the burden of disease will also increase. The ageing of the population will have an impact on health care, housing and community facilities, consumption patterns and also on social security costs. In response, health professionals, researchers and policymakers are increasingly concerned with healthy ageing, where ageing in place is used as a key concept. In this chapter, we first discuss the meaning of the concept of healthy ageing, and how sense of coherence contributes to this process. Next, we discuss the characteristics of the community in which older people live their lives and how the community can contribute to healthy ageing in place.

From Healthy Ageing to Salutogenic Ageing

The simple question, 'when is someone old?' is not easily answered. Up to now, the question is mainly answered from an exogenous, administrative and political perspective (Koelen, 2011). In many countries, 'becoming old' is defined by retirement (in countries where retirement exists) or chronological age (Cattan, 2009). Retirement age can however vary, from 55 to 75 years of age, depending on country and/or profession. Occasionally, people of ages 45 or 50 years are included under the label 'older' for policy or research purposes. At the same time, several countries seek to increase the paid work participation and to increase state-pension-age. Hence, defining 'old age' simply as chronological age can be rather misleading, particularly if we accept the social construct of old age. It is not possible, in this chapter, to explore the extensive debates, theories and research paradigms linked to ageing and old age, but suffice to say that the concept will continue to be redefined and refined as our perceptions and understanding of old age evolve. This is also true for the concept of healthy ageing. There are many definitions for 'healthy ageing', and the concept is often used alongside related concepts such as 'effective ageing', 'positive ageing', 'successful ageing' and 'ageing well'. Hanson-Kyle (2005, p. 52) summarized different definitions and, based on commonalities, defines healthy ageing as 'the process of slowing down, physically and cognitively, while

M. Koelen (✉)
Department of Social Sciences, Health and Society Group, Wageningen University, Wageningen, The Netherlands
e-mail: koelen@caiway.nl

M. Eriksson
Department of Health Sciences, University West, Trollhättan, Sweden

resiliently adapting and compensating in order to optimally function and participate in all areas of one's life (physical, cognitive, social and spiritual)'. The World Health Organization previously proposed to use the concept of 'active ageing', defined as 'the process of optimizing opportunities for health, participation and security in order to enhance quality of life as people age' (WHO, 2002; p. 12). In their 2015 World Report on Ageing and Health, WHO replaced the concept of active ageing by healthy ageing, defined as 'the process of developing and maintaining the functional ability that enables wellbeing in older age'. Functional ability is about having the capabilities that enable people to be and do what they have reason to value. It is made up of the intrinsic capacity of the individual, relevant environmental characteristic and the interaction between them (WHO, 2015). Intrinsic capacity is defined as the composite of all the physical and mental (including psychosocial) capacities that an individual can draw on at any point in time (Beard et al., 2016; Sadana and Michel, 2019).

The meaning attached to healthy ageing also depends on whether it is defined by professionals or by older people. Research reveals that older people have a different view from that of professionals, research scientists and policymakers. Older people may report that they experience good health and well-being, regardless of their clinical condition, impairment or disability (Young et al., 2009; Sadana and Michel, 2019). Professionals frequently focus on negatively phrased topics such as disability, disease, loneliness, overweight and falls, thereby emphasizing the problems and limitations that occur due to ageing. Older people focus more on supportive social environments, the ability to use resources, the ability to manage restrictions (Naaldenberg et al., 2011), the ability to make one's own decisions (Stephens et al., 2015) and on adaptation, meaningfulness and connectedness (Jeste et al., 2010). This perception relates to the increasingly accepted definition of health as 'the ability to adapt and self-manage' (Huber et al., 2011). Kennaugh (2016) explored how older Australian women experienced ageing. Using a salutogenic approach to ageing the focus in her doctoral thesis in philosophy, 'It's not how old we are; it's how we are old', was to understand the main issues that were reported by older women to be important, how they coped as they aged and how they adjusted following changes to their marital status. The women used multiple resources for strengthening SOC, which in turn enabled women to feel their life as comprehensible, manageable and meaningful. Despite the challenges of ageing, they found ways to manage the circumstances of life, and reported that they were indeed ageing well. In a systematic review on health assets in older age (n = 78,422 from more than 13 different countries), Hornby-Turner et al. (2017) evaluated an extensive range of health assets, highlighting the evidence for factors that positively influence health in older age. They found that higher scores of self-rated health, psychological well-being and life satisfaction were associated with better health in older age. Social network and contact with family and friends and engagement in leisure and social activities were important support mechanisms.

Life Course Perspective

Healthy ageing is a lifelong process, and it evolves through the lifespan from (pre-)conception, infancy, adolescence and young adulthood into old age. Lifespan is usually understood as the duration of a person's life history from conception to the end life. Genetic endowment, exposures to health enhancing or deteriorating occurrences in the physical and social environment at any moment in time influence health development across the lifespan (cf. Kuh and Ben Shlomo, 2004; Westendorp and Kirkwood, 2007; Kuh, 2019).

Older people are often seen as passive and frail, even though in reality a substantial number are quite resilient and active in managing the challenges they face as part of the ageing process. It should be recognized that older people do not constitute a heterogeneous group. People in their 60s and 70s are typically healthy and most continue to live independently. The dependency of those in their 80s and above is typically prone to increasing frailty and susceptibility to illness and disability (Stones and Gullifer, 2016, p. 450), but also the older old increasingly prefer to live independently. Indeed, individual diversity increases with age across the life course (Marcoen et al., 2007). Or, as Aldwin et al. (2006) put it, 'some individuals become severely disabled in midlife, whereas others are running marathons in their 70s and even 80s' (p. 85).

From a life course perspective, old age (65+) may be considered as the 'last season', or the third age, but reaching the age of 65 years is not the last transition. Increasingly, we also talk about 'the fourth age' or 'the oldest old', meaning people of ages 85 years and over. Life course in this context is taken to mean the social aspect of the lifespan which involves biological, social and psychological processes leading to planned or unplanned life transitions and/or events. Importantly, a life course approach recognizes that ageing experiences are influenced by factors relating to cohort effects (Hubley and Copeman, 2008; Phillipson and Baars, 2007). Some issues related to this are unique for later life; others are of greater relevance in later life.

With increasing age, many changes occur in the social environment, as a result of retirement (loss of role), death of a spouse, death of family members and friends and the onset of age-related sensory loss and mobility problems. It has sometimes been said that old age is an accumulation of losses forcing older people to adapt and adjust to constantly changing physical and social environments. For most part, older people demonstrate great ability to find a range of different strategies to deal with these changes. Over time, however, the available options become fewer as a result of declining resources and ability. This can have an impact on the older person's mental health and increase the risk of social isolation and loneliness (Dykstra, 2009). Research has shown that the availability of social contacts and the ability to engage in social interaction are important in maintaining healthy ageing and alleviating loneliness (Forte, 2009; Nyqvist et al., 2013). In adapting to changing circumstances, older people may use a range of 'tools' available to them to facilitate engagement. Results from a systematic review and meta-analysis suggest a significant relationship between the Internet use (through, for example, social media, email, Skype) and mental well-being in older people (Forsman and Nordmyr, 2015). Research on the facilitation of social participation and the stimulation of social interaction is ongoing, but there are still gaps in our knowledge and understanding of the processes involved. However, research in associated areas has shown that there is an accumulation of socioeconomic disadvantage with regard to disability over the life course, leading to morbidity and mortality inequalities in later life (Kingston et al., 2015) and also that high levels of physical capability is associated with mental well-being in older people (Cooper et al., 2014). Such findings suggest that investigations of the role of social interaction in maintaining health over the life course may need to consider the wider constructs of health in old age, including socioeconomic factors and physical capability.

Sense of Coherence and Its Three Dimensions

Sense of coherence (SOC) reflects a person's view of life and capacity to respond to stressful situations. It is a global orientation to view the life as structured, manageable and meaningful or coherent. It is a personal way of thinking, being and acting, with an inner trust, which leads people to identify, benefit, use and reuse the resources at their disposal (Antonovsky, 1987; Lindström and Eriksson, 2005; Eriksson, 2017). SOC consists of three elements: comprehensibility, manageability and meaningfulness. The original definition is as follows: 'a global orientation that expresses the extent to which one has a pervasive, enduring though dynamic feeling of confidence that: (1) the stimuli from one's internal and external environments in the course of living are structured, predictable, and explicable; (2) the resources are available to one to meet the demands posed by these stimuli; and (3) these demands are challenges, worthy of investment and engagement' (Antonovsky, 1987, p. 19).

Comprehensibility refers to the extent to which a person perceives the stimuli confronted with, deriving from the internal and external environments, as making sense as information that is ordered, consistent, structured and clear. The person scoring high on the sense of comprehensibility expects that stimuli they encounter in the future will be predictable, ordered and explicit. This is the cognitive component of the SOC. Manageability is the extent to which a person perceives that resources are at their disposal that are adequate to meet the demands posed by the stimuli that bombards them. 'At a person's disposal' refers to resources under the person's own control or to resources controlled by legitimate others. This is the instrumental/behavioural component of the SOC. Meaningfulness refers to the extent to which a person feels that life makes sense emotionally, that problems and demands are worth investing energy in, are worthy of commitment and engagement, seen as challenges rather than burdens. This is the motivational component of the SOC. The original name of the instrument to measure sense of coherence is 'the life orientation questionnaire'. The original SOC scales consist either of 29 items, or a shortened form of 13 items. There are also modified translations of the instrument with varying number of questions and scoring alternatives. Up to date it has been used in at least 51 different languages in at least 51 different countries around the world. For more details of the SOC questionnaire, see Chaps. 11 and 12 in this book.

Development of the SOC in the Life Course.

A person's SOC affects and is affected at each stage across the lifespan by the surrounding environment and people in the local environment. In the mid-1980s, Antonovsky wrote an article about the importance of the sense of coherence for mental health and related this to a life course perspective (Antonovsky, 1985). In a lecture he gave in Berkeley, he discussed the transition from adolescence to adulthood and ageing, and argued for the usefulness of the salutogenic perspective (Antonovsky, 1993). He positioned ageing persons in a context of a health continuum, the ease/dis-ease continuum, and argued that people are all constantly moving in this continuum. People, dependent on age, are in different positions in this continuum. In Antonovsky's words: 'I propose that all living human beings, at any point in time, are somewhere on a continuum between the two extreme poles. An elderly person with a thick medical folder is no less on the continuum than an active, hungry, screaming, and smiling infant or than a strapping adolescent. They are at different points on the continuum; the dynamic prognoses are different.'

Antonovsky considered ageing as a process of human development instead of just a biological and mental degradation of the body: 'Is it not possible that the 10 billion neurons in the human cortex can come up with some replacement for what has senesced? Whatever the case may be for the biological development of salutary factors till the very end of life ..., I can surely see the possibility of the growth of social-psychological salutary factors as one gets older' (Antonovsky, 1993). These thoughts can be related to Erikson's theory of human identity development and the need for full awareness of context, especially as one gets older (Erikson and Erikson, 1998).

According to Antonovsky (1987), the SOC is assumed to develop until the age of 30 years, to remain stable until retirement, and thereafter to decrease. However, this assumption has not been empirically supported in previous research. The SOC seems to be relatively stable over time, but not as stable as initially assumed (Eriksson and Lindström, 2011). Research findings show that the SOC develops over the entire lifespan; in other words, it increases with age (Wiesmann and Hannich, 2019; Lövheim et al., 2012; Feldt et al., 2007, 2011; Nilsson et al., 2010). Wiesmann and Hannich (2019) investigated the stability of SOC over a time span of four years in active older German individuals (n = 125) and long-term effects of this life orientation on three different indicators of positive ageing – subjective well-being, psychological health and physical health. This is the first study to explore associations between gain in sense of coherence and future positive ageing. They found that SOC increased over four years, disclosing a small effect size. The baseline SOC had a substantial predictive value for future subjective well-being and psychological health, but not for physical health. Analyses showed that both the baseline SOC and gain in SOC predicted future subjective well-being and psychological health.

Findings from additional longitudinal research (n = 19.629, response rate 80.2%) sheds light over how the development of the SOC from different age groups can be understood. Feldt et al. (2011) found that the strongest development (46–58%) was amongst those participants whose SOC was strong at baseline. A class of strong SOC with a decreasing trend and that of a weak SOC with an increasing trend was also found. Nilsson et al. (2010) were able to demonstrate on a sample of Swedes, aged 18–85 years (n = 43.598), that SOC increases with age in both men and women. In a longitudinal study amongst Japanese volunteers aged 65 and over, Murayama et al. (2014) investigated the effect of intergenerational programmes on the mental health amongst older adults. They found that the meaningfulness component of the SOC significantly increased for members of the intervention group at all terms, with no changes in the control group over time. Participation in the intergenerational programme was associated with a sense of manageability which was also significantly related to depressive mood.

SOC Contributes to Ageing Well

Research amongst older people shows, as during other periods of the life cycle, that a strong sense of coherence is related to good perceived health and quality of life (Tan et al., 2013; Eriksson and Lindström, 2005, 2006) and mediate the association between perceived stress and depression (Guo et al., 2018; Boeckxstaens et al., 2016). In the longitudinal Aichi Gerontological Evaluation Study (AGES), the relationships between social factors and depression amongst older Japanese were investigated (Misawa and Kondo, 2019). They found that of the study participants without mental illness or depression at Wave 1, 14% had become depressed by Wave 2 (3-year follow-up). In both men and women, life events predicted increased odds of depression, whilst SOC predicted reduced odds. In a German study amongst older people (n = 387, mean age 73.8 years), the role that the SOC and generalized resistance resources have for older people's experience of life satisfaction was investigated (Dezutter et al., 2013; Wiesmann et al., 2014). The results showed that the SOC – as the ability to cope in everyday life – social support and self-esteem were factors that contributed to older people's satisfaction with life. In a population-based prospective cohort study in 29 primary care practices throughout Belgium (n = 567, ages ≥80), subjects with strong SOC scores showed a higher cumulative survival than others (Log rank = 0.004) independent of other prognostic characteristics (adjusted hazard ratio 0.62 (95% CI, 0.38–1.00). Even very elderly persons with strong SOC scores were shown to have lower mortality rates and less functional decline. These effects were independent of multimorbidity, depression, cognition, disability and sociodemographic characteristics (Boeckxstaens et al., 2016). A selection of studies using SOC amongst older people is shown in Table 19.1.

A Singaporean qualitative study amongst 27 older adults, using focus group interviews, was conducted and appreciative inquiry was adopted as a strengths-based interviewing approach (Seah et al., 2020). Four themes emerged: (1) contending evolving vulnerabilities, (2) intrinsic value of health, (3) taking care of oneself is a personal responsibility and (4) taking one day at a time: outlook towards later part of life (ibid, p. 3). The authors suggest that SOC towards the pursuit of healthy ageing can be addressed by reducing the unpredictability of ageing-related processes and vulnerabilities (comprehensibility), supporting active adoption of actions which promotes physical, mental and social health (manageability) and individual reflection in making sense of old age to seek motivation in living each day purposefully (meaningfulness). In another review study, Tan et al. (2013, p. 497) found that a strong SOC amongst older people was correlated with better physical, social and mental health.

Table 19.1 A selection of studies using SOC amongst older people

Country	Sample	Variables	Study design and measures	Results and conclusions	First author
Singapore	Older adults ≥65 years	Perceptions of healthy ageing through SOC	Qualitative, focus groups, appreciative inquiry (AI)	The four emerging themes were: (1) contending evolving vulnerabilities, (2) intrinsic value of health, (3) taking care of oneself is a personal responsibility and (4) taking 1 day at a time: outlook towards later part of life. Older adults' underlying pathogenic orientation towards health contributed to their perceived unpredictable confrontations with vicissitudes including illness and death. This played a part to their short outlook towards old age. Consequently, this could limit their will and abilities to seek meaningful pursuits or valued aspirations and movement towards the salutogenic health pole. By reframing the definition of health to pursuing and fulfilling valued accomplishments, optimal health can be achieved regardless of physical health state. This study suggested that sense of coherence towards the pursuit of healthy ageing can be addressed by reducing the unpredictability of ageing-related processes and vulnerabilities (comprehensibility), supporting active adoption of actions which promotes physical, mental and social health (manageability) and individual reflection in making sense of old age to seek motivation in living each day purposefully (meaningfulness)	Seah (2020)
Republic of Korea	Literature review	Analysis of what works for whom, in what circumstances, focus on strategies/interventions, contexts, mechanisms and outcomes	Realist review methodology	Four key themes emerged: (1) maintaining personal identity, (2) maintaining social identity, (3) keeping a familiar environment and (4) sustaining daily activities. It is hypothesized that these four factors combine and interact to maintain continuity and ultimately lead to psychosocial benefits. Maintenance of identity, environment and activities is central to continuity for persons with dementia. The resulting model and programme theories respond to the need for a coherent approach to continuity maintenance	Lim (2020)
Germany	Elderly (mean age 71)	SOC, subjective well-being, subjective health	Longitudinal SOC-29, The Philadelphia Geriatric Centre Morale Scale, SF-36 Health Survey	The sense of coherence increased over 4 years, disclosing a small effect size. The baseline sense of coherence had a substantial predictive value for future subjective well-being and psychological health, but not for physical health. Stepwise hierarchical regression analyses showed that both the baseline sense of coherence and gain in sense of coherence predicted future subjective well-being and psychological health. With respect to future physical health, only gain in sense of coherence was significant. Consistent with gero-salutogenic theory, the baseline sense of coherence is an effective predictor of future positive ageing, and growth in sense of coherence within a time span of 4 years is reflected in improved positive ageing. It is important to encourage experiences in older age that cultivate the three components of the sense of coherence – feelings of comprehensibility, manageability and meaningfulness	Wiesmann (2019)

(continued)

Table 19.1 (continued)

Country	Sample	Variables	Study design and measures	Results and conclusions	First author
Japan	Elderly persons ≥65 years	Depression, social Factors, SOC, social support	Longitudinal Geriatric Depression Scale SRH, IADL, SOC-13	Of the subjects without mental illness or depression at Wave 1, 14% had become depressed by Wave 2. In both men and women, life events predicted increased odds of depression, whilst sense of coherence predicted reduced odds. The frequency of meeting with friends, hobbies and self-rated health predicted reduced odds of depression in men whilst age predicted increased odds in women. Social interaction is important for preventing depression in Japan, and that the establishment of a system capable of promoting social interaction and providing care to the elderly during life events may be a useful social policy approach to preventing depression	Misawa (2019)
China	Older stroke patients ≥60 years	SOC, perceived stress, depression	Cross-sectional Perceived Stress Scale (PSS), the Sense of Coherence Scale (SOC-13) and the Center for Epidemiologic Studies Depression Scale (CES-D)	The total score of the SOC and perceived stress showed a negative correlation ($r = -0.80$, $P < 0.01$), the total SOC and depression also resulted in a negative correlation ($r = -0.77$, $P < 0.01$) and the total score of the perceived stress and depression resulted in a positive correlation ($r = 0.82$, $P < 0.01$). The results of multiple regression analyses indicated that SOC mediated the association between perceived stress and depression, and the influence of perceived stress on depression was decreased by16.0% within the sense of being out of control dimension and was decreased by 12.3% within the feeling of tension dimension when sense of coherence was added to the model. The structural equation model confirmed that the sense of coherence had a partial mediation effect between perceived stress and depression. SOC is the mediating variable between perceived stress and depression and can reduce the influence of perceived stress on depression	Guo (2018)

Belgium	Caregivers of frail older patients (mean age 79.4)	Self-esteem, lack of family support, health problems, caregiver burden, SOC, depression	Cross-sectional Zarit Burden Inventory, SOC-13, Geriatric Depression Scale, Caregiver Reaction Assessment, Global Deterioration Scale, Neuropsychiatric Inventory	Caregivers with a high SOC and an older age reported a lower burden (odds ratio (OR) 0.18, 95% confidence interval (CI) 0.04–0.65 and OR 0.87, 95% CI 0.76–0.98, respectively). A higher burden was associated with patient functional limitations (OR 8.69, 95% CI 2.28–40.46). Having a high sense of coherence seems to be a protective factor against the burden. To support caregivers, health providers should recognize the expertise of the caregivers and the meaningfulness of this care situation	Potier (2018)
Iran	Elderly with chronic diseases (mean age 63)	Self-efficacy, SOC	Cross-sectional The Sherer's Self-efficacy Questionnaire, SOC-29	The mean change of the self-efficacy score in the intervention and control groups was 9.48 ± 5.32 and 1.68 ± 6.04, respectively (t[56] = 5.20, $P < 0.001$). The mean change of the SOC score in the intervention and control groups was 24.17 ± 12.05 and 0.10 ± 13.42, respectively, t[56] = 7.18, $P < 0.001$). The applied empowering self-management model led to an improved self-efficacy and SOC amongst the retired elderly with chronic diseases. This model can be used to empower the elderly to achieve comprehensibility, manageability and meaningfulness in their lives	Hourzad (2018)
Sweden	Older immigrants (mean age 74)	SOC	Longitudinal SOC-13	There was a significant improvement in total SOC scores for the intervention group at 6-month follow-up. Also, the ORs for the SOC components were higher in the person-centred intervention group. However, we found no significant between-group differences nor did the effect last until the 12-month follow-up. Persons who have lived a long time in a host country after migration seem to have an SOC similar to native-born persons. Interventions with a person-centred approach could support the SOC by capturing individual life situations. Such interventions could support older persons by making everyday life more comprehensible and manageable and helping them to cope with challenges in daily life caused by ageing	Arola (2018)
Belgium	Elderly ≥80 (mean age 84.7)	Depressive symptoms, cognitive dysfunction, mortality, hospitalization, ADL decline, SOC	Longitudinal Geriatric Depression Scale (GDS-15), Mini-Mental State Examination [MMSE], SOC-13	Subjects with high SOC scores showed a higher cumulative survival than others (Log rank = 0.004) independent of other prognostic characteristics (adjusted hazard ratio 0.62 (95% CI, 0.38–1.00), $P = 0.049$). For ADL decline, a high SOC was shown to be protective, and this effect tended to be independent from the covariates under study (adjusted odds ratio 0.56 (95% CI, 0.31–1.0), $P = 0.05$). Even very elderly persons with high SOC scores were shown to have lower mortality rates and less functional decline. These effects were independent of multi-morbidity, depression, cognition, disability and socio-demographic characteristics	Boeckxstaens et al. (2016)
Poland	Older adults (mean age 71.04)	Religiousness, SOC, coping	Cross-sectional Religious Meaning System Questionnaire, SOC-29, Coping Inventory for Stressful Situations	Findings showed that the religious meaning system had significant relationships with SOC and three coping styles: emotion-oriented coping, avoidance-oriented coping and social diversion. In addition, SOC mediated the relations between the religious meaning system and three coping styles: the emotion-oriented, avoidance-oriented and social diversion. The positive associations between meaning-oriented religiousness, SOC and coping styles imply that their underlying mechanisms are based on the structures of significance and comprehension. The character of mediational relations (i.e. mediator vs. suppressor) depended on the emotional and social coping strategies used by older adults	Krok (2015)

(continued)

Table 19.1 (continued)

Country	Sample	Variables	Study design and measures	Results and conclusions	First author
Norway	Cognitively intact nursing home residents	SOC	Cross-sectional SOC-13	In accordance with the salutogenic theory of sense of coherence, the three-factor model revealed the best fit to our data. In particular, item OLQ2, defined as 'concerns the experience of being surprised by the behaviour of people whom you know well', seemed troublesome. Removing this item resulted in good fit to the present data. Rewording or deleting item OLQ2 seems needed to get a reliable instrument measuring sense of coherence amongst nursing home residents	Drageset and Haugan (2015)
Norway	Nursing home residents	SOC, social support	Longitudinal SOC-13, Social Provisions Scale	SOC increased statistically significantly from baseline to follow-up. The social support sub-dimension reassurance of worth predicted change in SOC after adjustment for socio-demographic factors. When controlled for baseline SOC, attachment was associated with change in SOC, but reassurance of worth was not. The study indicates that the change in SOC over time during the 5 years of follow-up and the social support dimension attachment appear to be important components of change in SOC	Drageset et al. (2014)
Spain	Older adults (mean age 74.8)	SOC, posttraumatic stress disorder symptoms, daily life functioning, religious beliefs and practices and social support	Cross-sectional SOC-13, Severity of Posttraumatic Stress Disorder Symptom Scale, Daily Life Functioning Scale, Systems of Beliefs Inventory, Posttraumatic Growth Inventory	Older people may experience psychological growth following a life major event. The objective of this study was to analyse the degree of posttraumatic growth (PTG) developed by widowed and non-widowed older adults ($n = 103$) as well as the impact of possible predicting variables such as socio-demographic characteristics, experienced or witnessed life major events, religiosity and sense of coherence. The findings suggest that, in spite of widowhood, elder people develop PTG in the same way as non-widowed elder people. Therefore, the support of a religious community, age, life major events experienced and the subjective meaning given to them correlated with PTG	Lópes et al. (2014)
Japan	Volunteers >65 years old (mean age 69.1)	SOC, depressive mood	Longitudinal SOC-13, Geriatric Depression Scale-Short Version-Japanese (GDS-S-J)	Analyses of the simple main effects showed that sense of meaningfulness significantly increased for members of the intervention group at all terms, with no changes in the control group over time. Multiple mediation analysis revealed that participation in the intergenerational programme was associated with a sense of manageability which was also significantly related to depressive mood. However, given our limited sample size, generalizability was restricted and studies with larger cohorts are required to further validate our findings	Murayama et al. (2014)
Norway	Elderly caregivers (mean age 79)	SOC, cognitive decline (persons with dementia), caregiver burden, social support	Cross-sectional SOC-13, Informant Questionnaire on Cognitive Decline in the Elderly (IQCODE), Relative Stress Scale (RSS), Social Provision Scale (SPS)	With adjustments for socio-demographic variables, the association with burden of care was statistically significant for the sub-dimension attachment ($p < 0.01$) and for sense of coherence ($p < 0.001$). The burden of care was associated with attachment and with sense of coherence. Community nurses and other health professionals should take necessary action to strengthen attachment and sense of coherence among the caregivers of people with dementia	Stensletten et al. (2014)

Germany	Older persons (mean age 73.8)	SOC, self-esteem, generalized self-efficacy, optimism, social support, morbidity, bodily pain	Cross-sectional Bodily Pain subscale of the SF-36 Health Survey, SOC-29, Rosenberg Self-Esteem Scale, Life Orientation Test, Generalized Self-Efficacy Scale, Expected Social Support Scale	We found that morbidity and sense of coherence were the only significant predictors of pain, with morbidity showing the strongest effect. Using path analysis, the sense of coherence was a mediator of the relationship between resistance resources/deficits and pain. With respect to our analytical model, in which pain experience was the criterion variable, morbidity and the sense of coherence are important predictors of pain. Moreover, we found evidence for the salutogenic idea that the sense of coherence represents a mediator variable as it pools resistance/deficits influences on pain	Wiesmann et al. (2014)
Belgium	Flemish elderly (mean age 76.5)	Depressive symptoms, life satisfaction, SOC, ego-integrity, despair	Cross-sectional Centre for Epidemiological Studies Depression Scale (CES-D), The Satisfaction with Life Scale (SWLS), SOC-13, Ego-integrity and despair (Van Hiel & Vaansteenkiste)	A positive relationship between SOC and well-being was found. Elderly individuals with a strong SOC experienced less depressive symptoms and higher levels of satisfaction with their life. In addition, mediation analysis indicated that the relationship between SOC and depressive symptoms was partially mediated by the positive resolution of the integrity-despair crisis, whereas the relationship between SOC and life satisfaction was fully mediated by integrity and despair. Our findings indicate that SOC might be a resource for greater well-being in the elderly. Furthermore, our study offers a partial explanation for the relations found and points to the importance of finding integrity and resolving despair in this stage of life	Dezutter et al. (2013)
Sweden	Older Swedes (mean age 91.2)	Sense of coherence Negative life events	Longitudinal SOC-13, Barthel's index of activities in daily living (ADL), the mini-mental state examination (MMSE), Geriatric Depression Scale (GDS), The Philadelphia Geriatric Center Morale Scale (PGCMS), medical diagnosis, index of negative life events	For the whole group of subjects ($n = 56$), the SOC scores was higher (70.1 vs. 73.7, $p = 0.029$) at the second point measure. The most common negative life events at follow-up were loss of independence in activities in daily living and decrease in cognitive function. A significant correlation between the index of negative life events and changes in SOC over 5 years was found ($p = 0.025$). The more negative life events, the more decrease in SOC. We concluded that there is a risk of decreased SOC and thereby quality of life when negative life events accumulate among very old people. Nursing interventions might play an important role for maintaining and perhaps strengthening SOC among old people exposed to negative life events	Lövheim et al. (2012)
Sweden	75-year-old Swedes	General health, health behaviour, health problems, socio-demographic status, SOC	Cross-sectional SOC-3, VIPS-Well-being, Integrity, Prevention and Safety, The Health Index Questionnaire	Most 75-year-old persons reported their health as good or very good, but they also reported health problems such as pain, sleeping problems, memory failure, fatigue, poor understanding of their own health and illnesses, problems with elimination patterns and underweight and overweight. 75-year-old persons living alone, those with elementary school education and women reported worse health and well-being than other groups. This study contributes to the knowledge about health issues that concern persons of 75 years of age. It gives a suggestion as to what the district nurses should be aware of when performing preventive home visits	Sherman et al. (2012)

Gender differences are reported in terms of SOC and perceived health amongst older people. In a Norwegian study amongst 242 older people (mean age 84.6 years), examining how the SOC affected the perception of health (Saevareid et al., 2007), it was found that both men and women had health problems directly related to perceived health, whilst psychological symptoms were directly related to perceived health only in men. The gender difference reduced the effect of SOC on perceived health.

As pointed out earlier, ageing is a process, and concepts such as successful ageing and healthy ageing are frequently used (Lezwijn et al., 2011). Salutogenic research also uses the term 'resilient ageing' (Hicks and Conner, 2014) and 'ageing well' (Kennaugh, 2016). As a basis for an EU conference 'Salutogenesis and the promotion of positive mental health in older people' (19–20 April 2010, Madrid, Spain), Billings and Hashem (2010) conducted a review of studies amongst older people using a salutogenic approach to ageing. The review included concepts and theories closely related to SOC, such as resilience, hardiness and religiosity (religious beliefs). The authors highlighted different models for healthy ageing, including factors such as self-reliance, sense of control over life and a positive attitude to life, all to be important determinants of good ageing. They also noted that although the salutogenic approach provides a valuable contribution to maintain and develop health amongst older people, research and application in practice had not achieved the expected attention and impact. In a qualitative study on Irish healthy and active older people, Walsh (2014) examined the salutogenic theory within the context of later life and considered the value of salutogenesis as an analytical perspective applicable to understanding older people's health and well-being as they age in place. The analysis and the results demonstrated the potential value of the qualitative application of the SOC and incorporate context and place as central positions of analysis. This method contributes to a deeper understanding of the health-place relationship.

For a long time, research on SOC has been focused on testing the validity and reliability of the SOC questionnaire in a variety of samples, for example, older people. Thus, we have a good knowledge of how a strong SOC mediates and moderates perceived stress in different samples (Guo et al., 2018; Potier, 2018; Eriksson and Lindström, 2005, 2006). A new trend in salutogenic research is emerging, that is the development of salutogenically designed healthy ageing programmes, such as the AGES project in Japan (Misawa and Kondo, 2019), the SHAPE programme in Singapore (Seah et al., 2018), a health promotion intervention amongst ageing migrants (Arola et al., 2018) and finally an empowering self-management model on the self-efficacy and SOC in Iranian elderly (Hourzad et al., 2018). This is encouraging because research has moved from testing to implementation in practice.

GRRs and SRRs for Older People

Two important concepts in the salutogenic theory are *generalized resistance resources* (GRRs) and *specific resistance resources* (SRRs). *Generalized resistance resources* (GRRs) are those resources that help a person to avoid or to combat a wide variety of stressors (Antonovsky, 1979). GRRs arise from the cultural, social and environmental living conditions and early childhood upbringing and socialization experiences (see Chap. 7). GRRs can be found not only within people as resources bound to their person and capacity, but also within their immediate and distant environment and can be both material and non-material (Lindström and Eriksson, 2005). Examples of GRRs are genetic and constitutional qualities, knowledge, intelligence, ego-strength, control, social support, commitment, cultural stability and also material resources such as money. Importantly, it is not just that such resources are available, but that the individual has the capacity to recognize, use and reuse the resources for the intended purpose, which helps to increase health and well-being. GRRs are applicable in a wide variety of situations. SRRs on the other hand are particular resources, useful in specific situations. Or, as Mittelmark et al. put it, a GRR is a generality, an SRR is a particularity (Mittelmark et al., 2017, p. 75). In their words, '... SRRs ... are optimized by societal action in which public health has a contributing role, for example, the provision of ... health and social and protective (welfare) services, and supportive social and physical environments'.

The Community

Many of the 'prerequisites' to strengthen GGRs, SRRs and SOC are provided by or mediated through the community. But what constitutes a community? Even though the concept is used often in health promotion literature, there is no general understanding of the concept. However, two broad lines can be distinguished, that is, definitions in terms of geographical area and definitions in terms of shared characteristics (Koelen and van den Ban, 2004, p. 136). For the sake of simplicity, here we mean groups of people living in a certain geographical area, often sharing a common culture, values and norms, and who are placed in a social structure according to relationships which the community has developed over a period of time (based on Nutbeam, 1998).

At the centre of the community is the house, which is considered to be the primary setting for ageing in place (Felix et al., 2015; Orrell et al., 2013; Oswald and Wahl, 2005; Sixsmith and Sixsmith, 1991). Older people spend on average 80% of their time inside the house (Oswald et al., 2006; Windle et al., 2006). Studies by, for example, Felix et al. (2015), Oswald et al. (2006), Percival (2002), Rowles (1983), Sixsmith

(1986) and Smith (1994) show a variety of conditions that turn a house into a meaningful place in which to live. In the broader sense, 'home' refers to the constellation of both the built and social community within which the individual resides (Stones and Gullifer, 2016). The physical structure of the house functions as a stage for daily activities. Basic qualities of the house, like daylight, the level of thermal and sound insulation, and the ease of maintenance are valued for their physical comfort, as well as for providing feelings of privacy, safety, freedom and independence. A meaningful house enhances feelings of personal control, autonomy and responsibility, which seem to be pivotal to health development (Koelen and Lindström, 2005) and hence to healthy ageing. People who have a responsibility for day-to-day events, even seemingly small things such as watering plants, or caring for a little bird or dog, have more favourable psychological well-being and show higher health and activity patterns than people without such responsibilities (e.g. Rodin and Langer, 1977). In addition, the house provides a place for personal belongings, which are used to set priorities in life, to create a personal atmosphere and to keep memories of the past alive. As Rowles and Bernard (2013) argue, one's own home provides security, it holds memories and it provides the possibility to stay in proximity with friends, neighbours, kin and local services. As such, one's own home contributes to each of the SOC components: meaningfulness, comprehensibility and manageability.

The social dimension of the house is shaped through interaction with the surrounding community environment, which first of all includes the near social environment (family, friends, and neighbours). Social contacts are seen as an enrichment of life for all age groups: it is fun to do things together. It seems that, especially when people become older, social contacts become more and more important (Oswald and Wahl, 2005; Puts et al., 2007).

A key finding in a qualitative study by Felix et al. (2015), which focused on the experience of the house as a home, was that all participants mentioned the importance of the neighbourhood for feeling at home. Having contact with neighbours, the provision of help and care and the availability of facilities locally seem to be essential for people's sense of 'home'. Research shows that, irrespective of physical decline during older age, most older people prefer to continue living in their own homes amongst their own communities (Stones and Gullifer, 2016). Indeed, many aspects of the community environment are important for older people. This includes the social environment, which provides a feeling of belonging and social inclusion; features of the built environment, including services such as shops, restaurants, schools, churches and community centres, formal and informal health services and infrastructure and transportation; and features of the natural environment, such as availability of urban green space and recreation areas (Felix et al., 2015; Stephens et al., 2015). A study of Yu et al. (2019) showed that perceived neighbourhood environments were positively associated with sense of community and self-rated health. Especially 'transportation' and 'respect and social inclusion' were the physical and the social environmental domains most strongly associated with sense of community. Clearly, the physical and social environments interact. Spatial design of housing, proximity of shops, church and other services and infrastructure largely influence the mobility, self-reliance and social participation in the neighbourhood and larger community. A lack of facilities in each of these domains may negatively affect quality of life. Hence, the neighbourhood can provide important GRRs for older people. In their review study, Khoon-Kiat et al. (2013, p. 497) concluded that older people who have access to GRRs are more likely to have a strong SOC, relatively good health and quality of life.

Ageing in the Community

Important for healthy ageing is that people have the possibility to age in place. Ageing in place can be defined as 'the ability to live in one's own home and community safely, independently, and comfortably, regardless of age, income or ability level' (Centers for Disease Control & Prevention, 2009, p. 1). It enables older people to not only maintain autonomy and independence, but also connection to social support, family and friends. Assisting people to age in place implies that older people receive adequate support whilst they continue to live and be involved in the community. Attention needs to be given to housing options, health and care services, transportation, recreational opportunities and facilities for social interaction and cultural engagement. Over the past decade, the concept of 'age-friendly communities' has emerged. According to the WHO, 'in an age-friendly community, policies, services and structures related to the physical and social environment are designed to support and enable older people to "age actively", that is, to live in security, enjoy good health and continue to participate fully in society. Public and commercial settings and services are made accessible to accommodate varying levels of ability' (WHO, 2002). In line with this, in 2010 WHO established the Global Network for Age-friendly Cities and Communities (AFCC). The mission of the network is to stimulate and enable cities and communities around the world to become increasingly age-friendly. Currently, over 1000 cities and communities in 41 countries, covering over 240 million people worldwide, are connected to the network (WHO, n.d.) which shows the relevance that is assigned to facilitate healthy ageing. AFCC builds on the notion that the physical and social environment contribute to physical health, mental health and well-being (Menec and Brown, 2018), hence to quality of life. Menec et al. (2011) provided an interesting conceptualization of age-friendly communities (see Fig. 19.1).

According to the authors, age-friendly communities create connections between the older persons and the environ-

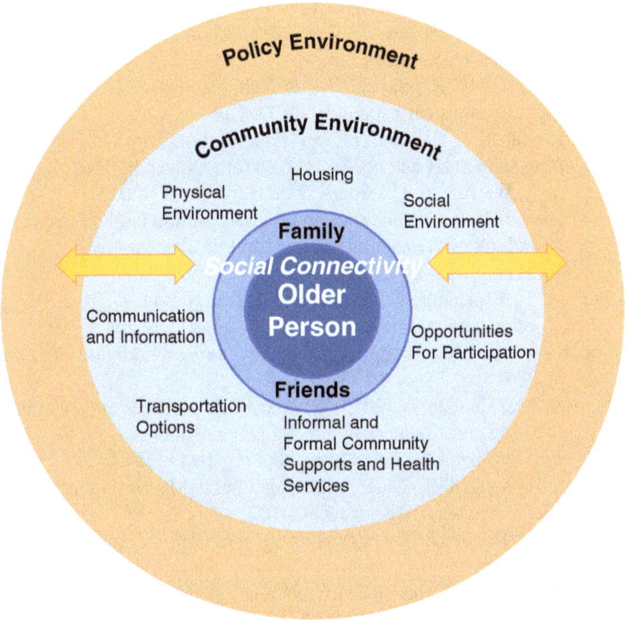

Fig. 19.1 Conceptualizing age-friendly communities . (Reprinted with permission from Cambridge University Press. Menec et al., 2011. This Figure cannot be reproduced, shared, altered or exploited commercially in any way without the permission of Cambridge University Press, as it is copyrighted material and therefore not subject to the allowances permitted by a CC licence)

ment in which they live and vice versa (p. 484). Without an extensive description of the seven identified community dimensions, we wish to emphasize the importance that is attached to conditions in both the physical and social environment contributing (or not) to healthy ageing. Housing is in fact a part of the physical environment but is considered in its own right. This relates to what we have mentioned before about housing and feelings of home. Also opportunities for participation are considered important. This includes social participation and employment, but also other forms of participation such as physical activity, spiritual activity and volunteer options.

From a life course perspective, perhaps an even more interesting concept is that of 'intergenerational communities'. In the age-friendly communities approach, the focus is foremost on how older people can be supported in the context of their environment. However, older people do not live in isolation but are part of the 'whole-life-cycle environment', which includes newborns, children, youth, young and older adults. Intergenerational communities address quality of life and physical and psychological needs for all age groups, with an additional consideration of how different generations interact and form relationships (Kaplan et al., 2016, p. 118). An intergenerational lens may also prevent communities to loose fit with its inhabitants. Communities are no static entities, but change over time, both in terms of population demography (e.g. from mainly young families to a mostly ageing population), the level of maintenance and quality of housing and the surroundings. In fact, communities with features which are important for older people might also be beneficial for children and young adults. For example, the quality of side-walks is important for both older people needing walking aids and young parents using a baby buggy. Moreover, intergenerational contacts are beneficial for all age groups, and, as pointed out before, healthy ageing is a lifelong process, evolving throughout the lifespan.

Intergenerational communities are age-friendly communities, creating connections between the older persons and the environment in which they live and vice versa. This very much relates to the SOC dimension of meaningfulness. The maintenance of social relationships and having the possibility to be physically and socially active is closely related to having a purpose in life (Takkinen and Ruoppila, 2001; Stones and Gullifer, 2016). It enables older people to recognize and use GRRs to strengthen one or more of the three dimensions of SOC – meaningfulness, manageability and comprehensibility – which in turn enables them to recognize, pick up and use SRRs as needed in specific encounters with stressors (see Chap. 8). The home and neighbourhood provide a basis for consistency (coherence) and GRRs, enhancing meaningfulness, comprehensibility and manageability. Intergenerational communities provide supportive environments for people whilst ageing. They provide resources for health in the social and physical environment which – combined with their personal resources – enable people to live their lives despite possible limitations. The model of intergenerational communities may provide a useful framework for future research and practice, towards the facilitation of independence, participation and well-being of older people.

Discussion and Implications for Salutogenic Research

Older people's perceptions of healthy ageing, that is, being independent, being connected, being able to use resources, being able to make one's own decisions (see the relation with the three dimensions of SOC), are related to the notion of ageing in place. Especially the availability of social contacts, the ability to engage in social interaction and the availability and accessibility of social and material resources (GRRs and SRRs) are important. The community, with home as a central place, offers many opportunities for maintaining or enhancing well-being and quality of life of older people.

Developing age-friendly, or preferably intergenerational communities, is more easily said than done. It requires input from a variety of disciplines, from the health, care and social sector, to architecture, city design and environmental planning. The fact that there is a difference in the perception of what constitutes healthy ageing and what is needed for ageing healthy by older people, professionals, researchers and policymakers emphasize the importance of active participation of older people in research and policy-making for healthy ageing, and also for environmental design. It can be expected that such differences in perceptions also exist between different age groups and between age groups and professionals. An intergenerational approach, hence, also requires input from the other age groups. Participation in decision-making and planning enhances feelings of control and empowerment, which, in turn, may contribute to a strong(er) SOC.

Societies are changing at a rapid pace, and ICTs are increasingly applied in all areas of society. The ability to use them is also increasingly essential for everyday life activities. The digitization of various activities in society can mean that new opportunities open up for older people to live an active life but can also be marginalizing for people who do not master the technology. Therefore, it becomes important when designing technological solutions for older people to take this notion into account. Another new innovation is that of artificial intelligence (AI), commonly known as robots with built-in human characteristics such as speech. So far, research of what the consequences of AI are for elderly is still scarce.

References

Aldwin, C. M., Spiro, A., III, & Park, C. L. (2006). Health, behaviour, and optimal aging: A life span developmental perspective. In J. E. Birren & K. W. Schaie (Eds.), *Handbook of the psychology of aging*. Elsevier Academic Press.

Antonovsky, A. (1979). *Health, stress and coping*. Jossey-Bass.

Antonovsky, A. (1985). The life cycle, mental health and the sense of coherence. *The Israel Journal of Psychiatry and Related Sciences, 22*(4), 273–280.

Antonovsky, A. (1987). *Unraveling the mystery of health. How people manage stress and stay well*. Jossey-Bass.

Antonovsky, A. (1993). The salutogenic approach to aging. A lecture held in Berkeley, 21 January 1993. Retrieved 24 Feb 2015, from http://www.angelfire.com/ok/soc/a-berkeley.html.

Arola, L. A., Barenfels, E., Dahlin-Ivanoff, S., & Häggblom-Kronlof, G. (2018). Distribution and evaluation of sense of coherence among older immigrants before and after a health promotion intervention – results from the RCT study promoting aging migrants' capability. *Clinical Intervention and Aging, 13*, 2317–2328.

Beard, J. R., Officer, A., Araujo de Carvalho, I., Sadana, R., Pot, A. M., Michel, J.-P., Lloyd-Sherlock, P., Epping-Jordan, J. E., Peeters, G. M. E. E., Mahanani, W. R., Thiygarajan, J. A., & Chatterji, S. (2016). The world report on ageing and health: A policy framework for healthy ageing. *The Lancet, 387*(10033), 2145–2154.

Billings, J., & Hashem, F. (2010). *Mental health and well-being in older people-making it happen*. Paper presented at the EU conference "Salutogenesis and the promotion of positive mental health in older people", Madrid, 19–20 April 2010.

Boeckxstaens, P., Vaes, B., De Sutter, A., Aujoulat, I., van Pottelbergb, G., Matbei, C., & Degryse, J. M. (2016). A high sense of coherence as protection against adverse health outcomes in patients aged 80 years and older. *Annals of Family Medicine, 14*(4), 337–343.

Cattan, M. (Ed.). (2009). *Mental health and well-being in later life*. Open University Press/McGraw-Hill.

Centers for Disease Control and Prevention. (2009). *Healthy places terminology*. Retrieved 27 May 2015, from http://www.cdc.gov/healthyplaces/terminology.htm.

Cooper, R., Hardy, R., Sayers, A., & Kuh, D. (2014). A life course approach to physical capability. In D. Kuh, R. Cooper, R. Hardy, M. Richards, & Y. Ben-Schlomo (Eds.), *A life course approach to healthy ageing* (1st ed., pp. 16–31). Oxford University Press.

Dezutter, J., Wiesmann, U., Apers, S., & Luyckx, K. (2013). Sense of coherence, depressive feelings and life satisfaction in older persons: A closer look at the role of integrity and despair. *Aging & Mental Health, 17*(7), 839–843.

Drageset, J., Espehaug, D., Halberg, I. R., & Natvig, G. K. (2014). Sense of coherence among cognitively intact nursing home residents—A five-year longitudinal study. *Aging & Mental Health, 18*(7), 889–896.

Drageset, J., & Haugan, G. (2015). Psychometric properties of the orientation to life questionnaire in nursing home residents. *Scandinavian Journal of Caring Sciences*. https://doi.org/10.1111/scs.12271

Dykstra, P. A. (2009). Older adult loneliness: Myths and realities. *European Journal of Ageing, 6*, 91–100.

Erikson, E. H., & Erikson, J. (1998). *The life cycle completed*. W.W. Norton.

Eriksson, M. (2017). The sense of coherence in the salutogenic model of health. In M. B. Mittelmark, S. Sagy, M. Eriksson, G. F. Bauer, J. M. Pelikan, B. Lindström, & G. A. Espnes (Eds.), *The Handbook of Salutogenesis*.

Eriksson, M., & Lindström, B. (2005). Validity of Antonovsky's sense of coherence scale—A systematic review. *Journal of Epidemiology & Community Health, 59*(6), 460–466.

Eriksson, M., & Lindström, B. (2006). Antonovsky's sense of coherence scale and the relation with health: A systematic review. *Journal of Epidemiology & Community Health, 60*(5), 376–381.

Eriksson, M., & Lindström, B. (2011). Life is more than survival: Exploring links between Antonovsky's salutogenic theory and the concept of resilience. In K. M. Gow & M. J. Celinski (Eds.), *Wayfinding through life's challenges: Coping and survival*. Nova.

Eurostat. (2013). Statistics explained archive. In *Vol. 2—Social statistics, December 2012*. Publications Office of the European Union.

Eurostat (2018). *Population structure and ageing*. Retrieved 6 Nov 2019 from https://ec.europa.eu/eurostat/statistics-explained/index.php.

Feldt, T., Leskinen, E., Koskenvuo, M., Suominen, S., Vahtera, J., & Kivimäki, M. (2011). Development of sense of coherence in adulthood: A person-centered approach. The Population-Based HeSSup Cohort Study. *Quality of Life Research, 20*, 69–79.

Feldt, T., Lintula, H., Suominen, S., Koskenvuo, M., Vahtera, J., & Kivimäki, M. (2007). Structural validity and temporal stability of the 13-item sense of coherence scale: Prospective evidence from the population-based HeSSup study. *Quality of Life Research, 16*, 483–493.

Felix, E., de Haan, H., Vaandrager, L., & Koelen, M. (2015). Beyond thresholds: Exploring the meaning of home for older people in the Netherlands. *Journal of Housing for the Elderly, 29*, 329–347.

Forsman, A. K., & Nordmyr, J. (2015). Psychosocial links between Internet use and mental health in later life: A systematic review of quantitative and qualitative evidence. *Journal of Applied Gerontology*, 1–48. https://doi.org/10.1177/0733464815595509

Forte, D. (2009). Relationships. In M. Cattan (Ed.), *Mental health and well-being in later life* (pp. 84–111). Open University Press/McGraw-Hill.

Guo, L.-N., Liu, Y.-J., McCallum, J., Söderhamn, U., Ding, X.-F., Yv, S.-Y., Zhu, Y.-R., & Guo, Y.-R. (2018). Perceived stress and depression amongst older stroke patients: Sense of coherence as a mediator? *Archives of Gerontology and Geriatrics, 79*, 164–170.

Hanson-Kyle, L. (2005). A concept analyses of healthy aging. *Nursing Forum, 40*(2), 45–57.

Hicks, M. M., & Conner, N. E. (2014). Resilient ageing: A concept analysis. *Journal of Advanced Nursing, 70*(4), 744–755. https://doi.org/10.1111/jan.12226

Hornby-Turner, Y. C., Peel, N. M., & Hubbard, R. E. (2017). Health assets in older age: A systematic review. *BMJ Open, 7*, e013226. https://doi.org/10.1136/bmjopen-2016-013226

Hourzad, A., Pouladi, S., Ostovar, A., & Ravanipour, M. (2018). The effects of an empowering self-management model on self-efficacy and sense of coherence among retired elderly with chronic diseases: A randomized controlled trial. *Clinical Interventions in Aging, 13*, 2215–2224.

Huber, M., Knottnerus, J. A., Green, L., van der Horst, H., Jadad, A. R., Kromhout, D., Leonard, B., Lorig, K., Loureiro, M. I., van der Meer, J. W., Schnabel, P., Smith, R., van Weel, C., & Smid, H. (2011). How should we define health? *British Medical Journal, 343*, d4163. https://doi.org/10.1136/bmj.d4163

Hubley, J., & Copeman, J. (2008). *Practical health promotion*. Polity Press.

Jeste, D. V., Depp, C. A., & Vahia, I. V. (2010). Successful cognitive and emotional aging. *World Psychiatry, 9*(2), 78–84.

Kaplan, M., Sanchez, M., & Hoffman, J. (2016). Intergenerational pathways to a sustainable society. In *Intergenerational strategies for sustaining strong communities* (pp. 109–139). Springer.

Kennaugh, R. (2016). *"It's not how old we are; it's how we are old": A salutogenic approach to how older Australian women experience ageing and respond to life stressors*. University of Newcastle, Australia, doctoral thesis.

Khoon-Kiat, T., Vehvilainen-Julkunen, K., & Wai-Chi-Chan, S. (2013). Integrative review: Salutogenesis and health in older people over 65 years old. *Journal of Advanced Nursing, 70*(3), 497–510.

Kingston, A., Davies, K., Collerton, J., Robinson, L., Duncan, R., Kirkwood, T. B. L., & Jagger, C. (2015). The enduring effect of education-socioeconomic differences in disability trajectories from age 85 years in the Newcastle 85+ Study. *Archives of Gerontology and Geriatrics, 60*, 405–411.

Koelen, M. A. (2011). *Health and society: New kid on the block*. Wageningen University.

Koelen, M. A., & Lindström, B. (2005). Making healthy choices easy choices: The role of empowerment. *European Journal of Clinical Nutrition, 59*(Suppl. 1), 10–16.

Koelen, M. A., & van den Ban, A. W. (2004). *Health education and health promotion*. Wageningen.

Krok, D. (2015). Sense of coherence mediates the relationship between the religious meaning system and coping styles in Polish older adults. *Aging & Mental Health, 19*, 1–8.

Kuh, D. (2019). A life course approach to healthy ageing. In J. P. Michel (Ed.), *Prevention of chronic diseases and age-related disability*. Practical issues in Geriatrics. https://doi.org/10.1007/978-3-319-96529-1_1

Kuh, D., & Ben Shlomo, Y. (2004). *A life course approach to chronic disease epidemiology*. Oxford University Press.

Lezwijn, J., Vaandrager, L., Naaldenberg, J., Wagemakers, A., Koelen, M. A., & van Woerkum, C. M. J. (2011). Healthy ageing in a salutogenic way: Building the HP 2.0 framework. *Health & Social Care in the Community, 19*(1), 43–51.

Lim, S. (2020). Strategies to improve continuity maintenance for people with dementia: A rapid realist review. *Public Health, 181*, 46–52.

Lindström, B., & Eriksson, M. (2005). Salutogenesis. *Journal of Epidemiology and Community Health, 59*(6), 440–442.

Lópes, J., Camilli, C., & Noriega, C. (2014). Posttraumatic growth in widowed and non-widowed older adults: Religiosity and sense of coherence. *Journal of Religion and Health, 53*(6). https://doi.org/10.1007/s10943-014-9876-5

Lövheim, H., Graneheim, U. H., Jonsen, E., Starndberg, G., & Lundman, B. (2012). Changes in sense of coherence in old age—a 5-year follow-up of the Umeå 85+ study. *Scandinavian Journal of Caring Science, 27*(1), 13–19.

Marcoen, A., Coleman, P., & O'Hanlon, A. (2007). Psychological ageing. In J. Bond, S. Peace, F. Dittman-Kohli, & G. Westerhof (Eds.), *Ageing in society* (pp. 38–67). Sage.

Menec, V. H., Means, R., Jeating, N., Parkhurst, G., & Eales, J. (2011). Conceptualizing age-friendly communities. *Canadian Journal on Aging, 30*(3), 479–493.

Menec, V., & Brown, C. (2018). Facilitators and barriers to becoming age-friendly: A review. *Journal of Aging & Social Policy*. https://doi.org/10.1080/08959420.20181528116

Mittelmark, M. B., Bull, T., Daniel, M., & Urke, H. (2017). Specific resistance resources in the salutogenic model of health. In M. B. Mittlemark, S. Sagy, M. Eriksson, G. F. Bauer, J. M. Pelikan, B. Lindström, & G. A. Espnes (Eds.), *The handbook of salutogenesis*. Springer. Open access. https://doi.org/10.1007/978-3-319-04600-6

Misawa, J., & Kondo, K. (2019). Social factors relating to depression among older people in Japan: Analysis of longitudinal panel data from the AGES project. *Aging & Mental Health, 23*(10), 1423–1432.

Murayama, Y., Ohba, H., Yasunaga, H., Nonaka, K., Takeuchi, R., Nishj, M., Sakuma, N., Uchida, H., Shinkai, S., & Fujiwara, Y. (2014). The effect of intergenerational programs on the mental health of elderly adults. *Aging & Mental Health*. https://doi.org/10.1080/136077863.136072014.136933309

Naaldenberg, J., Vaandrager, L., Koelen, M. A., & Leeuwis, C. (2011). Ageing populations' everyday life perspectives on healthy aging: New insights for policy and strategies at the local level. *Applied Gerontology*. https://doi.org/10.1177/0733464810397703

Nilsson, K., Leppert, J., Simonsson, B., & Starrin, B. (2010). Sense of coherence (SOC) and psychological well-being (GHQ): Improvement with age. *Journal of Epidemiology and Community Health, 64*(4), 347–352.

Nutbeam, D. (1998). *Health promotion glossary. WHO/HPR/HEP/98.1*. World Health Organisation.

Nyqvist, F., Cattan, M., Andersson, L., Forsman, A. K., & Gustafson, Y. (2013). Social capital and loneliness among the very old living at home and in institutional settings: A comparative study. *Journal of Aging and Health*. https://doi.org/10.1177/0898264313497508

Orrell, A., McKee, K., Torrington, J., Barnes, S., Darton, R., Netten, A., et al. (2013). The relationship between building design and residents' quality of life in extra care housing schemes. *Health & Place, 21*, 52–64.

Oswald, F., & Wahl, H. W. (2005). Dimensions of the meaning of home in later life. In G. D. Rowles & H. Chaudhury (Eds.), *Home and identity in late life: International perspectives* (pp. 21–45). Springer.

Oswald, F., Wahl, H. W., Naumann, D., Mollenkopf, H., & Hieber, A. (2006). The role of the home environment in middle and late adulthood. In H. W. Wahl, H. Brenner, H. Mollenkopf, D. Rothenbacher, & C. Rott (Eds.), *The many faces of health, competence and well-being in old age* (pp. 7–24). Springer.

Percival, J. (2002). Domestic spaces: Uses and meanings in the daily lives of older people. *Aging and Society, 22*, 729–749.

Phillipson, C., & Baars, J. (2007). Social theory and social ageing. In J. Bond, S. Peace, F. Dittman-Kohli, & G. Westerhof (Eds.), *Ageing in society* (pp. 68–84). Sage.

Potier, F. (2018). A high sense of coherence protects from the burden of caregiving in older spousal caregivers. *Archives of Gerontology and Geriatrics, 75*, 76–82.

Puts, M. T. E., Shekary, N., Widdershoven, G., Helders, P. J., Lips, P., & Deeg, D. J. H. (2007). What does quality of life mean to older frail and non-frail community-dwelling adults in the Netherlands? *Quality of Life Research, 16*, 263–277.

Rodin, J., & Langer, E. J. (1977). Long-term effects of a control-relevant intervention with the institutionalized aged. *Journal of Personality and Social Psychology, 35*(12), 897–902.

Rowles, G. D. (1983). Place and personal identity in old age: Observations from Appalachia. *Journal of Environmental Psychology, 3*, 299–313.

Rowles, G. D. R., & Bernard, M. B. (2013). The meaning and significance of place in old age. In G. D. R. Rowles & M. B. Bernard (Eds.), *Environmental gerontology: Making meaningful places in old age* (pp. 2–24). Springer.

Sadana, R., & Michel, J.-P. (2019). Healthy ageing: What is it and how to describe it? In J.-P. Michel (Ed.), *Prevention of chronic diseases and age-related disability*. Practical Issues in Geriatrics. https://doi.org/10.1007/978-3-319-96529-1_2

Saevareid, H. I., Thygesen, E., Nygaard, H. A., & Lindstrom, T. C. (2007). Does sense of coherence affect the relationship between self-rated health and health status in a sample of community-dwelling frail elderly people? *Aging & Mental Health, 11*(6), 658–667.

Seah, B., Espnes, G. A., Ang, E. N. K., Kowitlawakul, Y., & Wang, W. (2020). Achieving healthy ageing through the perspective of sense of coherence among senior-only households: a qualitative study. *Aging & Mental Health*, 1725805. https://doi.org/10.1080/13607863.2020

Seah, B., Kowitlawakul, Y., Chokkanathan, S., Fong, J. J. Y., Espnes, G. A., Ang, E., & Wang, W. (2018). Salutogenic Healthy Ageing Programme Embracement (SHAPE) for senior-only households: A study protocol. *Journal of Advanced Nursing, 74*, 946–956.

Sherman, H., Forsberg, C., Karp, A., & Törnkvist, L. (2012). The 75-year-old persons' self-reported health conditions: A knowledge base in the field of preventive home visits. *Journal of Clinical Nursing, 21*(21–22), 3170–3182.

Sixsmith, J. (1986). The meaning of home: An exploratory study of environmental experience. *Journal of Environmental Psychology, 6*, 281–298.

Sixsmith, A. J., & Sixsmith, J. A. (1991). Transitions in home experience in later life. *Journal of Architectural and Planning Research, 8*, 181–191.

Smith, S. G. (1994). The essential qualities of a home. *Journal of Environmental Psychology, 14*, 31–46.

Staehelin, H. B. (2005). Promoting health and wellbeing in later life. In M. L. Johnson, V. L. Bengtson, P. G. Coleman, & T. B. L. Kirkwood (Eds.), *The Cambridge book of age and ageing* (pp. 165–177). Cambridge University Press.

Stensletten, K., Bravik, F., Espehaug, B., & Drageset, J. (2014). Burden of care, social support, and sense of coherence in elderly caregivers living with individuals with symptoms of dementia. *Dementia*. https://doi.org/10.1177/1471301214563319

Stephens, C., Breheny, M., & Mansvelt, J. (2015). Healthy ageing from the perspective of older people: A capability approach to resilience. *Psychology and Health, 30*(6), 715–731. https://doi.org/10.1080/08870446.2014.904862

Stones, D., & Gullifer, J. (2016). 'At home it's just so much easier to be yourself': Older adults' perceptions of ageing in place. *Ageing & Society, 36*, 449–482.

Takkinen, S., & Ruoppila, I. (2001). Meaning in life in three samples of elderly persons with high cognitive functioning. *International Journal of Human Development, 53*(1), 51–73.

Tan, K.-K., Vehviläinen-Julkunen, K., & Chan, S. W.-C. (2013). Integrative review: Salutogenesis and health in older people over 65 years old. *Journal of Advanced Nursing, 70*(3), 497–510.

Walsh, S. (2014). Salutogenesis 2.0: An examination of healthy ageing-in-place using a qualitative application of the Sense of Coherence. Doctoral thesis. National University of Ireland Maynooth.

Westendorp, R. G., & Kirkwood, T. B. (2007). The biology of ageing. In J. Bond, S. Peace, F. Dittman-Kohli, & G. Westerhof (Eds.), *Ageing in society* (pp. 15–37). Sage.

WHO. (2002). *Global age friendly cities*. Retrieved 3 March 2015, from www.who.int/ageing/projects/age_friendly_cities/en/.

WHO. (2015). Ageing and lifecourse. Retrieved 6 Nov 2019 from: https://www.who.int/ageing/healthy-ageing/en/.

WHO. (n.d.). *About the Global Network for Age-friendly Cities and Communities*. Retrieved 3 March 2020 from: https://extranet.who.int/agefriendlyworld/who-network/.

Wiesmann, U., Dezutter, J., & Hannich, H. J. (2014). Sense of coherence and pain experience in older age. *International Psychogeriatrics, 26*(1), 123–133.

Wiesmann, U., & Hannich, H. J. (2019). A salutogenic inquiry into positive aging – a longitudinal analysis. *Aging & Mental Health, 23*(11), 1562–1568.

Windle, G. S., Burholt, V., & Edwards, R. T. (2006). Housing related difficulties, housing tenure and variations in health status: Evidence from older people in Wales. *Health & Place, 12*, 267–278.

Young, Y., Frick, K. D., & Phelan, E. A. (2009). Can successful ageing and chronic illness coexist in the same individual? A multidimensional concept of successful aging. *Journal of the American Medical Directors Association, 10*(2), 87–92.

Yu, R., Wong, M., & Woo, J. (2019). Perceptions of neighborhood environment, sense of community, and self-rated health: an age-friendly city project in Hong Kong. *Journal of Urban Health, 96*, 276–288.

20

Interventions over Life Course and their Impact on SOC

Eva Langeland, Lenneke Vaandrager, Anne Britt Vika Nilsen, Marco Schraner, and Claudia Meier Magistretti

Introduction

There is an extensive amount of publications about the Sense of Coherence (SOC), the main concept in salutogenesis (Eriksson and Lindström, 2005, 2006, 2007; Eriksson and Mittelmark, 2017). However, there is a lack of knowledge about studies investigating the effects of interventions, based on salutogenesis during the life course, on SOC (Bauer et al., 2019; Hochwälder, 2019). Besides, there is a call for reaching a consensus that defines what characterizes a salutogenic intervention and the minimal characteristics that a salutogenic intervention should follow (Álvarez et al., 2020).

Antonovsky (1979, 1987, 1992, 1996a) claimed that the Sense of Coherence is an internal experience that gradually develops during youth to a rather lasting and stable quality of an individual after 30 years of age. He emphasized that this is a hypothesis based on theoretical considerations and is not based on empirical evidence (Antonovsky, 1996a). However, Antonovsky made this tentative hypothesis in 1987, over 30 years ago. The world and societies have developed and changed since then. People live longer in general and experience major life changes after 30 years of age. They participate in different kinds of therapies or coaching, start a new partnership, parenthood, education, different kind of courses, and new jobs. In general, knowledge is much more available. Accordingly, the view that the SOC is stable after 30 years of age might be modified (Suominen, 1993). Research also indicates that the SOC may become stronger due to major life events such as childbirth (Lindström et al., 2017) or experiences in everyday life (Maass et al., 2017).

In the last two decades, there was an increasing research interest in the ability of tailored interventions to modify and strengthen the SOC of various target groups. Research emerged on therapies, training, or interventions aiming to strengthen the SOC (Langeland et al., 2006). However, an overview of empirical evidence on the SOC's changeability by health-promoting interventions is lacking. The main purpose of this chapter is to provide a synopsis of interventions over the life course and their effectiveness on the SOC. Besides, we aim to assess to what degree the content and methods of each intervention are salutogenic.

The Theory of Salutogenesis and Interventions

According to Antonovsky (1987), the salutogenic orientation does not view health as a dichotomous variable, but instead as an active process along a continuum. It focuses on the story of the whole person and life situation rather than on specific problems and diagnoses. It sees people as biological, psychological, social, and spiritual beings who are both proactive and reactive, and who make choices. Persons are perceived as actively involved in health-seeking and self-actualization. Further, salutogenesis understands tension and strain as potentially health-promoting, rather than as inevitably health-damaging. The use of potential and/or existing general and specific resistance resources (GRRs and SRRs) enhances the SOC, and the individual's active adaptation is emphasized as the ideal in treatment. This illustrates that the

E. Langeland (✉) · A. B. V. Nilsen
Department of Health and Caring Sciences, Faculty of Health and Social Sciences, Western Norway University of Applied Sciences, Bergen, Norway
e-mail: Eva.Langeland@hvl.no

L. Vaandrager
Department of Social Sciences, Health and Society, Wageningen University and Research, Wageningen, The Netherlands

M. Schraner · C. Meier Magistretti
Centre for Health Promotion and Participation, Lucerne University of Applied Sciences and Arts, Lucerne, Switzerland

theory of salutogenesis is a broad and comprehensive theory, and it provides a general understanding of how the SOC and well-being are created. Research shows that a strong SOC will also improve especially mental health (Eriksson and Lindström, 2006). The theory has been applied in several fields, such as nursing (Sullivan, 1989) and mental health care (Eriksson and Lindström, 2006; Griffiths, 2009; Langeland, 2007; Langeland et al., 2006; Langeland and Vinje, 2017). Salutogenesis has also been suggested as a suitable framework for public health development (Eriksson and Lindström, 2006; Super et al., 2016), health promotion (Antonovsky, 1996b; Garcia-Moya and Morgan, 2017), healthy aging (Lezwijn et al., 2011), workplace health promotion (Vaandrager and Koelen, 2013), mental health rehabilitation (Griffiths, 2009; Pijpker et al., 2019), mental health promotion (Langeland and Vinje, 2013), and maternity care (Downe, 2010; Meier Magistretti et al., 2016).

The main aim of salutogenic interventions is to create an environment with meaningful and attainable resources and thus arrange for that individuals and groups might come into a positive interplay between the use of internal and/or external resistance resources and the SOC. This means that there are many ways to possibly promote the SOC dependent on a person's or a group's needs and available resources. Yamazaki et al. (2011) have concluded that the first intervention program based on the salutogenic model of health (salutogenic orientation and main concepts) and aimed to strengthen Sense of Coherence as one main outcome was developed by Langeland et al. (2007), and this intervention program has been further developed in Langeland and Vinje (2013).

Up to present, we lack an overview of how much interventions based on salutogenic theory are effective to positively change the SOC.

Methods

This is a scoping review (Grant and Booth, 2009), including quantitative intervention studies with SOC as an outcome. We have systematically searched for, appraised, and summarized the existing research evidence on intervention studies with the SOC as a primary or secondary outcome.

Data Searches

We have carried out searches in the databases PubMed, PsycINFO, Ovid, ERIC, Embase, SocINDEX, Cochrane, Cochrane trials, Cochrane review, and Google Scholar. The inclusion criteria were English literature from 2005 to 2019, focusing specifically on intervention studies with the SOC as an outcome. We included RCTs, controlled clinical trials, and follow-up studies.

The data searches have been performed twice, where we included new search terms in the second search. The first search has been performed by an especially trained librarian and the fourth and the last author. The fourth author and last author also provided a first summary of all the retrieved articles to facilitate selection and further additions by the last author. Another librarian, trained specially in health disciplines, and the first author, have performed the second searches. The reference lists of all the papers retrieved have been examined for any paper missed with the other searches.

In the first searches, we identified 31 included articles. In the second search, we included an additional ten articles. Two articles were excluded because of insufficient reporting of the SOC scores. Thus, we finally considered 41 included articles (see Table 20.1 for an overview of the search process). Table 20.2 (Cf. The electronic supplementary file) shows a summary of the 41 articles, including authors, year of publication, country, title, method, sample, salutogenic intervention content, assessment points, and effect on the SOC.

Definition of the Criteria for Salutogenic Interventions

We developed five criteria based on salutogenic theory as well as on the work of Langeland et al. (2007), Langeland and Vinje (2013), and Polhuis et al. (2020). The criteria that designate an intervention salutogenic are defined as follows:

1. A focus on health-promoting factors: general resistance resources (GRRs) and/or specific resistance resources (SRRs).

Explanation: To promote health from a salutogenic perspective, the primary focus of the intervention must be on the dynamic interaction between GRRs, SRRs, and stressors in human life, thus facilitating the use of resistance resources and support the participants to move toward the healthy end of the health continuum.

Background: According to the theory of salutogenesis (Antonovsky, 1987), to increase awareness of internal and external resources and increase the ability to use them promotes the transformation of tension and stress into coping (Langeland et al., 2016; Langeland et al., 2007).

2. A whole-person approach (WPA).

Explanation: This perceives the participant as a whole person and includes the life course within the life circumstances of the participant. Understanding the unique life story and current life situation of people is important for providing meaningful interventions.

Background: In a salutogenic approach, the focus is on the history and experiences of human beings rather than

Table 20.1 Overview data searches

Database	Keywords	Number of hits	Inclusion criteria	Exclusions (title)	Exclusions (abstract) incl. duplicates	Number of suitable hits	Excluded (duplicates, theoretical, not intervention not relevant)	Included
PsycInfo Psyndex plus; ERIC	"Sense of coherence" AND intervention OR training AND increase OR strength* OR enhance*	298	English literature; from 2005 to 2019 /focuses specifically on interventions that should bring about a change in the SOC	189	68	41	Totally 79	**Totally 31**
Google Scholar	Sense of coherence; intervention; increase; strengthening; enhance	980	English literature; from 2005 to 2019 /focuses specifically on interventions that should bring about a change in the SOC	876	79	25		
PubMed	Sense of coherence; intervention; enhance	136	English literature; from 2005 to 2019 /focuses specifically on interventions that should bring about a change in the SOC	76	26	34		
Cochrane	"sense of coherence" AND intervention OR training AND increase OR strength* OR enhance*	73	English literature; from 2005 to 2019 /focuses specifically on interventions that should bring about a change in the SOC	31	32	10		
New search: December 4, 2019								
Oria	Salutogen*OR "Sense of coherence" AND intervention* AND effect*	102	English literature; from 2005 to 2019 /focuses specifically on interventions that should bring about a change in the SOC.	89	13	–	–	–
PubMed	"Sense of coherence" AND salutogen* AND intervention* AND effect*	8	English literature; from 2005 to 2019 /focuses specifically on interventions that should bring about a change in the SOC.		6	2		2
Embase	"Sense of coherence" AND intervention* AND effect*	118	English literature; from 2005 to 2019 /focuses specifically on interventions that should bring about a change in the SOC		111	7		7
Cochrane	Reviews "Sense of coherence"	28	2005–2019	13	14	1		1
								A total of 41 included articles

focusing solely on disease and physical health (Antonovsky, 1987). Health incorporates multiple aspects of well-being (Antonovsky, 1996b). Therefore, salutogenic interventions must take into account multiple aspects of health and well-being, including the physical, mental, social, and spiritual dimensions of participants.

3. Active adaptation (A).

Explanation: The focus is on the participant's ability to actively adopt or become actively involved in the interplay between the person or group and the internal and external environment. Adjusting intervention strategies to the individual's priorities, motivations, and capabilities increases the chance of accomplishing meaningful and active participation in the interventions. Active participation facilitates the successful change in comprehensibility, manageability, and meaning, as well as the implementation of newly adopted attitudes and behaviors in everyday life.

Background: Active adaptation is ideal in treatment (Antonovsky, 1987). This orientation leads us to the overall problem of active adaptation to an inevitably stressor-rich environment (Antonovsky, 1987). It is crucial that the participants experience appropriate challenges and thus develop the ability to use the resources (Langeland and Vinje, 2013; Langeland et al., 2007).

4. Stressors and Tension as potentially health-promoting (ST).

Explanation: This point is based on the understanding that stressors and tension are normal to experience. When demands or expectations are perceived as appropriate and challenging, the tension will be transformed into coping experiences (Antonovsky, 1987; Langeland and Vinje, 2013; Langeland et al., 2007). Magrin et al. (2006) define tension as "the salt of life."

Background: In the salutogenic model, stressors, tension, and strain are potentially health-promoting. Antonovsky (1987) distinguishes between tension and stress. When demands exceed a person's resources or a person's ability to use resources, then the tension created by the stressor leads to stress and the person moves toward the dis-ease end of the continuum.

5. A focus on the SOC as a learning process (L).

Explanation: To learn is to discover and use GRRs and SRRs, thus promoting a constructive self-identity, SOC, and health. A learning process focused on self-identity and social support may lead to the discovery of individual internal and external resources that can be used to facilitate coping with life challenges.

Background: In a salutogenic approach, health is understood as a lifelong process in which people learn to identify resources and to use them (Lindström and Eriksson, 2010). The process consists of: (a) experience life as being consistent, (b) to find an appropriate overload/underload balance, and (c) to participate in making decisions that are relevant to one's own life thus strengthening identity and other important resources (Antonovsky, 1987).

We rated the interventions according to the degree they fulfill the criteria for a salutogenic intervention. For each intervention, we assessed and determined the extent they matched the criteria. All authors did that individually by labeling each intervention as follows: specific resistance resources (SRRs) and/or general resistance resources (GRRs), whole person approach (WPA), active adaptation (A), stressors and tension as potentially health-promoting (ST), and learning (L). The labeling was then compared. Interventions that were assessed differently were studied again by the first, second, and last author individually and then discussed up to a consent agreement.

Some interventions combined salutogenic and pathogenic elements. Although the pathogenic elements might be in the description of the aim of the intervention such as prevent illnesses or stress and reduce burnout instead of describing what to promote such as promote coping and well-being, they have been defined as salutogenic if the content of the intervention fulfilled the criteria.

Findings

Search Outcomes

The search identified 41 articles that fulfilled the inclusion criteria. This includes 22 RCT studies, 11 follow-up studies with a control group, and 8 follow-up studies without a control group. Many of the included studies did not explicitly define whether the SOC was a primary or secondary outcome. In studies that have included several outcomes and that did not define primary and secondary outcomes, we defined the SOC as a primary outcome when it has been included in the title and/or mentioned first in the measure section of the article.

The SOC as the Outcome of the Studies: The Extent of Salutogenic Content in the Intervention and the Development of the SOC

Table 20.2 (Cf. The elctronic supplementary file) contains an overview of all included studies and the coded interventions as specific resistance resources (SRRs) and/or general resistance resources (GRRs), whole person approach (WPA), active adaptation (A), stressors and tension as potentially health-promoting (ST), and the SOC as a learning process (L)

The 41 articles have been classified according to their main target groups and are presented in the following paragraphs. The description of each study follows the structure: Specific target group, setting, content, length, frequency, the level of salutogenic content assessment, and the development of the SOC. The studies are described and discussed in the following paragraphs structured by the target groups of the interventions.

Young People

Nammontri et al. (2013) have performed a cluster RCT study, including a salutogenic intervention for enhancing oral health with the SOC as the primary outcome.

Students ages 10–12 years old participated in seven 40- to 60-minute sessions delivered by teachers over two months, focused on child participation and empowerment. The first four sessions were classroom activities involving didactic teaching, discussion, activities, and games. The last three sessions involved working on healthy school projects: brainstorming, planning, implementation, and evaluation. This intervention fulfilled four of the salutogenic intervention criteria: it addressed the participants with a whole-person approach (WPA), active adaptation (A), and enhanced an active learning process (L). They also received access to GRRs such as activities, games, and most likely social support. The SOC improved significantly in the experiment group ($n = 133$) compared to the control group ($n = 128$) both two weeks and three months after the intervention.

Another RCT study (Recabarren et al., 2019) included an intervention about stress prevention, quality of life, well-being, and psychological resources among university students with the SOC as a secondary outcome. The program included eight 2-hour weekly sessions with a salutogenic multidimensional stress prevention program, integrating mindfulness-based activities, cognitive and behavioral strategies, social skills exercises, and emotional regulation (A, GRRs, and L). Homework between sessions was also proposed (L). Participants performed written exercises, discussions, and role-playing in personal or fictive situations based on different types of material and triggers such as videos, audio, and visual supports (WPA). The program did fulfill four of the five criteria. The SOC improved significantly in the intervention ($n = 32$) after eight weeks (from before to after intervention) compared to the control group ($n = 32$).

Bronikowski and Bronikowska (2009) is a controlled clinical trial among adolescent boys aiming at improving the health resources of adolescent boys with the SOC as a secondary outcome. The program, which lasted 15 months, included regular moderate to vigorous physical activity (MVPA). During four lessons of physical education per week, the teacher used at least one activity per lesson including the following teaching strategies: teacher talk, modeling (being), reinforcement, reflection time, and student sharing to improve the levels of self-control, involvement, self-responsibility, and caring-responsibility of pupils. Additionally, a specially self-designed, personalized form "Planning of Leisure-time Physical Activity" was used. The program provided access to GRRs, active adaptation (A), and learning (L) related to physical training together with others. It did not fulfill the other criteria WPA and ST and was therefore considered to be a moderate salutogenic intervention. The pre- and post-intervention showed a significant difference between the groups on the SOC after a 15 months salutogenic program. However, the significant differences between the groups were due to decreased SOC in the control group ($n = 115$), and there was just a slightly SOC improvement in the experiment group ($n = 84$).

Davidson et al. (2012) have done an intervention study among first-year college students with the SOC as a secondary outcome. The participants were distributed in three groups (n = 14,15,14, respectively), all included salutogenic elements (promotion of hope, sense of coherence, and self-efficacy for enhancing students' academic adjustment), but one of these groups had an explicit focus on salutogenesis. The version of this workshop delivered to this group included a short lecture on the salutogenesis paradigm, including the SOC construct in addition to the short lecture on hope theory that the other groups received. In addition, they filled out a cognitive-mapping worksheet that was in line with the salutogenesis model and focused their attention on lessons they learned in the past and their future expectations. This intervention satisfies three of the five salutogenic criteria. The programs provided access to GRRs and their participation in workshops promoted their active adaptation (A) and learning process (L). At the times of measurement, just after the intervention one month after the conclusion of the program, there was a significant improvement in the SOC across the groups. However, there were no significant differences between the groups on the SOC.

A total of three of the four studies that have been performed among younger people showed a significant difference in the SOC in favor of the salutogenic intervention group. It includes two RCTs and two follow-ups with the control group(s), all with salutogenic elements in the interventions. The strongest salutogenic intervention seems to be Nammontri et al. (2013). It had the SOC as the primary outcome, it had the best design with adequate sample size, and it observed significant effects at two weeks and three months after the intervention. Recabarren et al. (2019) also has a strong design and good salutogenic content, but a much smaller sample and the significant effect are measured just after the intervention. The other two studies (Bronikowski and Bronikowska, 2009; Davidson et al., 2012) have weaker designs, salutogenic content, and effect. All the three latter had the SOC as a secondary outcome.

Occupational Health/Unemployed People

An RCT (Valtonen et al., 2015) among 234 occupational healthcare clients with depression with the SOC as a primary outcome consisted of a group intervention ($n = 134$) emphasizing the interaction between body and mind of 6 months and 31 active days. It consisted of four courses, the first two to understand the depression symptoms, and the third and fourth were focused on rehabilitation. It aimed at increasing the self-knowledge of depressive symptoms (SRRs), teach more effective coping with stressors (A and L), and provide peer and social support (SSRs). Thus it fulfilled three of the five salutogenic criteria. It found a significant improvement of the SOC in both the intervention and control group 6 months and one year after the intervention. However, there was no significant difference in the mean SOC scores between the groups at these follow-ups.

Another RCT (Viding et al., 2015) among 36 women with burnout with the SOC as a secondary outcome consisted of an intervention hosted by four healthcare centers and included a mixture of different cultural activities (a so-called Culture Palette): interactive theater, movie, vocal improvisation and drawing, dance, mindfulness training, and a musical show (GRRs). The intervention was based on the idea that cultural activities can enrich and enhance memory (L), stimulate connections among brain networks, and enable to accelerate learning (A) and differentiate feelings of meaning and context (SRRs and GRRs). It found no significant differences between the intervention and the control group after three and six months.

A controlled clinical trial of Kähönen et al. (2012) among employees suffering from severe burnout symptoms consisted of interventions of 16 separate days, over 9 months, with the SOC as the primary outcome. There were two intervention groups: one "psycho-dramatic" (n = 25) and one "action-based" (n = 24) and control group (n = 28). A common issue in both group methods was to investigate the balance between work, social life (including family life), and personal hobbies (A). Another common issue was to investigate participants' values, beliefs, attitudes, and patterns of behavior (WPA), especially those exposed to conflicts in their work (L). The "psycho-dramatic" method was based on a free discussion in several steps. In the beginning, group confidence and group cohesion were built up (SRRs). Cards and figures were used to help the group members express their feelings and ideas (GRRs). Drawing, music, and writing (GRRs) were used to investigate and express the group members' inner worlds. Muscle relaxation and exercises using the imagination (GRRs) were used in the last session of the day. During the intervention, every participant could be the protagonist of the day, that is, to use the whole group and coordinators to investigate through psychodrama something of crucial importance to him–/herself (A). Thus, it fulfilled four of the five salutogenic criteria. It found a significant increase in the SOC in favor of the intervention groups nine months after the intervention.

Another controlled clinical trial of Merakou et al. (2019), with the SOC as the primary outcome, among unemployed individuals with anxiety disorders, consisted of an intervention of a Progressive Muscle Relaxation (PMR) program (GRRs) and counseling services (SRRs). The participants were divided into four subgroups of six to eight people attending a two-month training course. The training (L) included four weekly sessions (45 min) facilitated by a professional PMR trainer. Participants were asked to practice at home (A). Thus it fulfilled three of the five criteria. Both groups received counseling services once a week during the entire period. It found a significant increase in the SOC after eight weeks in the intervention group (n = 30) and no significant changes in the control group (n = 20).

A follow-up study of Vastamäki et al. (2009) among 74 unemployed individuals, with the SOC as the primary outcome, consisted of a 6-month intervention program that provided support in the job-search process and personal life situations. The program combined three kinds of activities: labor market activities (i.e., vocational training and subsidized employment), personal guidance, and networking (SSRs) with other organizations providing support for the unemployed. After the start-up period, individual needs were assessed as a basis for further guidance processes, and different services were provided according to diverse needs (WPA). Through networking, healthcare services and financial support could also be provided (SSRs). At the beginning of the intervention, all participants took part in group counseling (L), which lasted two months. Participants' job-searching skills and activity (A) were improved, and their coping skills were strengthened to boost the job-search process and to make the process less stressful. It fulfilled four of the five criteria. It found a significant increase in the SOC over a 6-month period.

Another follow-up study (Gunnarsson and Bjorklund, 2013), with the SOC as a secondary outcome, among 35 persons with different mental health challenges consisted of an intervention of 5 sessions that included creative activities and occupational storytelling and was called "The Three Team Method" (TTM). The TTM implied that the clients draw and paint trees symbolizing various periods in their life (A). The pictures were then used as a starting point to tell their life story (L and WPA) to enhance their well-being and management of their everyday life (GRRs/SRRs). It showed a significant change in the SOC at three years' follow-up.

There are a total of six studies under this section of which all (Gunnarsson and Bjorklund, 2013; Kähönen et al., 2012; Merakou et al., 2019; Valtonen et al., 2015; Vastamäki et al., 2009; Viding et al., 2015) have SOC as a primary outcome except Gunnarsson and Bjorklund (2013) and Viding et al. (2015) that had the SOC as a secondary outcome. The strongest salutogenic interventions seem to be the controlled clinical trial of Kähönen et al. (2012) and the follow-up of Vastamäki et al. (2009) that also affected follow-up at nine months and six months, respectively. However, they included small sample sizes and had rather weaker designs. The follow-up study of Gunnarson and Bjørklund

(2013) included a rather strong salutogenic intervention and revealed significant change in SOC at three years' follow-up. However, this study applied a weak design and had a rather small sample size.

Health Professionals

An RCT consisted of medical personnel with burnout (Brooks et al., 2010) with the SOC as a secondary outcome. The intervention consisted of music and imagery experiences, 60–75 minutes a session per week, where the participants were guided through body relaxation and directed imagery experiences while listening to music (SRRs). Based on the needs of the participants, the research assistants selected pre-scripted directed imagery experiences. These directed music-guided imagery experiences typically included the participant interacting or relaxing in a nature scene (A and L). The intervention fulfilled three of the five criteria. The study showed that the experiment group ($n = 24$) and control group ($n = 23$) had no significant differences in the SOC after six weeks (before to after intervention).

A small clinical controlled trial of Sarid, Berger, Eckshtein, and Segal-Engelchin (2012) had the SOC as a primary outcome. The participants were nurses with occupational stress. The cognitive-behavioral intervention that was used in this study was based on a variety of cognitive-behavioral principles and techniques and not on a particular theory, thereby allowing them to choose the strategies that were most effective for them (A). Four-hour meetings took place once a week for 16 weeks. Behavioral interventions included teaching and practicing breathing techniques and progressive muscle training. Participants were taught to question their self-defeating thoughts by examining evidence, practicing the strategies to reduce psychophysiological aspects of stress, and rehearsing skills they acquired (L). Each meeting started with a theoretical presentation followed by the practice of and reflections on the relevant skills (GRRs). The intervention fulfilled three of the five criteria. There was a significant difference between intervention ($n = 20$) and control group ($n = 16$) in the SOC after four months (before to after intervention) in favor of the intervention group.

A pilot follow-up study among 38 nurses and midwives (Foureur et al., 2013) with the SOC as a secondary outcome, including a mindfulness-based program (GRRs) over eight-week daily practice (A and L) included knowledge of stress on the body, mind, emotion, and behavior (GRRs). Further, the content was daily meditation practice for 20 minutes, a repertoire of strategies for mindfulness on a day-to-day basis, and forming habits of daily mindfulness practice (L). The intervention fulfills three of the five salutogenic criteria. The study reveals significant positive strengthening of the SOC after eight weeks (before to after intervention).

This section consists of one RCT, one controlled clinical trial, and one follow-up. All the studies included relatively small samples and moderate salutogenic content (fulfilled three salutogenic criteria). Two of the studies (Foureur et al., 2013; Sarid et al., 2012) had positive development of the SOC before to after intervention. The study of Sarid et al. (2012) was the only one with the SOC as the primary outcome.

People with Disabilities, Psychosomatic, and Mental Health Problems

A three-armed RCT study among adults suffering from psychological stress (Arvidsdotter et al., 2015) with the SOC as secondary outcome consisted of two intervention groups: therapeutic acupuncture (TA) and integrative treatment (IT) ($n = 40$) and conventional treatment (CT). IT was a combination of a person-centered approach in a salutogenic dialogue and TA. The dialogue focused on the patients' understanding of meaning and resources to help them become aware of and mobilize their strengths and potential for managing their conditions (A, L, and WPA). The dialogue was exploratory and reflected on inner feelings, personal relationships, everyday activities (diet, exercise, relaxation, sleep habits) (L), and existential issues in an atmosphere that aimed to strengthen the therapeutic alliance (SRRs). It was performed once a week, 60 minutes per session, for 8 consecutive weeks. It fulfilled four of the five criteria for a salutogenic intervention. The results revealed significant improvements in the SOC in both intervention groups (most in the IT group) after eight weeks (before to after intervention) compared to CT.

An RCT (Forsberg et al., 2010) among persons with psychiatric disabilities with the SOC as a secondary outcome included a program for a healthy living, healthy diet, and physical activity. Each study circle comprised 5–13 participants, including between two to seven residents and three to seven staff members, and all circles had the same leader. They met twice a week for two hours for the duration of 12 months, once a week for diet sessions and once a week for physical activities (SRRs and L). The participants were encouraged to actively participate (A). The intervention fulfilled three of the five salutogenic criteria. The study revealed significant differences between the intervention ($n = 24$) and the control group ($n = 17$) in the SOC after 12 months (before to after intervention) in favor of the intervention group.

Another RCT (Langeland et al., 2006) among adults with mental health challenges with SOC as primary outcome consisted of a salutogenic group intervention program. The group intervention program targets people with various mental health problems who live at home but need support from the health system (see Langeland and Vinje 2013, 2021). The intervention was a talk-therapy group once a week, 16 times, each two hours, based on salutogenesis (the five basic salutogenic principles and core concepts the SOC and GRRs). The main objective of the group intervention in this study was to increase participants' consciousness of their potential, their internal and external resistance resources (GRRs, SRRs), and their ability to use them (L) in everyday life (Cf. Langeland et al. (2007)). Active adaptation (A) and tailoring and person-centeredness (WPA) was key. The intervention thus fulfilled all five salutogenic criteria. It revealed significant improvement in the intervention ($n = 56$) group compared to the control ($n = 42$) group from before to after intervention. At 12 months' follow-up, there were still differences between the groups in favor of the intervention group. However, the differences were not significant.

Among people with psychosocial disabilities, Sancassiani et al. (2017) have performed an RCT with the SOC as a secondary outcome. The intervention was a psychosocial rehabilitative intervention focused on sailing (SRRs). It was a structured course to learn sailing in a crew lasting (A and L) three months; two lessons a week, each almost four hours. The intervention met three of the five salutogenic criteria. There were no significant differences between the intervention ($n = 23$) and control ($n = 28$) group after three months (before to after intervention).

A pilot RCT (Schrank et al., 2016) among people with psychosis, with the SOC as a secondary outcome, included an intervention that targeted four areas of development: increasing positive experiences, amplifying strengths, fostering positive relationships, and creating a more meaningful self-narrative (A, L, and SRRs). These areas were addressed using ten exercises adapted from standard positive psychotherapy (PPT): positive introductions, savoring, good things, identifying personal strengths, personal strength activity, and strength activity with significant other, forgiveness, gratitude, and positive responding (L). Sessions begin and close with music savoring exercise. In contrast to standard PPT, WELLFOCUS PPT has a reduced focus on literacy and didactics but instead includes more experiential and interactive components. All exercises and homework tasks were tailored to the individual to be specific, attainable, and personally meaningful (WPA). Participants received a phone call between sessions to support them with homework and reflect on what they have learnt. The intervention was assessed to fulfill four of the five salutogenic criteria. The results showed significant development of the SOC in the intervention group ($n = 47$) from before to after intervention compared to the control group ($n = 47$).

A follow-up (Højdahl et al., 2015) among 534 women in correctional settings with the SOC as primary outcome consisted of an intervention called the "VINN" program. The program has been described in detail elsewhere (Højdahl et al., 2013; Højdahl et al., 2014) and is built on the program about salutogenic talk therapy groups (Langeland et al., 2006; Langeland et al., 2007). Briefly, two facilitators and four to eight women meet for up to 15 three-hour sessions over 6–12 weeks. Combined with homework exercises, relaxation exercises, and group work, the women were encouraged to identify something meaningful that they can engage within their personal lives (A and L). In the groups, each woman's personal motivation for and commitment to change behavior (L and ST) was purposefully stimulated, within an atmosphere of acceptance and compassion (WPA). The intervention fulfilled all the salutogenic criteria. The results revealed significant improvements in the SOC from before to after intervention.

This section included six studies (five RCTs and one follow-up) of which two had strong salutogenic content (Højdahl et al., 2013, 2015; Langeland et al., 2006, 2007). Both revealed significant effects from before to after intervention on the SOC that was the primary outcome. Langeland's study had the strongest design of these two. The four other studies had the SOC as a secondary outcome. A total of two studies (Arvidsdotter et al., 2015; Schrank et al., 2016) also had a rather strong salutogenic intervention content. Both were RCTs and revealed effects on the SOC from before to after intervention. The RCTs of Forsberg et al. (2010) and Sancassiani et al. (2017) both had moderate salutogenic content in the intervention. While Forsberg et al. (2010) showed a significant effect on the SOC from before to after intervention, the study of Sancassiani et al. (2017) did not affect SOC.

People with Physical Problems and Hospital Patients

An RCT (Bringsvor et al., 2018) among persons with chronic obstructive pulmonary disease used the SOC as a secondary outcome. The self-management intervention, "Better living with chronic obstructive pulmonary disease," aimed to increase the participants' consciousness of their potential, their internal and external resources, and their abilities to use them, and thus to improve their self-management capabilities in the context of everyday living. The intervention was ongoing once a week (2 hours) over 11 weeks and treatment as usual along with the new intervention. A salutogenic orientation was incorporated into group conversations. This orientation included a focus on the SOC; understanding, manageability, and meaningfulness (L), and on emphasizing health as a continuum focusing on resources for health (GRRs), the person's history (WPA), the understanding of tension and strain as potentially health-promoting (ST), and active adaption (A), as described by Langeland et al. (2007). Motivational interviewing (MI), congruent with improvement in self-efficacy, enhanced activation for self-management, and a salutogenic approach was used as interaction styles. All salutogenic criteria seem to be fulfilled. The intervention group ($n = 92$) had no significant changes in the SOC compared to the control group ($n = 90$) after 12 weeks.

Another RCT study (Graziano et al., 2014) among persons with multiple sclerosis, with the SOC as a secondary outcome, included intervention sessions held in a castle surrounded by a park (GRRs). The topics of the four sessions were as follows: identity change and redefinition following the diagnosis of multiple sclerosis (SRRs), life goals that gave people a sense of coherence before the diagnosis and life goals that might give a sense of coherence after the diagnosis (L), the definitions of new, realistic, and personally meaningful goals in life, strategies to reach goals and behavior evaluation (WPA); the promotion of self-efficacy over symptoms, the management of negative emotions related to the illness; positive, negative, and illusory thinking related to the illness; effective communication and the ability to ask for help (A) and also homework. Thus, a total of four of five of the salutogenic criteria seem to be fulfilled. The study found that the SOC increased in the intervention group ($n = 41$) compared with the control ($n = 41$) after six months from before to after intervention, though the differences were not significant.

Nøst, Steinsbekk, Bratas, and Gronning (2018) report on their RCT among adults with chronic pain with the SOC as a secondary outcome. It included an intervention group that was a group-based chronic pain self-management course with 2.5-h weekly sessions for six weeks comprising cognitive and behavioral strategies (SRRs) for pain management, movement exercises, group discussions, and sharing of experiences among participants (L). The course addressed central self-management skills such as goal setting, action planning, and problem-solving and focused on empowering the participants to play an active role in their healthcare (A). The course emphasized group discussions and sharing of experiences among participants. The salutogenic content fulfilled three of the five criteria. The study found no significant differences between the intervention ($n = 60$) and control ($n = 61$) group after 6 weeks (before to after intervention), 6 months, and 12 months.

An RCT (Jensen et al., 2016) among intensive care units survivors with the SOC as a secondary outcome included an intervention that was a nurse-led individualized intensive care units recovery program. The program was based on literature and theoretical approaches toward psychological recovery, including the salutogenic model, illness narratives, person-centered communication, and elements from guided self-determination and trauma-focused cognitive behavioral therapy (SRRs). The recovery program consisted of three consultations conducted by trained study nurses. The first consultation was conducted at the clinic with the patient and close relative at 1–3 months post-intensive care units. The dialogue focused on past and present as the patient was supported in constructing an illness narrative (A and L). A prerequisite for dialogue was the provision of patient photographs taken by intensive care units nurses during recovery. Second and third consultations at 5 months and 10 months post-intensive care units were conducted by telephone. Patients prepared by completing "Reflection sheets" indicating issues of importance to the individual (L). A total of three of the five were assessed to be fulfilled. The results revealed no significant changes between the intervention ($n = 136$) and control ($n = 196$) group in the SOC after 3 months and 12 months.

A cognitive behavioral therapy (CBT) program was investigated in an RCT (Malm et al., 2018) among atrial fibrillation (AF) patients where the SOC was a secondary outcome. The CBT program consisted of three 2.5-hour group sessions over nine weeks, with four to six AF patients, including spouses. In these sessions, participants were trained to be aware of their breathing, and heart rate variability biofeedback was demonstrated. In brief, patients in the first session tried to identify and stop unpleasant feelings and negative thoughts that led to cognitive distortions. Positive psychology (SRRs) was focused upon in the second session. In the final session, the patients were taught to work smarter rather than harder (L). Each subsequent session included at least a 15–20-minute mindfulness practice (SRRs) that targeted the different foci, for example, heart focus, and heart breathing guided by the therapist. This was followed by an inquiry about the participants' experiences during practice, as well as encouragement to practice at home daily (A and L). A total of three of the five Salutogenic criteria seems to be fulfilled. The study found that the SOC improved in the CBT group ($n = 56$) after the 12-month follow-up, compared to the TAU group ($n = 55$).

A controlled clinical trial (Dehnavi et al., 2019) among persons with MS and with the SOC as primary outcome included an intervention that was a 12-session unity-focused psychodrama therapy plan for six weeks. It consisted of a description of psychodrama and its techniques, unity-oriented psychology theory, rules, building confidence and training the participants to exercise talking skills, establishing a dialogue and presenting a problem (A), concentration exercises using nonverbal ways to express awareness of emotions, getting familiar with concepts of "unity in diversity" and "diversity in unity," getting familiar with the language of body and soul and the dialogue of soul and body in the form of psychodrama for unity-oriented connection to the universe (L and WPA), practicing death awareness for understanding the immortality of the soul, and emotional and mental linkage with the source of being (L). The intervention fulfills four of the five salutogenic criteria. The results revealed significant differences between the intervention ($n = 10$) and control ($n = 10$) group on the SOC two months after the completed intervention.

Another follow-up study with a control group (Hirsikangas et al., 2018) with the SOC as a secondary outcome included frequent attenders (FA) to their general practitioners. They had different physical diseases. The intervention included the following: FAs individualized care plans, assessment of FAs care needs and resources, coordination of multi-professional services, and support of FAs in self-management. The intervention emphasized the continuity of care and building a confidential care relationship (A). It also included a patient-oriented education (L), active self-management support (A), and patient's capabilities (SRRs). FAs had an individual, customer-oriented plan in two years, and FAs visited with their matron concerning all of their health-related issues. A total of three of the five salutogenic criteria seems to be fulfilled. There was no significant differences between the intervention (n = 285) and control (n = 177) groups and the SOC decreased after two years.

Among persons with type II diabetes mellitus, with the SOC as the primary outcome, Odajima, Kawaharada, and Wada (2017) have performed a follow-up study with a control group. The intervention comprised four 30-minute group sessions and was delivered by experienced nurses. The specific types of support were as follows: The educational goal of the first session included (1) promoting mutual understanding among participants (A), (2) sharing feelings during care (A), and (3) understanding the meaning of enhancing the SOC (L). The educational content of the first session covered: (1) feeling burdened by the disease and treatment, (2) how patients have managed their diabetes to date, (3) what patients learned after diabetes diagnoses (L), and (4) SOC. A total of three of the five salutogenic criteria seems to be fulfilled. The results revealed significant improvement in the SOC in the intervention group (n = 21) compared to the control group (n = 19) after two weeks.

A prospective intervention study with a control group (Norrbrink Budh, Kowalski, and Lundeberg 2006) among patients with spinal cord injury and neuropathic pain consisted of a pain management program that had the SOC as a secondary outcome. It included 20 sessions over ten weeks and with educational sessions, behavioral therapy, relaxation, stretching, light exercise, and body awareness training (SRRs). The sessions included training in mindfulness, attention-diverting strategies, cognitive reappraisal, social skills training, the pacing of activities, homework assignments, goal setting, and meeting with a role model (A and L). A total of three of the five salutogenic criteria seems to be fulfilled. The SOC increased significantly in the intervention group (n = 38) compared to the control group (n = 11) at 12 months' follow-up.

A one-year follow-up study (Fagermoen et al., 2015) among 68 persons with morbid obesity with the SOC as primary outcome consisted of a patient education course over a period over 9–12 weeks that consisted of 40 hours. The intervention was grounded in cognitive behavior theory and emphasized the participants to discover resources and strengthening self-image (A, L, and SRRs). It included life-style changes, individual action plans, guided reflections, self-help groups, and physical activity (L, SRRs, and WPA). A total of four of the five salutogenic criteria seems to be fulfilled. The results revealed a significant improvement in the SOC after one year.

Another follow-up study (Langeland et al., 2013) among 254 adults with psoriasis with SOC as the primary outcome was a study on 3-week climate-therapy patient education (healthy lifestyles) and sun treatment. The program consisted of both sun treatment and education (SRRs). Patients received, on average, 80 hours of sun therapy during the stay. Sun exposure was scheduled for each individual per skin type and UV index. Patients were encouraged to bathe frequently in saltwater and to use moisturizing creams. A dermatologist, nurses, and physiotherapist monitored patients and provided individual and group-based education, guidance, and daily training (A and L). The teaching program contained information/dialogue about psoriasis pathogenesis, manifestations, comorbidity, quality of life, and treatment options. The importance of lifestyle choices was emphasized, with a particular focus on physical activity and healthy eating (SRRs). Discussions in smaller groups focused on finding ways to manage psoriasis in daily life. A total of three of the five salutogenic criteria seems to be fulfilled. The results showed positive development of the SOC from before to after the intervention and after three months.

This section included five RCTs, four controlled clinical trials, and two follow-up studies. One of the RCTs (Malm et al., 2018) had a significant effect on the SOC at 12 months follow-up. This study has the strongest design with a good sample size, has a relatively long-term significant effect, and includes a moderate salutogenic intervention. A total of three (Dehnavi et al., 2019; Norrbrink Budh et al., 2006; Odajima et al., 2017), of the four clinical controlled trials, had significant improvements in the SOC. However, these studies have a weaker design and small sample sizes, and the effect was measured from before to after intervention except from the study of Norrbrink Budh et al. (2006) that included a 12 months follow-up and Dehnavi et al. (2019) that had a two months follow-up. Both the follow-up studies (Fagermoen et al., 2015; Langeland et al., 2013) showed significant improvements in the SOC at 12 and 3-months of follow-up, respectively. The studies of Dehnavi et al. (2019) and Fagermoen et al. (2015) had the strongest salutogenic content.

Elderly People

An RCT (Arola et al., 2018) among 131 older immigrants with the SOC as a primary outcome included an intervention aimed at creating regular encounters where participants support one another to make health-supporting decisions in daily life. It consisted of "senior meetings" with follow-up home visits. The meetings were organized by an interdisciplinary group of professionals, where each professional was responsible for one meeting and one follow-up home visit. A written booklet in the participants' native language supplied written information about health-related issues as a specific resistance resource (SSR). The topics and focus of the meetings were directed by the experiences and needs of the participants, such that the themes varied according to participants' preferences. This allows participants' active adaption (A). The interventions used a person-centered approach and focused on the person as an individual beyond any diagnoses or illnesses and thereby fulfill the criterion of the whole-person approach (WPA). Peer learning was adopted to support the awareness of health resources in daily life among participants. Social support, sharing of knowledge, and experiences about health further provided important resources (GRRs). Peer-learning and home visits created better opportunities for the individual to transfer knowledge in daily life. Thereby the intervention also fulfills the criterion of strengthening the SOC by learning processes (L). This program thus fulfills four of the five criteria of a salutogenic intervention.

The study found a significant change in the intervention group (n = 56) compared to the control group (n = 75) at six months and no significant differences between groups 12 months after the intervention.

A second RCT (Ericson et al., 2018) among healthy 32 women (ages 65–70 years) with the SOC as a primary outcome included resistance training (described in Strandberg et al. (2015)) in the intervention. It was conducted for 24 weeks. The exercises performed in the gym were squats, leg extensions, leg presses, seated rows and pulldowns, squat jumps, and core stability exercises. The intervention met two criteria of a salutogenic intervention: it provided access to physical activity and social support (GRRs) and it requested active participation (A). The results showed no significant difference between the intervention (n = 14) and control (n = 18) group on the SOC from before to after intervention.

Kekäläinen, Kokko, Sipila, and Walker (2018) report on their RCT among older adults with the SOC as a secondary outcome. The 9-month resistance training intervention consisted of different exercises for different muscle groups. In the first phase, all training groups attended supervised resistance training twice a week for three months. For the following six months, they continued training with different frequencies (1, 2, or 3 times per week). This intervention meets two criteria of salutogenic interventions. It provides active involvement of participants (A) and access to GRRs (physical well-being and activity, social contacts). The results revealed significant effects on the SOC in two of the three intervention groups (n = 26, 27, 28 respectively) compared to the control (n = 25) group from before intervention to after intervention.

Hourzad, Pouladi, Ostovar, and Ravanipour (2018) conducted an RCT among the elderly with chronic diseases using the SOC as a secondary outcome. The intervention, an empowerment self-management program, lasted eight weeks and aimed at improving participants' health, preventive behaviors, self-esteem, self-care behaviors, compliance with the long-term use of medication, the understanding of changes (in physical, mental, and social abilities), and the ability to manage stressful events. The intervention included five stages:

1. Self-awareness of changes, personal level of performance, and expectations: Participants evaluated the extent of changes in their physical, mental, and social abilities after retirement. They assessed the status of their performance, autonomy, adaptation to the existing conditions, and support resources, and they determined their expected level of performance after the intervention.
2. Goal setting: Participants defined a set of goals, the available supporting resources, and the possibilities for changing or modifying those resources toward the development of a set of strategies.
3. Planning: Based on the developed goals, a plan was drawn that incorporated the recommendations of the participants, available resources, and the program leader's expertise in an empowerment model. Stages 1–3 were conducted in two sessions of 45 minutes each.
4. Adjusting physical, psychological, and social structures: The participants were then requested to implement the defined strategies of their plan within six weeks during which the intervention team followed up their progress by phone on a weekly basis. Aims and strategies varied among participants and covered a wide range of topics, such as to learn how to receive timely information from the medical care system on various aspects of their disease, to learn new skills to compensate for their shortcomings, to learn how to handle available resources to maintain their health, to gain new empowerment skills (e.g., pottery, fishing, or other leisure activities), to preserve their role in the family, and to communicate effectively with those around them. In support of the implementation phase, the participants were advised to use the educational booklet and could freely call the intervention team by phone to clarify questions.
5. Evaluation: Program leaders conducted a follow-up evaluation over six weeks to ensure proper implementation of the proposed program and interventions. Participants who did execute less than 40% of the specified measures were excluded from the study program.

This intervention covers four criteria of salutogenic interventions, providing specific and general resistance resources (SRRs, GRRs), active involvement of participants (A), and a learning process (L). The intervention group (*n* = 29) revealed significant improvements in participants' SOC compared to the control group (*n* = 29) in routine care after eight weeks (before to after intervention).

An individually tailored, 12-week strength-power training program was investigated in an RCT (Pakkala et al., 2012) among 60- to 85-year-old people with hip fractures. The SOC was a primary outcome. The intervention consisted of resistance training for 12 weeks, conducted twice a week in a senior gym, and supervised by an experienced physiotherapist. Training intensity was adjusted individually and, when tolerated, increased progressively throughout the training period. The assessment was repeated in weeks 6–8 and training resistance adjusted accordingly. The assessment with the criteria for salutogenic interventions showed that two criteria were met: physical activity and individual support as GRRs and active participation in the intervention program (A). It found no significant differences between the intervention (*n* = 24) and control (*n* = 22) groups from before to after intervention.

An RCT (Sundsli et al., 2014) was conducted with 30 older home-living persons with the SOC as a secondary outcome. The intervention to improve self-care included a meeting with health professionals and additional five telephone talk sessions about self-care. The self-care talks captured topics such as practicing healthy habits, building self-esteem, focusing on the positive, communicating, and building meaning. It addressed GRRs (healthy habits, self-esteem, building meaning), fostered active participation (A), and induced a learning process (L). Accordingly, the intervention met three of the five salutogenic criteria. No significant differences between experiment (*n* = 15) and control (*n* = 15) groups after 19 weeks were found.

The Resource Enhancement and Activation Program (REAP) was investigated in an RCT (Tan et al., 2016) among older people in the community with the SOC as a primary outcome. The intervention included a 12-week (twice-weekly participation) program that was offered at community clubs and senior activity centers. REAP focuses on motivation, personal responsibilities, physical activity, and social and environmental impacts on health behavior. Through REAP, older people could review available external resources (e.g., public and health policies, neighborhood exercise facilities and groups, family and friends) and internal resources (e.g., values, assertiveness, self-efficacy skills). The rating with the salutogenic intervention criteria scored relatively high for this intervention since it addressed four salutogenic criteria: the person as a whole (WPA), fostered active involvement (A), facilitated a learning process (L) and it provided access to resources (GRRs, SRRs) such as motivation, personal responsibilities, physical activity, and social coherence. It promoted the understanding of external life challenges of older people (e.g., health, dependence care, and death) and the understanding of their personal beliefs, thoughts (e.g., new roles), and emotions (e.g., stress). The results showed significant differences between experiment (*n* = 32) and control (*n* = 32) groups from before intervention to after intervention.

The only intergenerational program related to the SOC (primary outcome) we found was reported in a follow-up study with a control group by Murayama et al. (2015). The intervention educated and engaged senior volunteers in picture book reading projects with preschool and school-aged children in educational settings. The rating based on the criteria showed access to GRRs (significant and meaningful contribution to society, social contacts, emotional and intellectual activation) and an active adaptation of participants (A). It found significant differences between the intervention (*n* = 26) and control (*n* = 24) groups in the SOC after nine months, one year, and two years after the intervention. However, the sample size was limited after two years (intervention group, *n* = 6, Control, *n* = 15).

Addressing self-management and following a similar proceeding as Hourzad et al. (2018), the intervention investigated by Musavinasab, Ravanipour, Pouladi, Motamed, and Barekat (2016) was addressed to a group of elderly with cardiovascular disease. The clinical trial conducted by the authors used the SOC as a primary outcome. The intervention (three to four months) consisted of five steps based on the self-management empowerment model. This included self-awareness of changes and an understanding of the levels of performance and expectations of themselves, the individuals, knowledge of changes in physical capacities in psychological and social capacities, the level of adaptation to the current situation, support resources, and the elderly's expectations of themselves (A, L and SRRs). Further, optimum goal setting, enhancing the autonomy to perform self-care behaviors, and improving the individual's understanding and knowledge of the changes in his/her physical, psychological, and social capacities (WPA) were given attention. The intervention fulfilled four of the five salutogenic criteria. The study revealed significant differences between the experimental group (*n* = 50) and control (*n* = 50) groups from before intervention to after intervention.

This section included seven RCTs and two controlled clinical trials. A total of four (Arola et al., 2018; Hourzad et al., 2018; Musavinasab et al., 2016; Tan et al., 2016) of the studies (three RCTs and one controlled clinical trial) fulfilled four of the five salutogenic criteria and all reported a significant effect on the SOC from before to after intervention. The controlled clinical trial (Murayama et al., 2015) fulfilled two of the criteria and showed effect after two years. However, the sample size was limited after two years and the design was weaker. The RCTs of Kekäläinen et al. (2018), Ericson et al. (2018), and Pakkala et al. (2012) included all two salutogenic criteria, and Kekäläinen et al. (2018) revealed significant effect and the two other no significant effect from before to after intervention. The RCT of Sundsli et al. (2014) included three salutogenic criteria in the intervention and revealed no significant effect on the SOC.

Interventions on Other Topics

A follow-up study (Edwards, 2006) among 26 exercisers at health clubs, with the SOC as a secondary outcome. The intervention was physical exercise for two to six months. Regular exercise was defined as meeting the criterion of exercising for an average of 30 minutes a day at least three times a week. The following salutogenic criteria are fulfilled: the GRRs (physical activity), active adaptation (A), and learning (L). The result shows significant improvement in the SOC from before to after intervention.

A follow-up study (Heggdal and Lovaas, 2018) among 108 people with different long-term physical and mental illnesses with the SOC as primary outcome found no significant changes in the total SOC score in the whole sample. The intervention, the Bodyknowledging Program, consisted of seven sessions stretched over four months. Bodyknowledging can be defined as a fundamental process for the development of personal knowledge about one's own body, coping skills, health, and well-being. It was conducted in 3-hour group sessions involving eight to ten persons living with different kinds of long-term conditions or in a 1.5-hour individual format with the same content. The following salutogenic criteria seem included: SRRs, WPA, A and L.

This section, including two follow-up studies, shows two different kinds of studies. Edwards (2006) has a rather simple intervention with a small sample and a rather weak salutogenic content and revealed significant improvement in the SOC. The study of Heggdal and Lovaas (2018) includes a rather strong salutogenic content in the intervention. However, there was no significant improvement in the SOC.

Discussion

This scoping review has included 41 intervention studies with SOC as the primary or secondary outcome. We developed and agreed upon five criteria for assessing the extent of salutogenically oriented content in the interventions. In addition, we explored the development of the SOC in all intervention studies.

The Extent of Salutogenic Content in the Interventions of the Different Studies

The analysis of the salutogenic orientation in the interventions was justified by the assumption that a match between the content of the intervention and the desired outcome will improve the latter (Coster, 2013). The outcome must be sensitive and compatible with the intervention to catch the eventually change among participants. It is reasonable to think that whether the SOC might change depends on the quality of the intervention such as fulfilling the criteria for salutogenic interventions, sample, duration and intensity, and the match with the outcome SOC.

Most of the studies have implemented interventions that have multiple strategies, including many different variables and might be defined as complex interventions (Bleijenberg et al., 2018). Accordingly, the interventions, therefore, represent a broad causal concept, including several elements, aims, and intentions.

Further, most interventions provided several GRRs/SRRs, and there was a broad range of different resources for promoting the SOC: for example, group climate, high quality of social support, physical exercise, sailing, music, cultural activities, relaxation exercises, emotional regulation, increased knowledge and ability to use it, increased meaning in life, the consciousness of and use of internal and external resources, and improved action competence.

Also, the included interventions vary in their topics, target groups, and duration. The longest intervention period was 15 months (Bronikowski and Bronikowska, 2009) and the shortest intervention period was two weeks (Odajima et al., 2017).

All the interventions in the included studies fulfilled at least two of the five criteria to be defined as salutogenic (Cf. Table 20.2). However, only three studies fulfilled all five salutogenic criteria. These studies explicitly describe and include the basic philosophical assumptions, the main concepts, and crucial spheres to keep or promote meaning (Bringsvor et al., 2018; Højdahl et al., 2015; Langeland et al., 2006). All interventions included the criterion of active adaptation. Although many of them did not mention active adaption explicitly, active adaption was included due to all interventions requiring active adaptation for people to participate. Had we adopted the criterion more strictly, in the sense that participants have to be allowed to influence the content of the intervention, fewer interventions would fulfill the requested level of active adaptation. The key to active adaptation and learning is that all human beings have to actively adapt to inevitable stressful rich environment and seek for useful inputs that create negative entropy and thus might promote coping (Antonovsky, 1987). All the interventions had a more or less strong focus on GRRs and/or SRRs.

Almost all interventions fulfilled the criteria of learning (L). If the participants experienced load balance or appropriate challenges, learning is key. It has, however, been difficult to assess to what degree participants have experienced appropriate challenges. In all interventions, participants have an active role and adapt, but it is unclear whether they experience load balance or appropriate challenges or overload/underload. The number of dropouts in the different studies might indicate overload. However, to systematically assess dropouts is beyond the scope of this review.

A few studies (Bringsvor et al., 2018; Højdahl et al., 2015; Langeland et al., 2006) have explicitly applied the salutogenic view of stressors that includes that stressors and tension might be salutogenic (Cf. criteria 4), neutral, or pathogenic.

Change and Development of the SOC in Different Life Situations

The periods of follow-up measures in the studies reviewed vary remarkably (cf. Table 20.2). A total of 29 of the 41 included studies just include measurements before and after the intervention. The follow-up periods varied between 2 weeks and 15 months. Studies accordingly did not report long-term follow-up measurements. A total of 24 studies report significant improvement in the SOC from before to after intervention. Of these, eight are RCTs (Arola et al., 2018; Arvidsdotter et al., 2015; Forsberg et al., 2010; Hourzad et al., 2018) (Kekäläinen et al., 2018; Langeland et al., 2006; Malm et al., 2018; Nammontri et al., 2013), nine follow-up studies with control group or another intervention group (Bronikowski and Bronikowska, 2009; Dehnavi et al., 2019; Kähönen et al., 2012; Merakou et al., 2019; Murayama et al., 2015; Musavinasab et al., 2016; Norrbrink Budh et al., 2006; Odajima et al., 2017; Sarid et al., 2012), and seven follow-up studies without a control group (Edwards, 2006; Fagermoen et al., 2015; Foureur et al., 2013; Gunnarsson and Bjorklund, 2013; Højdahl et al., 2015; Langeland et al., 2013; Vastamäki et al., 2009).

Further, we have expected that studies that have defined the SOC as the primary outcome would have a higher degree of match between salutogenic content and positive development of the SOC (Coster, 2013). Of the 26 studies that revealed a positive development of the SOC, 14 had the SOC as the primary outcome and 12 had the SOC as a secondary outcome. This might mean that being a primary or secondary outcome does not matter. However, only five studies with the SOC as primary outcome did not find a positive development of the SOC. This issue has to be further explored in future research.

The present review focused on possible changes in the SOC due to interventions. The SOC is conceptualized as a relatively stable, though changeable orientation that – as a consequence of learning processes – generally improves during life. It may be temporarily weakened or strengthened by major live events. Therefore, the possibility of temporary fluctuation of the SOC has to be taken into account: "If one tries to run short-term interventions the result may be confounded by such interventions" (Lindström and Eriksson, 2010, p.46). This might be true for some of the intervention studies described above, especially the follow-up studies without a control group and with short-time follow-up measures. The most solid intervention studies in this review with follow-ups longer than six months are the RCT studies of Arola et al. (2018), Jensen et al. (2016), Langeland et al. (2006), and Malm et al. (2018). However, only the study of Malm et al. (2018) revealed a significant effect on the SOC at 12 months' follow-up. The study included a CBT intervention program that consisted of three 2.5-hour group sessions over nine weeks, with four to six AF patients, including spouses. However, the change in the SOC was rather small.

Further, it is important to clarify what is meant by a major strengthening of the SOC. Antonovsky claims that if a substantial number of people experience a given mode of therapy and improve their SOC score by five points on the average "this is not to be sneezed at" (Antonovsky, 1996a, p.176). Moreover, he also suggests that practitioners can arrange for SOC-enhancing experiences and he writes: "This would be true for any therapeutic mode that facilitates a long-lasting, consistent change in real-life experiences that people undergo" (Antonovsky, 1987, p.126). Many of the interventions in the present study revealed significant changes above four points from before to after intervention (cf. Table 20.2). However, only one of the studies with the long-term positive development of the SOC revealed changes above five points (Fagermoen et al., 2015). However, the study of Fagermoen et al. (2015) had no control group.

The Effect on Participants' SOC According to the Interventions' Salutogenic Orientation

RCT studies based on Antonovsky's basic salutogenic orientation, in which the SOC is defined as the primary outcome, shows significant improvement will support the assumption that salutogenesis has contributed to the effect. In salutogenic intervention studies, the process that may lead to change the dependent variable, SOC, might, for example, be explained as follows: Through empowering dialogues, based on the salutogenic principles including comprehensibility, manageability, and meaning, with focus on crucial life spheres, resistance resources, and appropriate challenges (balance between overload and underload), the participants may increase their awareness of their potential, their internal and external resources (increased imaginable competence and manageability), and their ability to use them. Thus, they might learn to use salutogenic coping mechanisms more consciously and move toward more comfortable and creative inner adjustment and growth, productive use of emotional energy, more joy, generosity, and more reciprocal interaction with others. In this way, they may have developed their salutogenic capacity and, subsequently, their well-being.

Several recent in-depth studies have started to shed light on salutogenic processes demonstrating in detail how the activation of GRRs in everyday life contribute to strengthening the SOC (Langeland et al., 2016; Maass et al., 2017). For example, studies have found that incorporating sessions dedicated to self-examination and coping, such as through the use of narrative therapy may strengthen self-identity (Langeland and Vinje, 2013; Langeland et al., 2007). Further, studies show how professionals can improve the "Sense of Coherence" of the people they work with through the dimensions of the Sense *for* Coherence (Meier Magistretti et al., 2019; Meier Magistretti et al., 2016).

Some studies possibly are of special interest because they revealed positive development of the SOC six months or longer after the intervention was completed. The follow-up study of Fagermoen et al. (2015) revealed significant development of SOC 12 months after course completion. The intervention consisted of 40 hours for 9–12 weeks, with a sample of people suffering from morbid obesity. The intervention fulfilled four of the five salutogenic criteria. Further, the follow-up study of Gunnarsson and Bjorklund (2013), about adults with different psychiatric diagnoses, showed a significant positive change in the SOC three years after completed therapy and also included a strong salutogenic content (four criteria) in the intervention. In addition, a prospective intervention study with a control group of (Norrbrink Budh et al. 2006) among patients with spinal cord injury and neuropathic that included 20 sessions over 10 weeks, fulfilled 3 salutogenic criteria. The SOC increased significantly in the intervention group (n = 38) compared to the control group (n = 11) at 12 months of follow-up. However, the sample sizes were small and the significant difference was mainly due to the decrease of the SOC in the control group.

Furthermore, an RCT (Malm et al., 2018) among atrial fibrillation (AF) patients included a CBT intervention program consisting of three 2.5-hour group sessions over nine weeks. A total of three of the five salutogenic criteria seems to be fulfilled. The study found that the SOC significantly improved in the CBT group after the 12-month follow-up, compared to the TAU group. Murayama et al. (2015) follow-up study with a control group revealed significant differences between the intervention (n = 26) and control (n = 24) groups in the SOC after three months, one year, and two years after the intervention. However, the sample size was limited after two years (intervention group, n = 6, Control, n = 15). It fulfilled two of the salutogenic criteria.

The two RCT studies (Arola et al., 2018; Langeland et al., 2006) revealed a significant effect from before to after intervention that lasted for six months. The interventions in these studies had a strong salutogenic content fulfilling respectively four and five salutogenic criteria. However, at 12 months of follow-up, the positive change in the SOC was not significant any longer. It is important, though, to take into consideration the samples of older immigrants and people with long-term mental health challenges, respectively. It is reasonable to believe that these groups need follow-up interventions to keep and/or strengthen the improvement of the SOC.

Most of the interventions fulfill three of the five salutogenic criteria and preliminary we might suggest that it seems that there is not any strong relationship between the extent of salutogenic content and the effect on the SOC. However, we have based our assessment on what has been written about the interventions given and we do not know to what degree this has been implemented and how the participants have experienced the intervention.

Accordingly, we need more studies and knowledge on these issues by performing in-depth interviews among health professionals and participants.

Strengths and Limitations

Searches have been performed on different databases twice. To the best of our knowledge, all available English-language papers that fulfill the inclusion criteria have been included.

The present review has included articles in English. This means that papers with intervention studies with the SOC as an outcome in other languages such as German or Polish have been excluded.

Some methodological limitations need to be considered. The outcome of the SOC (cf. Table 20.2, last column) has been reported in different ways in the different studies. Most of the studies report the SOC-scale scores and p-values. However, others report only the change scores (difference) or CI or p-values. The degree of detail and accuracy of the descriptions of the interventions varied among the studies in this overview. Some interventions were explained in detail in a separate paper (cf. Table 20.2). It has also been challenging that the papers do not explicitly describe the content of the control group. Some describe it as treatment as usual and do not clarify what it is. Some do not comment on the control group. Besides, some RCTs and controlled clinical trials do not report whether the experiment group has received the intervention of the control group in addition to the new intervention.

We have assessed the different interventions according to our criteria for salutogenic interventions. To our best knowledge, only a few scholars (Álvarez et al., 2020; Polhuis et al., 2020) have tried to develop criteria, but we believe we have further elaborated existing criteria integrating the theory and findings of Antonovsky (1987), Langeland et al. (2006, 2007), and Langeland and Vinje (2013).

Implications for Further Research

This scoping review reveals that we need to further unravel what salutogenic interventions entail and study their effectiveness and develop salutogenic interventions that at least fulfill the five salutogenic criteria. It is reasonable to think that more specific salutogenic interventions, including health promotion aims, are likely to make the SOC and other relevant salutogenic outcomes more sensitive for change.

Also, we need several longitudinal salutogenic intervention studies with larger samples size and stronger research designs such as RCTs to increase the knowledge about the SOC's ability to change in the long run.

Conclusion

This overview indicates that it is possible to improve the SOC in the whole life course among different groups. Health promotion professionals (Cf. Langeland et al., 2021) should therefore work person-centered and resource-oriented with a focus on the SOC in different challenging life situations and thus arrange for people to come into a positive interplay between different resistance resources and the SOC to improve health (especially mental health) and well-being.

This review also reveals that there is a dearth of longitudinal RCT studies, including salutogenic interventions in the life course with SOC as an outcome. Overall, the chapter indicates that it is possible to improve the SOC in different challenging life situations if pre- and post-intervention states are compared. However, we lack studies measuring long-term outcomes, and we don't know if the progress in strengthening the SOC is long-lasting. The interventions aiming to strengthen the SOC seem to comprehend at least three qualities: they facilitate access and use of GRRs and/or SRRs, they foster active adaptation of participants, and they induce a learning process. To strengthen the salutogenic content, it is important to also include the whole person approach (WPA) and that stressors and tension (ST) might be potentially health-promoting.

References

Álvarez, O. S., Ruiz-Cantero, M. T., Cassetti, V., Cofino, R., & Alvarez-Dardet, C. (2020). Salutogenic interventions and health effects: A scoping review of the literature. *Gaceta Sanitaria*. https://doi.org/10.1016/j.gaceta.2019.12.002

Antonovsky, A. (1979). *Health, stress, and coping*. Jossey-Bass.

Antonovsky, A. (1987). *Unraveling the mystery of health: How people manage stress and stay well*. Jossey-Bass.

Antonovsky, A. (1992). Can attitudes contribute to health? *Advances, 8*(4), 33–49.

Antonovsky, A. (1996a). The sense of coherence: An historical and future perspective. *Israel Journal of Medical Sciences, 32*, 170–178.

Antonovsky, A. (1996b). The salutogenic model as a theory to guide health promotion. *Health Promotion International, 11*(1), 11–18.

Arola, L. A., Barenfeld, E., Dahlin-Ivanoff, S., & Haggblom-Kronlof, G. (2018). Distribution and evaluation of sense of coherence among older immigrants before and after a health promotion intervention - results from the RCT study promoting aging migrants' capability. *Clinical Interventions in Aging, 13*, 2317–2328. https://doi.org/10.2147/CIA.S177791

Arvidsdotter, T., Marklund, B., Taft, C., & Kylen, S. (2015). Quality of life, sense of coherence and experiences with three different treatments in patients with psychological distress in primary care: A mixed-methods study. *BMC Complementary and Alternative Medicine, 15*, 132. https://doi.org/10.1186/s12906-015-0654-z

Bauer, G., Roy, M., Bakibinga, P., Contu, P., Downe, S., Eriksson, M., Espnes, G. A., Jensen, B. B., Juvinya Canal, D., Lindström Mana, B. A., Mittelmark, M. B., Morgan, A. R., Pelikan, J. M., Saboga-Nunes, L., Sagy, S., Shorey, S., Vaandrager, L., & Vinje, H. F. (2019). Future directions for the concept of salutogenesis: a position article. *Health Promotion International*, 1–9.

Bleijenberg, N., Janneke, M., Trappenburg, J. C., Ettema, R. G., Sino, C. G., Heim, N., … Schuurmans, M. J. (2018). Increasing value and reducing waste by optimizing the development of complex interventions: Enriching the development phase of the Medical Research Council (MRC) Framework. *International Journal of Nursing Studies, 79*, 86–93.

Bringsvor, H. B., Langeland, E., Oftedal, B. F., Skaug, K., Assmus, J., & Bentsen, S. B. (2018). Effects of a COPD self-management support intervention: a randomized controlled trial. *International Journal of Chronic Obstructive Pulmonary Disease, 13*, 3677–3688. https://doi.org/10.2147/COPD.S181005

Bronikowski, M., & Bronikowska, M. (2009). Salutogenesis as a framework for improving health resources of adolescent boys. *Scandinavian Journal of Public Health, 37*(5), 525–531. https://doi.org/10.1177/1403494809105289

Brooks, D. M., Bradt, J., Eyre, L., Hunt, A., & Dileo, C. (2010). Creative approaches for reducing burnout in medical personnel. *The Arts in Psychotherapy, 37*(3), 255–263. https://doi.org/10.1016/j.aip.2010.05.001

Coster, W. J. (2013). Making the best match: selecting outcome measures for clinical trials and outcome studies. *American Journal of Occupational Therapy, 67*(2), 162–170. https://doi.org/10.5014/ajot.2013.006015

Davidson, O. B., Feldman, D. B., & Margalit, M. (2012). A focused intervention for 1st-year college students: Promoting hope, sense of coherence, and self-efficacy. *Journal of Psychology, 146*(3), 333–352. https://doi.org/10.1080/00223980.2011.634862

Dehnavi, S., Zadeh Mohammadi, A., & HassaniRaad, M. (2019). Effectiveness of Unity-Oriented Psychodrama on Sense of Coherence of MS Patients. *Iranian Journal of Psychiatry and Behavioral Sciences, 13*(1). https://doi.org/10.5812/ijpbs.5869

Downe, S. (2010). Towards Salutogenic Birth in the 21st Century. In D. Walsh & S. Downe (Eds.), *Essential Midwifery Practice: Intrapartum Care*. (pp. 289–295): Blackwell Publishing.

Edwards, S. (2006). Physical exercise and psychological wellbeing. *South Africa Journal of Psychology, 36*(2), 357–373.

Ericson, H., Skoog, T., Johansson, M., & Wahlin-Larsson, B. (2018). Resistance training is linked to heightened positive motivational state and lower negative affect among healthy women aged 65–70. *Journal of Women and Aging, 30*(5), 366–381. https://doi.org/10.1080/08952841.2017.1301720.

Eriksson, M., & Lindström, B. (2005). Validity of Antonovsky's sense of coherence scale: A systematic review. *Journal of Epidemiology and Community Health, 59*(6), 460–466.

Eriksson, M., & Lindström, B. (2006). Antonovsky's sense of coherence scale and the relation with health: A systematic review. *Journal of Epidemiology and Community Health, 60*(5), 376–381.

Eriksson, M., & Lindström, B. (2007). Antonovsky's sense of coherence scale and its relation with quality of life: a systematic review. *Journal of Epidemiology and Community Health, 61*(11), 938–944.

Eriksson, M., & Mittelmark, M. B. (2017). The sense of coherence and its measurement. In M. B. Mittelmark, S. Sagy, M. Eriksson, G. Bauer, J. Pelikan, B. Lindström, & G. A. Espnes (Eds.), *The handbook of salutogenesis* (pp. 97–106): Springer.

Fagermoen, M. S., Hamilton, G., & Lerdal, A. (2015). Morbid obese adults increased their sense of coherence 1 year after a patient education course: A longitudinal study. *Journal of Multidisciplinary Healthcare, 8*, 157–165. https://doi.org/10.2147/JMDH.S77763

Forsberg, K. A., Bjorkman, T., Sandman, P. O., & Sandlund, M. (2010). Influence of a life-style intervention among persons with a psychiatric disability: A cluster randomized controlled trail on symptoms, quality of life and sense of coherence. *Journal of Clinical Nursing, 19*(11–12), 1519–1528. https://doi.org/10.1111/j.1365-2702.2009.03010.x

Foureur, M., Besley, K., Burton, G., Yu, N., & Crisp, J. (2013). Enhancing the resilience of nurses and midwives: Pilot of a mindfulness-based program for increased health, sense of coherence and decreased depression, anxiety and stress. *Contemporary Nurse, 45*, 114–125. https://doi.org/10.5172/conu.2013.45.1.114

Garcia-Moya, I., & Morgan, A. (2017). The utility of salutogenesis for guiding health promotion: the case for young people's wellbeing. *Health Promotion International, 32*(4), 723–733. https://doi.org/10.1093/heapro/daw008

Grant, M. J., & Booth, A. (2009). A typology of reviews: an analysis of 14 review types and associated methodologies. *Health Information & Libraries Journal, 26*(2), 91–108.

Graziano, F., Calandri, E., Borghi, M., & Bonino, S. (2014). The effects of a group-based cognitive behavioral therapy on people with multiple sclerosis: a randomized controlled trial. *Clinical Rehabilitation, 28*(3), 264–274. https://doi.org/10.1177/0269215513501525.

Griffiths, C. A. (2009). Sense of coherence and mental health rehabilitation. *Clinical Rehabilitation, 23*(1), 72–78.

Gunnarsson, A. B., & Bjorklund, A. (2013). Sustainable enhancement in clients who perceive the Tree Theme Method((R)) as a positive intervention in psychosocial occupational therapy. *Australian Occupational Therapy Journal, 60*(3), 154–160. https://doi.org/10.1111/1440-1630.12034

Heggdal, K., & Lovaas, B. J. (2018). Health promotion in specialist and community care: how a broadly applicable health promotion intervention influences patient's sense of coherence. *Scandinavian Journal of Caring Sciences, 32*(2), 690–697. https://doi.org/10.1111/scs.12498

Hirsikangas, S., Kanste, O., Korpelainen, J., Bloigu, R., & Kyngäs, H. (2018). The effects of intervention on the quality of life, sense of coherence and daily activities of frequent attenders. *Journal of Nursing Education and Practice, 8*(2), 63–71. doi:DOI: https://doi.org/10.5430/jnep.v8n2p63

Hochwälder, J. (2019). Sense of coherence: Notes on some challenges for future research. *SAGE Open, 9*(2), 2158244019846687.

Hourzad, A., Pouladi, S., Ostovar, A., & Ravanipour, M. (2018). The effects of an empowering self-management model on self-efficacy and sense of coherence among retired elderly with chronic diseases: A randomized controlled trial. *Clinical Interventions in Aging, 13*, 2215–2224. https://doi.org/10.2147/CIA.S183276

Højdahl, T., Magnus, J. H., Hagen, R., & Langeland, E. (2013). " VINN"-An accredited motivational program promoting convicted women's sense of coherence and coping.

Højdahl, T., Magnus, J. H., & Langeland, E. (2014). A bridge to change: Experiences of participation in "VINN"—A motivational program for convicted women. A qualitative study. *EuroVista: Probation and Community Justice, 3*(2), 81–96.

Højdahl, T., Magnus, J. H., Mdala, I., Hagen, R., & Langeland, E. (2015). Emotional distress and sense of coherence in women completing a motivational program in five countries. A prospective study. *International Journal of Prisoner Health, 11*(3), 169–182. https://doi.org/10.1108/IJPH-10-2014-0037

Jensen, J. F., Egerod, I., Bestle, M. H., Christensen, D. F., Elklit, A., Hansen, R. L., ... Overgaard, D. (2016). A recovery program to improve quality of life, sense of coherence and psychological health in ICU survivors: a multicenter randomized controlled trial, the RAPIT study. *Intensive Care Medicine, 42*(11), 1733–1743. https://doi.org/10.1007/s00134-016-4522-1

Kähönen, K., Naatanen, P., Tolvanen, A., & Salmela-Aro, K. (2012). Development of sense of coherence during two group interventions. *Scandinavian Journal of Psychology, 53*(6), 523–527. https://doi.org/10.1111/sjop.12020

Kekäläinen, T., Kokko, K., Sipila, S., & Walker, S. (2018). Effects of a 9-month resistance training intervention on quality of life, sense of coherence, and depressive symptoms in older adults: Randomized controlled trial. *Quality of Life Research, 27*(2), 455–465. https://doi.org/10.1007/s11136-017-1733-z

Langeland, E. (2007). *Sense of coherence and life satisfaction in people suffering from mental health problems: An intervention study in talk-therapy groups with focus on salutogenesis*. University of Bergen.

Langeland, E., Ausland, L., Gunnarsdottir, H., Arveklev, S., & Vinje, H. F. (2021). Promoting salutogenic capacity in health professionals. In M. B. Mittelmark & M. Fere (Eds.), *Handbook of salutogenesis: Past, present and future.* (pp. x): Springer.

Langeland, E., Gjengedal, E., & Vinje, H. F. (2016). Building salutogenic capacity: A year of experience from a salutogenic talk-therapy group. *International Journal of Mental Health Promotion, 18*(5), 247–262. https://doi.org/10.1080/14623730.2016.1230070

Langeland, E., Riise, T., Hanestad, B. R., Nortvedt, M. W., Kristoffersen, K., & Wahl, A. K. (2006). The effect of salutogenic treatment principles on coping with mental health problems A randomized controlled trial. *Patient Education and Counseling, 62*(2), 212–219. https://doi.org/10.1016/j.pec.2005.07.004

Langeland, E., Robinson, H. S., Moum, T., Larsen, M. H., Krogstad, A.-L., & Wahl, A. K. (2013). Promoting sense of coherence: Salutogenesis among people with psoriasis undergoing patient education in climate therapy. *BMC psychology, 1*(1), 11.

Langeland, E., & Vinje, H. F. (2013). The significance of salutogenesis and wellbeing in mental health promotion: From theory to practice. In C. L. M. Keyes (Ed.), *Mental wellbeing: International contributions to the study of positive mental health* (pp. 299–329). Springer.

Langeland, E., & Vinje, H. F. (2017). The application of salutogenesis in mental healthcare settings. In M. B. Mittelmark & et.al *The handbook of salutogenesis* (pp. 299–305): Springer.

Langeland, E., & Vinje, H. F. (2021). The application of salutogenesis in mental health care settings. In M. B. Mittelmark & et.al (Eds.), *Handbook of salutogenesis: Past, present and future* (pp. x): Springer.

Langeland, E., Wahl, A. K., Kristoffersen, K., & Hanestad, B. R. (2007). Promoting coping: Salutogenesis among people with mental health problems. *Issues in Mental Health Nursing, 28*(3), 275–295. https://doi.org/10.1080/01612840601172627.

Lezwijn, J., Vaandrager, L., Naaldenberg, J., Wagemakers, A., Koelen, M., & van Woerkum, C. (2011). Healthy ageing in a salutogenic way: building the HP 2.0 framework. *Health & Social Care in the Community, 19*(1), 43–51. https://doi.org/10.1111/j.1365-2524.2010.00947.x

Lindström, B., Berg, M., Meier Magistretti, C., Perez-Botella, M., & Down, S. (2017). The salutogenetic approach to maternity care: from theory to practice and research. In *New thinking on improving maternity care*. Pinter & Martin Ltd..

Lindström, B., & Eriksson, M. (2010). *The hitchhiker's guide to salutogenesis: salutogenic pathways to health promotion.* Helsinki: Folkhälsan Research Centre, Health Promotion Research [etc.].

Maass, R., Lindström, B., & Lillefjell, M. (2017). Neighborhood-resources for the development of a strong SOC and the importance of understanding why and how resources work: a grounded theory approach. *BMC Public Health, 17*(1), 1–13.

Magrin, M. E., Bruno, C., Gheno, S., & Scrignaro, M. (2006). The power of stress: a salutogenic model of intervention. In A. D. Fave (Ed.), *Dimensions of well-being: Research and intervention* (pp. 470–488). FrancoAngeli.

Malm, D., Fridlund, B., Ekblad, H., Karlstrom, P., Hag, E., & Pakpour, A. H. (2018). Effects of brief mindfulness-based cognitive behavioural therapy on health-related quality of life and sense of coherence in atrial fibrillation patients. *Eur J Cardiovasc Nurs, 17*(7), 589–597. https://doi.org/10.1177/1474515118762796

Meier Magistretti, C., Topalidou, A., & Meinecke, F. (2019). The Sense FOR Coherence – an approach to a new concept. In C. Meier Magistretti, B. Lindström, & M. Eriksson (Eds.), *Knowing and understanding Salutogenseis*. Hogrefe (in German).

Meier Magistretti, C., Downe, S., Lindstrøm, B., Berg, M., & Schwarz, K. T. (2016). Setting the stage for health: Salutogenesis in midwifery professional knowledge in three European countries. *International Journal of Qualitative Studies on Health and Well-Being, 11*(0). https://doi.org/10.3402/qhw.v11.33155

Merakou, K., Tsoukas, K., Stavrinos, G., Amanaki, E., Daleziou, A., Kourmousi, N., ... Barbouni, A. (2019). The effect of progressive muscle relaxation on emotional competence: depression-anxiety-stress, sense of coherence, health-related quality of life, and well-being of unemployed people in Greece: An intervention study. *Explore (New York, N.Y.), 15*(1), 38–46. https://doi.org/10.1016/j.explore.2018.08.001

Murayama, Y., Ohba, H., Yasunaga, M., Nonaka, K., Takeuchi, R., Nishi, M., ... Fujiwara, Y. (2015). The effect of intergenerational programs on the mental health of elderly adults. *Aging & Mental Health, 19*(4), 306–314. https://doi.org/10.1080/13607863.2014.933309

Musavinasab, M., Ravanipour, M., Pouladi, S., Motamed, N., & Barekat, M. (2016). The effect of self-management empowerment model on the sense of coherence among elderly patients with cardiovascular disease. *Educational Gerontology, 42*(2), 100–108. https://doi.org/10.1080/03601277.2015.1078691

Nammontri, O., Robinson, P. G., & Baker, S. R. (2013). Enhancing oral health via sense of coherence: a cluster-randomized trial. *Journal of Dental Research, 92*(1), 26–31. https://doi.org/10.1177/0022034512459757

Norrbrink Budh, C., Kowalski, J., & Lundeberg, T. (2006). A comprehensive pain management programme comprising educational, cognitive and behavioural interventions for neuropathic pain following spinal cord injury. *Journal of Rehabilitation Medicine, 38*(3), 172–180. https://doi.org/10.1080/16501970500476258

Nost, T. H., Steinsbekk, A., Bratas, O., & Gronning, K. (2018). Twelve-month effect of chronic pain self-management intervention delivered in an easily accessible primary healthcare service - a randomized controlled trial. *BMC Health Services Research, 18*(1), 1012. https://doi.org/10.1186/s12913-018-3843-x

Odajima, Y., Kawaharada, M., & Wada, N. (2017). Development and validation of an educational program to enhance sense of coherence in patients with diabetes mellitus type 2. *Nagoya Journal of Medical Science, 79*(3), 363–374. https://doi.org/10.18999/nagjms.79.3.363.

Pakkala, I., Read, S., Sipilä, S., Portegijs, E., Kallinen, M., Heinonen, A., ... Rantanen, T. (2012). Effects of intensive strength-power training on sense of coherence among 60-85-year-old people with hip fracture: A randomized controlled trial. *Aging Clinical and Experimental Research, 24*(3), 295–299.

Pijpker, R., Vaandrager, L., Veen, E. J., & Koelen, M. A. (2019). A Salutogenic approach to understanding the potential of green programs for the rehabilitation of young employees with burn-out: protocol for a mixed method study on effectiveness and effective elements. *JMIR Res Protoc, 8*(10), e15303. https://doi.org/10.2196/15303

Polhuis, C. M. M., Bouwman, L. I., Vaandrager, L., Soedamah-Muthu, S. S., & Koelen, M. A. (2020). Systematic review of salutogenic-oriented lifestyle randomised controlled trials for adults with type 2 diabetes mellitus. *Patient Education and Counseling, 103*(4), 764–776. https://doi.org/10.1016/j.pec.2019.10.017

Recabarren, R. E., Gaillard, C., Guillod, M., & Martin-Soelch, C. (2019). Short-term effects of a multidimensional stress prevention program on quality of life, well-being and psychological resources. a randomized controlled trial. *Front Psychiatry, 10*, 88. https://doi.org/10.3389/fpsyt.2019.00088

Sancassiani, F., Cocco, A., Cossu, G., Lorrai, S., Trincas, G., Floris, F., ... Carta, M. G. (2017). "VelaMente?!" - Sailin in a crew to improve self-efficacy in people with psychosocial disabilities: A randomized controlled trial. *Clin Pract Epidemiol Ment Health, 13*, 200–212. https://doi.org/10.2174/1745017901713010200.

Sarid, O., Berger, R., Eckshtein, R., & Segal-Engelchin, D. (2012). Are cognitive-behavioral interventions effective in reducing occupational stress among nurses? *Applied Nursing Research, 25*(3), 152–157. https://doi.org/10.1016/j.apnr.2011.01.004

Schrank, B., Brownell, T., Jakaite, Z., Larkin, C., Pesola, F., Riches, S., ... Slade, M. (2016). Evaluation of a positive psychotherapy group intervention for people with psychosis: Pilot randomized controlled trial. *Epidemiology and Psychiatric Sciences, 25*(3), 235–246. https://doi.org/10.1017/S2045796015000141

Strandberg, E., Edholm, P., Ponsot, E., Wåhlin-Larsson, B., Hellmén, E., Nilsson, A., ... Kadi, F. (2015). Influence of combined resistance training and healthy diet on muscle mass in healthy elderly women: A randomized controlled trial. *Journal of Applied Physiology, 119*(8), 918–925.

Sullivan, G. C. (1989). Evaluating Antonovsky's salutogenic model for its adaptability to nursing. *Journal of Advanced Nursing, 14*(4), 336–342.

Sundsli, K., Soderhamn, U., Espnes, G. A., & Soderhamn, O. (2014). Self-care telephone talks as a health-promotion intervention in urban home-living persons 75+ years of age: A randomized controlled study. *Clinical Interventions in Aging, 9*, 95–103. https://doi.org/10.2147/CIA.S55925

Suominen, S. (1993). *Perceived health and life control. A theoretical review and empirical study about the connections between health and life control determined according to the strength of the sense of coherence.* (Research Report 26). Retrieved from Helsinki: http://www.julkari.fi/handle/10024/75715.

Super, S., Wagemakers, M., Picavet, H., Verkooijen, K., & Koelen, M. (2016). Strengthening sense of coherence: Opportunities for theory building in health promotion. *Health Promotion International, 31*(4), 869–878.

Tan, K. K., Chan, S. W., Wang, W., & Vehvilainen-Julkunen, K. (2016). A salutogenic program to enhance sense of coherence and quality of life for older people in the community: A feasibility randomized controlled trial and process evaluation. *Patient Education and Counseling, 99*(1), 108–116. https://doi.org/10.1016/j.pec.2015.08.003

Vaandrager, L., & Koelen, M. (2013). Salutogenesis in the workplace: Building general resistance resources and sense of coherence. In *Salutogenic organizations and change* (pp. 77–89): Springer.

Valtonen, M., Raiskila, T., Veijola, J., Laksy, K., Kauhanen, M. L., Kiuttu, J., ... Tuulio-Henriksson, A. (2015). Enhancing sense of coherence via early intervention among depressed occupational health care clients. *Nordic Journal of Psychiatry, 69*(7), 515–522. https://doi.org/10.3109/08039488.2015.1011230

Vastamäki, J., Moser, K., & Paul, K. I. (2009). How stable is sense of coherence? Changes following an intervention for unemployed individuals. *Scandinavian Journal of Psychology, 50*(2), 161–171. https://doi.org/10.1111/j.1467-9450.2008.00695.x

Viding, G. C., Osika, W., Theorell, T., Kowalski, J., Hallqvist, J., & Horwitz, E. B. (2015). The Culture palette - a randomized intervention study for women with burnout symptoms in Sweden. *British Journal of Medical Practitioners,* 8.

Yamazaki, Y., Togari, T., & Sakano, J. (2011). Toward development of intervention methods for strengthening the sense of coherence: suggestions from Japan. In *Asian perspectives and evidence on health promotion and education* (pp. 118–132): Springer.

Part IV

Salutogenic Model and its Core Concepts

21

Salutogenesis: Applications Beyond Health

Shifra Sagy

Aaron Antonovsky was my mentor in the long journey of writing my doctoral dissertation, which was the first to be written using the salutogenic paradigm framework. He was not only my academic advisor but also had a tremendous impact on my life. For me, the salutogenic model is not only a theoretical paradigm, whose genesis I witnessed and later on took an active part in its development. For me, this theory is the basis for a meaningful understanding of my life story, a story that has been embedded in the conflictual Jewish existence in Israel. Aaron and his salutogenic ideas have guided me in this difficult path too.

Aaron Antonovsky enriched us with a unique, challenging model, which had high levels of comprehensibility, manageability, and especially meaningfulness. When he passed away 25 years ago, I wondered whether, and perhaps how, the model would be developed after him. To witness today, the rich and active development of the model is deeply exciting. Thus, I am truly enthusiastic about taking part in this endeavor—the second edition of *The Handbook of Salutogenesis*—and especially pleased to edit this part dealing with new developments and creative advancements of the theory.

It was very tempting to continue Antonovsky's way by using his strict guidelines for salutogenic research. However, Aaron also taught me that "it is wise to see models, theories, constructs, hypotheses, and even ideas as heuristic devices, not only truths" (Antonovsky, 1996, p. 246). The chapters included in this part of the handbook represent good examples of following this advice.

In Chap. 22, my colleague Adi Mana and I ask how to broaden the salutogenic paradigm's scope into an interdisciplinary framework and include other social concepts in its research. As one example of such interdisciplinary research, we review some new studies in conflict areas investigating intergroup relations. By relating to such areas of research, we try to address not only the "classic" question—who copes successfully and stays healthy—but also other salutogenic questions such as "who expresses more openness to *the other*?"

In the 2017 edition of the *Handbook of Salutogenesis*, I suggested that these meaningful questions, stemming from our political and social reality, should be extensively discussed in the framework of salutogenesis. Indeed, since the 2017 edition of the handbook, there has been impressive advancement in this research direction, including the development of new concepts like the sense of national coherence.

The 2020 worldwide outbreak of the COVID-19 pandemic has shaken up lives and transformed perceptions about "normality." As of this writing, the pandemic is stimulating salutogenic-oriented interdisciplinary health research and social research—this chapter reviews some cutting-edge COVID-19 social studies *beyond* health.

In Chap. 23, Stephen Joseph and I propose integrating two paradigms—positive psychology and salutogenesis—and suggest a joint conceptual framework, which we term as "salutogenic positive psychology." Despite the differences between the two movements and their different theoretical roots, we believe that the integrative approach has greater utility in advancing psychological research on mental health and well-being.

The other three chapters in Part IV answer our call for interdisciplinary salutogenic-oriented research and discuss its possible application in three areas.

In Chap. 24, Maass, Kiland, Espnes, and Lillefjord thoroughly discuss the different possibilities of applying salutogenesis in politics and public policy. Politics is one of the upstream conditions that shape our individual lives as well as our society. Thus, asking about if and how salutogenesis can be applied to this field appears to be a most significant subject in Part IV of the handbook relating to salutogenesis beyond health. In all of his writing about his model, Antonovsky emphasized how politics and policies contribute to shaping individual and collective abilities to strengthen

S. Sagy (✉)
Martin Springer Center for Conflict Studies,
Ben-Gurion University of the Negev, Be'er Sheva, Israel
e-mail: shifra@bgu.ac.il

salutogenic resources. The authors of this chapter approach this issue from the opposite direction, asking, "how can salutogenesis contribute to outlining strategies and structural processes linked to politics and policy-making?" Their creative discussion succeeds in bringing the reader the utility of the salutogenic approach in addressing such issues.

In Chap. 25, Levasseur and Naud discuss some important aging factors that could increase the likelihood of a stronger SOC: aging at home, participation, and social support. In his last paper, Antonovsky (1996) highlighted an example of an intervention among older people, living in their homes, who refused to accept help. He suggested that if researchers had been guided by the salutogenic question of "how to strengthen the comprehensibility, manageability, and meaningfulness of elders," their intervention research could have been much more sophisticated and rich. Levasseur and Naud are addressing this call. In their chapter, they analyze how social support, active participation, mobility, and other factors can strengthen SOC in old age. They also bring some examples of individual and community programs that are already operating within this salutogenic orientation.

In Chap. 26, Golembiewski suggests adding another domain in our life to be viewed through the salutogenic lens: architectural design. In a creative and explorative discussion, the author analyzes detailed and concrete examples and offers ideas on how architecture can advance comprehensibility, manageability, and meaningfulness in our lives.

In Chap. 4 of this handbook, we wrote that Aaron taught us that the most meaningful advancement in scientific work is to ask good questions. I trust that our part of the handbook succeeds in relating to this challenge.

Reference

Antonovsky, A. (1996). The salutogenic model as a theory to guide health promotion. *Health Promotion International, 11*(1), 11–18.

22

Salutogenesis: An Interdisciplinary Framework

Shifra Sagy and Adi Mana

Introduction

Antonovsky's salutogenic model and its core concept "sense of coherence" (SOC) focus on the ability of individuals to cope with stressors in life and stay healthy. Accordingly, the relationship between SOC and health has received much attention and quite consistent results in research (see Chap. 9 of this book). However, since the paradigm of salutogenesis was introduced within the discipline of sociology of health, the relationships between salutogenesis and other social concepts have been mostly neglected. Unfortunately, until recently, the salutogenic model has almost never been broadened into an interdisciplinary framework. We believe that, at this stage of its development and its wide distribution in the scientific world, the salutogenic paradigm should broaden its scope. In proposing broadening the application of salutogenesis to interdisciplinary research, we may consider disciplines like social psychology, economics, geography, anthropology, or conflict studies. This chapter aims to raise new questions about applying the salutogenic paradigm to research in interdisciplinary fields and to review new studies that have already begun to do so.

S. Sagy (✉)
Martin Springer Center for Conflict Studies, Ben-Gurion University of the Negev, Be'er Sheva, Israel
e-mail: shifra@bgu.ac.il

A. Mana
School of Behavioral Science, Peres Academic Center, Rehovot, Israel

Dilemmas in Broadening Salutogenesis into an Interdisciplinary Framework

Broadening salutogenesis into an interdisciplinary framework raises several core dilemmas. First, we must deal with the questions: Does the salutogenic orientation enable us to deal with other concepts beyond the relationship with health? And if so, how? How can we ask salutogenic questions employing concepts embedded in other disciplines?

Let's start with the first question. In his writing about the development of SOC, Antonovsky wrote extensively about how one's life experiences can influence the strength of one's SOC (Antonovsky, 1987). Actually, in his dealing with this issue – *the origins of SOC* – Antonovsky expressed an interdisciplinary approach by relating to broad-ranging factors like culture, social forces, social position, gender, ethnicity, genetics, or even plain luck (Benz et al., 2014). Indeed, social factors have seldom been studied as predictors of SOC (e.g., Lam, 2007; Sagy & Antonovsky, 2000). Two aspects have mainly been studied: the experience of cultural integration vs discrimination due to being part of a minority group (Ying et al., 2001) and the experience of cultural stability vs instability (e.g., Antonovsky & Sagy, 1986).

Even though this body of research was mostly composed of correlational studies, which leave the direction of causality undetermined, in most of the studies, the suggested direction was that elements related to a variety of social factors should be considered as predictors of SOC.

However, while Antonovsky discussed the other direction of the equation, meaning how SOC can influence life situations, his answer was much less interdisciplinary. He clarified in his work that "a salutogenic orientation, no less than a pathologic one, defines health and disease only in terms of functioning and survival. All that it argues is that the stronger the SOC, the more likely the system, whether individual, family, or society, to function and survive" (Antonovsky, 1991, p. 8). What he meant was that SOC, whose development is influenced by social factors, cannot predict social concepts, which could have a positive or negative connotation.

Moreover, Antonovsky viewed such social factors as loaded by moral-philosophical problems and as such not inherently within the context of salutogenesis (Antonovsky, 1991). This original conviction of his can partly explain the focus of salutogenic research over almost four decades on the SOC/health hypothesis and why it has not been broadened to include other interdisciplinary concepts as well.

By raising this question, once again, we assume that salutogenesis, 40 years later, is challenged by the call of interdisciplinarity. We believe that researchers can ask salutogenic questions in different areas, not only health and well-being, and perhaps find other salutogenic answers. When we employ an interdisciplinary approach, the salutogenic question would not only be "Who copes successfully and stays healthy?" (Antonovsky, 1987) but also, for example, "Who expresses more openness to the other?", "Who is a social activist who pursues justice in the world"? Or "Who is a peacemaker?" If we broaden the level of our questions, we can ask about salutogenic schools, neighborhoods, or other social institutions, which enhance not only health and wellness but also justice, peace, and reconciliation. The definitions of these concepts can vary over different contexts and cultures, but the question remains a salutogenic one.

Toward Exploring Salutogenic Questions in an Interdisciplinary Framework

Now we arrive at the second part of our review: How can we ask salutogenic questions in an interdisciplinary framework? Relating to this "how" question, we will review some studies, which have already attempted to do so. Previous studies found positive interactions between SOC and the relationships between members of the same community (e.g., for reviews, see Koelen & Eriksson, and Vaandrager & Kennedy in this handbook; Maass et al., 2014; Morton & Lurie, 2013; Teig et al., 2009). This evidence was explained by the well-known relationship between strong social connection or connectivity and enhanced sense of health and well-being (Vaandrager & Kennedy, 2017). However, this explanation brings us back to the SOC/health equation, and we are looking for other equations as well.

Thus, in our attempt to move beyond the SOC/health equation, we decided to explore other equations like SOC/social relations or SOC/political orientations. Several studies have attempted to examine the relationship between SOC and personal traits which could facilitate social relations with out-group members. Feldt et al. (2007) analyzed the relations between SOC and the five-factor model of personality. The results indicate that a person with a strong SOC shows modest positive associations with extraversion, openness, conscientiousness, and agreeableness. Another study (Pålsson et al., 1996) found negative correlations between SOC and the personality traits of avoidance, detachment, hostility, and aggression and positive correlations between SOC and empathy.

In political psychology, SOC was measured as a predictor of different political orientations. No correlations were found, for example, between SOC and attitude scales measuring patriotism, nationalism, and authoritarianism (Renner et al., 2004). However, political attitudes toward peace were found in correlation with strong SOC (Braun-Lewensohn et al., 2015) in a study of Israeli adolescents during a political, violent event, in the context of the Israeli-Palestinian conflict. Adolescents who had a strong SOC had a strong tendency to view the conflict as another challenge in life with which to cope and perceived the conflict as manageable and as meaningful. This study, however, was a one-time, cross-sectional study and its causal interpretation could also be different.

The findings related to the equations of SOC/social relations or SOC/political orientation are quite ambiguous. We trust that more studies should be carried out to support their promising results. The prominent direction revealed in this body of research is that a strong SOC is connected with tendencies associated with positive values, at least in Western society. Are these conclusions that Antonovsky tried to avoid? Perhaps yes. In his lecture in Prague in 1991, he warned of the danger of defining health so that it becomes "...a catchall for anything that you think is good. Health then becomes not a scientific concept, but confused with a set of answers to moral-philosophical problems...the distinction must be made" (Antonovsky, 1991 p.9). Of course, when we broaden salutogenesis to include concepts other than health, we cannot avoid these moral-philosophical questions about values and science. Thus, we have to deal with them while fully recognizing our limitations in making such a distinction.

Sense of Coherence: From the Individual to the Collective Concept

Since attitudes and behaviors toward the other are developed within one's social context, the relationship between SOC and intergroup relations should be explored not only from the individual perspective but also in the supra-system context (Sagy, 2014, 2017). The global perception of the world as coherent does not necessarily mean that people must perceive the entire group they belong to as comprehensible, manageable, and meaningful. Relating to this question Antonovsky suggested: "Quite conceivably, people might feel that they have little interest in national government or international politics, little competence in manual (or cognitive or aesthetic) skills, little concern for local volunteer groups or trade union activity, and so on, and yet have a strong SOC" (Antonovsky, 1984, p. 119).

Van Breda (2001), in his review, based on the concept of "circle of concern and influence" (Covey & Merrill, 2006), explained that people draw boundaries within the objective world – provided those things which fall within the boundaries are considered coherent – the person will have a strong SOC, irrespective of the coherence of things outside the boundaries. Things outside of the circle of concern can be of no importance to that individual. Within the circle of concern is a smaller circle, the "circle of influence," which refers to those things which concern that individual and over which that individual has some influence. By focusing on the area between the two circles (i.e., those things that concern one but over which one has no influence), one creates SOC-reducing experiences, since the situation is not manageable. By focusing on issues within the circle of influence, one is assured of life experiences that are coherent, and in so doing, one can (theoretically) expand the circle of influence. There are cases when a person may have a very small circle of concern and an even smaller circle of influence, yielding a life that is very limited in scope, although potentially high in SOC. This question of boundaries within the objective world brings us to our second branch of research that deals with the role of sense of coherence in intergroup relationships.

The idea that the SOC concept should be broadened to larger levels than individuals has been suggested and discussed by Sagy and Antonovsky (Antonovsky, 1992; Sagy, 1990; Sagy & Antonovsky, 1992). It is beyond the scope of this chapter, however, to include this extensive discussion. Here, we will review some studies that link the SOC of the collective to intergroup and social relations.

Sense of Community Coherence

The concept of sense of community coherence (SOCC) was developed as related to a specific in-group and not to the "global orientation of the world" as it is defined for individual SOC. It constitutes the three components of SOC: comprehensibility, manageability, and meaningfulness (Braun-Lewensohn & Sagy, 2011; Elfassi et al., 2016; Peled et al., 2013; Sagy, 1998; Telaku et al., 2020). Community comprehensibility relates to the perception that life in one's community is predictable, safe, and secure and that one's community is a place that is known and understood. Community manageability relates to the perception that one's community can assist its members, is available to them, and meets their demands and needs. Lastly, community meaningfulness relates to the perception that the community gives meaning to its members, provides challenges, and is worthy of investment and engagement.

Most of the research which investigated the concept of SOCC has focused on its relationship with well-being and mental health, meaning the SOC/health equation. For example, positive relations have been found between a strong sense of community coherence and the level of resilience to stressful events (bomb attacks, a fire disaster) (e.g., Braun-Lewensohn et al., 2013; Braun-Lewensohn & Sagy, 2011). SOCC was found as negatively related to unhealthy behaviors. Elfassi et al. (2016) found significant negative correlations between SOCC and the levels of risk behaviors among Israeli adolescents and claimed that SOCC is a significant protective factor that could be related to decreased involvement in risk behaviors.

Just recently, however, several studies have attempted other equations, seeking to connect salutogenesis and SOC to other social concepts like intergroup relations, openness toward the other, and readiness to reconcile (Mana et al., 2019; Sagy, 2014; Sagy, 2017; Srour, 2015; Telaku et al., 2020). These studies connect the salutogenic paradigm with interdisciplinary models and concepts like social identity (Tajfel, 1981), acculturation (Berry, 1990), conflict studies (Bar-Tal, 1998), or peace and reconciliation (Nadler, 2012). The interdisciplinary salutogenic questions in these studies are: How does a collective with a strong SOC perceive, feel, or behave toward the other? Is the tendency of a group to perceive its world as comprehensible, meaningful, and manageable related to greater openness to the other, or does it involve clinging to rigid in-group identity and less openness toward the other? Is an individual, a group, a collective, or a system with a stronger SOC more likely to live in peace/justice/good relations with their surroundings?

Most of these new studies examined the relationship between SOCC and intergroup relations. The relations between the conflicted groups were examined by the levels of adherence to in-group collective narratives as well as acceptance of the out-group collective narratives. Some of the studies found a relationship between SOCC and acculturation attitudes (Somech & Sagy, 2019; Telaku & Sagy, 2018). One of the studies was conducted among Palestinian Muslims and Christians in Israel (Mana et al., 2016).

The results revealed that strong sense of community coherence (SOCC) was correlated with higher levels of acceptance of the in-group collective narrative and with lower levels of acceptance of the out-group collective narratives. Sense of community coherence was also related to higher levels of a tendency to adopt a separation strategy between the two groups in conflict.

The explanations for all these studies relied on a wide range of models in social psychology which suggest that group members who believe that their own group and its products are superior to other groups are prone to behaviorally discriminate against other groups (e.g., Bizumic & Duckitt, 2009). This notion was well established in the work of Tajfel (1981) who analyzed three cognitive aspects of prejudice:

the process of categorization, which gives shape to intergroup attitudes, the process of assimilation of social values and norms which provides their content, and as a main cognitive aspect which relates to the way individuals react to specific intergroup situations.

Following Tajfel's paradigm, we can interpret the strong SOCC as enabling group members to deal with changes that occur in intergroup situations. In order to deal with these changes, an individual must make constant attributions that help him deal with the new situations in a manner that appears consistent to him and preserves his self-image and integrity. The individual needs to build a cognitive structure which provides him with a satisfactory explanation of the causes of changes.

However, an improved group position is often achieved by using the group's capacity to put another group at a disadvantage and derives largely from biased comparisons on salient dimensions that are favorable to the in-group and unfavorable to the out-group (Brown, 2000; Tajfel, 1981).

Several studies focused on SOCC in the context of inter-religious group relations and international group relations in different social contexts. One was carried out in the context of two religious communities in Israel: ultra-Orthodox and national religious Jews (Somech & Sagy, 2019).

The results of this study indicated the same tendency of connection with openness to the other, while the ultra-Orthodox community exhibited stronger SOCC than their counterparts, as well as a stronger connection of SOCC with separation tendencies. Mana et al. (2020) suggested a mediation model in which the relationships between SOCC and the identity strategies of separation and competition are mediated by the tendency to reject or accept in-group and out-group collective narratives, in the context of intra- and inter-religious conflicts.

They compared the intra-religious conflict between ultra-Orthodox Jews and national religious Jews and the inter-religious conflict between Muslim and Christian Arabs who are Israeli citizens and found that the mediation model was stronger among those groups with a high SOCC (ultra-Orthodox Jews and Muslim Arabs) compared to groups with low SOCC (Christian Arabs and national religious Jews).

Another study (Telaku et al., 2020) related to SOCC and intergroup relations in the context of post-armed conflict between Serbs and Albanians in Kosovo. This study suggested that another factor – subjective experience of interpersonal power – mediates the relationships between SOCC and openness to the other, as measured by perceptions of collective narratives of the out-group and the in-group. The model was confirmed among both Serb and Albanian participants.

This review indicates that sense of coherence at the community level is indeed a salutogenic and health-promoting factor that has a significant role in the ability of community members to cope with threatening situations on the collective level (SOC/health equation). At the same time, however, the studies suggest SOCC as a barrier for positive intergroup relationships in different kinds of conflicts: intractable or periodic, political, ethnic, or religious conflicts.

In all of these conflicts, it appears that SOCC leads the community members to adhere to their own collective narratives and to reject the collective narratives of the out-group and to adopt strategies of separation from the out-group members. Although this process was explored as a linear process, it seems that it could also be circular, and the tendency of the in-group members to prefer their own group members, and their own collective narratives, while rejecting the others, may contribute to their perception of their own community as more comprehensive, manageable, and meaningful. Unfortunately, it seems that this pattern has a long-lasting effect even when the armed conflict is over, like in Kosovo. However, the preliminary evidence revealed that this pattern could be affected by other mediating factors like the subjective experience of interpersonal power. It has also been found to be more effective among groups with stronger SOCC. Exploring individual and group differences that enable group members to act differently could promote new insights to "break this chain" of the contribution of strong SOCC as a barrier to the possibility of openness to the other group and readiness to reconcile in intergroup relationships.

Sense of National Coherence

A wider concept recently suggested by Sagy (2014) relates to the national level, the sense of national coherence (SONC). The salutogenic concept of SONC reflects an enduring tendency to perceive one's national group as comprehensible, meaningful, and manageable.

The main assumption of the researchers who examined this concept is that SONC can provide a deeper understanding of political conflict situations. As such, SONC could be a resource of wellness and health, but, at the same time, it could serve as a potential barrier for a peace process in a conflict area. The first studies related to SONC were conducted in the context of the Israeli-Palestinian intractable conflict (Mana et al., 2020; Sarid et al., in press; Sarid & Sagy, 2015).

The initial results indicate a strong negative correlation between strong SONC and levels of openness to the narrative of the other group. Moreover, levels of SONC among Israeli students before and after a violent period (the Gaza war) indicated an increase in the level of SONC and a significant decrease in willingness to reconcile. The negative correlation between those two variables was stronger after the Gaza war than before it.

The findings suggest that the escalation in the conflict and in violence has an impact on the perceptions of the national sense of coherence and could be a potential barrier to reconciliation. Mana et al. (2019) explored SONC and its relationship with openness to the Palestinian collective narrative among Israeli-Jewish adults. SONC was found to be negatively related to level of legitimization toward the Palestinian collective narratives. This finding replicated previous studies related to SOCC. Moreover, SONC was found to be related to right-wing voting patterns and to religious groupings (Mana et al., 2019).

Research on SONC has moved in different directions beyond the political sphere to educational initiatives. For example, in a work submitted for publication, Agbaria, Mana, Bar-Gera, and Sagy et al., investigated levels of SONC with the aim of explaining behavioral intentions toward driving among young Israeli Jews and Arabs. The findings indicate strong correlations between SONC, behavioral intentions, and readiness to take risks while driving, and to the perceptions of the police as representing justice, especially among the minority group of Arab adolescents in Israel. The results suggest some implications for educational interventions among youngsters before their driving experience.

Salutogenesis and the COVID-19 Pandemic: Sociopolitical Considerations

We are writing this chapter in the midst of the COVID-19 pandemic, which has shaken up lives worldwide and is having strong economic, social, and political impacts in many countries. Naturally, the pandemic has led researchers to ask pathogenic questions about its pathogenic origins and the potential damage. This chaotic global pandemic, however, was also an opportunity to explore salutogenic concepts like SOC and SONC and to understand their roles not only in promoting health but also beyond health, as potential factors in increasing some order out of the chaos. Mana and Sagy, jointly with the Global Working Group on Salutogenesis, conducted some international research (Mana, Bauer, et al., 2021; Hardy et al., 2021; Mana, Super et al., 2021; Mana & Sagy, 2020). The theoretical basis of the salutogenesis, and its fundamental philosophical postulate that the world is chaotic in its nature, was an appropriate basis for these studies.

We revealed the important role of the salutogenic concepts of SOC and SONC in predicting higher levels of mental health and lower levels of anxiety in all of the countries involved in our research from Europe, Israel, and the USA. Beyond this, we sought to understand the social-political situation that has been developed while the acute stressor of the pandemic has become chronic. SONC, for example, was found to be highly related to level of trust in governmental institutions.

This relationship was even stronger among people who voted for the current government (Mana & Sagy, 2020; Super et al., 2020). However, low SONC, as well as low trust in the leadership, was strongly connected to lower levels of mental health. Our preliminary findings reveal that levels of SONC also decreased as the pandemic moved from acute to chronic stress, and the political stability in many countries has been eroded.

These studies could deepen our understanding of the theoretical basis of the salutogenesis. Moreover, these current studies reveal the relationships between sense of coherence at the personal and the collective levels and their role not only in the SOC/health equation but also in social relationships and political processes in the context of the chronic stress, which introduces entropy into the global system.

In conclusion, while there is a broad consensus regarding the contribution of SOC to health and well-being, the role of SOC – both of the individual or the collective – in social relations has been mostly neglected. We maintain that one of the reasons for this neglect is the initial excitement of Antonovsky and his followers about studying the SOC/health connection. Times have changed and interdisciplinarity seems to be the challenge of our era. In this chapter, we have attempted to review the small body of research, which asks other salutogenic questions about the relationship of SOC at the individual and the collective levels to other interdisciplinary concepts.

We believe that more research is needed in order to gain a deeper understanding of these initial answers. Moreover, interdisciplinarity can also lead to employing other salutogenic concepts – rather than SOC – to give answers to salutogenic questions. So we suggest that salutogenic researchers in the future not only ask new salutogenic questions but also develop new salutogenic concepts in the attempt to broaden and deepen our understanding of the paradigm. We hope that this chapter succeeds in posing this new challenge.

References

Agbaria, K., Mana, A., Bar-Gera, H., & Sagy, S. (Submitted). Personal and social factors related to behavioral intentions towards driving among teenagers: Comparing Israeli Arabs and Jews.

Antonovsky, A. (1984) The sense of coherence as a determinant in health. In: J.D. Matarazzo, (Ed.). *Behavioral health: A handbook of health enhancement and disease prevention,* (pp. 114-129) John Wiley.

Antonovsky, A. (1987). *Unraveling the mystery of health.* Jossey-Bass.

Antonovsky, A. (1991). The Salutogenic approach to family system health: Promise and danger. Lecture at European Congress on "Mental Health in European Families", Prague, Czechoslovakia,

5–8 May 1991. Retrieved from: http://www.angelfire.com/ok/soc/agolem.html.

Antonovsky, A. (1992). Can attitudes contribute to health? *Advances, 8*, 33–49.

Antonovsky, H., & Sagy, S. (1986). The development of a sense of coherence and its impact on responses to stress situations. *Journal of Social Psychology, 126*, 213–227.

Bar-Tal, D. (1998). Social beliefs in times of intractable conflict: The Israeli case. *International Journal of Conflict Management, 9*, 22–50.

Berry, J. W. (1990). Psychology of acculturation. In J. J. Berman (Ed.), *Nebraska symposium on motivation, 1989: Cross-cultural perspectives. Current theory and research in motivation, 37* (pp. 201–235). University of Nebraska Press.

Benz, C., Bull, T., Mittelmark, M., & Vaandrager, L. (2014). Culture in salutogenesis: The scholarship of Aaron Antonovsky. *Global Health Promotion., 21*(4), 16–23.

Bizumic, B., & Duckitt, J. (2009). Narcissism and ethnocentrism: A review. *Directions in Psychiatry, 29*, 99–109.

Braun-Lewensohn, O., Abu-Kaf, S., & Sagy, S. (2015). Attitudes toward war and peace and their relations with anxiety reactions among adolescents living in a conflictual area. *Journal of Youth Studies, 18*(1), 68–79.

Braun-Lewensohn, O., & Sagy, S. (2011). Salutogenesis and culture. Personal and community sense of coherence among adolescents belonging to three different cultural groups. *International Review of Psychiatry, 23*(6), 533–541.

Braun-Lewensohn, O., Sagy, S., Sabato, H., & Galili, R. (2013). Sense of coherence and sense of community as coping resource of religious adolescents before and after the disengagement from the Gaza strip. *Israeli Journal of Psychiatry & Related Sciences, 50*(2), 110–117.

Brown, R. (2000). Social identity theory: Past achievements, current problems and future challenges. *European Journal of Social Psychology, 30*(6), 745–778. https://doi.org/10.1002/1099-0992(200011/12)30:6<745::AID-EJSP24>3.0.CO;2-O

Covey, S. M. R., & Merrill, R. R. (2006). *The speed of trust: The one thing that changes everything*. CoveyLink.

Elfassi, Y., Braun-Lewensohn, O., Krumer-Nevo, M., & Sagy, S. (2016). Community sense of coherence among adolescents as related to their involvement in risk behaviors. *Journal of Community Psychology, 44*(1), 22–37. https://doi.org/10.1002/jcop.21739

Feldt, T., Metsäpelto, R.-L., Kinnunen, U., & Pulkkinen, L. (2007). Sense of coherence and five-factor approach to personality: Conceptual relationships. *European Psychologist, 12*(3), 165–172.

Hardy, L., Mana, A., Mundell, L., Benheim, S., Torres Morales, K., & Sagy, S. (2021). Living in opposition: How women in the United States cope in spite of mistrust of federal leadership during the pandemic of COVID-19. Journal of Community Psychology. 2021 Mar 17. https://doi.org/10.1002/jcop.22544. Epub ahead of print. PMID: 33729586.

Lam, B. T. (2007). Impact of perceived racial discrimination and collective self-esteem on psychological distress among Vietnamese-American college students: Sense of coherence as mediator. *American Journal of Orthopsychiatry, 77*(3), 370–376.

Maass, R., Lindström, B., & Lillefjell, M. (2014). Exploring the relationship between perceptions of neighborhood-resources, sense of coherence and health for different groups in a Norwegian neighbourhood. *Journal of Public Health Research, 3*(208).

Mana, A., Bauer, A., Meier Magistretti, C., Sardu, C., Juvinyà Canal, D., Hardy, L.J., Catz, O., Tušl, M., & Sagy, S. (2021). Order out of chaos: Sense of coherence and the mediating role of coping resources in predicting mental health during COVID-19 in 7 countries. SSM & Mental Health, 1. Online Advanced https://doi.org/10.1016/j.ssmmh.2021.100001.

Mana, A., & Sagy, S. (2020). Brief report: Can political orientation explain mental health in the time of a global pandemic? Voting patterns, personal and national coping resources, and mental health during the coronavirus crisis. *Journal of Social and Clinical Psychology, 39*(3), 187–193. https://doi.org/10.1521/jscp.2020.39.3.165

Mana, A., Sagy, S., & Srour, A. (2016). Sense of community coherence and inter-religious relations. *The Journal of Social Psychology, 156*(5), 469–482. https://doi.org/10.1080/00224545.2015.1129302

Mana, A., Sagy, S., & Srour, A. (2019). Sense of National Coherence and openness to the "other's" collective narratives: The case of the Israeli-Palestinian conflict. *Peace and Conflict: Journal of Peace Psychology, 25*(3), 226–233. https://doi.org/10.1037/pac0000391

Mana, A., Srour, A., & Sagy, S. (2020). Sense of community coherence, perceptions of collective narratives, and identity strategies in intra- and inter- religious group conflicts. In A. Mana & A. Srour (Eds.), *Israeli and Palestinian collective narratives in conflict: A tribute to Shifra Sagy and her work* (pp. 131–157). Cambridge Scholars.

Mana, A., Super, S., Sardu, C., Juvinya Canal, D., Neuman, M., & Sagy, S. (2021). Individual, social and national coping resources and their relationships with mental health and anxiety: A comparative study in Israel, Italy, Spain, and the Netherlands during the Coronavirus pandemic. Global Health Promotion. 18:1757975921992957. https://doi.org/10.1177/1757975921992957. Epub ahead of print. PMID: 33601955; PMCID: PMC7897541.

Morton, M. J., & Lurie, N. (2013). Community resilience and public health practice. *American Journal of Public Health., 103*(7), 1158–1160.

Nadler, A. (2012). Intergroup reconciliation: Definition, processes and dilemmas. In L. Tropp (Ed.), *Oxford handbook of conflict*. Oxford University Press.

Pålsson, M. B., Hallberg, I. R., Norberg, A., & Björvell, H. (1996). Burnout, empathy and sense of coherence among Swedish district nurses before and after systematic clinical supervision. *Scandinavian Journal of Caring Science, 10*(1), 19–26.

Peled, D., Sagy, S., & Braun-Lewensohn, O. (2013). Community perceptions as coping resource among adolescents living under rockets fire: A salutogenic approach. *Journal of Community Positive Practices, 4*, 681–702.

Renner, W., Salem, I., & Alexandrowicz, R. (2004). Human values as predictors for political, religious and health-related attitudes: A contribution towards validating the Australian value questionnaire (AVQ) by structural equation modeling. *Social Behavior and Personality, 32*(5), 477–490.

Sagy, S. (1990). *The family sense of coherence and adjustment to stressors*. Unpublished doctoral dissertation. Ben-Gurion University of the Negev.

Sagy, S. (1998). Effects of personal, family, and community characteristics on emotional reactions in a community stress situation: The Golan Heights negotiations. *Youth & Society, 29*(3), 311–329.

Sagy, S. (2014). Rak al atzmi l' saper yadati: M'yomana shel hokeret sichsuchim b'heder hamugan. (only about myself did I know to tell: From the diary of a conflict researcher). *Mifgash: Journal of social-educational Work, 40*, 9–26. (Hebrew). http://www.jstor.org/stable/24524253.

Sagy, S. (2017). Can we empathize with the narrative of our enemy? A personal odyssey in studying peace education. *Intercultural Education, 28*(6), 1–11. https://doi.org/10.1080/14675986.2017.1390889

Sagy, S., & Antonovsky, A. (1992). The family sense of coherence and the retirement transition. *Journal of Marriage and the Family, 54*, 983–993.

Sagy, S., & Antonovsky, H. (2000). The development of the sense of coherence: A retrospective study of early life experiences in the family. *International Journal of Aging & Human Development, 51*, 155–166.

Sarid, A., & Sagy, S. (2015). *National sense of coherence and openness to the other*. Conference of Kibbutz studies.

Sarid, A., Srour, A., & Sagy, S. (in press). Sense of national coherence and willingness to reconcile: The case of the Israeli- Palestinian conflict. In F. Ferrari, M., Leiner, Z. Barakat, & M. Sternberg (Eds.), Encountering the Suffering of the Other. Transdisciplinary Perspectives from the DFG Project "Hearts of Flesh-not Stone" Vandenhoeck and Ruprecht.

Somech, L., & Sagy, S. (2019). Perceptions of collective narratives and identity strategies as indicators of intergroup relations: The case of ultra-orthodox and National-Religious Jewish communities in Israel. *International Journal of Conflict Management, 30*(3), 290–308. https://doi.org/10.1108/ijcma-06-2017-0058

Srour, A. (2015). *Community sense of coherence, collective narrative perceptions and openness to the "other" group: The case of Muslims-Christians relations in Israel.* PhD thesis. Ben Gurion University of the Negev (Hebrew).

Super, S., Pijpker, R., & Polhuis, K. (2020). The relationship between individual, social and national coping resources and mental health during the COVID-19 crisis in the Netherlands. Health Psychology Report. https://doi.org/10.5114/hpr.2020.99028

Telaku, M., & Sagy, S. (2018). Community sense of coherence and openness towards the other group: The case of Albanians and Serbs in Kosovo. In L. Gardner-Feldman, R. Barash, & S. Goda (Eds.), *Societies in transition: The former Soviet Union and east Central Europe between conflict and reconciliation*. Vandenhoeck & Ruprecht. The Jena Center for Reconciliation Studies' (JCRS) series on research in peace and reconciliation (RIPAR).

Telaku, M., Mana, A., Srour, A., & Sagy, S. (2020). Sense of community coherence and perceptions of collective narratives in post-conflict context: The mediating role of subjective experience of interpersonal power. *Peace and Conflict: Journal of Peace Psychology*. https://doi.org/10.1037/pac0000525

Tajfel, H. (1981). *Human groups and social categories: Studies in social psychology*. Cambridge University Press.

Teig, E., Amulya, J., Bardwell, L., Buchenau, M., Marshall, J. A., & Litt, J. S. (2009). Collective efficacy in Denver, Colorado: Strengthening neighborhoods and health through community gardens. *Health & Place, 15*(4), 1115–1122. http://dx.doi.org/doi:%2010.1016/%20j.healthplace.2009.06.003

Vaandrager, L., & Kennedy, L. (2017). Communities and neighborhoods. In M. Mittelmark, S. Sagy, M. Eriksson, G. F. Bauer, J. M. Pelikan, B. Lindström, & G. A. Espnes (Eds.), *Handbook of Salutogenesis* (pp. 159–170). Springer International. https://link.springer.com/chapter/10.1007/978-3-319-04600-6_17

Van Breda, A. D. (2001). Resilience theory: A literature review (research report MPI/R/104/12/1/4). *South African Military Psychological Institute*. http://vanbreda.org/adrian/resilience/resilience_theory_review.pdf.

Ying, Y. W., Lee, P. A., Tsai, J. L., Hung, Y., Lin, M., & Wan, C. T. (2001). Asian American college students as model minorities: An examination of their overall competence. *Cultural Diversity & Ethnic Minority Psychology, 7*(1), 59–74.

23

Integrating Salutogenesis and Positive Psychology

Stephen Joseph and Shifra Sagy

Introduction

The advent of contemporary positive psychology can be traced back to Martin E.P. Seligman's Presidential Address in 1999 to the American Psychological Association (APA). In that address he told his own story of changing direction. Following a moment of epiphany when gardening with his daughter Nikki, he realised that psychology had largely neglected the latter two of its three pre-World War II missions: curing mental illness, helping all people to lead more productive and fulfilling lives and identifying and nurturing high talent. With this realisation, Seligman resolved to use his APA presidency to initiate a shift in psychology's focus towards a more positive psychology (Seligman, 2004). This presidential initiative was catalysed through a series of meetings with both junior and senior scholars who would become the leading voices of the new positive psychology movement, and who began to map out what they saw as a positive psychology research agenda. This was followed by the hugely influential January 2000 special issue of the *American Psychologist* on positive psychology in which Seligman and Csikszentmihalyi (2000) wrote:

> The aim of positive psychology is to begin to catalyze a change in the focus of psychology from preoccupation only with repairing the worst things in life to also building positive qualities. (Seligman & Csikszentmihalyi, 2000, p. 5)

S. Joseph (✉)
School of Education, University of Nottingham, Nottingham, UK
e-mail: Stephen.joseph@nottingham.ac.uk

S. Sagy
Martin Springer Center for Conflict Studies, Ben-Gurion University of the Negev, Be'er Sheva, Israel

That special issue provided a broad vista of topics that were deemed to be covered under the positive psychology umbrella and included articles on happiness, individual development, subjective well-being, optimism, self-determination theory, adaptive mental mechanisms, emotions and health, wisdom, excellence, creativity, giftedness and positive youth development. From these beginnings over 20 years ago, positive psychology has flourished.

Positive Psychology and Salutogenesis

The positive psychology movement has produced new conceptual frameworks, instruments to measure human strengths and increased interest in topics such as optimism, hope, locus of control, creativity, self-esteem, emotional intelligence, empathy, humour and gratitude (Linley et al., 2006; Lopez & Snyder, 2003). Positive psychologists have also endeavoured to apply this new work in educational, health and workplace contexts (Joseph, 2015a). Moreover, community researchers and public policy planners have suggested transforming positive psychology from an individual level to a societal level as well (Pavot & Diener, 2004).

However, despite the feeling of innovation, it has also become clear that positive psychology has had a much longer past and might even be traced back to the origins of psychology itself, like William James' writings on 'healthy mindedness' (James, 1902). Positive psychology also shares a common heritage with parts of humanistic psychology and the writings of Abraham Maslow and Carl Rogers, in particular. These alternative beginnings to positive psychology are now well recognised (Robbins, 2015). However, much less well acknowledged in positive psychology is the heritage of the salutogenic paradigm first suggested by Antonovsky in his book *Health, Stress and Coping* (Antonovsky, 1979).

At first glance, it would seem that the relatively new field of positive psychology had much in common with the earlier approach of salutogenesis. Interestingly, however, the concept of salutogenesis has received relatively little attention within the positive psychology literature. For example, in the 2004 edition of *Positive Psychology in Practice* (Linley & Joseph, 2004), there was no reference to salutogenesis in the book's subject index. Likewise, in the textbook *A Primer in Positive Psychology* (Peterson, 2006), it is similarly not indexed. There are exceptions – such as in Csikszentmihalyi and Csikszentmihalyi's (2006) edited book *A Life Worth Living: Contributions to Positive Psychology* – where a reference to salutogenesis comes half way through the book in the chapter by Antonella Delle Fave of the University of Milan on subjective experience and quality of life (Delle Fave, 2006). Delle Fave briefly notes the salutogenic approach. So it is not that the concept of salutogenesis has been invisible to positive psychologists, but rather that it has not achieved prominence as a framework for theory and research. How can this lack of attention to the concept of salutogenesis be explained? Our answer might be that the salutogenic theory originated in a different discipline than psychology: in medical sociology and – although subsequent applications have been more widespread – the concept has never been fully embraced by psychologists. Nonetheless, there are clear conceptual similarities between Antonovsky's ideas and some of those developed by the positive psychologists (Lutz, 2009).

In this chapter, however, we attempt to reflect on the conceptualisation of positive psychology in light of Antonovsky's theory of salutogenesis. Furthermore, we consider how Antonovsky's core concept, the sense of coherence, provides a new framework for understanding the operation of positive psychology constructs.

Both positive psychology and the salutogenic paradigm challenged mainstream thought about the pathological focus of sociology in the 1970s and psychology in the 2000s, respectively, to consider the resources of healthy functioning. In this regard, both approaches seem to be adopting the same view. However, there was a difference between the two approaches. As clinical psychology had traditionally adopted diagnostic language and a focus on pathology, positive psychology turned its attention to the normal category and positive functioning, and by doing so implicitly condoned the dichotomy between the normal and the abnormal (Joseph & Linley, 2006). Antonovsky's salutogenesis paradigm, on the other hand, offered a new definition of the ease–dis-ease continuum in the medical discipline, thus dissolving the dichotomy between illness and wellness (Antonovsky, 1979).

The argument of positive psychology was that insufficient attention had been paid to the positive side of human experience. The weight of psychological research had been on pathological functioning. This led researchers to turn their attention to strengths of character, talents and abilities and what makes for a healthy and happy life. This new focus challenged the mainstream to shift its attention so that new research would be conducted alongside traditional research. As Folkman and Moskowitz (2003) said:

> ...those who advocate the study of positive aspects of psychology do not intend that it replace concern with its negative aspects. What appears to be an overemphasis may instead be indicative of a catch-up phase for an area that has been underemphasised in recent years. (Folkman & Moskowitz, 2003, p. 121)

Such a position provided a clear vision for the investigation of the positive alongside the negative. Csikszentmihalyi (2003), referring to his and his collaborators' pioneering efforts, provided an argument for studying the positive relatively independently of the negative:

> Basically, we intended to do our best to legitimize the study of positive aspects of human experience in their own right—not just as tools for prevention, coping, health, or some other desirable outcome. We felt that as long as hope, courage, optimism, and joy are viewed simply as useful in reducing pathology, we will never go beyond the homeostatic point of repose and begin to understand those qualities that make life worth living in the first place. (Csikszentmihalyi, 2003, pp. 113–114)

Positive psychology has since developed into a distinct discipline in its own right. There have been new handbooks, textbooks and dedicated university-level courses in positive psychology. In addition, there are now biannual positive psychology conferences held by the *International Positive Psychology Association* and the *European Network for Positive Psychology*, together with a host of conference themes and sections dedicated to positive psychology. As such, the momentum of the positive psychology movement seems to be directed towards deliberately studying well-being in and of itself. Despite this, there are some who have expressed concern that to separate the positive aspects of human experience from the negative may be counterproductive (e.g. Pauwels, 2015).

What is potentially more valuable is to understand the relations between the positive and the negative, comprehending that the role of positive psychology should be to transform how we conceptualise human experience.

Indeed, the idea that human experience can be divided into positive and negative is problematic and the use of such terminology unhelpful. Some scholars have explicitly called for the integration of the positive and negative through the application of more humanistic ways of thinking (Joseph, 2015b). In this way, such a positive psychology could transform the agenda of mainstream psychology by looking for ways to dissolve the boundaries between the positive and the negative. In contrast, the danger of positive psychology now is that its existence serves to condone the separation of the positive and the negative. Thus, rather than serving as a transformational force, it maintains the status quo. Seen this way, it seems misleading to talk of positive psychology as challenging the mainstream pathological agenda of psychology. Moreover, by focusing on positive experiences only, it sends out a contradictory message that the positive is separable from the negative, and while worth studying in its own right, the necessity remains for disciplines of psychology committed to the negative. Thus, ironically, positive psychology strengthens the dichotomy between the positive and the negative.

In light of the above discussion of how it is problematic to think of human experience as either positive or negative, it becomes clear then that the concept of salutogenesis offers an alternative basic theory and conceptual framework. In his proposal, Antonovsky (1979) claims that health and illness should be viewed not as a dichotomy but as a continuum. Human environments by their very nature are stressor-rich, whether microbiological, personal, economic, social or geopolitical. As such, the human being inhabits a world in which it is impossible to avoid stressors and the normal state of the human organism is one of entropy, disorder and disruption of homeostasis.

The basic philosophical assumption of the salutogenic theory is that, instead of perceiving the human system as one which is sound unless it is attacked by some pathogen, the human system is viewed as basically unsound, continuously attacked by disturbing processes and elements which cannot be prevented. This basic assumption is different than the basic philosophical premises of much positive psychology.

Salutogenesis challenges the dominant pathogenic paradigm, but in a different way than the positive psychology movement. Rather than thinking about people as either healthy or diseased, it opens the way for thinking about health and disease along a continuum that goes from 'health ease' to 'dis-ease'. In such an approach, no one is categorised as healthy or diseased. All people are somewhere between the imaginary poles of total wellness and total illness. Even the fully robust, energetic, symptom-free, richly functioning individual has the mark of mortality: he/she wears glasses, has moments of depression, comes down with flu and may also have as yet non-detectable malignant cells. Even the terminal patient's brain and emotions may be fully functional. The great majority of us are somewhere between the two poles. Priority in service is justly given to those at the sicker end of the continuum, but all persons become the focus for research and intervention. Wherever they are on the continuum, there is the possibility of further movement towards the healthy pole.

Moreover, assuming that stressors are ubiquitous, and that there is a continuum of ease–dis-ease, our focus shifts from asking how to eradicate this or that stressor to how to facilitate becoming healthier. Thus, salutogenesis offers a brand new challenge to positive psychology to rethink its stance in relation to the negative. It might suggest that positive psychology consider the implementation of its concepts at all points along the spectrum of dis-ease to well-being. To deepen this direction, we turn to Antonovsky's concept of sense of coherence (SOC).

Sense of Coherence and Positive Psychology

Positive psychologists may be more familiar with the SOC concept than with the broader salutogenic theory itself. However, many of them misunderstand it as a personality disposition or as a coping style. Actually, the concept of SOC has been developed as a concept on a higher level of abstraction, as a worldview. It provides us with a powerful concept to predict health (Eriksson & Lindström, 2011), but yet underutilised. What positive psychology still misses is a theoretical framework for understanding how the range of positive psychological variables, such as optimism, gratitude, forgiveness, curiosity and others, that are routinely studied as predictors of health and happiness exert their effect.

It has become apparent in positive psychology that although some concepts seem to be more generally thought of as 'positive' than others, whether or not any such factor is related to well-being depends on the context. To illustrate, a trait such as optimism is generally considered a psychological ingredient that contributes to well-being. It may be that optimistic people are better able to cope with stress, for example. So, in a stressful context, optimism plays a beneficial moderating role. But, in another context, it could be that optimism impedes well-being. For example, more optimistic people may adopt more reckless investment strategies. As such, it is likely that many psychological traits and processes are neither inherently positive nor negative, but only positive or negative in their effect with regard to specific circumstances.

On a different level of abstraction, SOC refers not to a special set of traits or coping strategies but rather to the mediational mechanism through which all other factors exert their influence on health and well-being. Personal and social resources can build comprehensibility, manageability and meaningfulness of any given situation, allowing us to cope with the ubiquitous stressors of life, thus promoting well-being in the never-ending struggle against entropy. On the other hand, those factors that make demands on comprehensibility, manageability and meaningfulness leave us vulnerable to the effects of entropy.

Regarding the development of SOC, Antonovsy (1987) suggested that at a certain age (30 years), people have developed a fairly consistent SOC, although recent studies suggest that unexpected traumatic events can challenge our SOC, requiring us to rebuild a new SOC in light of our experiences (Antonovsky & Sagy, 1986; Bental-Israeli & Sagy, 2010).

In the past two decades, positive psychology has fuelled interest in post-traumatic growth (Joseph, 2011). Post-traumatic growth is a wide-ranging concept, still in development, but to date three broad domains of positive change have been noted that best describe the ways people often report that they have been changed following trauma. Firstly, relationships are enhanced in some way. For example, people describe that they come to value their friends and family more, feel an increased sense of compassion for others and a longing for more intimate relationships. Secondly, people change their views of themselves in some way, for example, that they have a greater sense of personal resiliency, wisdom and strength, perhaps coupled with a greater acceptance of their vulnerabilities and limitations. Thirdly, people describe changes in their life philosophy, for example, finding a fresh appreciation for each new day and re-evaluating their understanding of what really matters in life.

Positive changes are widely reported by people following trauma. Using psychometric measures and open-ended interviews, a large number of studies have shown that growth is commonly reported by survivors of various traumatic events, including transportation accidents (shipping disasters, plane crashes and car accidents), natural disasters (hurricanes and earthquakes), interpersonal experiences (combat, rape, sexual assault and child abuse), medical problems (cancer, heart attack, brain injury, spinal cord injury, HIV/AIDS, leukaemia, rheumatoid arthritis, multiple sclerosis and illness) and other life experiences (relationship breakdown, parental divorce, bereavement and immigration). Typically, 30–70% of survivors will say that they have experienced positive changes of one form or another (Joseph, 2011).

Moreover, research indicates that greater post-traumatic growth is associated with personality factors such as emotional stability, extraversion, openness to experience, optimism and self-esteem; ways of coping such as acceptance, positive reframing, seeking social support, turning to religion, problem solving; and social support factors (Joseph, 2011). Such a framework can be applied with the aim of understanding how positive psychological constructs may be beneficial, but the area where this framework seems most clearly applicable is in how people overcome and grow personally following adversity.

A Salutogenic Positive Psychology

The aim of this chapter is to promote bridge building between the paradigm of salutogenesis and the movement of positive psychology, and to suggest a joint conceptual framework of salutogenic positive psychology. We trust that despite the differences between the two paradigms, an integrative approach could contribute to deeper understanding of both approaches.

One contribution of the integrative approach relates to the role of sociological factors in explaining SOC development as well as other positive psychological concepts. In contrast to the common purely positive psychological view, Antonovsky (1991, 1993) attempted, within a systems theory framework, to analyse how *social structures* shape the strength of the SOC. He claimed that to disregard the power of history, the generational experiences of the macro-political events of war and depression, population shifts and revolutions are to disregard the context within which the strength of each of us is shaped. Indeed, early socialisation has been discussed in psychological theories, and experiences in the family have been considered as crucial. But these experiences are themselves shaped by the broader social structure which is usually ignored. Socioeconomic status and educational levels have been shown to be important factors in building strong SOC (Madarasova Geckova et al., 2010; Sagy & Antonovsky, 2000).

The implication of these analyses for salutogenically oriented clinicians could lead to interventions such as active participation in transforming environmental conditions. It certainly seems reasonable to hypothesise that one who sees life as comprehensible, manageable and meaningful is more likely to optimally exploit potential resistance resources. This approach can also help us to theoretically explain why some prevention programmes or health promotion plans tend to work well for some people but not as well for others (Sagy, 2014). Evidence from factor analysis suggests that SOC and well-being, although associated, are distinct constructs (Cilliers & Coetzee, 2003).

As such, we envisage that the relationship between well-being and commonly studied positive psychological constructs such as optimism, gratitude, forgiveness and hope is mediated by SOC. When this has been tested, the evidence is supportive (Lambert et al., 2009). But SOC is also influenced by life experiences and social systems, such that well-being is ultimately the product of trauma and other life events, positive psychology factors and the social structure. However, in each case, the relationship with well-being is mediated by SOC (see Fig. 23.1). Moreover, the possibility exists that each of these relationships is moderated by the other factors, such that, for example, positive psychological factors are only related to well-being in specific social structures or at particular levels of trauma.

Returning to the concept of posttraumatic growth, the salutogenic positive psychology framework could contribute especially well to the understanding of traumatic experience by the interaction of a variety of concepts related to personality, tendencies and strategies of coping together with sociological factors. These different factors could, for example, jointly predict post-traumatic growth, while the SOC could be the mediator/moderator in these interactions. For example, one line of investigation has been to study SOC in therapists who work traumatised clients, showing that those with higher SOC report more positive changes (Linley et al., 2005) and less compassion fatigue and burnout (Linley & Joseph, 2007).

From Fig. 23.1, one can hypothesise that trauma has a shattering effect on the person's SOC resulting in a process of breakdown of these foundational perceptions. It is though

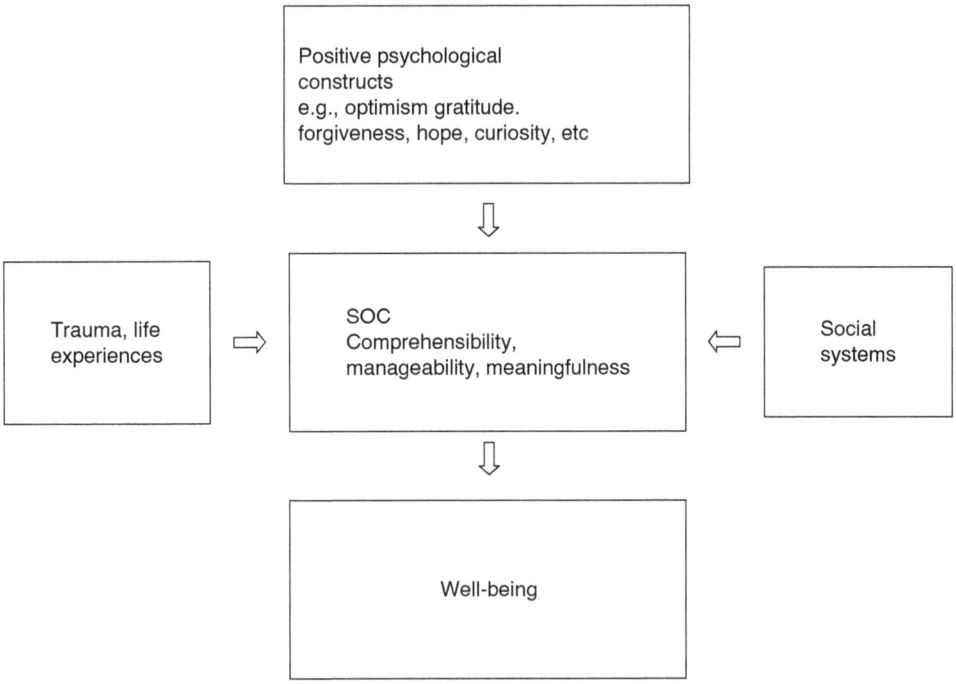

Fig. 23.1 The relationship between positive psychology constructs and well-being is hypothesised to be mediated by SOC

the influence of social systems external to the person and the development of positive qualities within the person that SOC can be re-established – but in ways that are accommodating of the changed circumstances. This process resulting in increased psychological well-being is post-traumatic growth.

Thus, we can view post-traumatic growth as a description of those positive changes that arise through the resolution and rebuilding of the person's SOC and the resultant post-traumatic distress that this process entails. The salutogenic positive psychology perspective allows us to develop an understanding of potential traumatic experiences which integrates post-traumatic distress and post-traumatic growth within a single conceptual framework. This new integrative perspective could also guide clinical practice to develop interventions which promote SOC amongst trauma survivors.

Our point is that SOC offers not so much an additional set of variables alongside those already studied by positive psychologists, but a larger theoretical framework within which to consider the operation of these variables. As others have also argued, SOC can be seen as an inclusive concept (Almedom, 2005).

Conclusion

It appears that despite their different theoretical roots, the integration of the two paradigms – salutogenesis and positive psychology – has stronger explanatory power in promoting health and well-being. We trust that positive psychologists will benefit from a deeper appreciation of the SOC construct in two ways: firstly, understanding how social structures shape the strength of SOC, and secondly, how SOC provides the cognitive mechanisms within the individual that mediates the relationship between positive psychology constructs such as hope, optimism, gratitude and well-being. Finally, there are two ways in which salutogenic researchers can benefit from positive psychology. Firstly, positive psychology offers a new and evidence-based means for putting salutogenesis into practice at both micro- and macro levels. However, the second and most important contribution of positive psychology is in reminding salutogenic researchers that their evaluation of outcomes related to SOC need not be pathological. We need to move beyond outcomes such as the absence of depression, reduction in hostility and the like, to include the presence of happiness, development of empathy and more. In this way, we begin to see greater convergence between the two disciplines and the emergence of salutogenic positive psychology.

References

Almedom, A. M. (2005). Resilience, hardiness, sense of coherence, and posttraumatic growth: All paths leading to "light at the end of the tunnel"? *Journal of Loss and Trauma, 10*(3), 253–265.

Antonovsky, A. (1979). *Health, stress, and coping*. Jossey-Bass.

Antonovsky, A. (1991). The salutogenic approach to family system health: Promise and danger. *European congress on "mental health in European families."* Retrieved from http://angelfire.com/ok/soc/agolem.html.

Antonovsky, A. (1993). The structure and properties of the sense of coherence scale. *Social Science and Medicine, 36*, 725–733.

Antonovsky, H., & Sagy, S. (1986). The development of a sense of coherence and its impact on responses to stress situations. *The Journal of Social Psychology, 126*, 213–225.

Antonovsy, A. (1987). *Unravelling the mystery of health. How people manage stress and stay well.* Jossey-Bass.

Bental-Israeli, A., & Sagy, S. (2010). Life experiences contributing to the development of a sense of coherence: Consistency and/or breakthrough experience. *Studies in education, 1*, 215–241. Hebrew.

Cilliers, F., & Coetzee, S. C. (2003). The theoretical-empirical fit between three psychological wellness constructs: Sense of coherence, learned resourcefulness and self-actualisation. *South African Journal of Labour Relations, 27*(1), 4–24.

Csikszentmihalyi, M. (2003). Legs or wings? A reply to R. S. Lazarus. *Psychological Inquiry, 14*, 113–115.

Csikszentmihalyi, M., & Csikszentmihalyi, I. S. (Eds.). (2006). *A life worth living: Contributions to positive psychology.* Oxford University Press.

Delle Fave, A. (2006). The impact of subjective experience on the quality of life: A central issue for health professionals. In M. Csikszentmihalyi & I. S. Csikszentmihalyi (Eds.), *A life worth living: Contributions to positive psychology* (pp. 165–181). Oxford University Press.

Eriksson, M., & Lindström, B. (2011). Life is more than survival: Exploring links between Antonovsky's salutogenic theory and the concept of resilience. In K. M. Gow & M. J. Celinski (Eds.), *Wayfinding through life's challenges: Coping and survival* (pp. 31–46). Nova.

Folkman, S., & Moskowitz, J. T. (2003). Positive psychology from a coping perspective. *Psychological Inquiry, 14*, 121–125.

James, W. (1902). *The varieties of religious experience: A study in human nature.* Longman, Green.

Joseph, S. (2011). *What doesn't kill us: The new psychology of posttraumatic growth.* Basic Books.

Joseph, S. (Ed.). (2015a). *Positive psychology in practice: Promoting human flourishing in work, health, education, and everyday life.* Wiley.

Joseph, S. (2015b). The future of positive psychology in practice. In S. Joseph (Ed.), *Positive psychology in practice: Promoting human flourishing in work, health, education, and everyday life* (pp. 823–828). Wiley.

Joseph, S., & Linley, P. A. (2006). Positive psychology versus the medical model?: Comment. *American Psychologist, 61*, 332–333.

Lambert, N. M., Graham, S. M., Fincham, F. D., & Stillman, T. F. (2009). A changed perspective: How gratitude can affect sense of coherence through positive reframing. *The Journal of Positive Psychology, 4*(6), 461–470.

Linley, A. P., & Joseph, S. (Eds.). (2004). *Positive psychology in practice.* Wiley.

Linley, P. A., & Joseph, S. (2007). Therapy work and therapists' positive and negative well–being. *Journal of Social and Clinical Psychology, 26*(3), 385–403.

Linley, A. P., Joseph, S., Harrington, S., & Wood, A. M. (2006). Positive psychology: Past, present, and (possible) future. *The Journal of Positive Psychology, 1*, 3–16.

Linley, P. A., Joseph, S., & Loumidis, K. (2005). Trauma work, sense of coherence, and positive and negative changes in therapists. *Psychotherapy and Psychosomatics, 74*(3), 185–188.

Lopez, S. J., & Snyder, C. R. (Eds.). (2003). *Positive psychological assessment: A handbook of models and measures.* American Psychological Association.

Lutz, J. (2009). Flow and sense of coherence: Two aspects of the same dynamic? *Global Health Promotion, 16*(3), 63–67.

Madarasova Geckova, A., Tavel, P., van Dijk, J. P., Abel, T., & Reijneveld, S. A. (2010). Factors associated with educational aspirations among adolescents: Cues to counteract socioeconomic differences? *BMC Public Health, 10*, 154–163.

Pauwels, B. G. (2015). The uneasy—And necessary—Role of the negative in positive psychology. In S. Joseph (Ed.), *Positive psychology in practice: Promoting human flourishing in work, health, education, and everyday life.* Wiley.

Pavot, W., & Diener, E. (2004). Findings on subjective Well-being: Applications to public policy, clinical interventions, and education. In P. A. Linley & S. Joseph (Eds.), *Positive psychology in practice* (pp. 679–692). Wiley.

Peterson, C. (2006). *A primer in positive psychology.* Oxford University Press.

Robbins, B. D. (2015). Building bridges between humanistic and positive psychology. In S. Joseph (Ed.), *Positive psychology in practice: Promoting human flourishing in work, health, education, and everyday life* (pp. 31–46). Wiley.

Sagy, S. (2014). Preventing drug abuse among children and adolescents: Where does the salutogenic approach direct us? *Health, 6*, 541–548.

Sagy, S., & Antonovsky, H. (2000). The development of the sense of coherence: A retrospective study of early life experiences in the family. *International Journal of Aging & Human Development, 51*, 155–166.

Seligman, M. E. P. (2004). Foreword. In P. A. Linley & S. Joseph (Eds.), *Positive psychology in practice* (pp. xi–xiii). Wiley: Hoboken.

Seligman, M. E. P., & Csikszentmihalyi, M. (2000). Positive psychology: An introduction. *American Psychologist, 55*, 5–14.

24

Implementation of Salutogenesis: Public Policy and Politics

Ruca Maass, Charlotte Kiland, Geir Arild Espnes, and Monica Lillefjell

Introduction

Politics can loosely be defined as the process of making and executing collective decisions (Hague & Harrop, 2010, p. 442). Political decisions affect every part of our lives, from the distribution of rights and resources, how institutions are run and which goals we pursue as a society, to regulating even personal relationships and family bonds. Thus, politics is one of the upstream conditions that shape our society and set the direction and the pace for how society is developing.

Salutogenesis is concerned about the relationship between societal conditions and health. According to the salutogenic model, health is created and maintained through repeated experiences with societal conditions (Antonovsky, 1987). Health is described along a continuum, ranging from ill-health to perfect health. An individual's position on this scale is heavily influenced by life experiences, shaped by biological, individual, societal and cultural forces sensitive to politics and policy-making (Antonovsky, 1979, 1987). Within public health, there has been a growing consensus that health is political, and that health issues need to be brought into the political arena to advance population health (Bambra et al., 2005; Kickbusch, 2015; Mackenbach, 2014). This is linked to the health determinants depending on political action. Health is understood as a critical dimension of human rights and citizenship (Bambra et al., 2005). Improving the upstream conditions for health demands to address social determinants and how they are shaped and negotiated through political processes (Marmot, 2005).

Within the field of political science and public administration, politics is understood as a continuous struggle for power amongst competing interests (Kickbusch, 2015). This power struggle might occur between and within countries. Politics is also about handling challenges at a societal level. A recent example of the importance of tackling challenges can be found in the Covid-19 pandemic (the Corona crisis); a global, collective threat. The crisis sparked a wave of political reactions, ranging from implementing far-reaching measures limiting people's possibilities and movements to an unprecedented extent, to political leaders denying and even ridiculing the threat. Besides yielding quite different results for the spread of, and the death toll from, the disease, do these variations in political actions also illustrate how competing interests (such as keeping the economy going vs. protecting the population from catching the disease) can hugely influence the outcome of political processes?

In turn, processes, and their interplay with media representations, influence coping at an individual as well as at a community level. On the one hand, trust in authorities and sense of coherence (SOC) emerged as crucial coping resources which reduced the risk of developing mental illness during the Covid-19 pandemic across countries (Généreux, David, O'Sullivan, et al., 2020; Généreux, Roy, O'Sullivan, & Maltais, 2020). On the other hand, false beliefs, mistrust in authorities, stigma, perceived threat and financial loss raised probabilities of ill mental health (Généreux, Roy, David, et al., 2020).

Simultaneously, regardless of what kind of measures were taken (or not taken) in the respective countries, there was protest. Some people in Germany, for example, protested what they perceived as exaggerated measures that deprived them of human rights. Meanwhile, some people in Brazil and the USA asked for more measures to protect the general public and to prioritise health above economic interest. This illustrates the power struggles inherent in political processes: competing interests need to be considered, and solutions that

R. Maass (✉) · M. Lillefjell
Department of Neuromedicine and Movement Science, Faculty of Medicine and Health Science, Norwegian University of Science and Technology (NTNU), Trondheim, Norway
e-mail: ruca.e.maass@ntnu.no

C. Kiland
Department of Political Science and Management, Faculty of Social Sciences, University in Agder, Kristiansand, Norway

G. A. Espnes
Center for Health Promotion Research, Department of Public Health and Nursing, Faculty of Medicine and Health Sciences, Norwegian University of Science and Technology, Trondheim, Norway

are in accordance with one group's interests might be at odds with other groups. Historically, collective challenges often resulted in conflict and division of societies. However, human history, often told as a recollection of catastrophe and conflict, also holds narratives of growth and hope, which helped to prevail and even evolve societies as well as individuals (Bregman, 2020). Also during the Corona crisis, examples of collective challenges bringing out 'the good' in people could be found: spontaneous acts of kindness and solidarity became visible, from theatre-playing outside of nursing homes to the upspring of neighbourhood help collectives that assisted vulnerable neighbours with shopping and other chores.

Moreover, the implemented measures contributed to speed up developments like digitalisation. In other words, resolving one collective challenge can sometimes fuel a positive development in society. Overcoming and growing with challenges is in line with a salutogenic perspective, and at the heart of the salutogenic process (Antonovsky, 1987; Généreux, Roy, O'Sullivan, & Maltais, 2020; Namihira, 2019).

This chapter explores if and how salutogenesis can be applied to the field of politics and policy-making. We start by giving a short overview of the field of political science, politics and policies. We then clarify the position of salutogenesis on politics and unravel potential links before we explore how salutogenesis could contribute to understand and inform politics.

Politics and Policies

Politics, as defined above, is about making collective decisions and negotiate power. Public policy-making relates to the actions of the government and the processes of articulating and matching actors' goals and means into decisions or non-decisions to affect and influence members of a national state or sub-national jurisdiction. Thus, whilst politics refers to the decision-making process, does public policy contribute to translate and implement these decisions into the various domains of societal life.

Within traditional administration, the political context is characterised by bureaucratic structures, separate spheres between politics and administration and a logic of rational–technical processes in which public policy-making take place. Those who are involved tend to follow some general procedures (Holmberg & Rothstein, 2012): (1) agenda setting helping policy-makers decide which problems to address; (2) policy formation where solutions to problems are shaped and argued; (3) policy legitimation to move the policy through a formal decision-making (or legislative) process; (4) policy implementation turning policies into action; (5) policy evaluation to determine if the policies they create are effective in achieving their goals; (6) policies resulting in their maintenance, succession or termination due to policy-makers' shifting goals, values, beliefs or priorities.

Critique of the rational–technical logic has underlined that the combination of traditional bureaucracy and interest-group politics led to a 'muddling through' approach (Lindblom, 1979). This resulted in fragmented politics creating 'silos' or 'stovepipes' within organisations (Wilson, 1989). Today, most major public policy problems are 'wicked', that is they are inherently resistant to a clear definition and an agreed solution (Head & Alford, 2015). As public health problems become more wicked, cutting across administrative levels, sectors and units, political and administrative leaders are challenged.

Since the late 1980s, two public reform waves have influenced the political-administrative system in European governments: that of New Public Management (NPM) and post-New Public Management (post-NPM) (Christensen, 2012; Christensen & Lægreid, 2007, 2011). NPM ideas focused on improving efficiency, horizontally specialisation of the political-administrative apparatuses, marketisation, private-sector management style, explicit performance standards and strengthened output/outcome control (Hood, 1991, Christensen, 2012, p. 1). Along with the increased need for more 'evidence-based' public policy-making and administrative expertise, this resulted in fragmented knowledge and understanding about factors that might cause or influence complex societal problems. It became difficult to address significant issues comprehensively and challenging to grapple the input and involvement of a broader range of actors in society. Generally, NPM practices have been unsuitable in dealing with complex problems (Christensen & Lægreid, 2011; Head & Alford, 2015). As a response to the failure in handling wicked and complex problems, the rise of so-called post- New Public Management ideas in the early 2000s called for more holistic approaches, arguing for whole-of-government approaches and lately whole-of-society approaches (Christensen, 2012; Christensen & Lægreid, 2007). They seek to improve the horizontal coordination of governmental organisations and to enhance coordination between government and other actors; for example, citizens, civil society actors, voluntary and private actors.

Within the context of representative democracy, processes to strengthen participation and influence between elections might be regarded as disturbing for the public policy-making processes (Østerud 2004). Still, the post-NPM reforms imply the focus of government to have increasingly shifted to horizontal coordination and collaboration. The organisational forms of public administration have become increasingly complex and hybrid (Christensen, 2012). We argue that these post-NPM ideas emphasising involvement and collaboration provide a new angle for the application of a more upstream and salutogenic perspective in public policy-making.

As a result of increased complexity and fragmentation of NPM reforms, there is now a widespread focus on the need for more "collaboration" and "coordination" (Agger &

Sørensen, 2018; Christensen, 2012). A commonly held notion is that working across organisational, jurisdictional and political-administrative boundaries will enable more efficient and effective policy development, implementation and service delivery. These ideas address the importance to think broadly about major social problems and possible ways of addressing them. However, collaboration across sectors carries it's own challenges, often rooted in the (politically defined) responsibilities, diverging values, fragmented knowledge and struggles over resources. As such, Head and Alford (2015) argue for new models of leadership that better appreciate the distributed nature of information, interests and power and can address these problems in a coordinated manner.

One challenge emerging from the fragmentation of knowledge and responsibility is that policies are developed to address specific problems, solutions or sectors. Accordingly, policies developed within one sector may fail to address important aspects in other sectors and result in incoherent policies. Policy coherence can be described as 'the systematic promotion of mutually reinforcing policy actions across government departments and agencies creating synergies towards achieving the agreed objectives' (OECD, 2019). Besides aiming to harmonise policies between sectors, policy coherence also touches into matters of implementing policies and ensuring that stakeholders receive the appropriate competence, resources and motivation to translate policies into effective action (Nilsson et al., 2012). Thus, policy coherence emerges as an important aspect in politics and policy-making and can be described horizontally (between sectors) and vertically (across different government levels and from decision-makers to the general public). Experiences of coherent structures have been linked to the ability to make compromises, participating in adapting and creating appropriate resources, and even develop trust in society and its institutions (Habermas, 2016; Kickbusch & Szabo, 2014; Marmot & Allen, 2013). Trust in the state and its governance emerged, in turn, as an important coping resource during the early stages of the Corona pandemic (Genereux et al., 2020; Généreux, David, O'Sullivan, et al., 2020; Généreux, Roy, David, et al., 2020). Thus, providing populations with a coherent understanding of what is going on contributes to stabilising society. Additionally, recent research suggests that populations which display more trust in their civic and political leaders are better equipped to handle collective challenges (Généreux et al., 2020; Sagy, 2015; Sagy & Braun-Lewensohn, 2009).

Linking Salutogenesis and Public Policy-Making

Salutogenesis aims at being an umbrella for a wide range of positive health and well-being-related concepts such as resilience, coping and quality of life (Lindström & Eriksson, 2010). Strümpfer (1995) attempted to broaden the term, to also include a general ability to meet hardship. He suggested to 'fortigenesis' (the origin of strength) as a term to include matters and outcomes beyond the health sector. Whilst the term itself did not reach widespread attention in the scientific community, researchers concerned with salutogenesis have increasingly applied salutogenic perspectives on matters beyond the health sector.

According to Antonovsky, the answer to the question 'what makes people healthy?' is 'a strong sense of coherence (SOC)'. The SOC describes an individual's outlook on life, based on individual experiences with societal forces (Antonovsky, 1979, 1987). A strong SOC indicates that the world is perceived as comprehensible, manageable and meaningful. A strong SOC helps to identify and adequately apply resources and to cope with stressors and resolve challenges in a health-promoting manner (Antonovsky, 1987; Maass, 2018).

The SOC is developed through overcoming challenges and the internalisation of resources. Specific resistance resources (SRRs) can be applied to resolve specific challenges. SRR play an important role in individual health promotion. For example, resources to support young families during the first weeks of a new baby's life can be crucial for this specific experience, whilst such specialised resources would not be applicable to resolve a wide range of other challenges.

On the other hand, resources can be internalised and turned into 'generalised resistance resources' (GRR). GRR can be found at any level, from the individual to the societal level, and can be applied flexibly to achieve various outcomes. GRR thereby become part of the individual's SOC. The internalisation of resources is fuelled by 'significant life events', which challenge established coping strategies. Significant life events touch into comprehensibility, manageability and meaningfulness simultaneously (Antonovsky, 1987).

Societal and political matters are thereby intertwined with individual SOC: they facilitate and order our experiences, pose challenges and distribute resources; they define our rights and responsibilities and the social position that again shapes our experiences and expectations. Developing society in a salutogenic direction might benefit populations, individuals and society itself. However, according to Antonovsky, 'no society [yet] (...) managed to avoid structural limitations, or (...) to provide structural access to the goals it has propagated' (Antonovsky, 1979, p.88).

Salutogenesis describes how matters of politics and policies contribute to shaping individual's and group's ability to cope. But how can salutogenesis contribute to outline strategies and structure processes linked to politics and policy-making? According to the above, salutogenesis can be understood and applied unto public policy-making in two distinct ways: as a global orientation towards a positive outlook on life, problem-solving and resource-focus; or as a distinct way to organise approaches in line with the more specific relationships between the 'upstream' conditions, resources and the three dimensions of SOC.

Salutogenesis as a Global Orientation Towards Positive Outcomes and Resources

Applying a salutogenic angle on politics and policy-making implies a focus on resources, possibilities and solutions. As outlined above, policies are often designed to resolve "wicked problems". Besides often leading to isolated and narrow measures, can this approach be described as problem-based. In a way, this mirrors the dominant approach in medicine, pathogenesis, which seeks to identify and isolate 'the cause of suffering' and then remove it. A salutogenic approach, on the other hand, challenges this starting point by posing the salutogenic question: "what makes people healthy?" As an equivalent in political science, one might ask, 'how can we tackle these challenges in a good way, by learning and growing?', or 'how can we create societies that bring out the good in people?'. This implies a focus on the questions 'what works?' and 'why and how does it work?', as starting points for developing policies.

Experiences from Various Settings

There are some examples of studies applying salutogenesis unto matters outside of the 'health' sector. For example, Kelly (2015) applies the salutogenic question unto the school context, turning the question from "why does it not work?" into "how can it work?", and proposes salutogenesis as a beneficial approach for framing new approaches for school leadership. Brolin et al. (2018) applied salutogenesis to develop a strength-based approach to health in a school. Students developed a narrative in which health was conceptualised as a collective, value-based asset, which implies that students are co-responsible for others' health outcomes. Students were more likely than teachers to include salutogenic factors and apply a value-based health discourse. This was also in contrast to the school health initiative, in which individualistic, pathogenic notions dominated. A similar finding was made by Dell' Olio, Vaandrager, & Koelen, (2018), who applied salutogenesis unto the specific context of students with disabilities and advocate changes in the academic services for these students. They found that the students were able to assess a number of both specific (such as institutional services and disease information) and generalised resistance resources (including social capital and awareness of one's strengths). Their findings suggest that policy-makers focus more on challenges and obstacles, whilst students themselves described some of these 'obstacles' as opportunities and even assets.

In salutogenesis, stressors and assets are described as 'two sides of the same coin'. Overcoming challenges is described as a salutary process (Antonovsky, 1979, 1987). A salutogenic orientation emphasises the importance of participatory approaches, the world views of stakeholders and target groups and applying empowering and enabling strategies. This turns the focus away from shortcomings which, in the long run, can contribute to further victimisation of vulnerable groups. Engaging in a positive process focused on strength and opportunities might in itself contribute to better health through a shift of focus and by experiences of mastery and learning along the way (Généreux, Roy, O'Sullivan, & Maltais, 2020). In the above examples, the desired outcome of the interventions is not at the level of individual health. Instead, the focus is on ways to organise the school environment to help students to cope with everyday challenges. They thereby illustrate the importance of organisation and policies to achieve a salutary process for collectives as well as individuals.

Similar findings from the work-sector support these notions. For example, Reid and Quayle (2008) apply a salutogenic perspective on occupational health and propose salutogenesis as a theoretical framework that could contribute to policy development and occupational assessments by bridging work-related and individual factors. Pijpker and colleagues (2019) investigated the role of learning with respect to SOC and GRR. They suggest promoting learning through both formal and informal ways as a mean to strengthen SOC through experiences from working life. Vaandrager and Koelen (2013) define a salutogenic workplace health as 'the ability of the workforce to participate and be productive in a sustained and meaningful way'. They describe a salutogenic organisation as an organisation that provides resources and offers coherent experiences. They advocate a salutogenic orientation to promote motivation and the experience of meaningfulness in the workforce, and to enable the organisation to focus on its strength and develop measures based on what works. Evidence suggests that users, in these cases, students and workers, apply a more salutogenic lens than do leaders and policy-makers, and emphasise structural and collective resources and outcomes above individual ones.

From 'Wicked Problems' to 'Healthy Societies'?

The above suggests that applying salutogenesis unto politics and policy-making implies to phrase positive goals, and emphasises the interplay between the individual and her supporting structures; society and societal institutions. A more consistent application of salutogenesis might benefit policy development in more than one way. To focus on growth and possibilities might in itself contribute to find solutions rather than dwell on challenges. Working together towards common goals might contribute to greater enthusiasm and commitment than working to prevent negative development (Elliot, 1999). It contributes to make possible benefits visible, instead of fostering fear and anxiety about what is to come. For policy-makers and implementers, it represents an opportunity to overcome the role as a 'fire extinguisher' rushing from challenge to challenge and trying to fight each crisis isolated. Instead, focusing on salutogenic solutions and societies might facilitate the development of desirable future scenarios and encourage visionaries to strive for a salutogenic society.

Policy-makers and politicians experience to be confronted with ever-new problems which have to be dealt with here and now to satisfy potential voters. However, this position is unfavourable to address the complexity and wickedness in such societal problems. For example, social inequality can contribute to increased crime, unemployment, drug abuse, raise levels of social conflict, exclusion and discrimination and even result in political instability and distrust. Trying to fight each of these adverse outcomes separately might contribute to diverting attention and effort from the inequality which is at the bottom of all these 'wicked' problems (Marmot, & Wilkinson, R. (Eds.)., 2005; Marmot & Allen, 2013).

A salutogenic approach would address these problems with a strategy of cooperative society development. It might thereby apply processes and produce solutions that contribute to level out social inequality. The above examples indicate that users (students and employees) often have a more salutary focus than policy-makers. This supports notions of citizen involvement throughout the whole process of policy-making: identifying shared goals and achieve shared understandings about what is going on is a crucial condition for cooperation. Simultaneously, acknowledging the experiences and aspirations of especially minority groups might be an important first step towards identifying resources and develop strength (Rappaport, 1995).

Politics and Policy Coherence

In salutogenesis, the origin of health is described as 'a sense of coherence', which is developed based on coherent experiences with the societal structures. Thus, aiming at creating coherent structures emerges as an important aim in politics and policy-making. Two main challenges arise from policy- and politics-making processes: cooperation and coherence both horizontally (between sectors and actors) and vertically (top-to-bottom within each sector, from decision-makers over implementers to the public).

Horizontal Coherence: Collaboration and Cooperation

Horizontal coherence addresses issues that arise from multi-sectorial collaboration. Collaboration and cooperation across sectors and actors are described as an important mean in respect to negotiating politics: solutions have to be found across spatial domains. However, this goal is challenged by structural elements within NPM, such as the fragmentation of responsibilities, silo-thinking and rigid input/output regimes which crave for effectiveness within each sector (Christensen, 2012; Wilson, 1989).

Collaboration processes thereby often illustrate the root problems within politics: struggles and negotiations about power and influence. Competing interests are not only driven by population groups. Even within public government and administration, conflict of interests arise. In politics, this is expressed by the political parties which are distributed power through an election. They depend upon and are sensitive to changes in public opinion. Within public administration, conflict of interest arises from divergent understandings and knowledge, shortness of staff and funding and the input/output regime, which leads each sector to prioritise their specific goals above common aims. These challenges can easily be described as incoherence, according to Antonovsky's framework: a lack of comprehensibility due to fragmented knowledge, a lack of manageability due to under-funding and time pressure and a lack of meaningfulness if common goals are perceived less important than sector-specific aims. As effectiveness is measured within each sector, contributing to achievements that are measured in other sectors might even be perceived to be contra-productive: if you or your sector cannot make your contributions visible, you might get distributed less resoruces next time budgets are negotiated.

To what extent the approaches of post-NPM endorse solutions to these common problems remains unknown. Post-NPM approaches build on extensive collaboration and imply a certain degree of citizen involvement (Christensen, 2012; Østerud, 2004). Instead of delegating power to market actors, cooperation with the third sector and involvement of civil society actors are at the forefront. However, solely emphasising the need for more collaboration is not enough, and might even be counter-productive, if it is perceived as yet another aim to live up to, without being equipped with the means to do so. To take a whole-of-government or even whole-of-society-approach seriously, it seems important that the aims of the approach indeed are rooted, and acknowledged as valid, by the whole of government/society (Kickbusch & Szabo, 2014). Likewise, common goals should be accompanied by a sound distribution of responsibilities and resources.

All in all, these notions emphasise the importance of establishing shared understandings and common goals across sectors. Such goals need to be phrased and incorporated into common both common strategic plans to ensure that they are perceived as valid across sectors. On an international level, the sustainable development goals (SDG) represent such common goals (UN, 2017). However, such overarching goals can sometimes be unclear, and stakeholders might lack insights about how they can address them within their sector and from their position. Thus, overarching goals should be translated into the various sectors, to ensure that all stakeholders have the motivation and the means to work towards the overarching, common goal within their field of responsibility. To achieve horizontal coherence, it seems crucial to a) ensure a shared understanding about what is going on, as well as increase understanding about the roles and responsibilities the different stakeholders can take in this regard; b) ensure that all involved stakeholders have the means and resources to take their responsibility and contribute to the common goal; and c) ensure that all stakeholders have the motivation to engage in working towards common goals, that is, by translating these goals into the sector-specific strategic plans and make the contributions of each sector visible throughout the process. Keeping an eye on these factors throughout decision-making and implementation might proof a beneficial way to establish and maintain coherence throughout the political process. Preferably, both the common aims that are established and the means applied to achieve them should be rooted in the population, which, according to the above, often phrases more salutogenic aims than professionals (Dell' Olio, Vaandrager, & Koelen, 2018; Reid & Quayle, 2008). Thus, besides horizontal collaboration, user involvement and participatory approaches emerge as important tools to achieve vertical coherence in politics.

Vertical Policy Coherence: From a Decision to Implementation

Vertical coherence in politics is about making decisions and implementing them in a way which adds to comprehensibility, manageability and meaningfulness for the targeted population. Here, the importance of policies and implementation processes emerges: often, valid goals can be translated into measures which are contradictive, add to the burden or are perceived as incoherent by those that are meant to be supported (Nilsson et al., 2012).

If policies are perceived as posing challenges without addressing the means to resolve these challenges, or if they are perceived as meaningless – or even a threat to what is perceived as meaningful – this might result in distrust towards decision-makers and their representatives (Genereux et al., 2020; Habermas, 2016; Marmot & Allen, 2013). Consequently, distrust and incoherence can result in destabilised societies, with fragmented sub-groups, and high levels of polarisation and conflict (Yeo, & Green, M. N. (Eds.)., 2017). During the past decade, we have seen a rise in 'fake news', conspiracy theories, decreasing trust in politicians and increasing polarisation in society, which, in its most extreme outcome, even can foster terrorism and violence. Could the root cause of this be collective experiences of incoherence with the political structures?

The SOC is built through accumulated experiences with coherent, societal structures. However, not only personal but also collective experiences can influence our perceptions and expectations. These are passed down to us across generations and communicated through cultural and social institutions and channels such as stories, movies and the educational system. However, members of different social groups can make profoundly different experiences with the same societal structures (Antonovsky, 1987; Rappaport, 1995). Thus, how society works for you also depends on matters of identity, status and group-belonging.

This also implies that members of minority groups sometimes experience that their expectations, developed through popular culture and learned values, are not met in real-life encounters with the resource. A recent example of this can be found in the "Black Lives Matter (BLM)" – demonstrations against police violence in the USA. They clearly illustrate that one of society's most crucial assets – the institution enforcing law and order and protecting citizens – is experienced more like a risk and a threat by large proportions of the population (Peck, 2015). Other examples include expectations of 'freedom of religion', but being met with ridicule and hatred based on religious clothing (i.e. Slettholm & Stokke, 2015), or expecting equal opportunities, but then experience geographical, ethnical or gender-based injustice that deprives people of crucial opportunities (Michelsen et al., 2017). Maass et al. (2014) suggest that members of minority groups experience this also in less-prominent contexts. Members of minority groups often experience incoherence regarding policies and their implementation. Such incoherence is reinforced by victim blaming, which fails to acknowledge the structural causes of social injustice (Marmot, 2004; Pascoe & Smart Richman, 2009; Rappaport, 1995). Examples can be seen in attempts to discredit the victims of police violence sparking the recent BLM protests, to distribute them (part of the) blame for their fate (compare, i.e. Jangar, 2020).

Incoherent experiences are, according to salutogenesis, characterised by a lack of comprehensibility, manageability and/or meaningfulness. Incoherent experiences result from repeatedly hearing that what you know about the world is not valid, realising that you cannot obtain the means to achieve your valid aspirations, discovering that a re-distribution of resources does not accompany promises of a better future or realising that your life lacks meaningfulness. Besides posing a risk for health and wellbeing, this can lead to feelings of alienation and powerlessness. For cultural or value-based groups, this can lead to diverging understandings, alienation and even open opposition to existing structures. A state of incoherence is in itself stressful, and individuals and groups will make efforts to re-establish coherence (Antonovsky, 1987).

Sharing experiences with your in-group can be a conscious-rising, empowering experience, which helps you to understand the structural components of your experience, and collectively seek solutions (Carr, 2003). The community emerges as an important coping resource in the face of disaster or conflict (Braun-Lewensohn et al., 2019; Braun-Lewensohn & Sagy, 2011; Braun-Lewensohn & Sagy, 2014; Généreux, David, O'Sullivan, et al., 2020; Généreux, Roy, David, et al., 2020; Généreux, Roy, O'Sullivan, & Maltais, 2020; Namihira, 2019). The community, and even national states, are crucial contexts for the experience of coherence in difficult times (Sagy et al., 2020; Sagy & Braun-Lewensohn, 2009; Sagy, 2015; Braun-Lewensohn et al., 2019; Ben David et al., 2017). Research in a European refugee camp suggests that individual and community SOC, together with time spent in the camp and appraisal of danger, explained more than half of the prevalence of anxiety (56%), depression (53%) and somatisation (58%) (Braun-Lewensohn et al., 2019).

On the other hand, individuals with a strong sense of community and national coherence (SOCC/SONC) are often also less open for out-group members, their experiences and interpretations (Mana et al., 2015; Mana et al., 2019; Ben David et al., 2017). A strong national sense of coherence affects willingness to reconcile and acceptance of out-group narratives negatively (Mana et al., 2019). Individuals with strong perceptions of community coherence are also found to be more supportive of separatist strategies and less supportive of integration strategies (Mana et al., 2015). This suggests that whilst the community can be an important coping resource, a strong emphasis on the community might worsen inter-group relations and contribute to shutting out other impulses and explanations. Thus, in-groups that contribute to re-establish coherence in a complex world can quickly develop into so-called echo chambers, in which one-sided information is endorsed, and challenging information is dismissed.

In this context, one might wonder if fake news and conspiracies are an expression of this quest for coherence. The struggle about 'the truth' has had a significant impact on political and social development in recent years and highlights the important role of the media concerning politics. Conspiracy theories are not a new phenomenon; however, in the last decade, they gained importance, partly because of social media. Social media are a crucial arena for people to come into touch with and can spread conspiracy theories to a greater audience. Moreover, due to the way social media work, beginning tendencies to get involved with conspiracies might be reinforced, as users are exposed to content similar to the content they engaged with earlier (Jones, 2016). However, also users themselves seek out information which reinforces, rather than challenges their beliefs. Especially consumers of right-wing populist news seem to have tendencies to shut out other impulses (Michelsen et al., 2017). In the long run, being exposed to one-sided information might result in a picture of the world that is only valid in socially confined spaces, where conflicting information is increasingly avoided or discredited (Jones, 2016). Achieved "coherence" would be built strictly on the in-groups world view, and new information has to be shut out or re-defined to fit the already established 'truth'.

Interestingly, Antonovsky describes a phenomenon he called 'fake' or 'rigid SOC'. A rigid SOC is characterised by high scores on all three dimensions but builds on a few specific strategies. Fake-SOC individuals display strong beliefs that they have found answers to 'everything', but these answers would continuously be challenged through everyday experiences involving the wider society (Antonovsky, 1987). Withdrawing into spaces that offer seemingly coherent explanations – such as so-called echo chambers on social media, distinct cultural sub-groups or even closed religious minorities – might seem beneficial in the short run. It can, however, damage SOC by spoiling for real comprehensiveness and flexible strategies (Antonovsky, 1987; Jones, 2016).

On a societal level, alternative explanations in various sub-groups can contribute to polarisation and distrust not only of officials but also other members of society (Mana et al., 2019; Mana et al., 2015; Ben David et al., 2017). To add to this notion, withdrawal into homogenous, deriving sub-groups often happens at the expense of a salutogenic lifestyle. Narratives from people that have been 'radicalised' indicate that the acceptance of the deviant world often is paired with a loss of relationships, of socially valued activities, and loss of meaningfulness. However, this influence might go both ways: accepting a 'new' explanation about society can lead to distrust and conflict in established relationships; or experiencing that relationships do not hold what they promised can lead to seeking acceptance and a new in-group elsewhere (Löf, 2018). Likewise, believing that the world is governed in secret by an all-powerful group of people (or reptiles) might damage for the experience of meaningfulness (after all, what's the point in trying if everything you do is orchestrated by 'the enemy'?). Simultaneously, gaining access to a group with information and a deeper understanding about 'what is really going on' might contribute to meaningfulness and purpose (after all, nothing better than being part of the exclusive groups battling the ultimate bad guys).

Increased political polarisation is a challenge for the development of a salutogenic society. For example, the importance of meaning-making dialogue to achieve shared understandings has been pointed out (Maass et al., 2017). Sharing experiences with out-group members can help to generalise resources beyond personal experiences and thereby gain a more coherent picture of how society works for everyone (Maass, 2018). Somewhat disappointingly have social media not contributed to this kind of dialogue. On the contrary, Internet debates are more likely to reinforce prior held beliefs than challenging them, thereby adding to simplified pictures of society and increasing polarisation (Bolsover, 2020). Combined with diverging values amongst sub-groups, finding common ground and a set of common goals for collaboration might prove difficult.

Thus, increased polarisation might even spoil for involvement and participatory processes, which were established to increase vertical coherence in the first place. Involvement and broad participation have become popular, and often even mandatory tools in policy development (Christensen, 2012). Participatory approaches seem to be compatible with the guiding values of western society, such as democracy and equality. On the other hand, participatory approaches that aim at fulfilling obligations rather than fostering real involvement are common. Notions of 'inclusive processes' can be utilised to defend and validate measures that do not really benefit those in question (Buanes et al., 2004).

Moreover, well-off people are more inclined to grasp chances for involvement and are better at making themselves heard than more deprived groups. Thus, participatory processes can even contribute to social inequality by reinforcing the majorities' world view at the expense of minorities (Buanes et al., 2004). If policies are developed through seemingly inclusive approaches, but in reality, dismiss the experiences of deprived groups, incoherence between expectations towards and experiences with the political processes itself emerges. Such experiences can be generalised unto the society as such and contribute to distrust and contempt towards politicians and political decisions.

Concluding Remarks

All in all, the picture emerges that salutogenesis can contribute to politics and policy-making by providing a framework that allows to take a step back from immediate, and often pressing, problems and establish a focus on positive outcomes, learning processes and opportunities. Political processes are often characterised by being evidence-based, with a strong emphasis on results and outcomes. Political representatives are concerned with the (short-time) effects of interventions, the "outputs" of politics. On the other hand, applying salutogenic approaches demands long-term and visionary strategies to meet complex challenges. One major challenge in this respect is that knowledge about cause and effectiveness of such appraoches is scarce, and long-time consequences of policies are hard to measure. However, we argue that recent developments, characterised by post-NPM and whole-of-governance approaches, highlight the need for a salutogenic perspective within politics and policy development. A salutogenic society can in this context be described as a society which phrases positive goals rooted in shared understandings about challenges and desirable outcomes. This might equip individuals, groups and stakeholders with necessary resources to resolve challenges and take part in decision-making from every position in society. A salutogenic society facilitates coherent experiences amongst its members and equips them with the necessary skills and resources to become active agents in their own life.

Salutogenesis can contribute to unravel the various influences on the processes of politics and policy-making and help to establish and maintain policy coherence, both vertically and horizontally. The framework of comprehensibility, manageability and meaningfulness might contribute to coherent processes as well as outcomes. 'Comprehensibility' highlights the importance of shared understandings, consistent messages and opportunities for inter-group dialogue. 'Manageability' emphasises the importance of distribution and design of resources in line with responsibilities and burdens, including the rights and the means to pursue one's goals. 'Meaningfulness' implies to apply inclusive strategies and ensure involvement of stakeholders. For multi-sector collaboration processes, linking specific and overarching goals could add meaningfulness and increase motivation to engage in common efforts across sectors.

References

Agger, A., & Sørensen, E. (2018). Managing collaborative innovation in public bureaucracies. *Planning Theory, 17*(1), 53–73.

Antonovsky, A. (1979). *Stress, health and coping. New perspectives on mental and physical Well-being*. Jossey-Bass.

Antonovsky, A. (1987). *Unraveling the mystery of health*. Jossey-Bass.

Bambra, C., Fox, D., & Scott-Samuel, A. (2005). Towards a politics of health promotion. *Health Promotion International, 20*, 87–93.

Ben David, Y., Hameiri, B., Benheim, S., Leshem, B., Sarid, A., Sternberg, M., ... Sagy, S. (2017). Exploring ourselves within intergroup conflict: The role of intragroup dialogue in promoting acceptance of collective narratives and willingness toward reconciliation. *Peace and Conflict: Journal of Peace Psychology, 23*(3), 269.

Bolsover, G. (2020). Black Lives Matter discourse on US social media during COVID: polarised positions enacted in a new event. arXiv preprint arXiv:2009.03619

Braun-Lewensohn, O., Abu-Kaf, S., & Al-Said, K. (2019). Women in refugee camps: Which coping resources help them to adapt? *International Journal of Environmental Research and Public Health, 16*(20), 3990.

Braun-Lewensohn, O., & Sagy, S. (2011). Coping resources as explanatory factors of stress reactions during missile attacks: Comparing

Jewish and Arab adolescents in Israel. *Community Mental Health Journal, 47*(3), 300–310.

Braun-Lewensohn, O., & Sagy, S. (2014). Community resilience and sense of coherence as protective factors in explaining stress reactions: Comparing cities and rural communities during missiles attacks. *Community Mental Health Journal, 50*(2), 229–234.

Bregman, R. (2020). *Humankind: A hopeful history*. Bloomsbury Publishing PLC.

Brolin, M., Quennerstedt, M., Maivorsdotter, N., & Casey, A. (2018). A salutogenic strengths-based approach in practice–an illustration from a school in Sweden. *Curriculum studies in health and physical education, 9*(3), 237–252.

Buanes, A., Jentoft, S., Karlsen, G. R., Maurstad, A., & Søreng, S. (2004). In whose interest? An exploratory analysis of stakeholders in Norwegian coastal zone planning. *Ocean & Coastal Management, 47*(5-6), 207–223.

Carr, E. S. (2003). Rethinking empowerment theory using a feminist lens: The importance of process. *Affilia, 18*(1), 8–20.

Christensen, T. (2012). Post-NPM and changing public governance. *Meiji Journal of Political Science and Economics, 1*(1), 1–11.

Christensen, T. & Lægreid, P. (2007). The whole-of-government approach to public sector reform. *Public Administration Review*, (November/December), 1059–1066.

Christensen, T., & Lægreid, P. (2011). Complexity and hybrid public administration – Theoretical and empirical challenges. *Public Organization Review, 11*(4), 407–423.

Dell' Olio, M., Vaandrager, L., & Koelen, M. (2018). Applying Salutogenesis to the experiences of students with disabilities in the Netherlands. *Journal of Postsecondary Education and Disability, 31*(1), 75–89.

Elliot, A. J. (1999). Approach and avoidance motivation and achievement goals. *Educational Psychologist, 34*(3), 169–189.

Généreux et al. (2020). One virus, four continents, eight countries: an interdisciplinary and international study on the psychosocial impacts of the COVID-19 pandemic among adults. *Submitted to the Lancet.*

Généreux, G., David, M.D., O'Sullivan, T., Carignan, M.E., Blouin-Genest, G., Champagne-Poirier, O., Champagne, E., Burlone, N., Qadar, Z., Herbosa, T., Hung, K., Ribeiro-Alves, G., Arruda, H., Michel, P., Law, R., Poirier, A., Murray, V., Chan, E., & Roy, M. (2020). Communication strategies and media discourses in the age of COVID-19: An urgent need for action. Submitted to *Health Promotion International.*

Généreux, M., Roy, M., David, M.D., Carignan, M.E., Qadar, Z., Blouin-Genest, G., & Champagne-Poirier, O. (2020). Psychological response to the COVID-19 pandemic in Canada: Main stressors and assets. *Submitted to Global Health Promotion.*

Généreux, M., Roy, M., O'Sullivan, T., & Maltais, D. (2020). A salutogenic approach to disaster recovery: The case of the Lac-Mégantic rail disaster. *International Journal of Environmental Research and Public Health, 17*(5), 1463.

Habermas, J. (2016). For a democratic polarisation: How to pull the ground from under right-wing populism. *Social Europe 17/11/2016*. Retrieved 10/08/2017 from https://www.socialeurope.eu/democratic-polarisation-pull-ground-right-wing-populism.

Hague, R., & Harrop, M. (2010). *Comparative government and politics. An introduction* (8th ed.). Palgrave Macmillan.

Head, B. W., & Alford, J. (2015). Wicked problems: Implications for public policy and management. *Administration & Society, 47*(6), 711–739.

Holmberg, S., & Rothstein, B. (Eds.). (2012). *Good governance*. Cheltenham.

Hood, C. (1991). A public management for all seasons? *Public Administration, 69*, 3–19.

Jangar, S. (2020). Georg Floyd criminal past record/arrest history/career timeline: Baggie, gun pregnant and all details. *The Courier Daily.*

Jones, A. (2016). *Talking to ourselves? Political debate online and the echo-chamber effect*. Demos.

Kelly, A. (2015). Introducing the concept of salutogenesis to school leadership research: Problematising empirical methodologies and findings. *International Journal of Leadership in Education, 18*(2), 167–177.

Kickbusch, I. (2015). The political determinants of health—10 years on. *BMJ, 350*, h81. https://doi.org/10.1136/bmj.h81

Kickbusch, I., & Szabo, M. M. C. (2014). A new governance space for health. *Global Health Action, 7*(1), 23507.

Lindblom, C. E. (1979). Still muddling, not yet through. *Public Administration Review, 39*, 517–526.

Lindström, B., & Eriksson, M. (2010). *The hitchhiker's guide to salutogenesis*. Salutogenic pathways to health promotion.

Löf, S. (2018). *Radicalisation and de-radicalisation in Finland-support needs in de-radicalisation process*. Diaconia University of Applied Science.

Maass, R., Lindstrøm, B., & Lillefjell, M. (2014). Exploring the relationship between perceptions of Neighbourhoodresources, sense of coherence and health for different groups in a Norwegian neighbourhood. *Journal of Public Health Research, 3*(1).

Maass, R., Lindström, B., & Lillefjell, M. (2017). Neighborhood-resources for the development of a strong SOC and the importance of understanding why and how resources work: A grounded theory approach. *BMC Public Health, 17*(1), 1–13.

Maass, R. E. K. (2018). *The neighborhood as a salutogenic setting: How can Salutogenesis contribute to the development of strategies for* promoting *health and strengthening SOC through a focus on neighborhood-resources?* Doctoral thesis, NTNU.

Mackenbach, J. P. (2014). Political determinants of health. *European Journal of Public Health, 24*(1), 2.

Mana, A., Sagy, S., Srour, A., & Mjally-Knani, S. (2015). On both sides of the fence: Perceptions of collective narratives and identity strategies among Palestinians in Israel and in the West Bank. *Mind & Society, 14*(1), 57–83.

Mana, A., Srour, A., & Sagy, S. (2019). A sense of national coherence and openness to the "other's" collective narrative: The case of the Israeli–Palestinian conflict. *Peace and Conflict: Journal of Peace Psychology, 25*(3), 226.

Marmot, M. (2004). Status syndrome. *Significance, 1*(4), 150–154.

Marmot, M., & Allen, J. (2013). Prioritising health equity. In K. Leppo, E. Ollila, S. Pena, M. Wismar, & S. Cook (Eds.), *Health in all policies-seizing opportunities, implementing policies*. Sosiaali-ja terveysministeriö.

Marmot, M. (2005). Social determinants of health inequalities. *The lancet, 365*(9464), 1099–1104.

Marmot, M., & Wilkinson, R. (Eds.). (2005). Social determinants of health. OUP Oxford.

Michelsen, D., Przybilla-Voss, M., & Luehrmann, M. (2017). *Rechtsextremismus und Fremdenfeindlichkeit in Ostdeutschland*. Goettinger Institut fuer Demokratieforschung.

Namihira, E. (2019). 'Salutogenesis' and the factors in natural disaster recovery: An essay of preventive measures to health damages caused by natural disaster. *Journal of the National Institute of Public Health, 68*(4).

Nilsson, M., Zamparutti, T., Petersen, J. E., Nykvist, B., Rudberg, P., & McGuinn, J. (2012). Understanding policy coherence: Analytical framework and examples of sector–environment policy interactions in the EU. *Environmental Policy and Governance, 22*(6), 395–423.

OECD, 2019. Policy coherence for sustainable development. Retrieved 20/08/21 from: https://www.oecd.org/gov/pcsd/#:~:text=The%20

OECD%20Recommendation%20on%20Policy%20Coherence%20for%20Sustainable,environmental%20goals%2C%20and%20accelerate%20progress%20towards%20the%20SDGs.

Østerud, Ø., Engelstad, F., & Selle, P. (2004). Makten og demokratiet. Gyldendal akademisk.

Pascoe, E. A., & Smart Richman, L. (2009). Perceived discrimination and health: A meta-analytic review. *Psychological Bulletin, 135*(4), 531.

Peck, J. H. (2015). Minority perceptions of the police: A state-of-the-art review. *Policing: An International Journal Of Police Strategies & Management.*

Rappaport, J. (1995). Empowerment meets narrative: Listening to stories and creating settings. *American Journal of Community Psychology, 23*(5), 795–807.

Reid, T., & Quayle, E. (2008). A salutogenic perspective on occupational health. *The Irish Journal of Psychology, 29*(1-2), 35–44.

Sagy, et al. (2020). Salutogenesis and Corona. *Work in progress, read more at* https://www.stars-society.org/coronaresearchcollab.

Sagy, S. (2015). Coping, conflict and culture: The salutogenic approach in the study of resiliency. *Resiliency: Enhancing Coping with Crisis and Terrorism*, 41–48.

Sagy, S., & Braun-Lewensohn, O. (2009). Adolescents under rocket fire: When are coping resources significant in reducing emotional distress? *Global Health Promotion, 16*(4), 5–15.

Slettholm, A., Stokke, O. (2015). Politiet: -Kvinner i hijab kan være spesielt utsatt for hatvold. *Aftenposten online, 08.08.2015,* retrieved 06/12/2017 from https://www.aftenposten.no/norge/i/gE8A/Politiet%2D%2D-Kvinner-i-hijab-kan-vare-spesielt-utsatt-for-hatvold.

Strümpfer, D. J. W. (1995). The origins of health and strength: From 'salutogenesis' to 'fortigenesis'. *South African Journal of Psychology, 25*(2), 81–89.

UN. (2017). Sustainable development goals. Retrieved 04/10/2020 from: https://sdgs.un.org/goals.

Vaandrager, L., & Koelen, M. (2013). Salutogenesis in the workplace: Building general resistance resources and sense of coherence. In *Salutogenic organisations and change* (pp. 77–89). Springer. WHO; 1946. Definition of health.

Wilson, J. (1989). *Bureaucracy: What government agencies do and why they do it.* NY, Basic Books.

Yeo, A. I., & Green, M. N. (Eds.). (2017). *Living in an age of mistrust: An interdisciplinary study of declining trust and how to get it back.* Routledge.

25

Promoting SOC: Aging at Home, Participation and Social Support

Mélanie Levasseur and Daniel Naud

Introduction

The world population is growing older; one person in five was aged 60 or over in 2017. According to projections, this proportion will be one in four by 2050 (United Nations, 2017). The majority of older adults reports living with chronic illnesses. Almost half have or will have disabilities at one point during their aging (Turcotte and Schellenberg, 2007), limiting their mobility within their home and community. Maintaining or improving the aging populations' health and well-being is an important challenge that can be addressed by targeted interventions on health determinants. It is important to plan and implement innovative and cost-effective population health interventions tackling modifiable determinants of health, including social support, participation, and mobility. Because it aims to generate, maintain, and promote health, rather than solving illness and pathology issues, a salutogenic framework is promising for healthy and active aging at home. Social support and participation are important factors that help older adults cope with stressful events and everyday life challenges. This chapter defines social support and participation, in contrast to social isolation and loneliness. Policies and programs are discussed to demonstrate the contribution of interventions using a salutogenic framework. Finally, opportunities and challenges in planning and evaluating policies and programs are addressed.

M. Levasseur (✉)
School of Rehabilitation, Université de Sherbrooke, Sherbrooke, Québec, Canada

Research Centre on Aging, Eastern Townships Integrated University Health and Social Services Centre, Sherbrooke, Québec, Canada
e-mail: Melanie.Levasseur@USherbrooke.ca

D. Naud
Research Centre on Aging, Eastern Townships Integrated University Health and Social Services Centre, Sherbrooke, Québec, Canada

Salutogenesis and Older Adults

From a salutogenic perspective, a person's health can be represented as a point on a continuum, located between illness and healthiness, or health "ease and dis-ease", using Antonovksy's terminology (1993b). Moving in the healthy direction of this continuum requires a person to have a global understanding of their individual and contextual situation and possess the capacity to know and use the available resources to help them cope with adverse life events and still move forward (Eriksson, 2017). Such understanding of one's situation is the sense of coherence (SOC) and, according to Antonovsky (1993a), is a global orientation a person has to the world, allowing them to perceive it as comprehensible, manageable, and meaningful. In other words, it is about feeling confident that life events that may negatively or positively impact health and well-being are worthy of investment and engagement and that there are resources that can be used to cope with them. The latter are referred to as generalized resistance resources (GRRs), found at the personal (e.g., material resources, personality traits, knowledge, experiences) or the community level (e.g., social support, culture, religion; Horsburgh and Ferguson, 2000). Research showed that GRRs, including social support, were associated with older adults' SOC and their location on the health continuum (Wiesmann and Hannich, 2010). If GRRs are available, individuals developing a stronger SOC can maintain or improve their health.

As it stabilizes by the end of young adulthood, shaped by personal and work experiences, social class, gender, and culture, Antonovsky (1993b) nevertheless suggested that older adults might be limited in developing their SOC. Reporting that "*those of us who are less fortunate will increasingly see the world as incomprehensible, unmanageable and meaningless*" (Antonovsky, 1993b; p. 9), such belief is not particularly optimistic for older adults with a lower SOC. Too many adverse late-life events could even worsen such perspective, as they were associated with a decreased SOC (Lövheim et al., 2013). Still, subsequent research showed that the SOC could be maintained or even developed, even at a very late age (Koelen et al., 2017).

From a health promotion point of view, maintaining or developing the SOC is important because it was associated with better physical health in young-old and old-old Canadians (Forbes, 2001). Antonovsky also believed that the retirement from employment is such a unique and radical transition that the person cannot rely solely on preexisting GRRs, but has to change previous mechanisms to cope with new challenges (Sagy and Antonovsky, 1994). For the Israeli cohort studied by Sagy and Antonovsky (1994), family ties and informal interpersonal engagement became the most meaningful life domains post-retirement. Indeed, older adults still have access to GRRs to cope and shape meaning for possibly very impactful later life events, such as retirement, death of loved ones, and disabilities. The promotion of social relationships could thus positively influence the development of SOC, especially for life meaningfulness (Wiesmann and Hannich, 2010). Allowing a person to benefit from experiences, family ties, or close and supportive relationships would provide meaning to the challenges and contribute to an inner strength to cope with late-life challenges (Tan, 2015). Social support and participation can help older adults in this coping.

Social Support and Participation

Social support and participation are important factors of active and engaged aging associated with favorable health outcomes (Bowling, 2005), notably because it allows older adults to stay integrated with their community. **Social support** can be defined as "*the social resources that persons perceive to be available or that are provided to them by nonprofessionals in the context of both formal support groups and informal helping relationships*" (Cohen et al., 2001, p. 4). This definition distinguishes perceived support (the belief that support is available from members of one's network) and received support (mobilization and expression; Gottlieb and Bergen, 2010). Antonovsky (1979) highlighted that social support and network contribute to the person's sense of coherence because it influences how one views the world and how the environment is perceived as meaningful and comprehensible (Eriksson and Lindström, 2005). Social support was identified as a GRR because relationships of trust can provide the right resources to meet older adults' specific challenges (Bryant et al., 2001). While sometimes mentioning social ties, Antonovsky mostly addressed the role of family ties when transitioning between labor and retirement (Antonovsky et al., 1990; Sagy and Antonovsky, 1994). More recently, researchers investigated social relationships and their contribution to the SOC among older adults. For example, higher levels of social support in older adults were found associated with superior self-efficacy and problem-solving (Trouillet et al., 2009), which was linked to the manageability domain of the SOC by Antonovsky (1993a), helping a person cope with stressful life events. Although not exclusively in older adults, the strengthening of social support was also shown to contribute to improving or restoring the SOC for people with mental health problems (Langeland and Wahl, 2009). Social support contributes to a person's social integration and provides opportunities to assist others, improving self-esteem.

Additionally, different forms of social support were also found to be associated with health and well-being. Greater perceived social support was associated with better self-perceived health (Smith et al., 2013). Received support also influences older adults' self-esteem and community belonging (Krause, 2007). Still, it could revive conflicts with close ties or be interpreted as a threat to older adults' sense of independence and control, which is possibly detrimental to their health and well-being (Uchino, 2009). In addition to the number and quality of social ties, active involvement in community activities was shown to be linked to health and SOC.

Social participation can be defined as the "*person's involvement in social activities that provide interactions with others in society or the community*" (Levasseur, Richard, Gauvin, and Raymond, 2010, p. 2144). These social activities can be formal, such as volunteering or being engaged in a community organization, or informal, such as helping a neighbor, visiting friends, or attending a cultural event (Couton and Gaudet, 2008). Social participation is associated with many health-protective effects, notably fewer disabilities (Lund et al., 2010) and depressive symptoms (Glass et al., 2006), greater well-being (Gilmour, 2012), and self-perceived health (Lee et al., 2008), the preservation of cognitive functions (Glei et al., 2005), shorter hospital stays (Newall et al., 2014), and lower risk for all-cause mortality (Holt-Lunstad et al., 2015). Social participation fosters the development of relationships and engagement with others in the community, which were shown to be associated with the feeling of attachment to others (Grewal et al., 2006). When older adults have regular interactions with younger people, they report better self-reported health, plausibly because they feel more valued, included, and appreciated (Ronzi et al., 2018). When social activities enable the sharing of resources and expertise within a group, they are meaningful and contribute to providing purpose in the older person's life, which is a fundamental domain of SOC (Antonovsky, 1993b).

Social Isolation and Loneliness

Social support and participation, including their associations with positive health outcomes, are different than social isolation and loneliness. Older adults in a situation of **social**

isolation have fewer fulfilling social ties, social interactions of inferior quality, and a weaker sense of belonging and social engagement (Nicholson, 2009). Older adults are at higher risk of being isolated when living alone, having a low income, presenting poorer health or restricted mobility, and having no children or close family members (Keefe et al., 2006). Life events were also found to be associated with social isolation, such as the loss of a loved one, retirement, driving cessation, or relocation to a long-term care facility (Keefe et al., 2006). Although it was found to be associated with limited social support (Tomaka et al., 2006), fewer social interactions, and lower participation in social activities (Cornwell et al., 2009), the association of social isolation to adverse health outcomes differ from those of low social support and participation. Older adults in a situation of isolation often report more health-risk behaviors such as smoking and being physically inactive than those who are socially integrated (Cornwell et al., 2009). Social isolation has been associated with poorer self-rated physical and mental health (Cornwell et al., 2009), as well as a greater risk of dementia (Fratiglioni et al., 2000), cardiovascular disease in response to stress-related events (Grant et al., 2009), and suicide (Rapagnani, 2002). From a salutogenic and health promotion perspective, reducing social isolation can have different outcomes than fostering social participation, which is more likely to be regarded as a GRR, potentially contributing to the SOC (Ronzi et al., 2018).

Loneliness is a negative subjective state experienced when a person's social ties are not sufficiently fulfilling (Cornwell et al., 2009). Because some people may prefer to be alone without experiencing negative feelings, it is recommended not to study social isolation independently of loneliness. Loneliness was more common in older women than men and was associated with living alone or being widowed (Victor et al., 2006). However, men were less likely than women to report being lonely, plausibly because of the risk of stigmatization (Borys and Perlman, 1985). Compared to reduced social support, loneliness was more strongly associated with lower self-perceived mental health and the presence of depressive symptoms (Cornwell and Waite, 2009). As for social isolation, loneliness is associated with adopting multiple health-risk behaviors, such as physical inactivity and smoking (Shankar et al., 2011). Both social isolation and loneliness may contribute to adverse health effects through these health-risk behaviors.

In summary, higher social support and participation do not only diminish the risk of illnesses associated with social isolation and loneliness. Indeed, social support and participation have a distinct and positive contribution to the older adults' sense of coherence and health. Aging at home allows older adults to keep relationships built over the years within their community and facilitate the preservation of their SOC.

Environment and Salutogenesis for an Active and Engaged Aging at Home

Inspired by Antonovksy's salutogenesis and Lawton's ecological model of aging (Lawton and Nahemow, 1973), researchers showed that SOC, health, and well-being are associated with several characteristics of the local environment, which facilitate mobility and participation in community activities (Stokols, 1992; Wister, 2005). For example, safer environment, urban revitalization programs, accessible and safe public transportation, reduction of noise and air pollution, and availability of walking pathways influence the health and well-being of aging adults (Wister, 2005). According to the ecological model of aging (Lawton and Nahemow, 1973), the person, including his cognitive, physical, and mental competencies, interact with the environmental characteristics, facilitating or hindering these competencies. This interaction provokes an adaptive behavior and emotion (satisfaction if successful, stress otherwise). Lower competence increases the likelihood that the person's behavior will be dependent on the environmental factors and may not be able to operate within the environment without assistance (Lawton, 1990).

Environments that promote health can be developed or encouraged through **aging at home** strategies. Wished by most of them (Farber et al., 2011), strategies related to aging in place can help older adults remain in their homes, despite increasing difficulties (Fry, 2012; Iecovich, 2014). An aging at home strategy promotes important environmental characteristics such as physical accessibility, service proximity, security, recreational resources, housing, and transportation (Plouffe and Kalache, 2010), aimed at improving the mobility, health, and well-being of older inhabitants and their communities. The SOC may be stronger in older adults living in their homes than in communal-care facilities (Haak et al., 2011; Tan, 2015). Aging at home may provide a sense of security, help preserve memories, and provide better proximity to friends, neighbors, and kin (Rowles and Bernard, 2013). Aging at home contributes to all three domains of the SOC, that is, meaningfulness, comprehensibility, and manageability (Koelen et al., 2017). For example, attachment to a place might help individuals maintain a sense of control (Rowles, 1983), which is important for comprehensibility and manageability. Maintaining access to GRRs, such as social support and participation, increases the likelihood of a stronger SOC and health and well-being (Tan, 2015).

Aging at home is partly about providing access to GRRs, notably the retention of social support within the community (Iecovich, 2014), which helps older adults cope with stressful events and contribute to their SOC. To participate socially and maintain social network and support, older adults must be able to move within their community, regardless of their physical disabilities. Understood as a cornerstone to the social integration of the persons into their community, **mobility** is defined as "*the ability to move oneself (e.g., by walking, by using assistive devices, or by using transportation) within community environments that expand from one's home, to the neighborhood, and regions beyond*" (Webber et al., 2010, p. 1). Older adults with reduced mobility reported lower participation in social activities (Rosso et al., 2013), which put them at a higher risk of social isolation. Limited mobility restricts the life space, that is, the "extent of travel into the environment, regardless of how one gets there" (Stalvey et al., 1999, p. 472). Mobility is affected by factors such as physical abilities, gender, culture, and income (Webber et al., 2010) and can deteriorate with driving cessation in areas with limited alternative transportation options (Marottoli et al., 2000). Also, an inferior SOC in older adults was found to increase the risk of reduced mobility (Avlund et al., 2003), suggesting the importance of providing equal access to GRRs within a community. Because the life space encompasses the potential GRRs that older adults can rely on, it has strong SOC and health implications.

Mobility is important in enabling social participation, especially for adults with a disability (Verdonschot et al., 2009). Accessibility in the physical neighborhood environment is also essential for older adults with a disability (Richards et al., 1999; Verbrugge et al., 1997) or frailty (Fairhall et al. 2011). In Canada, rural women that wished to participate more were more likely than rural men to be constrained by transportation problems (Naud et al., 2019), illustrating that mobility options are not equally distributed across the aging populations. In general, older adults in rural areas are more dependent on private car use or on informal support (Davis and Bartlett, 2008), which may be a limiting factor in their social participation within the community.

Older adults' SOC, relying notably on GRRs made available through their social support and participation, is thus associated with the local environment. By modifying factors that can foster social support and participation and decrease social isolation and loneliness, SOC, health, and well-being could be enhanced (Bowling, 2005). Moreover, because they are associated, interventions targeting one dimension could potentially affect others (Dickens et al., 2011). For example, social isolation is associated with reducing social support and participation (Hombrados-Mendieta et al., 2013). These interventions, provided with a relatively modest cost compared to health infrastructure and equipment, could reduce healthcare spending (Kaye et al., 2009). Thus, policies and programs should be planned, implemented, and evaluated to facilitate aging at home. Improving older adults' ability to identify and use the community's GRRs may also strengthen their sense of meaningfulness, manageability, and comprehensibility.

Aging in Place Policies and Programs Fostering Mobility and Social Support

Over the past decades, aging in place policies and programs addressing social support, participation, isolation, loneliness, and mobility have shown varying degrees of effectiveness. On the one hand, policies are defined as contextual interventions, coming from consensus-based negotiations between multiple actors, intended to be implemented into practices that create conditions in which the scope of options available in deciding what to do is reduced or altered (Ball, 1993). On the other hand, a program can arise from policies and an organized and planned effort to ameliorate social conditions (Rossi et al., 2018). Considering that the SOC is a disposition orientation that can be developed over time (Read et al., 2005), the following sections introduce examples of policies and programs that had an objective of increasing the levels of SOC in older adults by promoting social support, participation, and mobility, which facilitate aging at home.

Policies

Over the last three decades, health promotion policy frameworks were elaborated using an ecological model to facilitate social participation and reduce the risk of isolation. Evaluating policy trends, Lui et al. (2009) found that the current discourse on aging has redirected the major determinants from economic or welfare issues to matters of social inclusion, engagement, and community development, which are in line with salutogenesis. In their policy review, Eriksson and Lindström (2008) showed that before the 1980s, health promotion was mostly about reducing risk behaviors by health education. Although not explicitly addressing older adults, the seminal *Ottawa Charter for Health Promotion* (World Health Organization, 1986) aimed at providing individuals and communities more control over the health determinants (Eriksson and Lindström, 2008), notably by promoting supportive environments, community action, and leisure as a source of health and well-being. More extensive than the Charter, the WHO's *Active Aging Policy Framework* (World Health Organization, 2002) emphasized the process of active aging as a multidimensional key mechanism for healthy aging, aimed at "continuing participation in social, economic, cultural, spiritual and civic affairs, not just the ability to be physically active or to participate in the labor force" (p. 12). The framework promoted environments that contribute to increase older adults' autonomy, by alleviating environmental barriers (e.g., inaccessible transportation, discontinuous sidewalks, and heavy traffic) and increasing opportunities for resource acquisition, such as social participation. Most importantly, it recommended that decision-makers strengthen community initiatives, voluntarism, peer mentoring and visiting, family caregivers, intergenerational programs, and outreach services. Finally, the framework introduced mobility as a key factor for a full participation in the community, regardless of the person's abilities and highlighting specifically the contextual differences between rural and urban environments (World Health Organization, 2002).

More recently, the guide *Global Age-Friendly Cities* (World Health Organization, 2007) proposed a framework to implement easily applicable age-friendly policies and programs at the national and regional levels, which was recognized by many governing bodies (Rémillard-Boilard, 2018). Defining mobility as a key factor for active aging, the framework highlights the importance of available and affordable transportation options. This is especially vital for older adults with a disability or frailty, allowing them to reach their chosen destinations and participate in community activities. Indeed, mobility allows older adults in the formal and informal life of their communities. Universal accessibility, affordability, and diversity of the activities are also highlighted in the framework. Simultaneously, the framework addressed the various reasons that could lead older adults to social isolation and recommends outreach programs to provide them with social connections with the community. The implementation of social programs may be facilitated and oriented by the models of governance suggested by policies (i.e., top-down or bottom-up) and emphasizing either the physical or the social environment (Lui et al., 2009).

Programs

Several health promotion programs aim to develop access and knowledge to resources, notably by facilitating social interactions and mobility for older adults living in their community. Although not necessarily developed from a salutogenic theory, the programs can plausibly enhance the SOC and, subsequently, older adults' health and well-being. The following paragraphs present: (1) three programs relying on passive social involvement; (2) five programs relying on active social involvement, and (3) two programs targeting the community rather than the individuals. These programs provide opportunities for social activities and build social support within the older adults' communities, aiming to maintain or improve health and well-being.

Some programs encourage older adults to gather outside the participants' homes but mostly in passive social gatherings, such as educational programs promoting healthy behaviors. Such programs may enhance SOC by improving the knowledge and use of local resources available to older adults. Still, these programs do not necessarily increase social participation or decrease social isolation. For example, Tan (2015) evaluated a Resource Enhancement and Activation Program, a self-care program facilitating aging at home or in the community, helping older adults develop resilience and use resources optimally to maintain health. The 12-week program involved 64 aging Singaporeans, who participated in 24 group activities about nutrition, physical activity, mental health, social capital, preventive health services, injury prevention, and environment, contributing to all three domains of the SOC (Tan et al., 2014). Following the program, the participants reported a better knowledge of available resources, developed new skills, and enjoyed sharing their experiences with others. Compared to a control group that did not receive an intervention, the participants improved their overall SOC, specifically in the comprehensibility and manageability domains, but did not differ in loneliness (Tan, 2015). In a sparse rural area in Galicia, Spain, older adults were recruited for 9 months to participate in three weekly mobility workshops: cognitive stimulation, craft with others, and exercise (Dumitrache et al., 2017). After the intervention, the participants considered they had more opportunities for leisure activities than before. Additionally, older participants showed lower risks of cognitive impairment, which contributed to a more positive perception of their quality of life and mental health (Dumitrache et al., 2017). The *University of Queensland Driver Retirement Initiative*, in Australia, held weekly meetings for 6 weeks with urban older adults that stopped driving (Liddle et al., 2014). The meetings involved information sharing, group discussion, speakers, practical exercises, and outings. Compared to a control group, the participants had more activities outside the home, regardless of their self-perceived health (Liddle et al., 2014). They also used alternative transportation options (e.g., walking, public transit, volunteer driver programs, and paratransit) more often than adults in the control group and were more satisfied with their transport situation. The participants to the meetings felt more confident of staying involved within their community and in meaningful activities without driving (Liddle et al., 2014), which demonstrates that informing and providing relevant practical mobility exercises can plausibly positively influence the manageability domain of SOC.

Other programs emphasize an active social involvement of older adults through social activities and workshops. While such programs are not aimed at increasing knowledge about available local GRRs, they help older participants build social support and increase their social participation, improving their sense of manageability and meaningfulness, two domains of the SOC. For example, the *Volunteer Friendly Visitor Program* in Ontario, Canada, peered voluntary undergraduate students with older adults in a situation of isolation, to socialize for about 3 hours every week (MacIntyre et al., 1999). Activities mutually chosen included short walks, talking or listening, assisting with care activities, reading aloud, and writing letters. Compared to a control group receiving no visitor, the program was shown to foster health promotion in many aspects, notably the participants' self-worth, social support, and life satisfaction increased. In the Canadian province of Quebec, the

Personalized citizen assistance for social participation peered a trained volunteer with an older adult with a disability for 6 months (Levasseur et al., 2016). The volunteer assisted the older adult with social and leisure activities self-reported as challenging to accomplish (such as walking inside or outside the home or playing games requiring cognitive abilities). Their participation in social and leisure activities was improved, in addition to their mobility, and they perceived fewer barriers in their social environment (Levasseur et al., 2016). The *Men's Shed* is a growing social activity intervention, providing a communal space for older men to meet, socialize, learn new skills, and participate in practical activities with other men (Milligan et al., 2016). In Winnipeg, Manitoba, a Men's Shed program housed in a seniors' center recruited older male participants to engage in activities such as woodcarving, cooking, game playing, or gardening (Reynolds et al., 2015). The program successfully increased the participants' social network, improved their mental health, and generated stronger bonds with other men. The Finnish initiative *Volunteering, Access to Outdoor Activities, and Well-being in Older People* assigned retired trained volunteers with older adults with severe difficulties accessing the outdoors independently (Rantanen et al., 2015). Together, they had weekly out-of-home activities (e.g., running errands or recreational activities) for 3 months. The intervention effectively improved the participants' satisfaction with their physical capacity, notably by identifying, facing, and solving barriers for outdoor activities, making the outdoors more accessible (Rantanen et al., 2015). Lastly, in a Japanese intergenerational program, older trained volunteers were recruited for reading picture books every week to children at school or kindergarten (Murayama et al., 2015). Such activities allow older adults to care for others by transferring knowledge and wisdom to a younger generation, positively affecting their meaningfulness. After the 3-month program and compared to a control group that did not engage in intergenerational activities, participants reported higher levels of their overall SOC and all three domains. Additionally, superior meaningfulness was found to mediate lower levels of depressive mood (Murayama et al., 2015).

Finally, some programs target the community rather than the individual. These programs provide older adults with new resources or increase their accessibility to improve their SOC. In a rural region in Quebec, Canada, a community development initiative combined with an action research program was instigated by local community partners (Clément et al., 2018). Public consultations were held to identify the needs of the community's older residents at risk of social isolation and define the most relevant initiatives. They developed the *Benevolent Community*, aimed at locating older adults in a situation of social isolation and assisting them in developing social connections. A website was created to provide information on social activities and services, and transportation opportunities were increased for older adults with disabilities and lacking transportation options (Levasseur et al., 2021). The American *Naturally occurring retirement communities (NORC) supportive services program* (Bedney et al., 2010) promotes age-friendly transformations of housing developments not planned for older adults (e.g., apartment buildings, condominiums, neighborhoods, small towns, or rural areas). In hundreds of housing developments across the United States, older residents, building managers, and community partners cooperated to create a network of services and volunteer opportunities that promote aging in place. For example, building managers and community partners coordinate the efforts of voluntary support systems, promote social support among older residents, and enhance the accessibility and affordability of existing services (Greenfield et al., 2013). Bedney et al. (2010) surveyed the residents of the NORC. They found that the majority of them talked to more people and increased their participation and social network than before their participation. The NORC program also increased older residents' engagement in out-of-home activities and used of community services. Asked to self-rate their health, almost three residents in four reported that they felt healthier than before their participation in the program (Bedney et al., 2010).

In summary, individual or community programs aimed at increasing access or knowledge to local GRRs, notably through mobility, social support, and participation, can positively impact older adults' SOC, health, and well-being. By improving older adults' capacities and knowledge of GRRs, these programs can help them cope more easily with challenges of the daily life within their community, which can be facilitated by a stronger SOC (Tan, 2015), but simultaneously also contributes to strengthening the SOC (Koelen et al., 2017). An active and socially integrated aging allows older adults, with or without disabilities, to continue to live in their community and gain benefits from their long-standing assets. Still, intervening on older adults and their communities requires researchers, community partners, and decision-makers to tackle several challenges.

Opportunities and Challenges Related to Planning and Evaluation

The current policy trend, which targets health promotion, social inclusion, and engagement within the community (Eriksson and Lindström, 2008; Lui et al., 2009), offers many opportunities to plan and implement salutogenic programs for older community dwellers. Challenges have nevertheless to be addressed, notably the scarcity of evaluated salutogenic programs aimed at older adults, the adaptation of health promotion interventions to their geographical context, and the elaboration of a more inclusive discourse about aging in place.

There is an abundance of recent studies interested in aging populations, using a salutogenic framework, which provides the theoretical grounds required to plan and evaluate such initiatives. Indeed, longitudinal studies have demonstrated that older adults' SOC can be improved, even at later ages (Lövheim et al., 2013; Murayama et al., 2015). Such demonstration and potential replications are essential in justifying future interventions. Other studies have found associations between superior SOC and positive health outcomes in older adults (Borglin et al., 2006; Eriksson and Lindström, 2005; Koelen et al., 2017), but mostly cross-sectionally (Tan, 2015). Tan's (2015) synthesis of published salutogenic empirical evidence showed the scarcity of literature evaluating older community dwellers' interventions. Using the lenses of salutogenesis, such evaluations are important to provide measurements of the SOC and access to GRRs (Antonovsky, 1993a). Consequently, evaluations measuring the impacts of the intervention on health outcomes and well-being are also needed. Fortunately, there are promising community-based research protocols published (Levasseur et al., 2017; Seah et al., 2018), which could provide further evidence for the effectiveness of the salutogenic framework.

Programs well-tailored to their environmental context, for example, rural neighborhoods, could be effective for health promotion. Rural older dwellers may be further at risk of social isolation due to a lack of transportation options and resources (Keefe et al., 2006). Indeed, rural communities' declining resources reduce older rural community dwellers' access to GRRs because they are less mobile (Milne et al., 2007), which can limit their SOC's level and lower their capacity to cope with daily life activities and stressful events. The improvement of social support and the promotion of social participation for older adults living in a rural setting is particularly important because they can increase GRRs accessibility, health, and well-being. As evidence of policy and program effectiveness is still equivocal and fragmented, improved knowledge on adapted interventions may help facilitate aging in place strategies, especially in rural context (Milne et al., 2007). Unlike rural areas, suburban municipalities are not addressed in the World Health Organization's frameworks (World Health Organization, 2002, 2007), and very few ecological interventions were held in this setting (Lord and Luxembourg, 2007). As American suburbs have the most rapid growth in adults aged 65 and over, growing by 39% since 2000 (Igielnik and Brown, 2018), the lack of interventions for these areas could be a challenge in the following decade. Indeed, suburban areas have specific characteristics (e.g., high rates of car ownership, neighborhoods designed for families) that may be constraining to older adults' mobility without a driving license (Brook Lyndhurst Ltd, 2005). The private car's reliance increases the risk of mobility limitations and social isolation for older suburban dwellers (Stjernborg et al., 2015). Aging in place strategies should be promoted regardless of the living context.

Aging in place strategies were shown to be compatible with salutogenic and health promotion approaches, mainly by improving GRRs accessibility through social support and mobility options. A better comprehension of the person-environment interactions and the development of indices to predict potential mismatches (e.g., older adults with mobility limitations living in resource-scarce neighborhoods), notably in relation to social needs (Oswald et al., 2005), could provide further opportunities for health promotion interventions. However, aging at home strategies have been criticized as not well adapted for all aging populations, notably low-income and frail older homeowners (Golant, 2008). Discourses about aging and healthcare strategies should be more inclusive of older adults with limited abilities or lower socioeconomic status. Home maintenance in older adults may incur considerable financial costs and increase stress and risk of injuries (Coleman et al., 2016). There are promising avenues for effective communal-care facilities, such as the NORCs and the Green Houses program (Greenfield et al., 2013; Kane et al., 2007). Tan's (2015) review showed that older adults in communal-care facilities had a lower SOC than those living in the community. Because living in the community is not accessible to all, salutogenic interventions aimed at improving the SOC for older adults living in communal-care facilities should also be of interest to researchers.

Conclusion

The current health and aging policy context are favorable to applied salutogenic research, especially for older adults living in the community. Indeed, interventions targeting both the individuals and the communities can enhance the SOC of older adults by providing them opportunities for social interactions and increasing their life space with new mobility options. By increasing their SOC, which predicts health and well-being, older adults can cope more easily with daily life activities and adverse life events, such as retirement, deaths of loved ones, and disabilities. Better coping strategies can allow older adults to live longer at home, surrounded by their peers, and maintain meaningful activities. Opportunities to increase accessibility to GRRs through social interactions and mobility options are numerous. Still, challenges need to be addressed to provide evaluated and effective interventions, regardless of their abilities, environmental context, or culture. Researchers, decision-makers, and community partners can apply a salutogenic framework to policies and interventions by improving knowledge and access to social resources that help seniors cope with everyday life challenges.

References

Antonovsky, A. (1979). *Health, stress, and coping*. Jossey-Bass.

Antonovsky, A. (1993a). The structure and properties of the sense of coherence scale. *Social Science & Medicine (1982), 36*(6), 725–733. https://doi.org/10.1016/0277-9536(93)90033-z

Antonovsky, A. (1993b). The salutogenic approach to aging. http://www.angelfire.com/ok/soc/a-berkeley. Html.

Antonovsky, A., Sagy, S., Adler, I., & Visel, R. (1990). Attitudes toward retirement in an Israeli cohort. *The International Journal of Aging and Human Development, 31*(1), 57–77. https://doi.org/10.2190/A937-BUU4-DDHW-2CAU

Avlund, K., Vass, M., & Hendriksen, C. (2003). Onset of mobility disability among community-dwelling old men and women. The role of tiredness in daily activities. *Age and Ageing, 32*(6), 579–584. https://doi.org/10.1093/ageing/afg101

Ball, S. J. (1993). What is policy? Texts, trajectories and toolboxes. *The Australian Journal of Education Studies, 13*(2), 10–17.

Bedney, B. J., Goldberg, R. B., & Josephson, K. (2010). Aging in place in naturally occurring retirement communities : Transforming aging through supportive service programs. *Journal of Housing for the Elderly, 24*(3–4), 304–321. https://doi.org/10.1080/02763893.2010.522455

Borglin, G., Jakobsson, U., Edberg, A.-K., & Hallberg, I. R. (2006). Older people in Sweden with various degrees of present quality of life : Their health, social support, everyday activities and sense of coherence. *Health & Social Care in the Community, 14*(2), 136–146. https://doi.org/10.1111/j.1365-2524.2006.00603.x

Borys, S., & Perlman, D. (1985). Gender differences in loneliness. *Personality and Social Psychology Bulletin, 11*(1), 63–74.

Bowling, A. (2005). *Ageing well: Quality of life in old age*. McGraw-Hill Education.

Brook Lyndhurst Ltd. (2005). *Sustainable cities and the ageing society*. Office of the Deputy Prime Minister.

Bryant, L. L., Corbett, K. K., & Kutner, J. S. (2001). In their own words : A model of healthy aging. *Social Science & Medicine, 53*(7), 927–941. https://doi.org/10.1016/S0277-9536(00)00392-0

Clément, A.-P., Djilas, D., Vinet, T., Aubin, A., Demers, K., & Levasseur, M. (2018). Identification and feasibility of social participation initiatives reducing isolation and involving rural older Canadians in the development of their community. *Aging Clinical and Experimental Research, 30*(7), 845–859.

Cohen, S., Gottlieb, B. H., & Underwood, L. G. (2001). Social relationships and health : Challenges for measurement and intervention. *Advances in Mind-Body Medicine, 17*(2), 129–141.

Coleman, T., Kearns, R. A., & Wiles, J. (2016). Older adults' experiences of home maintenance issues and opportunities to maintain ageing in place. *Housing Studies, 31*(8), 964–983.

Cornwell, E. Y., & Waite, L. J. (2009). Social disconnectedness, perceived isolation, and health among older adults. *Journal of Health and Social Behavior, 50*(1), 31–48.

Couton, P., & Gaudet, S. (2008). Rethinking social participation : The case of immigrants in Canada. *Journal of International Migration and Integration/Revue de l'integration et de la migration internationale, 9*(1), 21–44.

Davis, S., & Bartlett, H. (2008). Review article : Healthy ageing in rural Australia: Issues and challenges. *Australasian Journal on Ageing, 27*(2), 56–60. https://doi.org/10.1111/j.1741-6612.2008.00296.x

Dickens, A. P., Richards, S. H., Greaves, C. J., & Campbell, J. L. (2011). Interventions targeting social isolation in older people : A systematic review. *BMC Public Health, 11*(1), 647. https://doi.org/10.1186/1471-2458-11-647

Dumitrache, C. G., Rubio, L., Bedoya, I., Rubio-Herrera, R., Dumitrache, C. G., Rubio, L., Bedoya, I., & Rubio-Herrera, R. (2017). Promoting active aging in rural settings : An intervention program implemented in Orense, Spain. *Universitas Psychologica, 16*(3), 112–123. https://doi.org/10.11144/javeriana.upsy16-3.paar

Eriksson, M. (2017). The sense of coherence in the Salutogenic model of health. In M. B. Mittelmark, S. Sagy, M. Eriksson, G. F. Bauer, J. M. Pelikan, B. Lindström, & G. A. Espnes (Éds.), The handbook of Salutogenesis. Springer. http://www.ncbi.nlm.nih.gov/books/NBK435812/

Eriksson, M., & Lindström, B. (2005). Validity of Antonovsky's sense of coherence scale : A systematic review. *Journal of Epidemiology & Community Health, 59*(6), 460–466. https://doi.org/10.1136/jech.2003.018085

Eriksson, M., & Lindström, B. (2008). A salutogenic interpretation of the Ottawa charter. *Health Promotion International, 23*(2), 190–199. https://doi.org/10.1093/heapro/dan014

Farber, N., Shinkle, D., Lynott, J., Fox-Grage, W., & Harrell, R. (2011). Aging in Place: A State Survey of Livability Policies and Practices. American Association of Retired People.

Fairhall, N., Sherrington, C., Kurrle, S. E., Lord, S. R., & Cameron, I. D. (2011). ICF participation restriction is common in frail, community-dwelling older people : An observational cross-sectional study. *Physiotherapy, 97*(1), 26–32. https://doi.org/10.1016/j.physio.2010.06.008

Forbes, D. A. (2001). Enhancing mastery and sense of coherence : Important determinants of health in older adults. *Geriatric Nursing, 22*(1), 29–32. https://doi.org/10.1067/mgn.2001.113532

Fratiglioni, L., Wang, H.-X., Ericsson, K., Maytan, M., & Winblad, B. (2000). Influence of social network on occurrence of dementia: A community-based longitudinal study. *The Lancet, 355*(9212), 1315–1319

Fry, C. L. (2012, Novembre 12). Social structure and successful aging. *Healthy & successful aging: A public health mandate*. https://healthyandsuccessfulaging.wordpress.com/2012/11/12/paper-4-social-structure-and-successful-aging/.

Gilmour, H. (2012). Social participation and the health and Well-being of Canadian seniors. *Health Reports, 23*(4), 23–32.

Glass, T. A., De Leon, C. F. M., Bassuk, S. S., & Berkman, L. F. (2006). Social engagement and depressive symptoms in late life longitudinal findings. *Journal of Aging and Health, 18*(4), 604–628.

Glei, D. A., Landau, D. A., Goldman, N., Chuang, Y.-L., Rodriguez, G., & Weinstein, M. (2005). Participating in social activities helps preserve cognitive function : An analysis of a longitudinal, population-based study of the elderly. *International Journal of Epidemiology, 34*(4), 864–871.

Golant, S. M. (2008). Commentary : Irrational exuberance for the aging in place of vulnerable low-income older homeowners. *Journal of Aging & Social Policy, 20*(4), 379–397. https://doi.org/10.1080/08959420802131437

Gottlieb, B. H., & Bergen, A. E. (2010). Social support concepts and measures. *Journal of Psychosomatic Research, 69*(5), 511–520.

Rapagnani, G. (2002). Suicide in the elderly. *Revue Médicale de Liège, 57*(2), 91–96

Rowles, G. D., & Bernard, M. A. (2013). *Environmental gerontology : Making meaningful places in old age*. Springer Publishing Company.

Rosso, A. L., Taylor, J. A., Tabb, L. P., & Michael, Y. L. (2013). Mobility, Disability, and Social Engagement in Older Adults. *Journal of Aging and Health, 25*(4), 617–637.

Grant, N., Hamer, M., & Steptoe, A. (2009). Social isolation and stress-related cardiovascular, lipid, and cortisol responses. *Annals of Behavioral Medicine, 37*(1), 29–37. https://doi.org/10.1007/s12160-009-9081-z

Greenfield, E. A., Scharlach, A. E., Lehning, A. J., Davitt, J. K., & Graham, C. L. (2013). A tale of two community initiatives for promoting aging in place : Similarities and differences in the National Implementation of NORC programs and villages. *The Gerontologist, 53*(6), 928–938. https://doi.org/10.1093/geront/gnt035

Grewal, I., Lewis, J., Flynn, T., Brown, J., Bond, J., & Coast, J. (2006). Developing attributes for a generic quality of life measure for older people : Preferences or capabilities? *Social Science & Medicine, 62*(8), 1891–1901. https://doi.org/10.1016/j.socscimed.2005.08.023

Haak, M., Malmgren Fänge, A., Iwarsson, S., & Dahlin-Ivanoff, S. (2011). The importance of successful place integration for perceived health in very old age : A qualitative meta-synthesis. *International Journal of Public Health, 56*(6), 589–595. https://doi.org/10.1007/s00038-011-0282-4

Holt-Lunstad, J., Smith, T. B., Baker, M., Harris, T., & Stephenson, D. (2015). Loneliness and social isolation as risk factors for mortality a

Meta-analytic review. *Perspectives on Psychological Science, 10*(2), 227–237.

Hombrados-Mendieta, I., García-Martín, M. A., & Gómez-Jacinto, L. (2013). The relationship between social support, loneliness, and subjective Well-being in a Spanish sample from a multidimensional perspective. *Social Indicators Research, 114*(3), 1013–1034. https://doi.org/10.1007/s11205-012-0187-5

Horsburgh, M. E., & Ferguson, A. L. (2000). Salutogenesis: "origins of health" and sense of coherence. In Virginia Hill Rice (Éd.), Handbook of stress coping and health. Implications for nursing research, theory and practice (p. 175–194). Sage.

Iecovich, E. (2014). Aging in place : From theory to practice. *Anthropological Notebooks, 20*(1), 21–33.

Igielnik, R., & Brown, A. (2018). 5 facts about U.S. suburbs. *Pew research Center*. https://www.pewresearch.org/fact-tank/2018/10/02/5-facts-about-u-s-suburbs/.

Kane, R. A., Lum, T. Y., Cutler, L. J., Degenholtz, H. B., & Yu, T. C. (2007). Resident outcomes in small-house nursing homes: A longitudinal evaluation of the initial green house program. *Journal of the American Geriatrics Society, 55*(6), 832–839. https://doi.org/10.1111/j.1532-5415.2007.01169.x

Kaye, H. S., LaPlante, M. P., & Harrington, C. (2009). Do noninstitutional long-term care services reduce Medicaid spending? *Health Affairs, 28*(1), 262–272. https://doi.org/10.1377/hlthaff.28.1.262

Keefe, J., Andrew, M., Fancey, P., & Hall, M. (2006). *A profile of social isolation in Canada. Report submitted to the F/P/T Working Group on Social Isolation*. Province of British Columbia and Mount Saint Vincent University.

Koelen, M., Eriksson, M., & Cattan, M. (2017). Older people, sense of coherence and community. In M. B. Mittelmark, S. Sagy, M. Eriksson, G. F. Bauer, J. M. Pelikan, B. Lindström, & G. A. Espnes (Éds.), The handbook of Salutogenesis. Springer. http://www.ncbi.nlm.nih.gov/books/NBK435844/.

Krause, N. (2007). Longitudinal study of social support and meaning in life. *Psychology and Aging, 22*(3), 456–469.

Langeland, E., & Wahl, A. K. (2009). The impact of social support on mental health service users' sense of coherence : A longitudinal panel survey. *International Journal of Nursing Studies, 46*(6), 830–837. https://doi.org/10.1016/j.ijnurstu.2008.12.017

Lawton, M. P., & Nahemow, L. (1973). Ecology and the aging process. In *The psychology of adult development and aging* (pp. 619–674). American Psychological Association. https://doi.org/10.1037/10044-020

Lawton, M. P. (1990). An Environmental Psychologist Ages. In I. Altman & K. Christensen (Eds.), Environment and Behavior Studies: Emergence of Intellectual Traditions (pp. 339–363). Springer US.

Lee, H. Y., Jang, S.-N., Lee, S., Cho, S.-I., & Park, E.-O. (2008). The relationship between social participation and self-rated health by sex and age : A cross-sectional survey. *International Journal of Nursing Studies, 45*(7), 1042–1054.

Levasseur, M., Dubois, M.-F., Généreux, M., Menec, V., Raina, P., Roy, M., Gabaude, C., Couturier, Y., & St-Pierre, C. (2017). Capturing how age-friendly communities foster positive health, social participation and health equity : A study protocol of key components and processes that promote population health in aging Canadians. *BMC Public Health, 17*(1), 1–11.

Levasseur, M., Lefebvre, H., Levert, M.-J., Lacasse-Bédard, J., Desrosiers, J., Therriault, P.-Y., Tourigny, A., Couturier, Y., & Carbonneau, H. (2016). Personalized citizen assistance for social participation (APIC) : A promising intervention for increasing mobility, accomplishment of social activities and frequency of leisure activities in older adults having disabilities. *Archives of Gerontology and Geriatrics, 64*, 96–102.

Levasseur, M., Richard, L., Gauvin, L., & Raymond, E. (2010). Inventory and analysis of definitions of social participation found in the aging literature : Proposed taxonomy of social activities. *Social Science and Medicine, 71*(12), 2141–2149.

Levasseur, M., Naud, D., & Routhier, S. (2021). Community development by and for older adults. In I. Rootman, P. Edwards, M. Levasseur, & F. Grunberg (Eds.), Promoting the Health of Older Adults: The Canadian Experience (pp. 206–220). Canadian Scholars' Press.

Liddle, J., Haynes, M., Pachana, N. A., Mitchell, G., McKenna, K., & Gustafsson, L. (2014). Effect of a group intervention to promote older adults' adjustment to driving cessation on community mobility : A randomized controlled trial. *The Gerontologist, 54*(3), 409–422. https://doi.org/10.1093/geront/gnt019

Lord, S., & Luxembourg, N. (2007). The mobility of elderly residents living in suburban territories : Mobility experiences in Canada and France. *Journal of Housing for the Elderly, 20*(4), 103–121.

Lövheim, H., Graneheim, U. H., Jonsén, E., Strandberg, G., & Lundman, B. (2013). Changes in sense of coherence in old age – A 5-year follow-up of the Umeå 85+ study. *Scandinavian Journal of Caring Sciences, 27*(1), 13–19. https://doi.org/10.1111/j.1471-6712.2012.00988.x

Lui, C., Everingham, J., Warburton, J., Cuthill, M., & Bartlett, H. (2009). What makes a community age-friendly : A review of international literature. *Australasian Journal on Ageing, 28*(3), 116–121. https://doi.org/10.1111/j.1741-6612.2009.00355.x

Lund, R., Nilsson, C. J., & Avlund, K. (2010). Can the higher risk of disability onset among older people who live alone be alleviated by strong social relations ? A longitudinal study of non-disabled men and women. *Age and Ageing, 39*(3), 319–326.

Mac Intyre, I., Corradetti, P., Roberts, J., Browne, G., Watt, S., & Lane, A. (1999). Pilot study of a visitor volunteer programme for community elderly people receiving home health care. *Health & Social Care in the Community, 7*(3), 225–232.

Marottoli, R. A., de Leon, C. F. M., Glass, T. A., Williams, C. S., Cooney, L. M., & Berkman, L. F. (2000). Consequences of driving cessation : Decreased out-of-home activity levels. *The Journals of Gerontology: Series B, 55*(6), S334–S340. https://doi.org/10.1093/geronb/55.6.S334

Milligan, C., Neary, D., Payne, S., Hanratty, B., Irwin, P., & Dowrick, C. (2016). Older men and social activity : A scoping review of Men's sheds and other gendered interventions. *Ageing & Society, 36*(5), 895–923.

Milne, A., Hatzidimitriadou, E., & Wiseman, J. (2007). Health and quality of life among older people in rural England : Exploring the impact and efficacy of policy. *Journal of Social Policy, 36*(3), 477–495. https://doi.org/10.1017/S0047279407001055

Murayama, Y., Ohba, H., Yasunaga, M., Nonaka, K., Takeuchi, R., Nishi, M., Sakuma, N., Uchida, H., Shinkai, S., & Fujiwara, Y. (2015). The effect of intergenerational programs on the mental health of elderly adults. *Aging & Mental Health, 19*(4), 306–314. https://doi.org/10.1080/13607863.2014.933309

Naud, D., Généreux, M., Bruneau, J.-F., Alauzet, A., & Levasseur, M. (2019). Social participation in older women and men : Differences in community activities and barriers according to region and population size in Canada. *BMC Public Health, 19*(1), 1–14.

Newall, N. E., McArthur, J., & Menec, V. H. (2014). A longitudinal examination of social participation, loneliness, and use of physician and hospital services. *Journal of Aging and Health, 27*(3), 500–518.

Nicholson, N. R. J. (2009). Social isolation in older adults : An evolutionary concept analysis. *Journal of Advanced Nursing, 65*(6), 1342–1352.

Oswald, F., Hieber, A., Wahl, H.-W., & Mollenkopf, H. (2005). Ageing and person–environment fit in different urban neighbourhoods. *European Journal of Ageing, 2*(2), 88–97. https://doi.org/10.1007/s10433-005-0026-5

Plouffe, L. A., & Kalache, A. (2010). Towards global age-friendly cities : Determining urban features that promote active aging. *Journal of Urban Health, 87*(5), 733–739. https://doi.org/10.1007/s11524-010-9466-0

Rantanen, T., Äyräväinen, I., Eronen, J., Lyyra, T., Törmäkangas, T., Vaarama, M., & Rantakokko, M. (2015). The effect of an outdoor activities' intervention delivered by older volunteers on the quality of life of older people with severe mobility limitations : A randomized controlled trial. *Aging Clinical and Experimental Research, 27*(2), 161–169. https://doi.org/10.1007/s40520-014-0254-7

Read, S., Aunola, K., Feldt, T., Leinonen, R., & Ruoppila, I. (2005). The relationship between generalized resistance resources, sense of coherence, and health among Finnish people aged 65-69. *European Psychologist, 10*(3), 244–253. https://doi.org/10.1027/1016-9040.10.3.244

Rémillard-Boilard, S. (2018). The development of age-friendly cities and communities. In T. Buffel & H. Sophie (Éds.), Age-friendly cities and communities : A global perspective (p. 3–12). Policy Press.

Reynolds, K. A., Mackenzie, C. S., Medved, M., & Roger, K. (2015). The experiences of older male adults throughout their involvement in a community programme for men. *Ageing & Society, 35*(3), 531–551.

Richards, J. S., Bombardier, C. H., Tate, D., Dijkers, M., Gordon, W., Shewchuk, R., & DeVivo, M. J. (1999). Access to the environment and life satisfaction after spinal cord injury. *Archives of Physical Medicine and Rehabilitation, 80*(11), 1501–1506.

Ronzi, S., Orton, L., Pope, D., Valtorta, N. K., & Bruce, N. G. (2018). What is the impact on health and wellbeing of interventions that foster respect and social inclusion in community-residing older adults? A systematic review of quantitative and qualitative studies. *Systematic Reviews, 7*(1), 26. https://doi.org/10.1186/s13643-018-0680-2

Rossi, P. H., Lipsey, M. W., & Henry, G. T. (2018). *Evaluation : A systematic approach*. Sage Publications.

Rowles, G. D. (1983). Place and personal identity in old age : Observations from Appalachia. *Journal of Environmental Psychology, 3*(4), 299–313. https://doi.org/10.1016/S0272-4944(83)80033-4

Sagy, S., & Antonovsky, A. (1994). The reality worlds of retirees : An Israeli case-control study. *Journal of Psychology; Provincetown, Mass., Etc, 128*(1), 111–128.

Seah, B., Kowitlawakul, Y., Chokkanathan, S., Fong, J. J. Y., Espnes, G. A., Ang, E., & Wang, W. (2018). Salutogenic healthy ageing programme embracement (SHAPE) for senior-only households : A study protocol. *Journal of Advanced Nursing, 74*(4), 946–956. https://doi.org/10.1111/jan.13502

Shankar, A., McMunn, A., Banks, J., & Steptoe, A. (2011). Loneliness, social isolation, and behavioral and biological health indicators in older adults. *Health Psychology, 30*(4), 377.

Smith, R. J., Lehning, A. J., & Dunkle, R. E. (2013). Conceptualizing age-friendly community characteristics in a sample of urban elders : An exploratory factor analysis. *Journal of Gerontological Social Work, 56*(2), 90–111. https://doi.org/10.1080/01634372.2012.739267

Stalvey, B. T., Owsley, C., Sloane, M. E., & Ball, K. (1999). The life space questionnaire : A measure of the extent of mobility of older adults. *Journal of Applied Gerontology, 18*(4), 460–478. https://doi.org/10.1177/073346489901800404

Stjernborg, V., Wretstrand, A., & Tesfahuney, M. (2015). Everyday life Mobilities of older persons—A case study of ageing in a suburban landscape in Sweden. *Applied Mobilities, 2*(2), 134–150.

Stokols, D. (1992). Establishing and maintaining healthy environments : Toward a social ecology of health promotion. *American Psychologist, 47*(1), 6.

Tan, K. K. (2015). *Enhancing health resources among older people in the community using a salutogenesis-based intervention programme*. University of Eastern Finland. http://epublications.uef.fi/pub/urn_isbn_978-952-61-1952-6/index_en.html

Tan, K.-K., Chan, S. W.-C., & Vehviläinen-Julkunen, K. (2014). Self-care program for older community-dwellers : Protocol for a randomized controlled trial. *Central European Journal of Nursing and Midwifery, 5*(4), 145–155. https://doi.org/10.15452/CEJNM.2014.05.0010

Tomaka, J., Thompson, S., & Palacios, R. (2006). The relation of social isolation, loneliness, and social support to disease outcomes among the elderly. *Journal of Aging and Health, 18*(3), 359–384.

Trouillet, R., Gana, K., Lourel, M., & Fort, I. (2009). Predictive value of age for coping : The role of self-efficacy, social support satisfaction and perceived stress. *Aging & Mental Health, 13*(3), 357–366. https://doi.org/10.1080/13607860802626223

Turcotte, M., & Schellenberg, G. (2007). *A portrait of seniors in Canada, 2006*. Statistics Canada.

Uchino, B. N. (2009). Understanding the links between social support and physical health : A life-span perspective with emphasis on the separability of perceived and received support. *Perspectives on Psychological Science, 4*(3), 236–255.

United Nations. (2017). *World population ageing, 2017 highlights* (United Nations).

Verbrugge, L. M., Rennert, C., & Madans, J. H. (1997). The great efficacy of personal and equipment assistance in reducing disability. *American Journal of Public Health, 87*(3), 384–392.

Verdonschot, M. M. L., de Witte, L. P., Reichrath, E., Buntinx, W. H. E., & Curfs, L. M. G. (2009). Impact of environmental factors on community participation of persons with an intellectual disability : A systematic review. *Journal of Intellectual Disability Research, 53*(1), 54–64.

Victor, C. R., Scambler, S. J., Marston, L., Bond, J., & Bowling, A. (2006). Older people's experiences of loneliness in the UK: Does gender matter? *Social Policy and Society, 5*(1), 27–38.

Webber, S. C., Porter, M. M., & Menec, V. H. (2010). Mobility in older adults : A comprehensive framework. *The Gerontologist, 50*(4), 443–450. https://doi.org/10.1093/geront/gnq013

Wiesmann, U., & Hannich, H.-J. (2010). A Salutogenic analysis of healthy aging in active elderly persons. *Research on Aging, 32*(3), 349–371. https://doi.org/10.1177/0164027509356954

Wister, A. V. (2005). The built environment, health, and longevity : Multi-level Salutogenic and pathogenic pathways. *Journal of Housing for the Elderly, 19*(2), 49–70. https://doi.org/10.1300/J081v19n02_04

World Health Organization. (1986). *Ottawa charter for health promotion*. World Health Organization.

World Health Organization. (2002). *Active ageing : A policy framework*. World Health Organization.

World Health Organization. (2007). *Global age-friendly cities : A guide*. World Health Organization.

26

Architectural Design and Salutogenesis

Jan A. Golembiewski

Introduction

Following many years of effort of Alan Dilani and the International Academy of Design and Health (Dilani, 2006, 2008), the term 'salutogenic' has made inroads to hospital design, and it is creeping into the architectural design of aged care, schools, workplaces and correctional care – at least at first as a buzzword for marketing. The term was coined to describe Antonovsky's model for socio-environmental influences on health. However, in most designers' hyperbole it means little more than fuzzy intentions to create restorative environments by providing views that represent nature: whether it be vegetation (designed parkland, grassy areas, trees, etc.), views of the sky or even photographic representations of these things. The theory is thus often bleached of its full potential, like an apothecary that only stocks aspirin. The architectural design industry can take a great deal more from salutogenic theory than it currently does.

But to do so, it needs to dig deeper into the theory to be better informed about how their ideas and interventions are likely to be helpful on a case-by-case basis, and perhaps more importantly, to reach beyond the axiom of 'views of nature' and locate other ways to use the environment to improve health outcomes – especially in conditions where views into natural woodland just are not possible, are inappropriate or simply insufficient. The marketer's sense that salutogenic theory is a powerful tool for determining design impacts on health is well-placed; as Antonovsky suggested, salutogenesis might be the only comprehensive theory of health promotion (1996), and it is certainly one that can be used in diverse disciplines as this handbook attests. In short, it is something the architectural industry needs for the design process itself, not just for marketing spin.

J. A. Golembiewski (✉)
Psychological Design, Sydney, Australia

Interior Architecture and Environmental Design, Bilkent University, Ankara, Turkey
e-mail: jg@psychological.design

This chapter is about how we can bring salutogenic theory to (literally) concrete reality using architectural design. The following sections look at salutogenesis as a model – comparing it with other models of health-oriented architecture, then it looks at salutogenesis in general terms before looking at how it can be applied by addressing each of the Specific Resistance Resources (SRRs – more about them later).

Limitations of Previous Theories Linking Aesthetic Design and Health

Substantial evidence shows aesthetic design interventions can affect health. Several theories have been offered to explain these effects – but most of them are limited to the specific interests of the theorists. Examples include an evolutionary hypothesis to explain the restorative effects of nature (The Biophilia Hypothesis (BH) of Wilson, 1984); the influence of 'views of nature' (The Stress Reduction Theory (SRT) of Ulrich, 1991); the very similar Attention Restoration Theory (ART) of Kaplan and Kaplan (1989); and the Ecological Theory (ET) of Lawton and Nahemow (1973), which argued that there is a 'sweet spot' to be found in a trade-off between designing for comfort and designing for mental and physical challenges. In addition to these, architectural and urban layouts have been found to indirectly affect a person's biology. For instance, natural light-filled structures will influence sunlight-dependent Vitamin D, serotonin, melatonin and L-Dopa levels (Deguchi & Axelrod, 1972).

Of the bodies of research the designed environment on health, BH (Wilson, 1984), its architectural twin, SRT (Ulrich, 1991) and close relative, ART (Kaplan & Kaplan, 1982), have been the pre-eminent models for translating design to health – largely because these theories have been subject to half a century of study, and also because the first scientific health + design studies drew on these 'low-hanging fruit' as a theoretical premise. ART, SRT and BH involve designing closer relationships with naturalistic elements like views into vegetation and the presence of pet animals. BH makes this explicit, whereas the ART acknowledges all 'fascinating' environments for the way they allow people to rest their cognitive processes. In effect the way these theories are translated into means that most health design research is not actually about designing better buildings, but turning away from the environments we build, and towards the ones we plant – or better still, totally natural environments. Again, the question is, are BH and ART sufficient to explain the salutogenic effects we see in bio-oriented designs?

The BH, SRT, ART, Medical and salutogenic approaches are not mutually exclusive, but any health benefits we see from ART, SRT or BH approaches are better understood using the salutogenic framework than from within their paradigms, or even using the Medical paradigm, because of all these models, only the salutogenic theory has broad enough scope to encompass them all.

Overview of Salutogenic Theory and its Relevance to Architecture

While these theories are all important, they ignore the elephant in the room – that architecture can be psychologically manipulative, for better or for worse. Architecture does this by providing *a narrative context*. It continually tells *a story*, which affects people's behaviour, how they are treated by others and how they feel about themselves. The story further influences neural and endocrine systems through the biochemical correlates of these emotions (Sapolsky, 2017). It is evident then that architecture can directly influence health (Golembiewski, 2016), but how can architects plan for these effects? Antonovsky's salutogenic theory provides an accessible overarching logic for determining the health and well-being benefits of design (Golembiewski, 2012b), beyond the basics covered by Environmental Medicine[1,2] and without the need to understand any illnesses suffered by the environment's users. The theory does this by modelling how a person's milieu enables action in the ceaseless endeavour of the betterment of one's life and circumstances. The milieu is both social and physical – and this chapter is concerned by the latter. Does the environment enable physical actions? Does it provide clarity? Does it provide for emotional support? Or does the environment block action, frustrate plans and make people feel exasperated? These are the questions to be asked when assessing how 'salutogenic' a design is.

The salutogenic theory is not a model of disease, rather it is a model of health (Mittelmark & Bull, 2013). As a theory, it has a scope and perspective that other ways of understanding health lack (Antonovsky, 1996), yet it is not an alternative to Medicine[3] or Public Health interventions. Salutogenesis looks the opposite direction, towards a more vibrant sense of well-being; towards better and more robust health; health-promotion and recovery-orientation, rather than to the illnesses that threaten life. But salutogenesis is not the opposite of orthodox Medicine, rather it is complementary, in the true sense of the word. Because they are health-oriented, salutogenic interventions are largely general in nature and are therefore best used to support common-sense health initiatives. Salutogenic interventions work because they inform systems and environments design to speed the natural process of recovery, provide insight into social approaches to complex health problems and promote health before disease or infirmity ever takes hold. But this does not mean they are not powerful – a strong salutogenic disposition may mean survival against impossible odds, as witnessed by Frankl (1963), a psychiatrist and prisoner in the concentration camps of World War II.

Salutogenesis is a way of understanding the entire spectrum of wellness and illness, regardless of specificity and detail. The salutogenic theory does not only seek to improve health but to assist in all other human endeavours because that is the level on which it works. Thus, salutogenic interventions do not make people better, they make architectural and other interventions better, and in that way, salutogenic interventions help people to help themselves, to get the most out of their lives and to be their best selves. Salutogenic approaches, therefore, reach beyond Medicine, to maximise our endeavours, help us fulfil our desires and provide for our constantly evolving needs to improve our circumstances. This broad effort is understood as the basis for maintaining and supporting one's health (Golembiewski, 2013b).

Salutogenic theory explains how generalised factors affect well-being wherever we find ourselves on the health/illness spectra. As such, it is useful for managing indirect, complex, obscure or unknown factors of health such as our general motivations and frailties, including those that lead us to fall prone to illness.[4] Because salutogenic theory has this higher-level validity, it continues to make sense beyond the specific findings of experiments and singular design interventions (Strümpfer et al., 1998a, 1998b). Salutogenic theory provides a basis for informed decision making in the absence of specific knowledge or whenever circumstances are too complex to suggest easy solutions, such as design choices that must be made now for an unknown future. In short, salutogenesis is an excellent model to provide insight and inspire health professionals

[1] Environmental Medicine is a field of Public Health focusing on environmental toxicity and other specific risks to somatic health.

[2] Medicine, Medical and Health are capitalised to refer to the prevalent health paradigm, rather than to individual treatments, endpoints and goals.

[3] Antonovsky makes it clear that Salutogenic Theory does not advocate abandoning Medicine (1987, p.13).

[4] This kind of complexity typifies the way the physical environment affects health.

to provide intangible help in addition to just prescriptive treatments, and for non-health professionals (like architects and urban designers), Salutogenic theory helps recognise that they too can bring a health dimension to their work just by making spaces and places easier to negotiate and more human.

Relationships Between General Resistance Resources and Stressors

The theory of salutogenesis asserts that good social/emotional, psychological, and physical/somatic health is maintained through a dynamic ability to adapt to life's changing circumstances. The opposite is also true – challenges that are too great to overcome or adapt to exert an aetiological influence on illness. One 'succumbs to illness', when demands exceed one's capacity to cope with them (Antonovsky, 1972), that is when the salutogenic resources are not sufficient to support ones' needs and desires in the face of adversity and challenges. So, a germ on its own is insufficient to cause a disease – it needs to be cultured in an environment that lacks the capacity for resistance. Models that accept 'multiple causation' typically describe the specific influences that cause maladaptivity as 'stressors': but these must include everything from intensely joyous events to life's tragedies and banal concerns (Antonovsky, 1987). In effect, everything can be considered a stressor unless there is a model that can predict which stressors will cause failure and which will be successfully negotiated – or even be celebrated. The 'stress' concept, as it is widely accepted, is therefore useless except in post hoc reflection. The forces at work to improve adaptability, on the other hand, are specific enough to allow practical, buildable and highly bespoke solutions.

When applying salutogenesis to architecture, it is a useful conceit to picture GRRs and GRDs as opposing forces in a zero-sum equation. On the one hand, the combined support (the generalised resistance resources or GRRs) stack up (and must be stronger than) life's challenges, whatever they may be, which we can also imagine as deleterious forces (the generalised resistance deficits or GRDs[5]). Where GRRs are stronger, a person will be left with a robust, flexible and buoyant sense of coherence (SOC), which will maximise ones' resistance to illness, or (at the least) enable a prompt and full recovery. Where GRRs are low, adaptive failures will occur, and these lead to decline and even death.

[5]GRDs are not actually forces, much less deleterious ones called 'stressors' in most health promotion literature. Antonovsky observes that 'stressors' are 'omnipresent, …not necessarily pathological and may be salutary' in some instances (1987, p.12). They tend to be random and agnostic. The only danger is that there are absences of the resources needed to deal with them. The desert sun is an example. If you have photovoltaic panels, the same energy that can so easily kill can equally supply valuable power.

The GRRs fall into three domains, each of which relates to one of the dimensions in Antonovsky's description of the SOC in his 1987 book: '…the extent to which one has a pervasive, enduring though dynamic feeling of confidence that;

1. … one's environments… are structured, predictable and explicable;
2. The resources are available to meet … demands…; *and*
3. These demands are challenges, worthy of investment and engagement' (pp. 18–19).

The GRRs then, are those resources that enhance the cognitive domain – comprehensibility [1]; those that enhance the domain of action and physical resources – manageability [2]; and those that enhance the affective domain – meaningfulness [3]. The adverse forces, on the other hand, are any challenges to the resistance resources. In salutogenic theory, these are usually lumped together because they are ubiquitous, arising as they do from natural entropy and the relentless inevitability of eventual death. And much as we like to personify these negative forces as vindictive and aggressive, at least in his later work (1987 onwards), Antonovsky sees the GRDs simply as insufficiencies; as deficits that exert a continuous disintegrative force, allowing illnesses to overcome a person when the GRRs are too weak to support a robust and dynamic SOC (Antonovsky, 1996). But on occasion, the resource deficits can be very specific and vulnerable to specific antagonists, in which case the deficits are called the SRDs (the specific resource deficits) (Mittelmark et al., 2017). Scurvy, for instance, is caused by a lack of vitamin C. In this instance, no alternative resource will suffice. But at this level of specificity, the SRRs are inseparable from the treatments and preventions that fuel the Medical paradigm, so an important point can be made here: salutogenic interventions can be as specific as any medical intervention to address specific resistance deficits but are usually very generalised to fortify a person holistically.

When one is unable to adapt to circumstances and experiences, people cannot manage even the simplest tasks. This causes a 'breakdown' (Antonovsky, 1972: 64), and illness follows shortly thereafter. But with knowledge of the GRR/GRD (SRR/SRD) dynamics, a scaffold emerges that can be readily applied to tailor resources for just about all endeavours – including architectural and urban design. SOC-supportive design can help liberate the other GRRs to work together to enable resistance to disease and reduce the disintegrative forces that cause maladaptation in the first instance.

A useful way to illustrate salutogenesis is through metaphor (Fig. 26.1). A person regards adversity and challenges much as a knight who goes out daily to slay dragons. The knight finds meaning in fighting dragons (the meaningfulness salutogenic resource) – in protecting the society she loves so much, in the ribbon from her beaux that is tied to

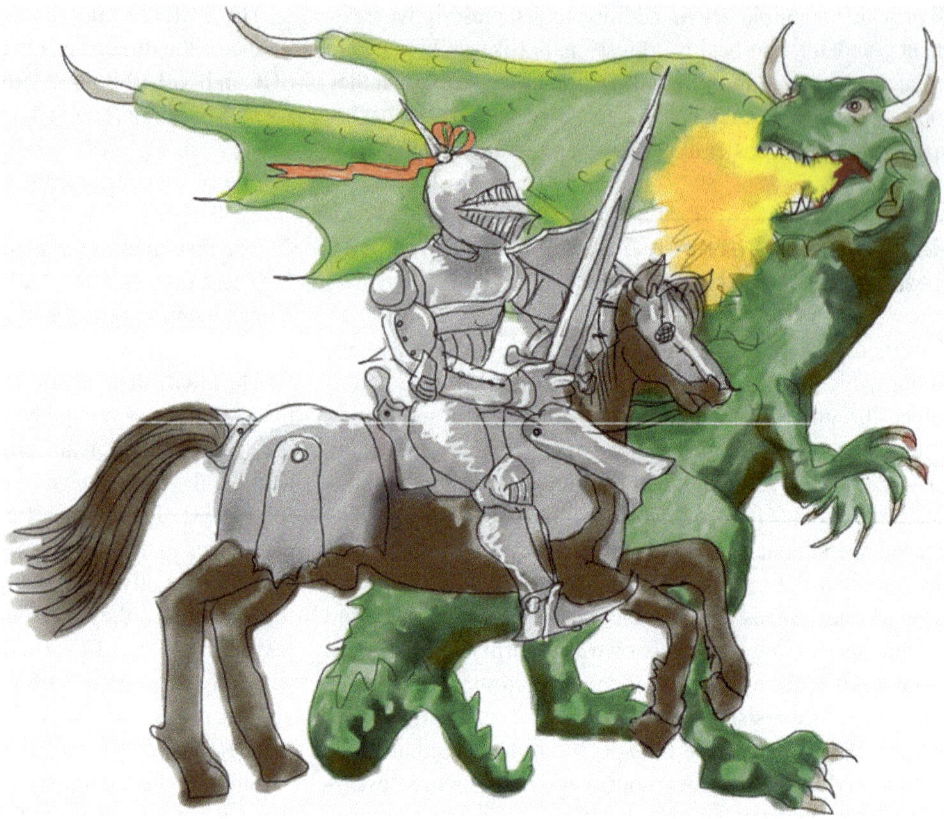

Fig. 26.1 A useful way to understand salutogenesis is through metaphor. (Illustration courtesy of the author by J Golembiewski)

her helmet, in the heroism of her actions. But the knight also needs to act, and protection and tools to do so: it is in her armour, shield and sword the knight finds her manageability resources. Finally, she also needs knowledge. The knight needs to know how dragons move and attack; she needs tactics, plans and skills – and knowledge about how to communicate to her horse. Here the knight finds comprehensibility resources. These resources are the specific resistance resources (SRRs) – collectively known as the generalised resistance resources (GRRs). Deficits in any of these resources (generalised resistance deficits – GRDs) are dangerous and potentially fatal – holes in her armour, insufficient knowledge about dragons, and most critically, a lack of desire to fight them in the first place, lead to severe losses and possibly even death. Success on the battlefield, on the other hand, is rewarded by life – the knight returns triumphant, to a hero's welcome. The overall feeling the knight has, that she will ultimately either fail or triumph, is called the sense of coherence (SOC). A strong SOC improves the chances of success and makes health more robust. A weak one makes the night more vulnerable to any surprise turns from the dragons. The dragon metaphor distinguishes between GRDs and stressors: the dragon is just as much a malign force as it is essential to the SOC of the knight. Without the dragon, the knight cannot battle and return victorious. The SOC then is dependent on both adversity and the capacity to resist it.

The Three SOC-Related Categories of Generalised Resistance Resources

'Comprehensibility' resources are those of the cognitive domain. These help to make sense of one's life narrative, one's context and current circumstances, and without this fundamental knowledge and associated skills, people have little capacity to make the most of life's circumstances or to negotiate its challenges (Golembiewski, 2012c). In essence, comprehensibility is a person's sense of 'agency'. The ability to negotiate most of circumstance is an essential resource; people feel terrible frustration when they just cannot get what they want because they do not know how or other reasons. Because of the dissonance a failure of comprehensibility might cause, an extreme failure is often patched with an untested or improvised epistemic scaffolding, precipitating delusional ideas and magical thinking (Keinan, 1994), the worst of which might present as symptoms or predictors of paranoia (Antonovsky, 1987) or even psychosis (Mason et al., 2004).

'Manageability' resources are of the domain of action and are thus about physical resources and real actions. These are personified by the words, '*I do.*' Manageability resources are those a person needs to act. Mostly this activity relates to day-to-day physical realities like staying warm, dry, clean, rested, nourished and other the maintenance requirements of their physical lives. Many manageability actions involve critical processes such as cooking, cleaning and working. There is little question that these are basic concerns of architecture. But over the last few decades, concern for users' manageability has shifted to be more inclusive – to consider the needs of people with generic disabilities. Now manageability resources in architecture include requirements for *universal accessibility* – reachability, controllability, liveability comfort and staying safe – even for people who are deaf, blind or use wheelchairs.

In architecture, there is also a current trend to advance accessibility to the realm of *inclusive design*. Where universal accessibility aims to make the environment generically barrier-free for everyone but ends up making it easier for many users (with such things as the implementation of ramps for wheelchairs, strollers and skateboards), inclusive design attempts to *solve* accessibility problems for specific extreme cases, with the understanding that the solution will have side benefits for everyone (Clarkson et al., 2003) – for example, a designer might look at how buildings are used by people born with *amelia* (missing limbs). The architect might specify sound- or movement-activated light switches, which will provide the general benefits of making switches more sanitary and potentially even invisible. As advanced as it is, inclusive design is still largely concerned with enabling action and is, therefore, an approach to improve the manageability of architecture.

Manageability is mostly about doing things. And for the best part, this involves looking after one's self and others in your care. Failure to manage these tasks exemplify the traditional pathogenic definition of stress (Sapolsky, 2004), and total failure can easily lead to death.

'Meaningfulness': according to Antonovsky (1979) and Frankl (1963), meaningfulness is the principal reason for life. Meaningfulness resources are those of the emotional ('affective') domain. Meaningfulness provides the will to resist adversity, challenges, the entropic pull of illness and fears about death's inevitability. As such, it is (in so many ways) the most important of the salutogenic resources. Meaningfulness is also the most elusive because it is difficult to define and is intrinsically personal.

Meaningfulness is found in the intensity of personal connections, responsibilities and desires with the outside world: 'Profound ties to concrete, immediate others... and between an individual and his community are decisive resistance resources' (Antonovsky, 1972, p. 542). People find meaning in different social groupings, in different causes and concerns, and continually disagree wholeheartedly about how such concerns should be prioritised. Yet it is in these distinctions that people find the basis of a sense of identity and purpose (Frankl, 1963; Searles, 1966). Without meaningfulness, people find themselves utterly bereft of any desire to act and subsequently fall prey to somatic or mental illness (particularly the depressive signs and anhedonia) (Frankl, 1963; Searles, 1960, 1966), both of which can be fatal.

Aesthetics of the Built Environment Influencing Health

Salutogenesis is expressed in architecture through *affordances* – the opportunities that are structured into the environment that stimulate action; cause us to reflect on how we feel; or stimulate thought. Some of these affordances are aesthetic. They are thus 'regarded' as sensory information, rather than as things that directly manipulate us or vice versa. But this is a mistake. The idea that aesthetic concerns have an impact on health can be challenging because it could mean that where we thought about aesthetic decisions as ultimately empty opinions, these could prove to be therepeutic or deleterious.

For millennia humans have customised their accommodation as a resource to protect against danger, discomfort, wildlife, social threats and the deleterious effects of weather. Architecture's role in these protective purposes is fundamental. However, the supportive effect of architecture is not only physical but psychological too – if people cannot find respite from the pressures of life at home, the resulting compounding mental and emotional strain may be enough to cause debilitating mental illness, possibly even without an underlying biological or genetic dysfunction (Golembiewski, 2013a). But all shelter is not equal: even once we have achieved the basic need for shelter from the weather, the wild and other dangers, we continue to customise the environment on an aesthetic level (Fig. 26.2), in what appears to be an attempt to make the environment better on a psychological level. People have decorated their surroundings in all parts of the world since at least Neolithic times. Much of this effort is thought to be to create a sense of meaning and perhaps even to entreat gods to moderate circumstances that are otherwise beyond human control (Harari, 2015).

Perhaps because of these ancient origins, the correlation of aesthetics and health (and even on mortality) appears to be superstitious and occult and is thus not nearly as widely accepted as evidence suggests it should (Golembiewski, 2016). But the impact of aesthetics (such things as views and presence of potted plants) on health has been scientifically tested thousands of times, including dozens of studies against a null hypothesis (a statistical method used to demonstrate causality). In 2005, a systematic review located and analysed 30 peer-reviewed articles that showed this effect to be significant and reliable (Dijkstra et al., 2006), with findings that sometimes defy belief – for example, 30.8% faster recovery and 38% lower mortality were found when patients recovering in hospital were given sunlit rooms for psychiatric

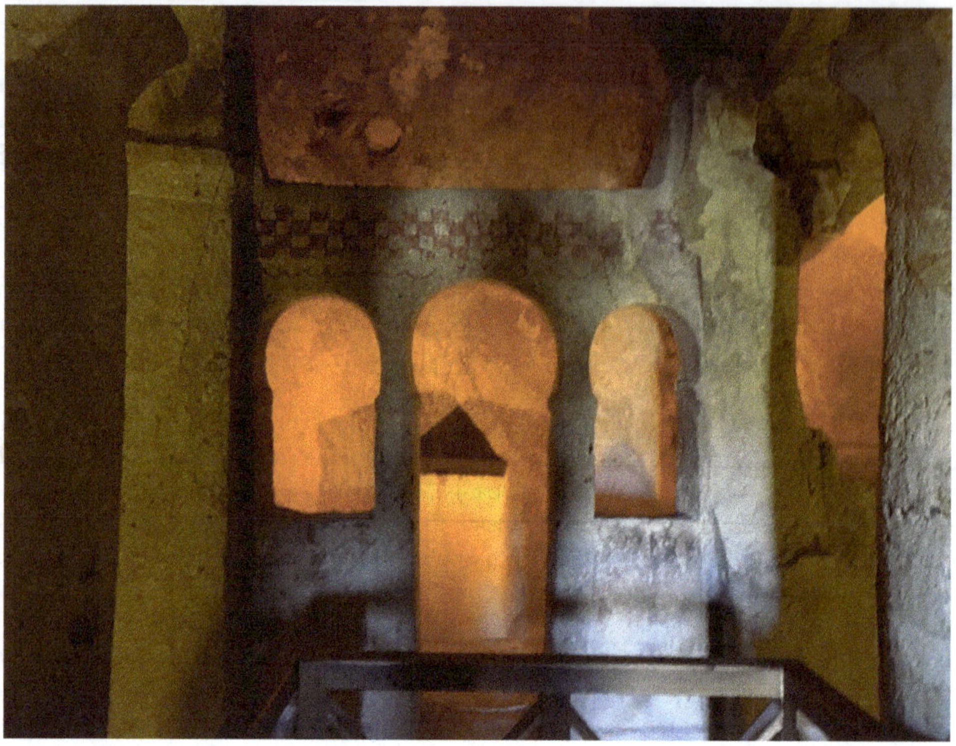

Fig. 26.2 A 1400-year-old prayer niche in a cave in Göreme (Turkey) has been painstakingly carved and painted for apparently no functional purpose except to improve the space on a psychological level. (J. Golembiewski, Photograph courtesy of the author)

disorders (Beauchemin & Hays, 1996, 1998) (an effect size that cannot be reasonably traced to vitamin D deficiencies!)

From a salutogenic perspective, such findings are of immense importance: when people are healthy, they demonstrate a theoretical surplus of resistance resources, so for many people, aesthetic improvements are nice, but are not essential, unless they seek extraordinary levels of wellness. Maslow (1962) described these people as 'peakers' – the highly creative souls who maximise the human experience and thrive in a state of self-actualisation. These people have an insatiable desire for the greater states of well-being. But many people are not concerned for peak experience and are happy to get on being simply 'well' (Maslow, 1962) This means that many people who do not currently suffer from disease can too easily dismiss the impact of aesthetics. But when people are ill, they suffer in the balance between deterioration and recovery, so any genuine influences (whether for better or worse) are likely to reflect in their SOC, and because of that, their ability to recover. As an example, two cohorts of severe psychiatric patients (each n = 10) and 10 matched healthy controls were shown emotionally manipulative imagery whilst undergoing fMRI of their frontal lobes. When the observed inhibitory potential was subtracted from the activation caused by the images, the differences between the cohorts were extreme – especially when it came to negative images, where the psychiatric patients showed greater surplus excitation than the controls. The implication is that the healthy controls had the resources they required to process the negative images fully, and therefore barely noticed and change. Whereas the psychiatric patients did not have the resources to reprocess this information. The surplus triggered symptoms, therefore adding to the diagnosable criteria of disease, thereby making the patients only sicker (Golembiewski, 2012a).

When Antonovsky speaks of the outside world, he uses the term 'stimulus' to refer to the neurological effect the environment evokes (as observed in scientific studies like the one just mentioned). This way of referring to the environment typifies scientific attitudes, but the term denigrates the omnipresent and immersive quality of the environment, which is as fundamental to existence as the three dimensions of SOC. Certainly, the environment is replete with stimuli, but it is so much more than that because our bodies, minds and emotions simply cannot exist without context. The built environment is full of opportunities and restrictions – aesthetic ones (as above) and physical ones like fences and walls, and opportunities like pathways, bridges or windows. All of these determine the choices we make. Some are insignificant – for example, there is little phenomenological difference between a left or right turn, even though they are opposites. But many physical restrictions and opportunities are deliberately there to moderate our behaviour (Golembiewski, 2016). Consider the design of shops, for instance, where every detail is assessed on its capacity to improve sales (Turley & Milliman, 2000). The manipulative possibilities of the physical environment can be used to directly improve 'factors' which are thought to affect health outcomes also: cities around the world are compiling 'fit city' design guidelines to encourage people to take the stairs and leave the car behind, and walk or cycle instead (City of New York, 2013; Jackson & Sinclair, 2012). Physical interventions like these are often assumed to be the most the built environment can do to improve health – if only because the therapeutic pathways between aesthetics and health outcomes are difficult to trace or predict. This is of course where salutogenesis is most useful. Salutogenesis groups supportive factors (GRRs, SRRs), and deficits (GRDs, SRDs), and when deficits outweigh resistance resources, people will fall sick in the way they are genetically, physiologically, biologically, mentally and socially most vulnerable.

When designing at an urban scale, models like the 'fit city' initiatives make axiomatic sense – with greater fitness, comes better health. And people mistakenly believe this to be the basis for the salutogenic effect (e.g. Mazuch, 2017). Although there is a relationship, it is not only because of increased fitness levels of residents. It is more because the 'fit city' architecture provides good things to do, positive choices and pleasant experiences, including exposure to urban green spaces, all of which support resistance resources. The 'fit city' choices have a broad psychological benefit to the whole community that far outweighs the physical fitness benefit that is conferred only to a few individuals. Perhaps the greatest generalised benefit is from having choices. The possibility of something healthy to do provides everyone with a sense of meaningfulness, regardless of whether the affordance is accepted and acted on. Of the impressive results reviewed by Dijkstra et al. (2006), none of the health improvements of persons in healthcare institutions was because the hospitals had more steps or longer corridors. Most salutogenic factors of causation are not directly somatic, but aesthetic – they are largely psychological rather than physical.

Promoting Manageability, Comprehensibility and Meaningfulness in Architecture

As pointed out early in this chapter, the traditional lens for understanding the impact of the built environment on health is focused on how well it provides basic functionality, shelter and whether it exposes users to toxins. The built environment is thus relevant to Medicine only in as much as it provides shelter, ease of cleaning and other basic functionality. This understanding has been somewhat updated to include views of nature to improve Medical outcomes, but still, it is a low bar. However, salutogenic architecture is not Medicine oriented; it is geared to support peoples' lives by helping them to cope with whatever life throws at them. It helps with manageability, comprehensibility and meaningfulness, and their collective synthesis: the sense of coherence (SOC). In other words, salutogenesis is a way of understanding the diverse ways a person can be helped through the natural process of recovery and development of positive health.

Manageability in Architecture

Perhaps one of the most obvious tests of the quality of architecture is manageability. Architecture is after all, the domain of the physical and tangible actions – and the built environment is nothing if not present in concrete reality. To understand what manageability is in architectural terms, we can look at the misery and impotence we feel when it is absent: the powerlessness we have when we cannot stop the weather (be it cold and penetrating rain, wind and snow or the opposite; unchecked heat and humidity) getting to us when we need something else – such as sleep or an environment where we can work. Poor design for manageability might be apparent in a building that requires you to bend over to reach things if you have arthritis, or again a chic home with white surfaces that never look or feel clean despite hours of effort.

In architecture, manageability resources are improved by:

- Functionality, 'fit-for-purpose' design
- Safety by design
- Barrier-free accessibility and design to enable action
- Person-centred design
- The design of positive affordances
- Forgiving design

Regarding *functionality and fit-for-purpose* design, the question is: does the design of your home/ workplace/school/ city/institutions enable you to *do* whatever it is that needs to be done or is the environment just a hindrance? Do not assume that the law or the good sense of architects have pre-empted these things for you. Do not expect that architects will ensure that a new home (which is surely a place to let go and relax) will be designed for that, and therefore fit-for-purpose. The responsibility for designing a building that actively fosters well-being can only be enforced by specific agreements to address this issue because fit-for-purpose design (bizarrely) is not considered a reasonable expectation of an architect (Cooke, 2001) – even if they are commissioned to design a family home, a school or hospital. On the other hand, that the design is *physically safe* is legally enforceable (and has been since the laws of Hammurabi of Babylon in 1792 BCE), and so too are specific access and egress provisions, especially for emergencies. But when armed with salutogenic theory to provide insight, manageability in architecture can mean so much more than just protection from the elements, safety and accessibility.

When talking about *accessibility and enabling action*, thoughtful consideration needs to be given to functionality and to the needs of anticipated users of the space over time.

The way salutogenesis looks to peoples' needs, and not only to the needs of any illness they may suffer ('the person needs care' vs 'the wound needs dressing'), makes the salutogenic paradigm intrinsically *person-centred.* Person-centred (and its industry-specific equivalents: patient-centred for healthcare; student-centred for education; customer-centred for retail, etc.) design pays attention to the details that make living life easier: door-handles that are easily manipulated and will not stress weak or arthritic limbs; a well-defined and distinctive front door for someone with Alzheimer's disease; low-contrast, low reflectivity interiors for ageing eyes, lecture halls that do not draw attention to late students, etc. Some features are more universal: Why design shelves above 150 cm (5′) for children, short males, most females or people who will one day grow old or might suffer a permanent or temporary disability?

These considerations improve the scope of manageability in design hugely. But manageability can be richer still. The most valuable tool designers can employ is *positive affordance design.* As mentioned earlier, we live an immersive experience of the world, and have an ecological relationship to it: the environment is not just 'stimulus'. We perceive the world around us through opportunities to act rather than through a rational cognitive process (Bargh, 1994; Gibson, 1979). These opportunities are called *affordances.* Mostly we sense affordances unconsciously. We walk down paths without thinking; 'Hey, how cool is it that this path is here, that it leads to where I want to go, and that the ground is stable and there's no poison ivy…' And yet we create paths like these all the time, and without them, we make entirely different choices. We sense affordances of all kinds – objects that inspire action, signs that tell us to do things and the calming aesthetic impacts of the natural environment (now there's where ART fits in!) (Golembiewski, 2013b). We are constantly presented with affordances, but the choice about whether to accept or deny the affordance is far more subject to our mood and outlook than most people can imagine. When we are feeling down or are ill, we are far less likely to notice positive things and far more likely to perceive negative ones (Golembiewski, 2012a). We are therefore more susceptible to make bad choices – that is, we are more likely to reject good choices and pick up on negative affordances than when we are healthy, happy and thriving (Golembiewski, 2014). But even when we are gloomy and in a space where we reject the best the world has to offer, having those good affordances present is nevertheless critical because the choice alone can make us feel better, *whether we accept them or not.*

Forgiving design improves manageability – a home that is designed to look great, even when it is a mess (Fig. 26.3); a building that is optimally positioned and ventilated to feel comfortable, even when the heating and air-conditioning are turned off (Brager & de Dear, 1998) (Fig. 26.4); an urban layout that is of a human scale, which enables you to walk to your destination (Zook & Ewing, 2010) (Fig. 26.5). All these affordances improve manageability.

Manageability is good and more manageability is better, but sometimes people find that decisions that are made to improve manageability can block the development of

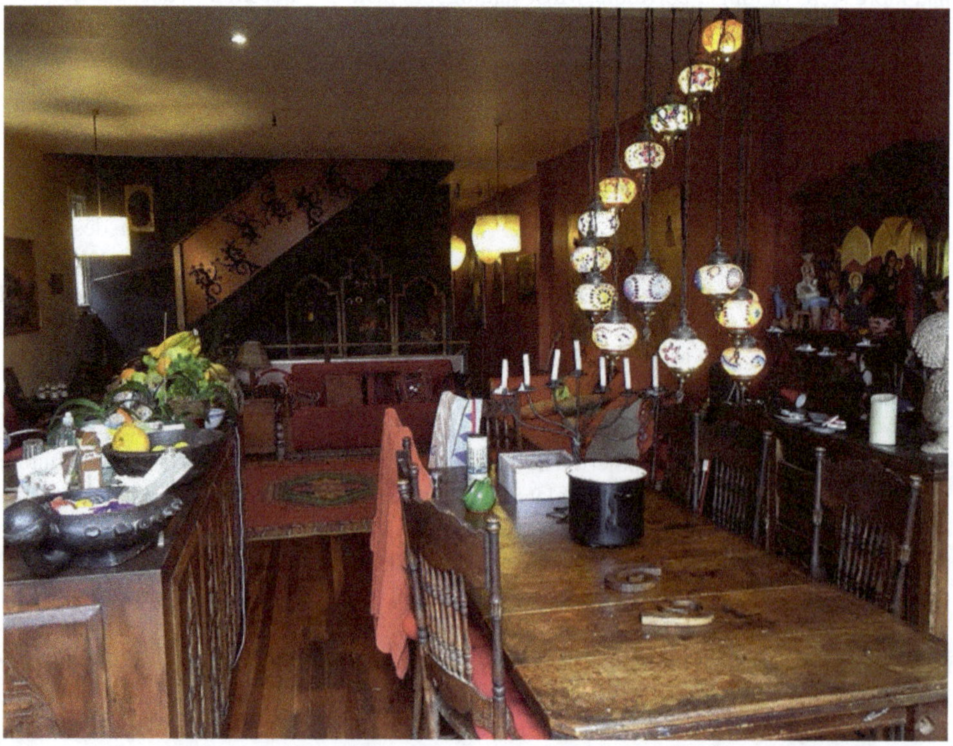

Fig. 26.3 A home that is designed to look good, even when it is a mess. (J. Golembiewski, Photograph *courtesy of the author*)

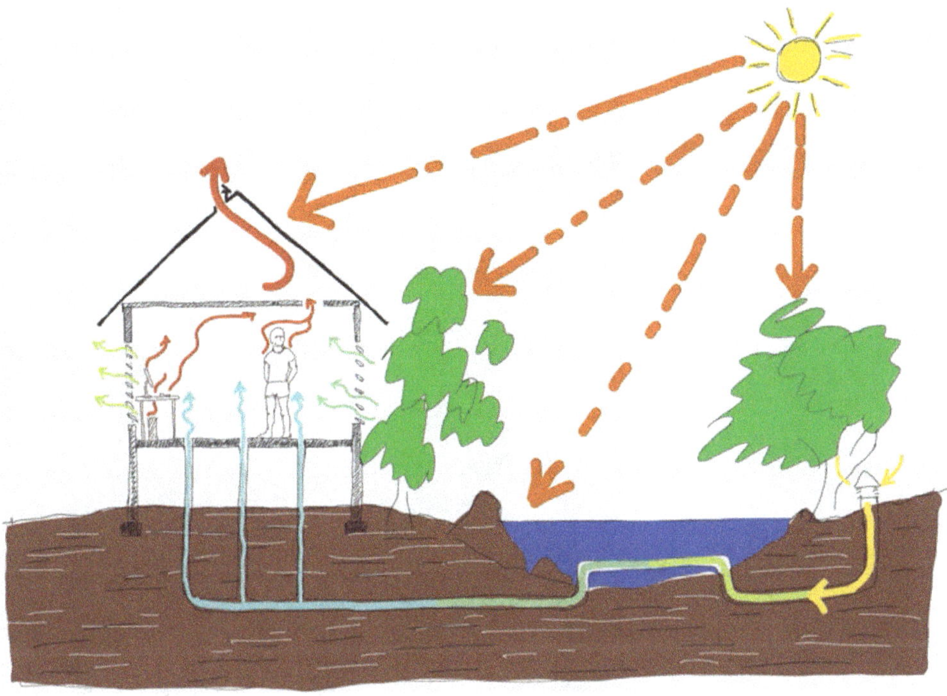

Fig. 26.4 A building that is optimally positioned and ventilated to feel comfortable, even when the heating and air-conditioning is turned off. (J. Golembiewski, Diagram *courtesy of the author*)

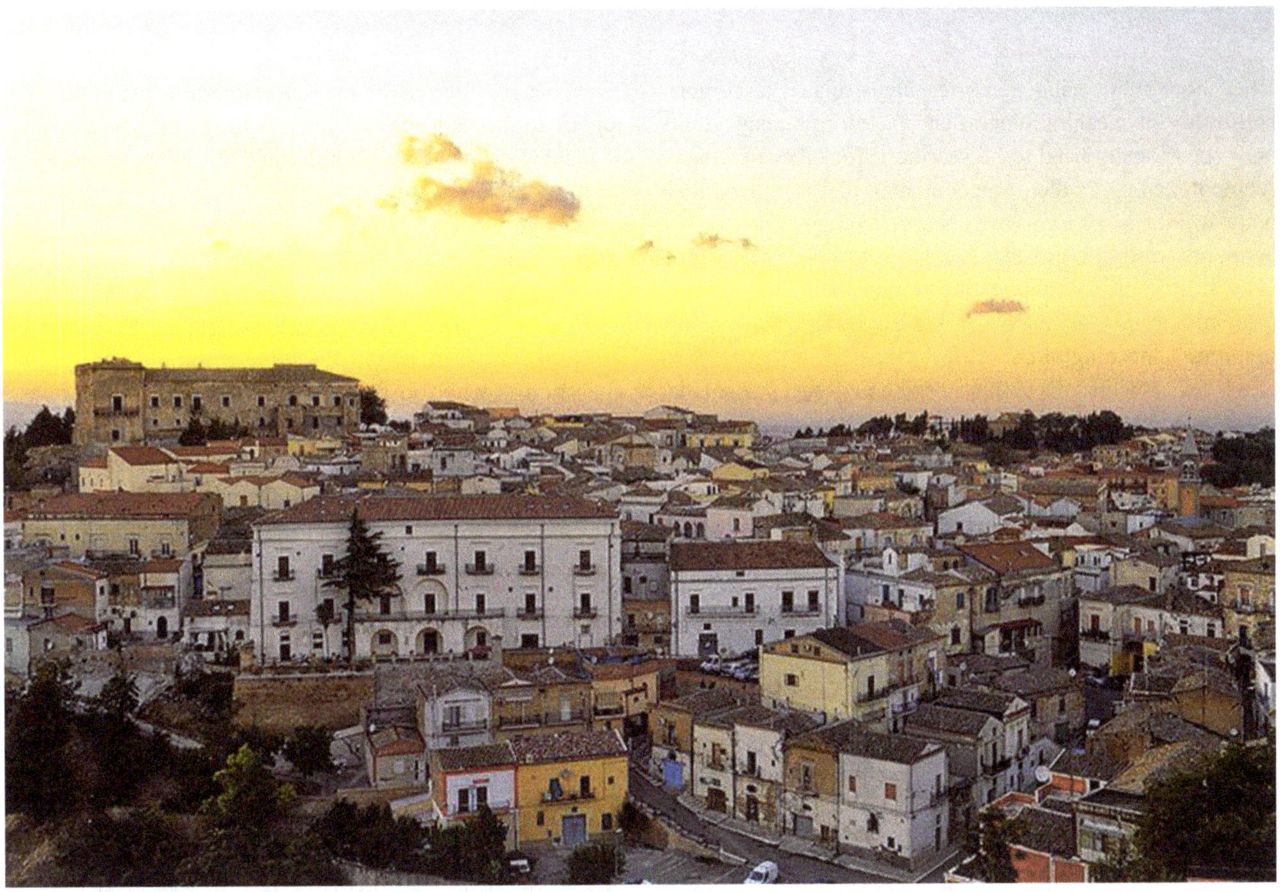

Fig. 26.5 An urban layout that is of a human scale, which enables you to walk to your destination – such cities are common in Europe. (Photograph of Ascoli Satriano courtesy of Giuseppe Valvano, under a CC Share-alike licence)

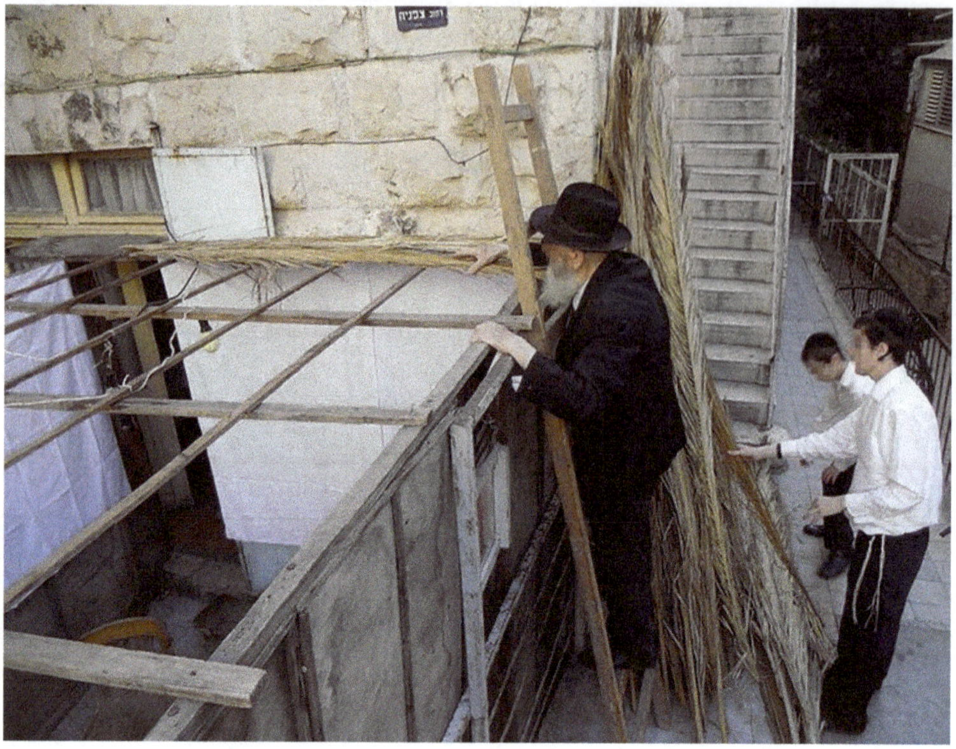

Fig. 26.6 During the Jewish festival of Sukkot, people sleep rough outdoors in improvised shacks to deny comforts for greater spiritual gains. (Photograph courtesy of ציון הלוי, under a CC Share-alike licence)

other more subtle salutogenic resources related to comprehensibility or meaningfulness, and therefore manageability may occasionally need to be sacrificed for other outcomes. A good example is diet. Someone may diet to reduce their body weight and to improve their self-image. Dieting is a deliberate restriction of manageability to improve comprehensibility because comprehensibility is about mental states (like self-image). Dieting may also be religious and therefore to improve meaningfulness. How this may apply to architecture is less obvious, but perhaps people may accept a smaller home to reduce their carbon-footprint or give part of their home over to others? There is a religious practice called Sukkah on the Jewish festival of Sukkot, where people sleep in a shack outside so they can feel the frailty of existence and acknowledge their dependence on the divine (Rubenstein, 1994) (Fig. 26.6). This is an architectural sacrifice of manageability for greater meaningfulness, although it is only temporary.

Comprehensibility in Architecture

Comprehensibility is the domain of the mind. It is 'the extent to which… the internal and external environments [make] cognitive sense… are orderable and explicable' (Antonovsky, 1987, pp. 16–17). An understanding of the rules, laws and the limits of the circumstances we find ourselves in gives us a foundation for improvement, should we wish to negotiate changes for our betterment. Comprehensibility, as it applies to the built environment, is therefore about a sense of agency: our capacity to understand, negotiate and customise the contexts we find ourselves in. It is about having the knowledge we need to get what we want out of life and to progress with certainty. Comprehensibility is structured into design through the following design values: readability, simplicity and predictability.

Of all these values, *predictability* is the most important. The brain is wired to feel uncomfortable with uncertainty, in a parallel way that the body is wired to react against hunger. If uncertainty is prolonged or significant, it will trigger the amygdalae, causing a fight/flight response, which in turn blocks frontal processes (which relate mostly to meaningfulness), the normal hormone and endocrine cycle is virtually abandoned while the brain secretes adrenocorticotropic hormones, glucocorticoids and beta-endorphin instead. This is good news if you are being chased by a bear because your blood pressure will increase to feed your muscles while you bolt. It also means the blood is more likely to clot just in case the bear gets a little taste. Various relevant psychological effects are also observed, including increased fear and paranoia. But unless you are genuinely being chased by a carnivore, these responses are more likely to kill you than uncertainty (Sapolsky, 2017). A lack of comprehensibility makes us feel like we are in a Kafkaesque trap: uncertainty is exhausting, frustrating and can feel like it will never end – in other words, it carries such a significant cognitive cost, many people will make decisions that involve self-harm, rather than wait out uncertainty (Berns et al., 2006).

Predictability is enhanced in architecture and urban design by the other virtues – simplicity and readability. But the main risks to predictability in the built environment are not architectural (unless there is a risk of collapse), they are housing insecurity and unpredictability of a warm and welcome atmosphere. With unstable housing (bad rental agreements and risks of foreclosure) health (particularly Mental Health) outcomes are also at risk (Libman et al., 2012). The atmosphere in the city, at work or home, can also be subject to sudden change, especially in overcrowded situations where the actions of a few can radically affect the well-being of others (Ittelson, 1978), and the fear that this might happen can be more disruptive than the actions themselves (as demonstrated in the rat studies of Calhoun, 1952).

Simplicity aids a sense of predictability. It is the reason why Robert Browning's 'less is more' adage is so popular among architects (Browning, 1856- quoted by architect, Mies Van Der Rohe in 1947). Surprisingly, simplicity is not easy to achieve in architectural and urban design and is often the hallmark of experience. While simplicity is desirable because it carries a lower cognitive and somatic burden, it is also empowering because it renders the environment easily subservient to a person's needs. Wayfinding, for instance, is easy in a simple layout. In a simple layout, you can go from A to B without having to rely on signage or directions – the very typology, landmarks and locations of buildings, spaces or rooms will tell you their purpose. One can navigate a simple street layout or simple building layout easily, without frustration, getting lost or trying to remember tricky directions. Simple buildings are also flexible by nature. They lend themselves to customisation easily, which means they make good tools, helping people do whatever it is that needs doing, simply by getting out of their way.

Again, *readability* assists in *way-finding*. People should be able to tell from a distance what space, room or building is used for based purely on prior experience, memory or knowledge of familiar patterns (Albright, 2015). But we read more into our buildings than just purpose. We can also read the intentions that are embodied through design. We read the materials, the lighting and other details and make all kinds of assessments about who we are when we are in the space. 'Is the space for me or against me? Am I welcome here?' Architects and their clients should be certain that buildings are designed to give positive, generous and uplifting answers to questions like these.

The premise of inclusive design is that we should design for the minority who need special considerations, and the majority will benefit. For those people who suffer from confusion, hallucinations and paranoia, the importance of making sense of the environment cannot be underestimated (Woodbury & Woodbury, 1969). For this reason, it is important to provide familiar environments in all conditions where users are expected to relax, take respite and comfort (so that definitively excludes experiences which are designed to be extraordinary, such as rides in Disneyland). Familiarity will take on cultural hues, but familiar concepts, languages, objects, forms, materials, textures, typologies, emotions and expectations will all improve this sense provided that they are essentially regarded as positive (Golembiewski, 2010, 2013c). These things speak to authenticity in design, material choice and intent.

The authenticity of symbolism, intent and materiality speaks to the universal virtue of honesty, and again to predictability. On some level, honest design using natural materials, predictable typologies and other features of straight-forward design demands a reciprocal response from inhabitants and reflects on the behaviour of inhabitants also – as if the architecture calls us to ask, 'Is this place authentic, and does it demand an authentic response from me?' Although little formal research has been conducted to link this approach to health outcomes, this design property and its relationship with honesty and virtue has been long recognised by the Shakers of Maine, USA (Vincent, 2012).

Meaningfulness in Architecture

Constant action is required even to maintain homeostasis – you must breathe, eat, find shelter and so much more. This is because life is entropic: do nothing and you will die. Life is always an uphill battle. Even with constant attention and care, one will always have struggles and demons to fight, and a degree of failure is inevitable. At a point, the ultimate failure is assured because life itself is fatal. Having sufficient physical abilities and resources (manageability) helps, as does knowledge (comprehensibility) – but why would anyone even bother, except for an innate sense that life itself is worth it? This picture is depressing because what is being described here is what causes depression: find someone with no sense of meaning and they will be a portrait of the most distressing symptoms mood disorders. They will feel anhedonia (emotional flatness), avolition (disinterest in action) and may even present with alogia (where people stop bothering complete thoughts, validate assumptions and make sense).

The missing ingredient is meaningfulness: the thing that not only makes life worth living but can even turn hopeless adversity into joy. It is meaningfulness, the motivational power that drives us 'to get out of bed in the morning'. With a strong sense of meaningfulness, the salutogenic resource of affect (emotion) provides the capacity to turn ones' attention away from the uncertainties, negatives and difficulties of life and instead to focus instead on positive desires and what is otherwise good and purposeful.

Of all the salutogenic resources, meaningfulness is the most abstract. Indeed, the more abstract our concerns are, the more meaningful. Meaningfulness starts with concerns for ‘the other’ and expands into abstractions that are indistinguishable from fantasies; beliefs in non-physical entities, metaphysics and commitments to heroism that override any kind of logic (comprehensibility), our basic instincts for the preservation of life (manageability) and even our primal abhorrence of atrocities (Kruglanski et al., 2009) (Fig. 26.7). Meaningfulness is thus exemplified by heroic acts where concerns for the self are sacrificed for the greater good – the good, that is, of whatever it is that a person believes is worth living for. For most people, this means family and friends, the good of greater society, of culture, perhaps the well-being of the planet or ecosystem or even of metaphysical concerns built of myths, religious beliefs and quite possibly even delusions. (Why not? This level of abstraction is the zone of untethered imagination.) Against these haughty aspirations, the demands of the physical world (the domain of manageability) can all too easily sing like sirens, ready to dash the hero’s boat on all-to-physical rocks: the demands that one focus on bills, leaks, dinner or sleep instead of ones’ *magnum opus*.

The abstract nature of meaningfulness poses difficulties for architects who wish to foster it because architects are required to be concerned with concrete realities (literally). Where building materials, methods and compliance might preoccupy the architect, their clients’ sense of meaningfulness is linked to symbolic and fleeting representations of personal narratives. In a sense, concrete concerns are for architects the equivalent of pathologies for Medicine. How and why should doctors focus on what patients’ think and believe when there is an infection to treat? But just as Medicine is well advised to turn around and take an expanded salutogenic perspective, so too is architecture.

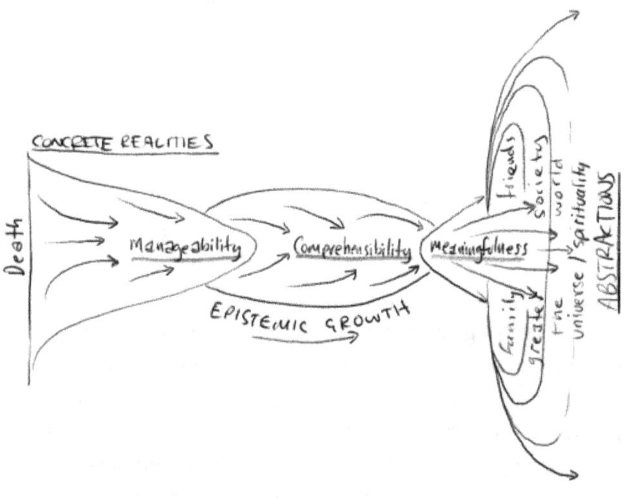

Fig. 26.7 Meaningfulness occurs most powerfully where concerns transcend self-interest and become more abstract – in connections, inspirations and metaphysical concerns. (Diagram J. Golembiewski, *courtesy of the author*)

In architecture, meaningfulness resources are improved by:

- Design for the greater good
- Setting the stage for positive narratives
  (Often this means finding and eradicating meaninglessness-in-design)
- Embodying meaningful symbolic expressions
- Providing for meaningful engagement
- Design for positive choices

Design for the Greater Good

What is good and bad depends on perspective – but as the dragon metaphor illustrates, salutogenesis is a broad enough theory to allow for contradictions. It does not matter what ‘good’ is, provided people feel it. The greater good (as it is addressed by architecture) traditionally means designing buildings that are harmonious with their surroundings (the decorousness and eurythmy of Vitruvius). More recently the fashion for expressing common ‘good’ has been in environmentally sensitive and low-carbon-impact design or civic-minded functionality.

Setting the Stage for Positive Narratives

Affect is processed using the limbic areas of the brain: the area of the brain that processes and deciphers narrative (Le Hunte & Golembiewski, 2014). Emotions and narratives are neurologically interwoven. When we feel, it is because our endocrine chemistry changes in response to the narratives we experience. And for this reason, the most direct way to design for meaningfulness and to elicit positive emotions is to create architecture using the language of storytelling: to design as if buildings, precincts, rooms and other spaces were stage-sets. By asking ‘what does this “set” say to the user? And how does it deliver meaning?’ architects can use the commonalities of language and culture to purposefully establish appropriate meaning. Similarly, the salutogenic architect can be surgical, addressing and designing for the SRDs that speak of undesirable narratives: the features of the built environment that say the wrong things and speak to meaninglessness as surely in real life as they do in a play: environments that are creepy or are difficult to negotiate are especially problematic – as are ones that use electronic surveillance, have disturbing acoustics, smells, textures or lighting in buildings and car-centric wastelands and dead-ends in urban design.

Embodying Meaningful Symbolic Expressions

Architectural stage sets can be designed with universal or near-universal symbols of the greater good, such as hope, growth and attainment. These symbols should be implicit, rather than applied. (A prison-like environment with the words 'hope, freedom and safety' emblazoned on the walls by an interior designer (it happens!) is more likely to cause frustration than a sense of release (Golembiewski, 2013d).) The same goes for inaccessible views of nature through impenetrable walls. But the quality of finish and construction on the other hand cannot be easily dismissed. There is no doubt that culturally some styles will fit better than others, especially in the domestic milieu, but *quality* transcends these differences because it says, 'we care about you' even beyond the mannerisms of style. Natural environments that are so cherished by advocates of ART, SRT and the BH serve a key role here. Good views generally are salutogenic, and more so if they reinforce our place as part of something bigger than ourselves like the natural environment. This effect is enormous. In a German city, people were cued to rate their subjective experience about 10 times/day over a week on a phone app. When asked, they rated subjective measures of wellness and happiness. This data was correlated to a map showing where the participants were, and how much greenery (a generic positive aesthetic affordance) was around them when they gave their ratings. Results showed that even a little greenery positively and robustly impacted on all health and happiness measures (Tost et al., 2019). The study was replicated with a neuroimaging study and a twist: Visible urban greenery made people feel on average 9–10 points better (on a 0–100 visual analogue scale), even when the subject was also exposed to salient emotionally aversive cues. Meanwhile, the greenery caused a significant *deactivation* of the dorsolateral prefrontal cortex (DLPFC) during this negative exposure, suggesting that negative social affordances were cancelled out by the green aesthetic experience. This makes sense – at least in as much as people care about the environment (and the recent wave of interest that catapulted Greta Thunberg to fame suggests that the green issue is more important to many people than religion.) And if there is validity in the ART, SRT and BH, then to at least a lesser extent, in everyone else also. So buildings that look out into nature or make an effort to reduce the carbon footprint (Fig. 26.8) naturally make people feel they are doing something meaningful for the environment and therefore improve meaningfulness.

Providing for Meaningful Engagement

Meaningfulness in architecture is improved whenever the design enables engagement in the things that create meaning and joy. The things we engage in are personal, and for this reason, meaningfulness is a shifting goalpost, changing with life-experience and circumstance. But humans are fundamentally alike. Humanity is at shared at familial, cultural, societal and even universal levels. If we consider the places people find meaning at these levels, then we can design spaces that afford those activities (without detracting from them) (Table 26.1).

Design for Positive Choices

Providing opportunities for engagement makes for good salutogenic interventions. But better still, is a *choice* of good things to get engaged in. A sense of abundance removes the pressures of poverty to make way for a sense of happiness (Cook, 2017), and there is no better way to impress a sense of abundance on people that by providing irresistible, positive choices. Over the history of mankind – or even of life itself, people have had few opportunities to sit back and make such choices, tethered as we tend to be by the demands of daily life whether it be filing tax returns to escape an audit from tax department trolls, or tilling fields to make sure there's stock for winter. If this sense of abundance and quality can be anchored by the architecture, there is little left for the architecture to do to create meaning. But the individual needs that are at the heart of meaningfulness are more important than choices alone: 'positive choices' do not always mean decadent indulgence - to some individuals the best choice may be to just 'be'. There is a salutary lesson in the myth of Prince Siddhartha, who rejected the trappings of the palace to sit naked under a mango tree to become the enlightened Buddha. Just as manageability sometimes needs to be sacrificed for comprehensibility of meaningfulness, so too the trappings of meaningfulness may need to be sacrificed for the thing itself – but that is no longer the domain of architecture.

Discussion

Since Dilani (2006) brought the concept of salutogenesis to healthcare design, he has led the International Academy for Design and Health to promote salutogenic theory in healthcare architecture throughout the world, even offering an annual prize for excellence in salutogenic architecture. As

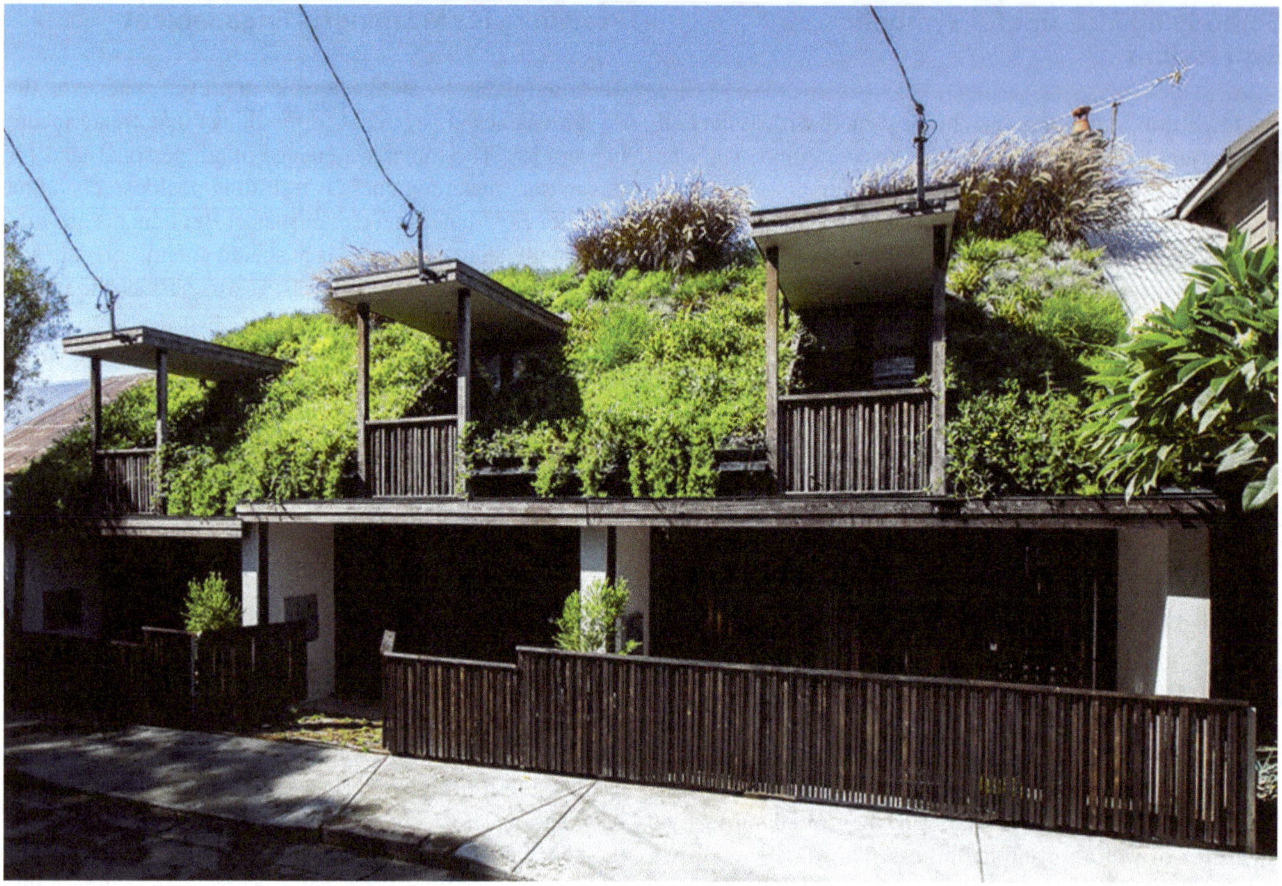

Fig. 26.8 88 Angel, by Steele Associates Architects, is a stage-set that makes a clear statement about meaningfulness. This terrace of low-energy houses not only provides 'views of nature' it is buried by it and it also gives views away to neighbours and passers-by. It is also located near the heart of Sydney so it is the perfect place to establish social connections. (Photograph © Steele Associates Architects, courtesy of Steele Associates Architects)

Table 26.1 Some generic architectural solutions to encourage the discovery and maintenance of meaning in life

Area of engagement	Practical solutions
Interests: Creative, intellectual works, sports.	Studios, halls rooms and spaces designed for specific activities (that do not detract by being too noisy/too quiet, too difficult to keep clean etc. See manageability).
Animals	Design for pets. Is there sufficient space? Are there open areas? Are the surfaces going to limit the inconvenience of fur, feathers, poo and animal noises?
Family and friends	Good spaces for entertaining. Fun provisions for visitors (got a swimming pool?) Kitchens that are in the heart of the action, spaces for kids to play safely, etc..
Greater society	Good locations, urban living, good transport connections, appropriate typologies and decorous designs.
World	Views of nature, natural materials, low-carbon footprint.
Universe	Bespoke religious affordances and symbols, 'sacred' architectural forms.

a result, the concept has grown in popularity at least as a buzzword. The result is that salutogenesis is now a respected and encouraged design goal. The downside is that the term 'salutogenic' is overused by architects, most of whom do not know what it means. As a result, at times, the term can mean nothing more systematic than 'friendly-looking' or 'leafy'. This is not to criticise those designs – after all, 'nice looking' and 'leafy' are often the outcomes of more systematic salutogenic approaches, but there is so much more unexplored potential in the concept. There are now systematic methods to bring salutogenic principles in many areas of institutional design: healthcare design (Golembiewski, 2010, 2015) and emergency care (Golembiewski, 2012b) and aged care (Golembiewski, 2017a, 2017b) and dementia care (Chap. 48 of this volume). And when adopted appropriately, salutogenic architecture is invariably exemplary. Some of these projects reach beyond the accepted evidence basis for health-promoting design (generic factors like views of nature and allowances for natural daylight) and explore the realms of story-making, psychology, neuroscience and endocrinology. It is now time for salutogenesis in design to be deployed outside of institutions, in workplaces, in urban designs and in people's own homes. But for this to happen, it is time to wrestle the term from the clutches of marketeers, and for solid salutogenic theory to become part of the architects' tool-bag.

Challenges for the Future

Salutogenic principles are a practical way to integrate the dynamics of health and experience with architecture. But for people in praxis, challenges abound: in most countries the procurement systems are conservative, and led by precedents and guidelines, and controlled by stakeholder groups who struggle to save capital, often with little regard for on-going healthcare costs. The decision-makers are usually poorly informed or simply do not believe in the capacity of aesthetics to influence health. To add to this, the pathogenic model of health is dominant in the healthcare sector, a field with enormous inertia, which will not reorient towards health promotion easily. As a result, stakeholders may place a greater stake in 'keeping it normal' than on real benefits of change. Belief in the value of functional efficiencies, traditional finishes and approaches are not changing fast. Although some groups (particularly in the private sector) are beginning to understand how salutogenic values can lift their game when faced with shrinking budgets, tight deadlines, constricted sites and profit-oriented project managers, the question is will they have the courage to go beyond generic 'views of nature' tropes?

References

Albright, R. (2015). Neuroscience for architecture. In S. Robinson & J. Pallasmaa (Eds.), *Mind in architecture: Neuroscience, embodiment and the future of design* (pp. 197–219). MIT Press.

Antonovsky, A. (1972). Breakdown: A needed fourth step in the conceptual armamentarium of modern medicine. *Social Science & Medicine, 6*(5), 537–544.

Antonovsky, A. (1979). *Health, stress, and coping*. Jossey-Bass.

Antonovsky, A. (1987). *Unravelling the mystery of health: How people manage stress and stay well*. Jossey-Bass.

Antonovsky, A. (1996). The salutogenic model as a theory to guide health promotion. *Health Promotion International, 11*(1), 11.

Bargh, J. A. (1994). The four horsemen of automaticity: Awareness, intention, efficiency, and control in social cognition. *Handbook of social cognition: Basic processes, 1*, 1ñ40.

Beauchemin, K. M., & Hays, P. (1996). Sunny hospital rooms expedite recovery from severe and refractory depressions. *Journal of Affective Disorders, 40*, 49–51.

Beauchemin, K. M., & Hays, P. (1998). Dying in the dark: Sunshine, gender and outcomes in myocardial infarction. *Journal of the Royal Society of Medicine, 91*, 352–354.

Berns, G. S., Chappelow, J., Cekic, M., Zink, C. F., Pagnoni, G., & Martin-Skurski, M. E. (2006). Neurobiological substrates of dread. *Science, 312*(5774), 754–758. https://doi.org/10.1126/science.1123721

Brager, G. S., & de Dear, R. J. (1998). Thermal adaptation in the built environment: A literature review. *Energy and Buildings, 27*(1), 83–96. Retrieved from http://www.sciencedirect.com/science/article/B6V2V-3SYXHRY-9/2/4d52df91215e9c9e0401d0cfb21da59b

Browning, R. (1856). Andrea Del Sarto. In *Men And Women*. Ticknor and Fields.

Calhoun, J. (1952). The social aspects of population dynamics. *Journal of Mammalogy*, 139–159.

City of New York. (2013). *Active design: Shaping the sidewalk experience*. NYC.

Clarkson, J., Coleman, R., Keates, S., & Lebbon, C. (2003). *Inclusive Design: Design for the whole population*. In: J. Clarkson, R. Coleman, S. Keates, & C. Lebbon (Eds.).

Cook, D. (2017). The ART of Hope: Healing the Wounded City. In R. Phillips & C. Wong (Eds.), *Handbook of community well-being research* (pp. 39–68). Springer Nature.

Cooke, J. (2001). *Architects, engineers and the law* (3rd ed.). Federation Press.

Deguchi, T., & Axelrod, J. (1972). Control of circadian change of serotonin N-acetyltransferase activity in the pineal organ by the ß-Adrenergic receptor. *PNAS, 69*(9), 2547–2550.

Dijkstra, K., Pieterse, M., & Pruyn, A. (2006). Physical environmental stimuli that turn healthcare facilities into healing environments through psychologically mediated effects: A systematic review. *Journal of Advanced Nursing, 56*(2), 166–181. https://doi.org/10.1111/j.1365-2648.2006.03990.x

Dilani, A. (2006). A new paradigm of design and health in hospital planning. *World Hospitals and Health Services, 41*(4), 17–21.

Dilani, A. (2008). Psychosocially supportive design: A salutogenic approach to the design of the physical environment. *Design and Health Scientific Review, 1*(2), 47–55.

Frankl, V. E. (1963). *Man's search for meaning: An introduction to Logotherapy*. Pocket Books.

Gibson, J. J. (1979). *The ecological approach to visual perception*. Houghton Mifflin Company.

Golembiewski, J. (2010). Start making sense; applying a salutogenic model to architectural design for psychiatric care. *Facilities, 28*(3/4), 100–117. https://doi.org/10.1108/02632771011023096

Golembiewski, J. (2012a). All common psychotic symptoms can be explained by the theory of ecological perception. *Medical Hypotheses, 78*, 7–10. https://doi.org/10.1016/j.mehy.2011.09.029

Golembiewski, J. (2012b). Moving from theory to praxis on the fly; introducing a salutogenic method to expedite mental healthcare provision. *Australian Journal of Emergency Management, 27*(1), 42–47. Retrieved from http://www.em.gov.au/Publications/Australianjournalofemergencymanagement/Pastissues/Pages/AJEM27TWO/Moving-from-theory-to-praxis-on-the-fly-introducing-a-salutogenic-method-to-expedite-mental-health-care-provision-in-disas.aspx

Golembiewski, J. (2012c). Salutogenic design: The neural basis for health promoting environments. *World Health Design Scientific Review, 5*(4), 62–68.

Golembiewski, J. (2013a). Are diverse factors proxies for architectural influences? A case for architecture in the aetiology of schizophrenia. *Curēus, 5*(3), e106. https://doi.org/10.7759/cureus.106

Golembiewski, J. (2013b). Determinism and desire: Some neurological processes in perceiving the design object. *International Journal of Design in Society, 6*(3), 23–36.

Golembiewski, J. (2013c). Lost in space: The role of the environment in the aetiology of schizophrenia. *Facilities, 31*(9/10), 427–448.

Golembiewski, J. (2014). Introducing the concept of reflexive and automatic violence: a function of aberrant perceptual inhibition. *Archives of Psychiatry and Psychotherapy, 16*(4), 5–13. https://doi.org/10.12740/app/33358

Golembiewski, J. (2015). Salutogenic architecture in health care settings. In G. Bauer & M. Mittelmark (Eds.), *Handbook of Salutogenesis: Past, present and future* (pp. 267–276). Springer Nature.

Golembiewski, J. (2016). The designed environment and how it affects brain morphology and mental health. *HERD, 9*(2), 161–171. https://doi.org/10.1177/1937586715609562

Golembiewski, J. (Writer). (2017a). Salutogenic approaches for dementia care. In Dementia Training Australia Training Webinars. Dementia Training Australia.

Golembiewski, J. (Producer). (2017b, 12/12/2017). Salutogenics for Dementia Care. *Dementia Training Australia*. [Webinar] Retrieved from https://www.youtube.com/watch?v=5v_UOakjUoI

Harari, Y. N. (2015). *Sapiens: A brief history of humankind*. HarperCollins.

Ittelson, W. H. (1978). Environmental perception and urban experience. *Environment and Behavior, 10*(2), 193.

Jackson, R., & Sinclair, S. (2012). *Designing healthy communities*. Jossey-Bass.

Kaplan, R., & Kaplan, S. (1989). *The experience of nature: A psychological perspective*. Cambridge University Press.

Kaplan, S., & Kaplan, R. (1982). *Cognition and environment*. Praeger.

Keinan, G. (1994). The effects of stress and tolerance of ambiguity on magical thinking. *Journal of Personality and Social Psychology, 67*(1), 48–55.

Kruglanski, A. W., Chen, X., Dechesne, M., Fishman, S., & Orehek, E. (2009). Fully committed: Suicide Bombers' motivation and the quest for personal significance. *Political Psychology, 30*(3), 331–357.

Lawton, M. P., & Nahemow, L. (1973). Ecology and the aging process. In C. Eisdorfer & M. Powell Lawton (Eds.), *Social environment of aging* (pp. 619–673). American Psychological Association.

Le Hunte, B., & Golembiewski, J. (2014). Stories have the power to save us: A neurological framework for the imperative to tell stories. *Arts and Social Sciences Journal, 5*(2), 73–77. https://doi.org/10.4172/2151-6200.1000073

Libman, K., Fields, D., & Saegert, S. (2012). Housing and health: A social ecological perspective on the US foreclosure crisis. *Housing, Theory and Society, 29*(1), 1–24. https://doi.org/10.1080/14036096.2012.624881

Maslow, A. H. (1962). Lessons from the peak-experiences. *Journal of Humanistic Psychology, 2*(1), 9–18. https://doi.org/10.1177/002216786200200102

Mason, O., Startup, M., Halpin, S., Schall, U., Conrad, A., & Carr, V. (2004). Risk factors for transition to first episode psychosis among individuals with 'at-risk mental states'. *Schizophrenia Research, 71*(2–3), 227–237. https://doi.org/10.1016/j.schres.2004.04.006

Mazuch, R. (2017). Salutogenic and Biophilic design as therapeutic approaches to sustainable architecture. *Architectural Design*.

Mittelmark, M. B., & Bull, T. (2013). The salutogenic model of health in health promotion research. *Global Health Promotion, 20*(2), 30–38. https://doi.org/10.1177/1757975913486684

Mittelmark, M. B., Bull, T., Daniel, M., & Urke, H. (2017). Specific resistance resources in the salutogenic model of health. In M. B. Mittelmark, S. Sagy, M. Eriksson, G. F. Bauer, J. M. Pelikan, B. Lindström, & G. A. Espnes (Eds.), *The handbook of Salutogenesis* (pp. 71–76). Springer.

Rubenstein, J. L. (1994). The symbolism of the sukkah. *Judaism, 43*(4), 371.

Sapolsky, R. (2004). *Why zebras Don't get ulcers: An updated guide to stress, stress related diseases, and coping* (3rd ed.). Henry Holt and Company.

Sapolsky, R. M. (2017). *Behave: The biology of humans at our best and worst*. Penguin Press.

Searles, H. F. (1960). *The non-human environment in normal development and in schizophrenia*. International Universities Press.

Searles, H. F. (1966). Concerning the development of an identity. *Psychoanalytic Review, 53*(4), 7–30. Retrieved from http://www.pep-web.org

Strümpfer, D., Gouws, J., & Viviers, M. (1998a). Antonovsky's sense of coherence scale related to negative and positive affectivity. *European Journal of Personality, 12*(6), 457–480.

Strümpfer, D., Gouws, J., & Viviers, M. (1998b). Item phrasing in Antonovsky's sense of coherence scale related to negative and positive affectivity. *Personality and Individual Differences, 24*(5), 669–675.

Tost, H., Reichert, M., Braun, U., Reinhard, I., Peters, R., Lautenbach, S., … Meyer-Lindenberg, A. (2019). Neural correlates of individual differences in affective benefit of real-life urban green space exposure. *Nature Neuroscience*. https://doi.org/10.1038/s41593-019-0451-y

Turley, L. W., & Milliman, R. E. (2000). Atmospheric effects on shopping behavior: A review of the experimental evidence. *Journal of Business Research, 49*(2), 193–211.

Ulrich, R. S. (1991). *The Effects of Interior Design on Wellness; Theory and Recent Scientific Research*. Paper presented at the Journal of Health Care Interior Design; Proceedings from the National Symposium on Health Care Interior Design.

Vincent, N. C. (2012). Shaker Furniture. *Heilbrunn Timeline of Art History*. Retrieved from http://www.metmuseum.org/toah/hd/shak/hd_shak.htm

Wilson, E. O. (1984). *Biophilia: The human bond with other species*. Harvard University Press.

Woodbury, M., & Woodbury, M. (1969). Community centered psychiatric intervention: A pilot project in the 13th arrondissement, Paris. *American Journal of Psychiatry, 126*(5), 619–625.

Zook, J. B., & Ewing, R. (2010). *Active design guidelines: promoting physical activity and health in design*. Retrieved from New York:

Permissions

All chapters in this book were first published in THS, by Springer; hereby published with permission under the Creative Commons Attribution License or equivalent. Every chapter published in this book has been scrutinized by our experts. Their significance has been extensively debated. The topics covered herein carry significant information for a comprehensive understanding. They may even be implemented as practical applications or may be referred to as a beginning point for further studies.

The contributors of this book come from diverse backgrounds, making this book a truly international effort. We would like to thank all the contributing authors for lending their expertise to make the book truly unique. They have played a crucial role in the development of this book. Without their invaluable contributions this book wouldn't have been possible. They have made vital efforts to compile up to date information on the varied aspects of this subject to make this book a valuable addition to the collection of many professionals and students.

This book was conceptualized with the vision of imparting up-to-date and integrated information in this field. To ensure the same, a matchless editorial board was set up. Every individual on the board went through rigorous rounds of assessment to prove their worth. After which they invested a large part of their time researching and compiling the most relevant data for our readers.

The editorial board has been involved in producing this book since its inception. They have spent rigorous hours researching and exploring the diverse topics which have resulted in the successful publishing of this book. They have passed on their knowledge of decades through this book. To expedite this challenging task, the publisher supported the team at every step. A small team of assistant editors was also appointed to further simplify the editing procedure and attain best results for the readers.

Apart from the editorial board, the designing team has also invested a significant amount of their time in understanding the subject and creating the most relevant covers. They scrutinized every image to scout for the most suitable representation of the subject and create an appropriate cover for the book.

The publishing team has been an ardent support to the editorial, designing and production team. Their endless efforts to recruit the best for this project, has resulted in the accomplishment of this book. They are a veteran in the field of academics and their pool of knowledge is as vast as their experience in printing. Their expertise and guidance has proved useful at every step. Their uncompromising quality standards have made this book an exceptional effort. Their encouragement from time to time has been an inspiration for everyone.

The publisher and the editorial board hope that this book will prove to be a valuable piece of knowledge for students, practitioners and scholars across the globe.

Index

www.ingramcontent.com/pod-product-compliance
Lightning Source LLC
LaVergne TN
LVHW082121200926
848484LV00008B/1989